W9-CMB-914

MAYO CLINIC | Guide to Women's Cancers

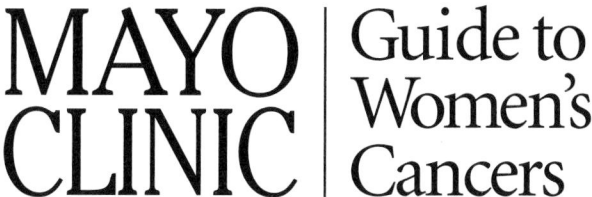

MAYO CLINIC | Guide to Women's Cancers

Lynn C. Hartmann, M.D.

Charles L. Loprinzi, M.D.

Editors in Chief

Bobbie S. Gostout, M.D.
Associate Editor

MAYO
CLINIC

Published by Mayo Clinic Health Information, Rochester, Minn. Distributed to the book trade by Kensington Publishing Corp., New York, N.Y.

Photo credits: Photos on pages 33, 273 and 497 are from PhotoDisc. The individuals pictured in these photos are models, and the photos are for illustrative purposes only. There is no correlation between the individuals portrayed and the condition or subject being discussed.

Library of Congress Control Number: 2004104238

ISBN 1-893005-33-X

Printed in the United States of America

First Edition

1 2 3 4 5 6 7 8 9 10

Preface

If you've picked up this book, you've likely been touched by breast cancer or a type of gynecologic cancer. So many women have. Each year in this country alone, 350,000 women are diagnosed with one of these cancers. And that doesn't take into account the women at risk of such cancers, or family or friends of a woman who has received a breast or gynecologic cancer diagnosis.

Given that there are already multiple books on cancer, what does one more book add in this information-rich age? Because there are many different options for treating women's cancers, accurate and reliable information is essential. This book contains the best information available at this time, reflecting recent improvements in both the understanding and treatment of breast and gynecologic cancers.

We chose to combine breast and gynecologic cancers in the same book because they share many features, including similar risk factors, genetic predispositions, treatment approaches and survivorship issues. In addition, the psychological and emotional challenges for women with these cancers, and for their families, are very similar.

Mayo Clinic Guide to Women's Cancers is intended to provide you with information you need as you face a cancer diagnosis, to help you deal with the challenges that can accompany treatment for these cancers, and to help you cope with the emotional impact of living with cancer. The book addresses multiple aspects of cancer, including risk factors, prevention, early detection, treatment and coping.

Mayo Clinic Guide to Women's Cancers is rich in hope, with stories of women who have navigated the same waters. It is also realistic. When a cure may not be possible, the book provides guidance for redirecting hope and priorities toward goals other than cure, such as prolonged survival, comfort and a good death.

Each chapter was reviewed by multiple experts at Mayo Clinic with a wide variety of expertise. We have tried to provide you with a balanced account of where things stand with each cancer — similar to the guidance Mayo Clinic doctors provide to their individual patients. Nonetheless, the information in this book is no substitute for the one-on-one relationship between patient and doctor. The purpose of this book is to allow you to discuss treatment options with your doctors in a more informed manner so that together you can make the best choices for your medical care.

This book is a tribute to many. First and foremost, it's a tribute to the many women and men who have taught us about these diseases. Many people helped us with suggestions for content, with their own personal stories and with reviews of the text. In addition, the book is a tribute to our colleagues who provided input, taking time from their busy schedules to assist us. Special thanks go to our managing editor, Karen Wallevand, who provided the high standards and staying power to make this book what it is, and to Bobbie Gostout, M.D., who provided special expertise with the gynecologic cancer chapters. Particular thanks go to our families and loved ones who supported us during our efforts to bring this book forward.

Lynn C. Hartmann, M.D.
Charles L. Loprinzi, M.D.

Editorial Staff

Editors in Chief
Lynn C. Hartmann, M.D.
Charles L. Loprinzi, M.D.

Associate Editor
Bobbie S. Gostout, M.D.

Managing Editor
Karen Wallevand

Assistant Editors
Mary Gallenberg, M.D.
Yolanda Garces, M.D.
Sandhya Pruthi, M.D.

Creative Director
Daniel Brevick

Art Director
Paul Krause

Medical Illustration
Michael King

**Illustration and
Photography**
Joseph Kane
Kent McDaniel
Rebecca Varga
Randy Ziegler

Contributing Writers
Mary Amundsen
Rachel Bartony
Lee Engfer
Jennifer Jacobson
Kelly Kershner
Regina Martinez
Amy Michenfelder
Robin Silverman

Copy Editor
Mary Duerson

Proofreading
Miranda Attlesey
Louise Hutter Filipic
Donna Hanson

Indexing
Steve Rath

**Editorial Research
Manager**
Deirdre Herman

**Editorial Research
Librarians**
Anthony Cook
Danielle Gerberi
Michelle Hewlett

MMV Editorial Director
Sara Gilliland

**MMV Editor in Chief,
Books/Newsletters**
Christopher Frye

Mayo Medical Ventures
Marne Gade
Daniel Goldman, J.D.
James Hale Sr.
Vicki Moore
Carol Olson
Gary Peterson
S. Rebecca Roberts
Richard Van Ert

Literary Agent
Arthur Klebanoff

Additional Contributors & Reviewers

Contributors

Brigitte Barrette, M.D.

Ann Bartlett, R.N.

Debra Barton, Ph.D.

Brent Bauer, M.D.

Kathleen Brandt, M.D.

James Cerhan, M.D., Ph.D.

Matthew Clark, Ph.D.

William Cliby, M.D.

Amy Degnim, M.D.

Jill Dowdy

Sean Dowdy, M.D.

David Farley, M.D.

Tom Fitch, M.D.

Marlene Frost, Ph.D.

Gail Gamble, M.D.

Karthik Ghosh, M.D.

Jean Girardi, P.T.

Matthew Goetz, M.D.

Clive Grant, M.D.

Axel Grothey, M.D.

Michele Halyard, M.D.

James Ingle, M.D.

Aminah Jatoi, M.D.

Chaplain Mary Johnson

Monica Jones, M.D.

Kimberly Kalli, Ph.D.

Judith Kaur, M.D.

Jeffrey Korsmo

Harry Long, M.D.

Margie Loprinzi, R.N.

Jacqueline Luong, M.D.

Javier Magrina, M.D.

Paul Magtibay, M.D.

Cathy Marks, M.D.

Betty Mincey, M.D.

Timothy Moynihan, M.D.

V. Shane Pankratz, Ph.D.

Prema Peethambaram, M.D.

Edith Perez, M.D.

Karl Podratz, M.D., Ph.D.

Julie Ponto, R.N., A.O.C.N.

S. Vincent Rajkumar, M.D.

Carol Reynolds, M.D.

Deborah Rhodes, M.D.

Paula Schomberg, M.D.

Bernd-Uwe Sevin, M.D., Ph.D.

Jeffrey Slezak

De Anne Smith, C.N.P.

Robert Stanhope, M.D.

Celine Vachon, Ph.D.

Janet Vittone, M.D.

Katie Zahasky, C.N.P.

Reviewers

Loyce Brown

Margaret Gilseth

David Jackman Jr.

Jenise Roberts

Shirley Ruedy

Michael Samaniego

Organizational Reviews

Minnesota Ovarian Cancer Alliance

Ovarian Cancer National Alliance

Y-ME National Breast Cancer Organization

Contents

Part 3: Living With Cancer

When Cancer Strikes

"When I was not only called back for more mammogram films, but scheduled for an ultrasound, my anxiety began to skyrocket."

Mary Amundsen
Breast Cancer Survivor

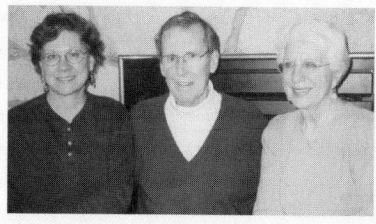

Mary Amundsen, right, with her daughter and husband. All three are in remission from cancer.

A cancer diagnosis can be a lightning bolt. Once the word *cancer* is spoken, life stops — or seems to. Normal routines unravel. Emotions are laid bare. Concentration is lost. Things that once were so important no longer are.

With the lightning, comes the rain — a pelting of information, statistics, questions and tests. At a time when all you may seek is warmth and shelter, you can't get out of the storm. Appointments need to be scheduled. Decisions need to be made. Steps need to be taken.

Sometimes, it's difficult to know where to begin or which way to turn for guidance. This book was written to provide reliable and easy-to-comprehend information to help you better understand your cancer, make informed decisions regarding your care, and cope with the emotional and physical effects of cancer treatment.

The focus of the book is on cancers that primarily affect women — breast and gynecologic cancers. Men also get breast cancer, but the disease is rare in them. Together, breast cancer and gynecologic cancers — cancers of the ovaries, fallopian tubes, uterus, cervix, vagina and vulva — represent about 45 percent of all

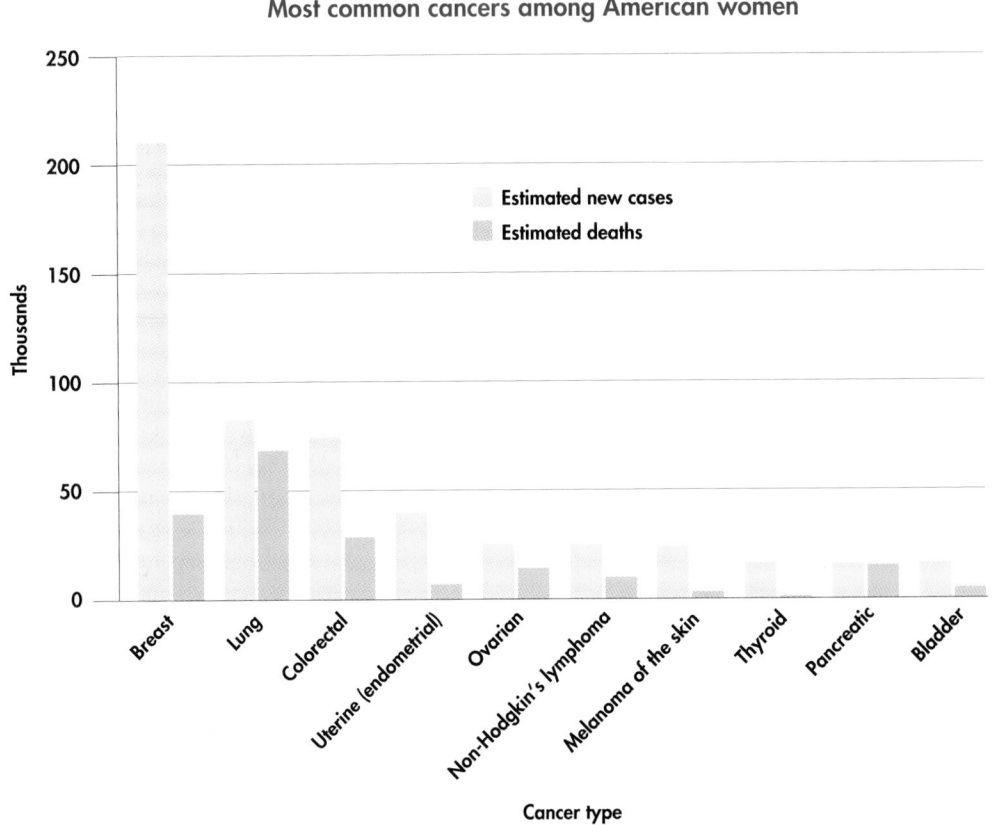

Most common cancers among American women

Source: American Cancer Society, "Cancer Facts and Figures 2004"

new life-threatening cancer cases diagnosed in American women. Invasive breast cancer is the most common life-threatening cancer among women, with an estimated 216,000 new cases in the United States in 2004. Uterine cancer is the fourth most common cancer in women, with more than 40,000 new cases expected in 2004, and ovarian cancer is fifth, with about 25,000 new cases.

Breast and gynecologic cancers share many genetic and reproductive characteristics, and they can have a similar effect on women emotionally and socially. They touch deeply personal aspects of the female body and psyche — body image, sexuality, identity as a woman and, possibly, fertility. The cancers can alter how you feel about yourself, how you relate to others and how you think others perceive you.

The following chapters provide a wealth of information about cancers unique to women. Part 1 covers breast cancer, and Part 2 discusses gynecologic cancers. Part 3 offers strategies for dealing with the emotional and physical challenges after cancer treatment, as well as information on quality-of-life issues. The book also contains personal stories from women who have been diagnosed with breast or a gynecologic cancer — the decisions they faced, the choices they made, and their lives today.

We begin this book with Mary's story. A registered nurse and licensed psychologist, Mary Amundsen has not only confronted — and weathered — cancer herself, but also witnessed firsthand the fears, concerns and courage of many women facing the same struggle. Mary offers her story and shares her advice, to reassure you that you aren't alone in your journey.

Mary's Story

My annual mammogram. I didn't feel particularly anxious, although in the past I had been called back for additional films, which had reassured me that the radiologists were very precise. Because I was over age 50, I was at increased risk of breast cancer, even though I didn't have a family history of it. No one in my family had had breast cancer, but our daughter had been treated for ovarian cancer. So, when I was not only called back for more mammogram films, but scheduled for an ultrasound, my anxiety began to skyrocket.

Summoning my husband, to give me support and to provide an extra listening ear, we met with the radiologist. He explained the finding of clustered microcalcifications on my mammogram and suggested that I could get another mammogram in six months. No one, not even I, could feel a lump, and the mammogram films didn't show a suspicious mass. But did I want to

wait until a lump developed? The questions, ambivalence and fear were just beginning. We asked for a second opinion. The second radiologist explained that the microcalcifications had been present on previous films but now were clustered, suggestive of cancer. He recommended a biopsy, although I still had the choice of waiting six months for another mammogram. That was decision point number 1.

At the time I was faced with this decision seven years ago, I thought of my years as a nurse and of my leadership of a breast cancer support group. The stories of others waiting too long for a biopsy and not having enough information to make an informed decision gave me a sense of urgency. It suddenly felt like my life was spinning out of control once again. It had been only six years since our daughter, at age 30, was diagnosed with ovarian cancer. At that time, I had desperately wished it were me instead of her. Four years after that, my husband had gone through extensive surgery and radiation for a sinus cancer. I felt our family had paid its dues to the "Big C," and I was angry that we might be facing this ordeal again.

The radiologist tried to assure us that most breast biopsies are benign, but the experience with our daughter and my husband, whose cancer shocked even the surgeon, made us very uneasy. The biopsy wasn't an emergency requiring an overnight decision, so I had some time to gather information and talk with supportive people, but by now I knew I didn't want to wait six months for another mammogram.

A possible cancer diagnosis seems to bring up every emotion and bad outcome you've ever heard. I knew literally hundreds of women who had had breast cancer and were still alive, but my mind jumped to those who had died of it.

An even stronger reaction was the grief and guilt I felt in putting our family through this again. Our daughter was doing very well six years after her two surgeries and chemotherapy treatment, and we were anxiously waiting out each checkup for my husband to reach the five-year cancer-free mark. My reactions felt familiar, and although I knew I could get through this, my heart was heavy.

Once I made the decision to have the biopsy sooner rather than later, I was faced with another decision point. If the biopsy did show cancer, what type of surgery would I want, if I had a choice? Did I want the surgeon to proceed with a mastectomy, if indicated, and what about reconstruction? By this time I had talked with two radiologists, a surgeon and my internist. What I found, and now tell others, is that you must be your own advocate and gather as much information as you need to feel comfortable with your decisions.

Although it may feel like a burden to be involved in the decision-making process, we're fortunate that there are choices. You likely will be given treatment options that will require you to make decisions. As much as you might wish for the old days when a doctor made all of the decisions, times have changed.

My surgeon was very patient with all of my questions and my desire to be involved in the decision making. Even though I preferred to keep my breast, I wasn't going to put my future at risk. We discussed the research findings of lumpectomy and radiation versus mastectomy. This information

conflicted with my gut reaction to have my breast removed and be done with it.

I was very lucky. My cancer was discovered early, which increased my chances of a good outcome. Surgery showed a small, slightly invasive cancer, and the surgeon removed only a small part of the breast. A lymph node dissection was negative, so only radiation, not chemotherapy, was recommended as part of my treatment.

After I was finished with radiation, I wondered what was next. I wasn't comfortable doing nothing, so I contacted an oncologist to discuss the drug tamoxifen. There had been news articles about promising results from research studies involving the drug, and I knew others who were taking it. I felt like I needed to pursue every avenue. The oncologist, after reviewing my records, didn't recommend it, though, because my prognosis was extremely favorable without it. At this point, I needed to trust the opinion of my doctor but also keep myself informed as new research results were published.

The decision of whether to have additional treatment once primary treatment is complete is another major decision point for many women. Learning more about possible therapies is essential to prepare yourself for this phase of your recovery. If your doctor recommends additional treatment, knowing why he or she is recommending that particular treatment can help to alleviate the anxiety. During this time, your relationship with your medical team needs to be one of support, understanding and patience by all involved. Your physical recovery may be progressing, but the emotional aspects of cancer now are beginning to surface. The changes cancer has brought to your family and your life are now being realized.

When cancer involves the reproductive and sexual organs, it strikes at the very core of a woman's identity. Your physical appearance and physiology may be significantly altered very abruptly. The gradual changes of adolescence and menopause allow a woman to adjust psychologically over a period of time. Cancer, however, often brings sudden changes. The changes are not only sudden but also unwanted and uncomfortable. Your feelings of femininity may be challenged, and you may feel insecure about your most intimate relationships. Future dreams and plans may never be realized in ways you had hoped.

It's a time of grief and loss and a time of coping, often in new ways. Cancer can bring out a creativity never realized. A friend of mine started to write a poem about her breasts and what they had meant to her. The poem became many poems as her feelings poured out onto the paper. Others have used art and sculpture to evoke their deepest emotions, and music to ease some of the difficult times during sleepless nights or chemotherapy treatments. My daughter played meditation tapes during her chemotherapy treatments. Quilting or fiber art can express our darkest times and our birth of hope. To view one of these creations is to know the deeper connection with others who have walked this path of cancer.

Keeping a journal of your experience is a way to express fears and feelings that are difficult to speak aloud. Humor can provide some relief to the seriousness we live with every day. I keep a folder of cartoons for those times. Just the physical act of a smile changes the way I feel, for a short time at least. You can choose how you deal with this crisis in your life.

Is cancer a life-changing event? You may read about those who radically altered their lives after a cancer diagnosis and wonder if you need to think about major changes. Cancer does change your life in many ways as you learn a new language (medical), meet new people (the medical team), fill up your calendar (with appointments) and, perhaps, see a different body in the mirror. Many women in my support group have expressed feeling a sense of urgency to do things now, instead of later. As a cancer survivor, you become very tuned in to news reports of cancer research, new treatments and statistics of survival. Every ache and pain is viewed with new concern, and checkups are approached with anxiety. So, yes, cancer is a life-changing event. But then, any major life-threatening diagnosis will change a person's life. You are face to face with your vulnerability. The illusion of an open-ended future has been shattered and reality can be harsh.

One of the biggest fears, of course, is that of recurrence — that the treatment didn't work. It's a fear all people who've had cancer live with and don't want to think about. However, some preparation can help you cope if that day comes. Think about what information you would want to know, who would be most helpful to you, and how you coped with your initial diagnosis. The courage and strength of those I have known with cancer is a continuous source of hope and inspiration for me during anxious times. If others can get through it with grace, then so can I.

In addition to my daughter, husband and me, cancer has been diagnosed in my brother (melanoma) and daughter-in-law (bladder). We are now all considered cancer-free, or in remission, although we know that at any time our status could change. What factors made a difference in our outcomes? There was no doubt some luck and other factors beyond our control that contributed to our successful treatments. But we also did some things that probably made a difference. I had a routine mammogram, which found the cancer at a very early stage. My daughter had some unusual abdominal discomfort and had a checkup. My husband pursued increasing pain in his sinus area, which he considered unusual. I noticed a mole on my brother and urged him to see a dermatologist. Our daughter-in-law sought attention for intermittent episodes of urinary bleeding. In other words, we were aware of body changes, and we were persistent in having those changes evaluated. You do have to be assertive and an advocate for yourself when you feel that something is physically wrong in your body. No one else can truly know how you feel.

Many people made a difference in the quality of our lives during those months and years, for those of us with cancer and for our family as a whole. Cancer is a family affair and everyone needs support and understanding. It's not a journey to travel alone. A burden shared is easier to carry.

No doubt all of you have experienced difficult times in your lives, and managed to get through them. Think back to those times and what you did that was the most helpful. Draw on those strengths now. Educate yourself, select a skilled medical team, find support and proceed with hope.

Chapter 2: Cancer Basics

Understanding Cancer

Thirty-five years after the U.S. government declared war on cancer, the disease remains a formidable foe. Each year in the United States, more than a million people are diagnosed with cancer. It's the second-leading cause of death, after heart disease. Each year, more than 560,000 people in the United States die of cancer.

Despite those somber statistics, there's growing cause for optimism. Much has changed since President Richard Nixon signed the National Cancer Act in 1971, providing federal funding for cancer research. At the time, cancer was poorly understood and usually deadly. Today, thanks to improvements in detection and treatment of many forms of cancer, and even prevention of some, the death rate from all cancers combined is declining. In 1974, the five-year survival rate for women diagnosed with breast cancer was approximately 75 percent. Today, it's closing in on 90 percent. For women diagnosed with ovarian cancer, five-year survival has increased from 37 percent in the early '70s to just more than 50 percent today.

Scientists now have a far better understanding of how cancer develops and progresses. Unprecedented growth in the area of biomedical research along with an explosion in sophisticated technologies such as gene sequencing and supercomputing have resulted in a new era of molecular oncology — the study of cancer at the submicroscopic, molecular level.

Although total elimination of all cancers likely isn't possible, some are increasingly being seen as longer-term, manageable conditions, such as heart disease and diabetes. Regular screening can result in early detection of many types of cancer. Most cancers are curable if found early. With prompt treatment, regular monitoring, and social and psychological support, many people with cancer can live productive, satisfying lives for many years. Today, there are about 9 million cancer survivors in the United States.

Scientific discoveries of the last few decades have given researchers a better understanding of just how complex cancer is. They know more about what makes cancer such a difficult enemy — and more about how to fight it.

This chapter is an overview of what's known about the biology of cancer and how that knowledge has been gained. The chapter goes into a fair amount of scientific detail and, therefore, might provide more information than you wish to learn right now. Feel free to move on to other chapters that follow, and then come back to this chapter in the future.

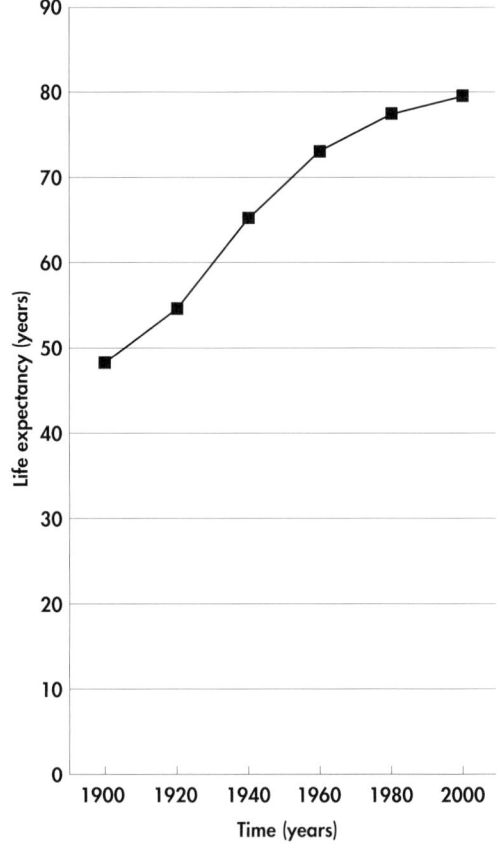

Increases in life expectancy of American women

Because of improved sanitation and medical advances, including advances in cancer detection and treatment, American women today are living significantly longer than their grandmothers and great-grandmothers.

Source: National Vital Statistics Reports, 2002

What Is Cancer?

Although *cancer* is often thought of as a single disease, the term actually refers to a group of related diseases that begin in cells, the body's basic units of life.

The human body is made of trillions of cells, categorized into about 200 different types that combine to form human tissues, such as skin, muscle, bone, breast, blood and others. To understand how cancer develops, it's helpful to know something about how healthy cells behave.

Normal cell behavior

Normally, cells grow and divide to produce more cells only when the body needs them. This process takes place according to genetic programs and instructions that are unique to each type of cell. As a cell grows, it takes its proper place among the other cells. When the cell matures, it performs the task it's genetically programmed to do. Eventually, the cell dies and is replaced by a new, younger cell. This orderly process keeps the body healthy and functioning.

Cells are also equipped with controls designed to prevent them from making too many copies of themselves, or from making flawed copies of themselves. For instance, cells are programmed to die after a certain number of divisions, a process known as programmed cell death (apoptosis).

No cell is an island unto itself. Each cell is regularly bombarded at its surface by nutrients and by hormonal and chemical signals, including signals from neighboring cells. To remain alive and healthy, cells must decode, filter and respond properly to many such molecular "conversations." For example, normal cells are stimulated to divide by molecular messages called growth signals. They also receive anti-growth signals when it's time to stop growing. If you cut yourself, skin cells around the wound divide to replace the injured cells. When the gap is filled properly, cell growth is turned off.

Some researchers compare this intricate network of cellular signaling pathways with a computer chip, in which the interconnected components are each responsible for receiving, processing and sending signals according to specific rules. Cellular pathways involve interactions among thousands of diverse molecules within and outside the cell. These interactions regulate cell growth.

Cancer cells

Cancer results from the loss of control of the intricate system of normal cell growth. Cancer is characterized by the overgrowth of abnormal cells. The development of these abnormal cells is a complex, lengthy, multistep process called carcinogenesis. It starts with the transformation of one normal cell into an abnormal one. Over time, the abnormal cells multiply out of control and accumulate into a mass of tissue — called a growth, or tumor — that can invade and destroy nearby normal tissue. The cancer cells can also spread throughout the body.

Even though cancer cells arise from normal body cells, they change so that they don't look or act like normal cells. Normal body cells, like law-abiding citizens, follow the rules set out for them by their genetic instructions. They grow when told to and stop growing when they get such a signal.

Cancer cells, however, are biological anarchists. They stop following the rules. Not only are there too many of them, but they have new and different characteristics. Their growth is disorderly, and they don't mature properly. Unlike normal cells, which tend to form exact copies of themselves when they divide, cancer cells are more likely to change when they divide. Tumor cells often look different

Cancer development and progression

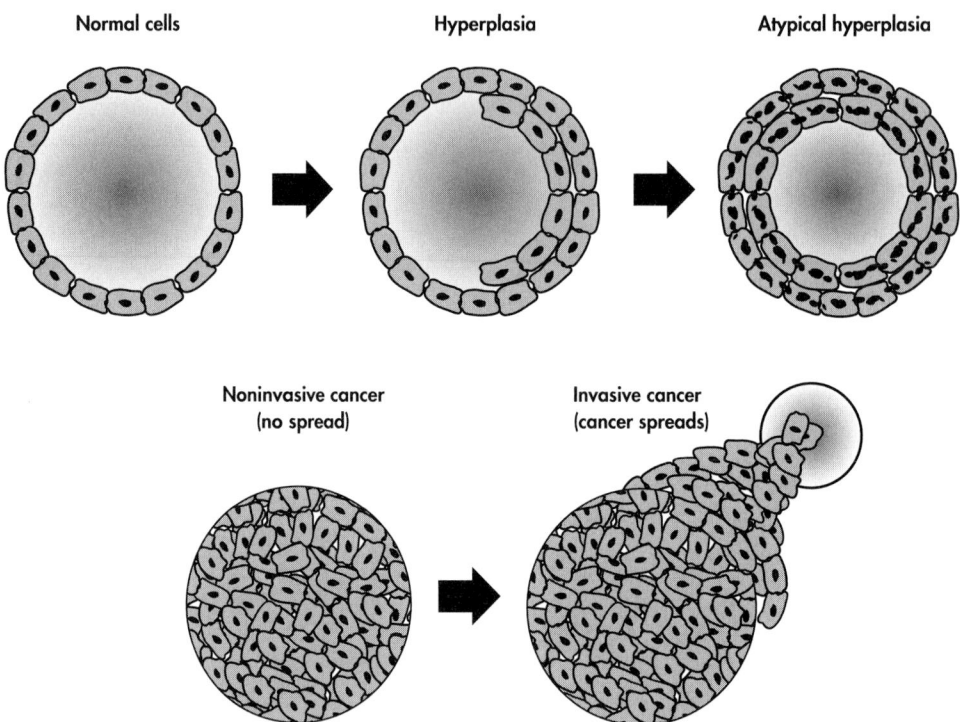

Normal cells

Hyperplasia

Atypical hyperplasia

Noninvasive cancer
(no spread)

Invasive cancer
(cancer spreads)

Cancer development first begins when there's excess production of cells. This is known as hyperplasia. Over time, the excess cells may begin to change in appearance and become abnormal. This is known as atypical hyperplasia. As the cells continue to change and multiply, cancer develops. If the abnormal cells stay contained within normal borders and don't invade neighboring tissue, the condition is known as noninvasive cancer. When the cells invade deeper into surrounding tissue, it's called invasive cancer.

from one another, and they can be highly disorganized. The abnormal cells tumble over each other, and they stack up on neighboring cells.

Characteristics of cancer cells

Cancer cells have many genetic differences from normal cells. Important regulatory genes within cancer cells become mutated or lost. Genes that slow growth in a normal cell are shut off in cancer cells. Other genes that in a normal cell stimulate growth are duplicated many times in cancer cells. Cancer genes often become unstable, meaning that they can change rapidly and acquire additional deadly features as they multiply.

By studying the molecular makeup of cells, researchers have identified specific characteristics that cancer cells acquire as they develop that allow them to grow out of control.

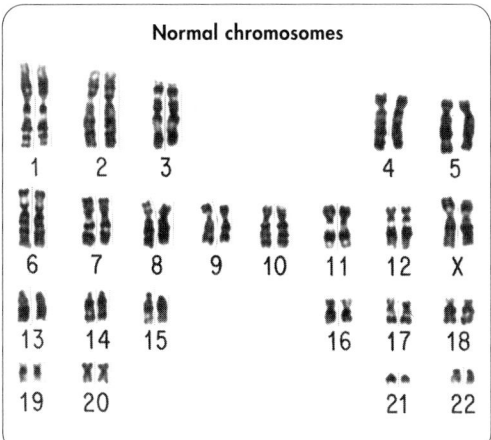

Normal chromosomes

The extent of genetic changes in cancer cells can be seen in this comparison of the chromosomes in a woman's normal blood cells (left) and in her ovarian cancer cells (below).

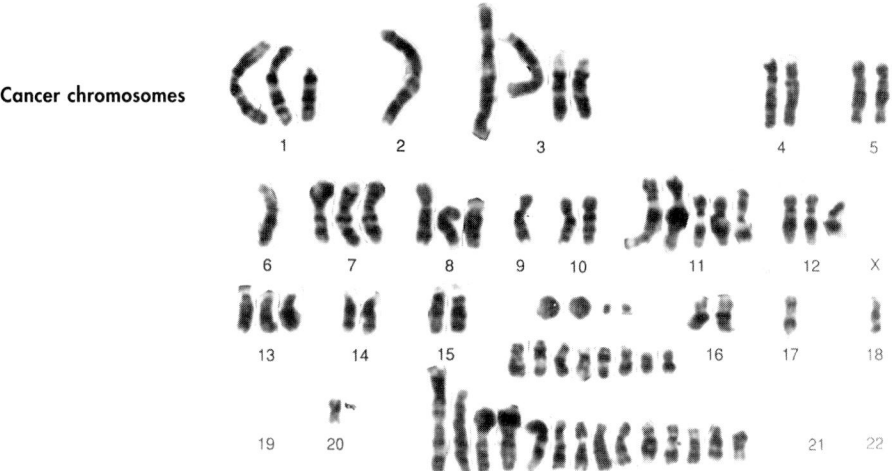

Cancer chromosomes

For example, cancer cells:
- **Supply their own growth signals.** Normal cells receive growth signals mainly from neighboring cells or hormones, but cancer cells generate many of their own growth signals. They also coerce their neighbors to make growth factors that stimulate their growth.
- **Stop responding to anti-growth signals from neighboring cells.** Cancer cells don't obey the molecular messages that normally stop cell growth to maintain a balanced cell growth cycle.
- **Develop their own blood supply.** A tumor gets the nutrients and oxygen it needs by developing new blood vessels in a process called angiogenesis. Normally, angiogenesis is tightly regulated, but cancerous tumors don't follow this regulation.
- **Don't self-destruct.** Normal cells have a natural life cycle — they age and

Genetics 101

Each cell in the body, except for mature red blood cells, has a control center called the nucleus. The nucleus houses your DNA, a long, double-stranded structure composed of sugar and phosphate molecules that are joined together by paired chemicals called nucleotide bases. DNA is tightly packed into structures called chromosomes. There are two sets of 23 chromosomes in the cell nucleus, for a total of 46 chromosomes. One set comes from each parent. The only cells that don't contain two sets of chromosomes are the sex cells — eggs and sperm. These contain only one set of chromosomes. Thus, when an egg and sperm join together to form what's called a zygote, the zygote contains a new, complete set of 46 chromosomes.

A gene is a defined segment of DNA on a chromosome. Genes are the blueprints for the cells of your body. They provide instructions for making proteins that, in turn, do the business of a particular cell. Many kinds of proteins play various roles in the body. They control how cells divide, grow and function.

Genes determine characteristics such as how tall you are and what color your eyes are. They tell your body to repair tissue that has been injured and to keep tumors from growing. Your genes also influence your susceptibility to diseases such as cancer.

Genetics is the study of genes and the diseases caused by genetic defects.

When a cell divides, each gene must be copied so that the two resulting cells each has a complete set of genes. Mistakes in this process can and do occur. Quite often these mistakes are harmless and easily repaired, but sometimes they can lead to the development of cancer or other diseases.

Not all genes are active all the time. Some genes continuously produce proteins for basic cell function, and other genes are switched on (activated) only when their protein-coding information is needed. Each cell's function is largely determined by which of its approximately 40,000 genes are activated.

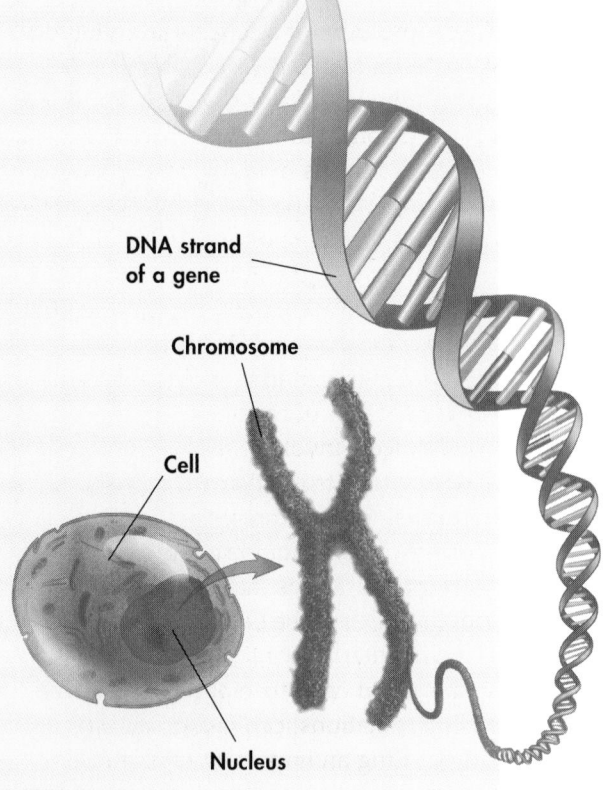

DNA strand
of a gene

Chromosome

Cell

Nucleus

eventually they die. Cancer cells become seemingly immortal. This resistance toward programmed cell death is a hallmark of most, if not all, types of cancer.

Although the life-threatening properties cancer cells acquire may seem daunting, these properties also can serve as targets for treatment. The illustration on page 29 shows how scientists are taking advantage of cancer cell characteristics in designing new drugs.

How Does Cancer Occur?

A key question for scientists studying cancer is to understand what causes the transformation of a normal cell into an abnormal one. How does cancer begin?

Major progress in understanding this process came in the 1950s with the discovery of the structure of deoxyribonucleic acid (DNA) and the advent of molecular biology. Since then, powerful new technologies for studying DNA and genes have led to breakthroughs in understanding the biology of cancer.

All cancers involve the malfunction of genes that control cell growth and division. The order (sequence) of molecules in each gene spells out instructions for producing the proteins that carry out a cell's activities. When the chemical sequence of a gene is altered, it's like a genetic misspelling that can cause problems. These errors (mutations) can result in a cell either losing an important regulatory function or gaining an abnormal function.

Over time, as more cell divisions occur, the chance for mutations increases. Although there are genes that control orderly cell division (replication) and others that check for errors, these too can become damaged, allowing cells to pass along mutations. In fact, the change from a normal cell to a cancerous cell requires several separate, different genetic alterations.

Alterations in the following genes important to cell growth play a critical role in the development of cancer:

- **Tumor suppressor genes.** These genes are responsible for restraining cell growth. They can slow cell division, increase programmed cell death and repair DNA. Defects (mutations) in these genes can make them inactive, allowing a cell and its offspring to divide rapidly and grow out of control. These defects may be passed on from one generation to the next (inherited), or they can develop during a person's lifetime.
- **Oncogenes.** Oncogenes are genes that normally stimulate cell division, but in a properly regulated way. When these genes become altered, they allow for excessive cell growth.
- **Mismatch repair genes.** When DNA is duplicated — a part of the normal process of cell division — errors can occur. There's a complex apparatus, known as the DNA mismatch repair system, that's designed to detect and repair these mistakes. Individuals who inherit defects in this mismatch repair system have a higher likelihood of developing certain cancers, such as colon, uterine or ovarian cancer.

A long process

Cancer development is a process — it has a beginning and a number of steps that must occur for the cancer to progress and become a lethal threat. The first stage, called initiation, involves damage to critical areas of a cell's DNA. The cell can then reproduce abnormal versions of itself.

As cancer cells reproduce, they can become very adaptable. New generations acquire properties that give them an advantage in growth, helping them compete with normal cells for nutrients, so the tumor becomes larger and more destructive. These properties allow cancer cells to evade recognition by the immune system, develop their own blood supply and spread to distant areas of the body.

Several years often pass between the time a single abnormal cell divides and a cancer is detectable. By the time a tumor is large enough to be felt as a lump or seen on an imaging test, it probably contains at least 1 billion cells.

Typical tumor growth

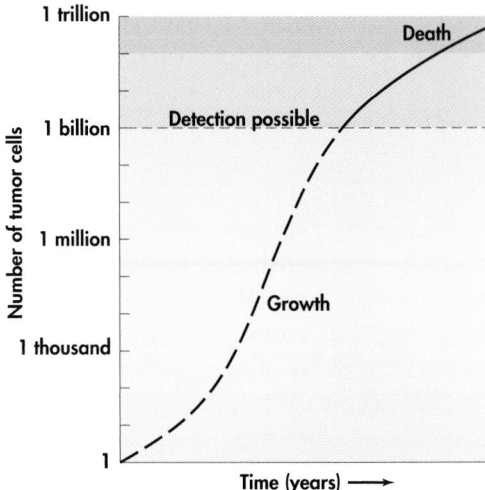

Initially, cancer cells grow rapidly. Even so, it takes several years before a tumor is large enough to be detected with medical tests. At this point — when it contains approximately 1 billion cells — the tumor may grow more slowly because it's outgrowing its nutrient or oxygen supply or because the cells are so abnormal they can no longer divide properly.

Causes

Most cancers don't have one single cause but result from a complex, long-term process. The exact causes of many cancers aren't yet known.

In general, the causes of the majority of cancers can be divided into external and internal factors.

- **External factors.** These are outside influences on the body, including lifestyle and environmental factors. External factors associated with cancer include tobacco use, excessive use of alcohol, an unhealthy diet, a sedentary lifestyle, radiation from the sun and other sources, and exposure to certain chemicals, such as benzene or asbestos. Some cancers are caused by infections. For example, the human papillomavirus (HPV) contributes to cervical, vaginal and vulvar cancers.
- **Internal factors.** These include hormone levels, inherited genetic mutations and immune conditions.

Researchers estimate that 50 percent to 75 percent of all cancers in the United States result from lifestyle factors, including tobacco and alcohol use, an unhealthy diet, and sexual behaviors that may lead to certain sexually transmitted infections.

Risk factors

Factors that increase a person's chance of developing cancer are called risk factors. Identifying risk factors points the way to possible causes of cancer. For example, the observation that lung cancer occurs more frequently among smokers led to research that identified cancer-causing agents (carcinogens) in cigarette smoke.

A number of risk factors for cancer have been identified, although it's not known exactly how some of these factors cause cells to become cancerous.

Having a risk factor or a combination of risk factors means you have a greater than average chance of getting cancer, but it doesn't mean that you'll definitely get it. Many people who develop a type of cancer don't have any of the known risk factors for it, while other people who do have risk factors never get cancer.

Following are some of the common risk factors for cancer.

Age

For the large majority of cancers, age is the most significant risk factor. Simply stated, the older you are, the more likely you are to get cancer. People older than age 55 develop 80 percent of all new cancer cases.

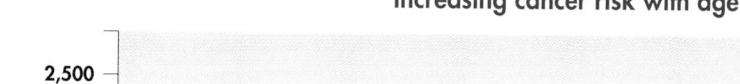

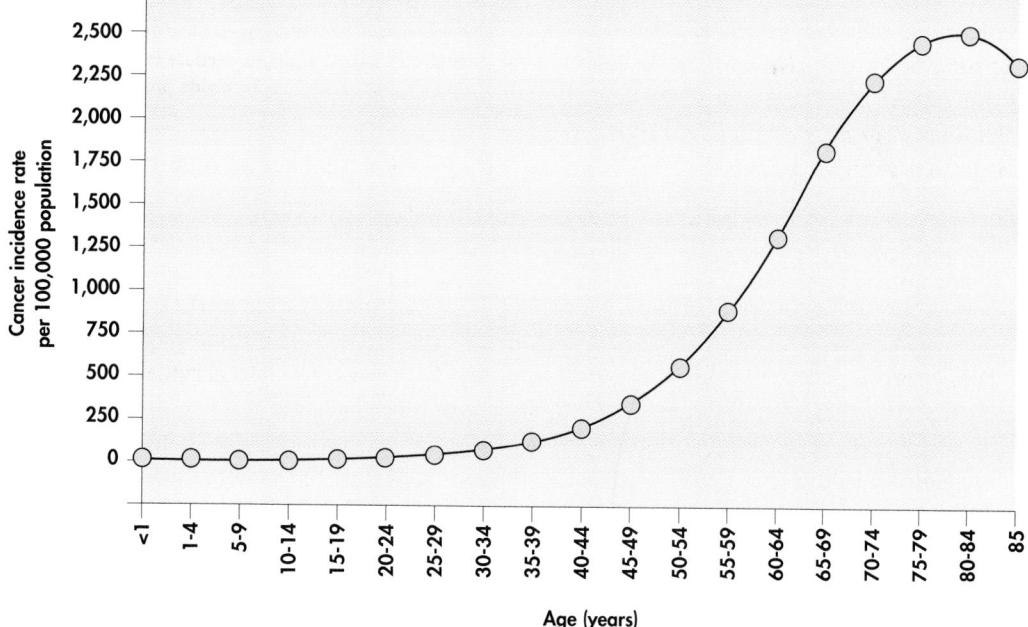

Increasing cancer risk with age

Cancer incidence rate per 100,000 population vs *Age (years)*

Cancer is relatively uncommon in young adults. It becomes considerably more common once people reach age 70.

Source: Surveillance, Epidemiology, and End Results (SEER) Statistics Review, 1975-2000

Age might contribute to cancer for several reasons:

- The natural process of aging leads to changes in the body's cells. Over time, as cells divide, problems with the replication of genetic material may occur. Some genes may mistakenly be turned off, and others may be altered in a way that changes how they function, allowing cancer cells to form and take hold.
- Another theory suggests that immune function declines with age, so people may lose some of their natural ability to fight cancer.
- Yet another factor may be that as people live longer, they're exposed to cancer-causing substances for a longer period of time.

Family history

People who have close relatives with cancer may be at higher risk of the disease. For example, a woman whose mother or sister had breast cancer is about twice as likely to develop the disease.

In some families, cancer is linked to an inherited mutation in a specific gene. But families with such gene mutations are rare. Cancer risk is more likely to be familial, or spontaneous, rather than inherited. *Familial* simply means that something occurs more commonly in a particular family but isn't the direct result of the passage of a single cancer-causing gene. Familial cancer may be due to environmental or lifestyle similarities shared by family members or more subtle genetic effects.

Others

Other risk factors associated with cancer include smoking, obesity, a sedentary lifestyle, exposure to radiation, excessive alcohol use, use of hormones after menopause, exposure to certain chemicals, race, socioeconomic status, certain health conditions, and reproductive and sexual behaviors. Risk factors for the cancers discussed in this book are described in more detail in subsequent chapters.

QUESTION & ANSWER

Q: **Does *genetic* mean the same thing as *inherited*?**

A: The word *genetic* is sometimes used to mean "inherited." In that sense, the two words have the same meaning. But *genetic* can also have a different meaning — it isn't always synonymous with *inherited*. Most of the gene alterations that lead to cancer aren't inherited — that is, they're not passed from one generation to another. Rather, they're spontaneous (acquired) genetic changes that occur in the body's cells during an individual's lifetime.

About 5 percent to 10 percent of cancers are clearly hereditary — a faulty gene inherited from a parent predisposes the descendants to a high risk of a particular cancer. The other 90 percent to 95 percent of cancers stem from damage to a cell's genes that occurs throughout a person's life.

Advancing Our Knowledge of Cancer

"Without research, there is no hope," wrote Paul Rogers, sponsor of the legislation that launched the War on Cancer in 1971. Since the passage of the National Cancer Act that same year, more than 1 million research papers about cancer have been published. This growing body of scientific knowledge has resulted in major strides in our basic understanding of cancer and its detection and treatment, offering hope for even more discoveries and improvements in the future.

Many different types of scientists are engaged in cancer research. They include individuals who study the molecules that make up living matter (molecular biologists) and scientists who study the chemical makeup of living matter (organic chemists). Physiologists study the functions and vital processes of organisms, and biochemists conduct research in the chemistry of life processes. Epidemiologists examine the frequency and distribution of cancer within populations along with certain factors that appear to influence those particular patterns. Pharmacologists study how drugs work. Clinical researchers move basic fundamental discoveries into the clinical setting.

The research process is complicated, time-consuming and costly, and the outcome is never known at the outset. Along the way, as basic research is translated into specific interventions, new technologies and tools are developed. These advances make it possible to put theory into practice.

QUESTION & ANSWER

Q: **What types of radiation exposure contribute to cancer?**

A: Some forms of radiation exposure are linked to a higher risk of cancer. One familiar example is ultraviolet (UV) radiation from sunlight or tanning lamps. UV radiation exposure is a risk factor for skin cancer, especially in light-skinned people.

Being exposed to large amounts of X-ray (ionizing) radiation also can increase cancer risk. For example, women who received radiation to the chest area to treat Hodgkin's disease or tuberculosis have an increased risk of breast cancer. This is particularly true for women who received radiation to their chests during their teenage and young adult years when breast tissue was developing.

In comparison, the small amount of X-ray exposure you get from occasional dental exams or ordinary diagnostic exams, such as chest X-rays or mammograms, doesn't appear to pose a significant health risk.

Basic research

Basic research lies at the heart of scientific discovery. Research independently conceived and developed by scientists has often been the driving force behind medical advances. Basic research provides insights into how cancer starts, and it offers clues regarding key steps involved in cancer progression.

Through basic research, scientists can:

- Explore how errors in genes and proteins disrupt normal cellular communication and regulation and lead to uncontrolled growth of abnormal cells
- Learn which genes and proteins play key roles in cancer invasion and spread
- Identify the ways neighboring cells and tissues contribute to tumor growth
- Develop and test new technologies to detect and monitor cancer
- Develop new drugs and technologies for treating cancer
- Conduct laboratory and animal tests of new drugs

Epidemiologic studies

Epidemiologists look at trends in cancer incidence and death (mortality) rates and study patterns of cancer in the population to identify risk factors and protective factors. They compile statistics, such as the number of estimated new cases of cancer, annual deaths from cancer, the most common cancers in men and women, cancer rates among various age groups, and cancer occurrence in various racial and ethnic groups. The findings from this research provide important clues about what contributes to the development of cancer.

Epidemiologists conduct studies that may be either retrospective or prospective in nature. A retrospective study goes back in time and evaluates a group of people who previously had a procedure or a type of exposure. A prospective study evaluates participants going forward in time and follows them for certain outcomes of interest. Both types of studies have different strengths and limitations.

Clinical trials

Clinical trials are research studies in humans that test new approaches for diagnosis, treatment and prevention. These studies are used in all specialties of medicine.

Today's cancer treatments are based on the results of past clinical trials. Doctors all over the world conduct many types of clinical trials to study ways to prevent, detect, diagnose and treat cancer, as well as to understand and treat the psychological effects of the disease and to improve comfort and quality of life.

The importance of clinical trials can be seen in how surgery is used to treat breast cancer. In 1970, the treatment for virtually all women with localized breast cancer was the same: radical mastectomy. Clinical trials then compared that approach with less extensive surgery. Results were comparable, proving that lumpectomy combined with radiation therapy is equally effective. Clinical trials also showed that shorter durations of chemotherapy were just as effective as the yearlong treatment that women with breast or ovarian cancer used to receive.

All clinical trials begin with a basic ethical question: Do the potential benefits of a particular treatment outweigh the potential harm from it? The approaches tested in clinical trials are potential therapies — they're not established therapies or generally accepted treatments until they've been proved to be effective. But a clinical trial is conducted only when researchers have reason to believe that the treatment or prevention being studied may be valuable to the patient.

How new cancer drugs work

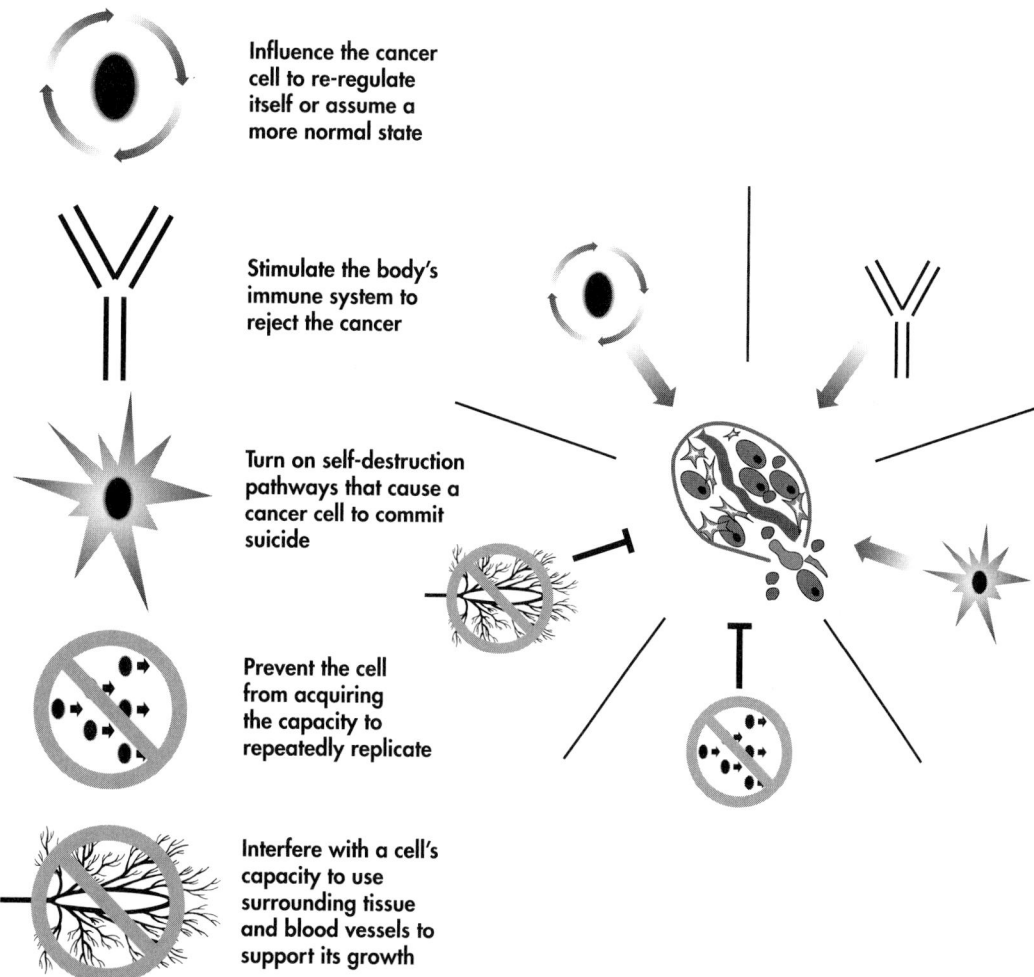

Influence the cancer cell to re-regulate itself or assume a more normal state

Stimulate the body's immune system to reject the cancer

Turn on self-destruction pathways that cause a cancer cell to commit suicide

Prevent the cell from acquiring the capacity to repeatedly replicate

Interfere with a cell's capacity to use surrounding tissue and blood vessels to support its growth

Researchers foresee a day when cancer treatment will be based on a set of characteristics unique to an individual's tumor. New drugs can now be designed that target specific molecular characteristics that may be causing or stimulating cancer development.

Modified from "The Nation's Investment in Cancer Research, A Plan and Budget Proposal for Fiscal Year 2004," National Institutes of Health

Enrolling in a Clinical Trial

By taking part in a clinical trial, you may have the first chance to benefit from new approaches to cancer prevention and treatment. And you'll be making a contribution to medical science while taking an active role in your own health care.

If you're in a well-designed trial, you'll receive excellent care, with a team of experts examining you and monitoring your progress.

There are some risks, though. No one involved in the study knows in advance whether the new treatment will work or exactly what side effects or adverse reactions might occur. In addition, the trial may require some extra time for trips to the study site, treatments, hospital stays or complex dosage requirements. Participants may be required to keep detailed records of any symptoms they may experience and to follow certain schedules and guidelines.

The best place to start in finding a clinical trial is to talk with your doctor. Doctors are usually aware of investigational drugs that might benefit their patients and clinical trials involving these drugs. You can also get a list of current clinical trials by calling the National Cancer Institute's Cancer Information Service at (800) 4-CANCER, or (800) 422-6237, or by visiting its Web site: *www.cancer.gov.*

Phases of clinical trials

A clinical trial involves a long and careful research process. Before a new treatment or preventive approach can be administered to humans, researchers must conduct preclinical experiments under controlled circumstances in a laboratory, using test tubes and animals. Scientists analyze a treatment's physical and chemical properties in the lab and study its pharmacologic and toxic effects in animals to determine its possible effectiveness and harm. This type of evaluation, which can take several years, is called preclinical research.

If the preclinical research shows promising results, the sponsor of the trial may request permission to begin clinical trials by filing an application with the Food and Drug Administration. If the application is approved, researchers can begin to investigate the new therapy in people. A new treatment is normally studied in three phases of clinical trials.

Phase I

Phase I trials are the first tests of a new treatment in humans. The goal is to gather information on the safest and most effective dose and the schedule for giving it. Doctors watch participants carefully for any harmful side effects. These trials generally last several months to a year and involve a small number of patients, usually no more than 20 to 40.

Phase II

Once the appropriate dose and schedule are known, a phase II trial of the new therapy is done for specific cancer types. Phase II trials are designed to see if a

RESEARCH UPDATE

Genomics and proteomics

Two important areas of ongoing cancer research are genomics and proteomics.

Genomics is the study of the human genome — the complete set of approximately 40,000 genes in a human being. The completion of the Human Genome Project was an enormous advance in genomics. It resulted in a map that details the sequence of chemical base pairs (nucleotides) that make up the 6 feet of tightly coiled DNA contained in each human cell. The map shows genetic landmarks along each of the chromosomes, including the locations of genes that are altered in various cancers. Information about particular genes can help identify key molecular targets for cancer diagnosis and treatment.

As work continues on refining the map of the human genome, the next frontier is proteomics, the study of human proteins. The word stems from the term *proteome*, which refers to the complete array of human proteins.

Although genes carry the instructions for making proteins, proteins are the actual players that carry out the cell's activities. Proteomics aims to evaluate the structure, function and expression of proteins. This is a huge task. There are about 40,000 genes, but there may be as many as 10 million proteins. Only a small percentage of them have been identified to date.

A major goal of proteomics is to diagram the "protein wiring" (signaling) pathways that control cell growth and activity.

---

therapy has a biologic effect in treating a specific cancer. In addition to testing for effectiveness, researchers also gather more detailed information about safety. Phase II trials take about two years and usually include 20 to 40 participants. At times, multiple phase II trials are done for a promising new agent.

Phase III

The goal of phase III trials is to compare a promising new approach with the most accepted current treatment. Researchers want to learn if the new treatment is more effective, less toxic, less expensive or can be given over a shorter period of time. Phase III trials involve large numbers of

individuals, sometimes thousands of people from hundreds of research centers around the country or the world.

Participants in phase III trials are randomly assigned (randomized) into one of two or more groups. One group, the control group, receives the standard treatment. The other, the intervention group, receives the investigational treatment.

In double-blind trials neither the participant nor the doctor knows which treatment the person is receiving, to avoid bias. In other clinical trials, however, both the participant and doctor know which treatment the participant is receiving.

Researchers try to ensure that individuals in the treatment and control groups

MYTH vs. FACT

Myth: **Cancer rates are soaring.**

Fact: From 1992 to 1999, death rates from cancer in the United States declined by 1.5 percent a year for men and 0.6 percent a year for women. Since 1950, cancer death rates, excluding lung cancer, declined 16 percent.

Incidence rates of cancer in women did increase from 1987 to 1999. Incidence rates refer to the number of new diagnoses per 100,000 individuals of a defined age. But the increase was slight, just 0.3 percent, while incidence rates of cancer in men have stabilized. However, the total number of people living with cancer is expected to rise because the U.S. population is aging, and cancer is more common in older people.

are as similar as possible in characteristics that could affect treatment outcomes. For instance, in most studies, all patients in both groups should have the same type and stage of cancer.

Once an agent has been proved successful in phase III trials, the new approach becomes part of the standard treatment.

Patient safety

Patient safety is of utmost priority in clinical trials. Investigators must follow strict guidelines. Clinical trials are subject to a rigorous review and oversight process designed to protect the rights and safety of people who enroll.

Several groups have to approve the protocol for many clinical trials. These groups may include the study's sponsor, such as the National Cancer Institute or the American Cancer Society, and the participating institution's institutional review board (IRB). An IRB is an independent committee of doctors, statisticians, community advocates and other experts. All institutions that conduct or support medical research involving humans must have

an IRB. These committees of experts and laypersons also review the research as it progresses.

In addition, all participants in clinical trials must provide informed consent. When an individual inquires about a particular clinical trial, he or she is provided key facts about the study, including its possible risks and benefits. Before that individual can enroll in the study, he or she needs to indicate, in written form, that he or she is aware of the possible risks and benefits involved.

Participants are free to leave a clinical trial at any time.

PART 1

Breast Cancer

Chapter 3: Breast Cancer

An Overview

Perhaps no other disease has a greater hold on a woman's fears than does breast cancer. It's not the deadliest cancer women can get — lung cancer is. And it's not the most common life-threatening illness to affect women — that's heart disease. But ask a group of women what disease they worry about most, and the majority will likely say breast cancer.

This fear isn't unfounded. Breast cancer is the most common life-threatening cancer among women in the United States. It's the second most common cause of cancer death in women and the main cause of cancer death in women ages 40 to 55. Most women know someone who has had breast cancer — a friend, sister, mother, other relative or an acquaintance.

The disease strikes close to home in other ways as well. It can affect how a woman looks and feels about her femininity and sexuality. Many women who have breast cancer are afraid that changes in their bodies will affect not only their appearance but also the way other people perceive them.

Yet there's more cause for optimism with regard to breast cancer than ever before. In the last 35 years, scientists have learned much more about how and why breast cancer develops and have made tremendous strides in diagnosis and treatment. Research has led to better treatments, a lower chance of death from the disease and an improved quality of life for women living with breast cancer.

In 1970, breast cancer was more likely to be diagnosed at a late stage, and treatment usually involved a radical mastectomy — removal of the entire breast along with underarm lymph nodes, skin and muscles underneath the breast. Chemotherapy after surgery typically lasted a whole year.

Today, breast cancer is often detected early through mammography, and a radical mastectomy is rarely performed. Many women receive breast-sparing treatments, such as lumpectomy and radiation, and they go through a shorter course of chemotherapy. In addition, a growing network of agencies and other resources exists to help women who have just received a diagnosis of breast cancer, are facing treatment decisions or are living with a history of breast cancer.

If you've been diagnosed with breast cancer, take heart that what used to be a dismal diagnosis often no longer is. Yes, breast cancer is a serious illness, and, yes, it can be fatal. But in larger numbers than ever before, women are beating the disease and living productive lives.

This chapter provides an overview of what's known about breast cancer, its causes and women who develop it. Subsequent chapters look at risk factors, prevention, diagnosis and treatment.

Benign Breast Conditions

A lump or thickening in the breast is the most common sign of breast cancer. But most breast lumps (masses) are benign, meaning they're not cancerous. These benign lumps don't spread outside the breast, and they aren't life-threatening. A variety of conditions other than breast cancer can cause lumps in your breasts and can cause your breasts to change in size or feel. Common benign breast conditions include:

- **Fibrocystic breast changes.** Fibrocystic breast changes are common, occurring in at least half the women in the United States. *Fibro* refers to the presence of fibrous connective tissue, and *cystic* refers to cysts, which are fluid-filled sacs. You may feel a bumpy texture or lumpiness in your breasts, along with swelling, tenderness or pain, most likely just before your menstrual period. You may also experience fibrocystic changes if you're postmenopausal and taking hormones.

  If your breasts are quite lumpy, performing a breast self-exam is more challenging. Becoming familiar with what's normal for you through monthly self-exams may make it easier to detect any new lumps or changes.

- **Cysts.** These are fluid-filled sacs that feel like a soft lump or tender spot. They're found most often in women ages 35 to 50. Cysts can range from tiny to about the size of an egg. They may increase in size or become more tender just before your period and disappear completely after it.

- **Fibroadenomas.** These are solid, noncancerous tumors that often occur in

Your Breasts

Breasts are composed mainly of connective and fatty tissues. Suspended within the tissues of each breast is a network of milk-forming lobes. Within each lobe are many smaller lobules, each of which ends in dozens of tiny bulbs that can produce milk. Thin tubes called ducts connect the bulbs, lobules and lobes to the nipple, which is surrounded by an area of dark skin, called the areola. No muscles are in the breasts themselves, but muscles covering your ribs lie underneath each breast.

Blood vessels and lymph vessels run throughout your breasts. Blood nourishes breast cells. Lymph vessels carry a clear fluid called lymph, which contains immune system cells and drains waste products from tissues. Lymph vessels lead to pea-sized collections of tissue called lymph nodes. Most of the lymph vessels in the breast lead to lymph nodes under the arm, called axillary nodes.

Breast Cancer

Breast cancer is the common term for a cancerous (malignant) tumor that starts in cells that line the ducts and lobes of the breast. If the cancerous cells are confined

women during their reproductive years. A fibroadenoma is a firm, smooth, rubbery or hard lump with a well-defined shape. It moves easily under your skin when touched and is usually painless. Fibroadenomas are more common among younger women and black women.

- **Infections.** Infection of the breast (mastitis) typically affects women who are breast-feeding or who recently stopped breast-feeding, although it's also possible to develop mastitis that's not related to breast-feeding. Your breast will likely be red, warm, tender and lumpy, and the lymph nodes under your arms may swell. You may also feel slightly ill and may have a low-grade fever.
- **Trauma.** Sometimes, a blow to the breast or a bruise can cause a lump. This doesn't mean you're more likely to get breast cancer.

- **Calcium deposits (microcalcifications).** Tiny deposits of calcium can appear anywhere within your breast and often show up on mammograms. Most women have one or more areas of calcium deposits. Cellular secretions and debris, inflammation, trauma or prior radiation may cause them. Microcalcifications don't result from taking calcium supplements.

  The majority of calcium deposits are harmless, but a small percentage may be associated with cancer. Microcalcifications associated with cancer typically have a particular appearance on mammography X-rays. If these are found, your doctor will likely recommend additional tests.

  If you're concerned about a lump in your breast or a change in how your breast feels, see your doctor.

Breast anatomy

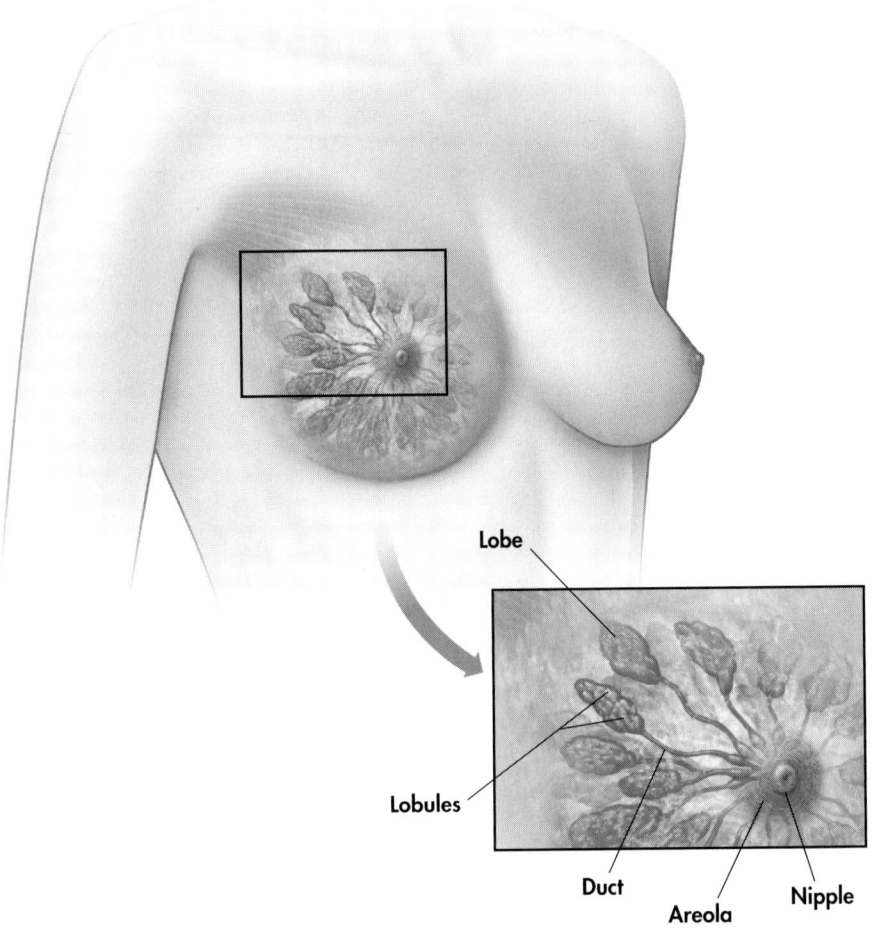

Lobe

Lobules

Duct

Areola

Nipple

The female breast has between 15 and 20 milk-forming units (lobes). Each lobe is made up of many smaller structures (lobules) that end in tiny bulbs that can produce milk. The lobes, lobules and bulbs are linked by a network of thin tubes called ducts. Ducts carry milk from the bulbs and eventually empty at the nipple.

Normal breast tissue

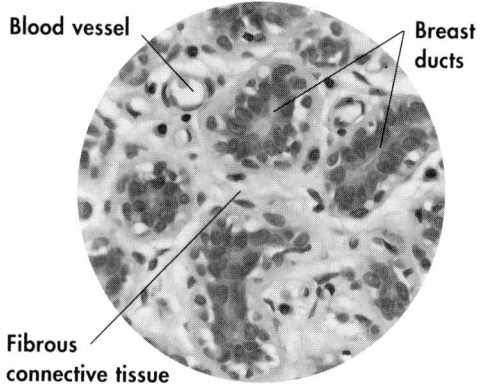

Blood vessel

Breast ducts

Fibrous connective tissue

Noninvasive cancer

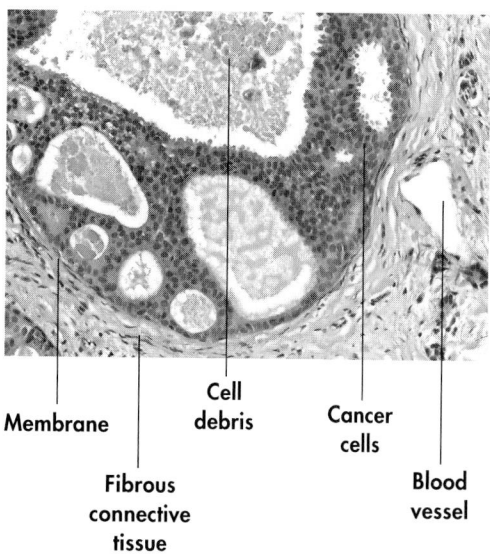

Membrane

Cell debris

Cancer cells

Fibrous connective tissue

Blood vessel

Invasive cancer

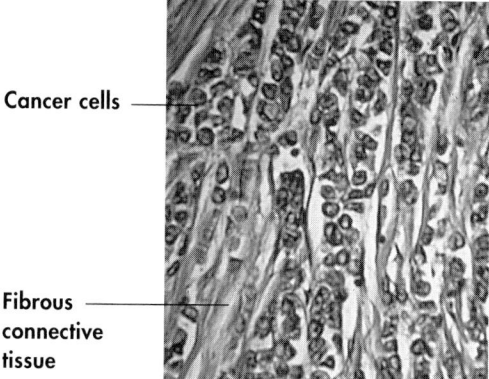

Cancer cells

Fibrous connective tissue

The slide at upper left shows several normal breast ducts surrounded by fibrous connective tissue. The slide at upper right shows noninvasive cancer (ductal carcinoma *in situ*). A large duct in the center containing cell debris is expanded by layers of cancer cells. Importantly, the membrane around the duct is intact — there's no spread into the surrounding fibrous connective tissue. The slide at bottom left shows invasive cancer. Breast cancer cells are highly disorganized. They're too large, and they've invaded through the fibrous connective tissue of the breast.

to the ducts or lobules and haven't invaded surrounding breast tissue, the cancer is called noninvasive or *in situ*. Cancer that has spread through the walls of the ducts or lobules into connective or fatty tissue is referred to as invasive or infiltrating.

Types of breast cancer

Breast cancer is categorized by the microscopic appearance of the cancer cells and whether the cancer has invaded surrounding tissue. Following is a list of the most common types of breast cancer:

• **Invasive ductal carcinoma (IDC).** This cancer begins in a duct, breaks through the duct wall and invades the connective or fatty tissue of the breast. There, it can gain access to blood vessels and can spread to other parts of the body. Invasive ductal carcinoma is the most common type of breast cancer. It

Rising Rates of Invasive Lobular Cancer

In recent years, the incidence of invasive lobular carcinoma (ILC) in the United States has increased steadily. ILC is a less common form of cancer that begins in the milk-producing glands (lobules) of the breast. Meanwhile, rates for the more common form of breast cancer, invasive ductal carcinoma (IDC), have remained about the same.

Historically, ILC represented about 5 percent to 10 percent of all breast cancers in the United States. But from 1987 to 1999, the proportion of all breast cancers that had a lobular component — either lobular carcinomas or mixed ductal-lobular carcinomas — rose to 16 percent.

Increased rates of ILC were most pronounced among women older than age 50. Use of hormone replacement therapy — the hormones estrogen and progestin — during and after menopause has been shown to increase the risk of ILC.

Use of hormone replacement therapy (HRT) increased in the United States at the same time that the rates of ILC rose, leading researchers to suspect a possible link between hormone replacement therapy and this type of cancer. Now that HRT isn't as widely recommended as it once was, researchers will be looking to see if future ILC rates decline.

represents about 75 percent of all invasive breast cancers.

- **Invasive lobular carcinoma (ILC).** This cancer starts in the lobules, breaks through to the connective or fatty tissue of the breast and can spread to other parts of the body as well. ILC accounts for about 15 percent of invasive breast cancers.
- **Other invasive cancers.** In addition to IDC and ILC, there are several less common types of breast cancer, including medullary, mucinous, tubular and papillary. These cancers account for the last 10 percent of invasive cancers.
- **Ductal carcinoma *in situ* (DCIS).** This is the most common type of noninvasive breast cancer. The abnormal cells have not spread through the walls of the ducts into the connective and fatty tissues of the breast. But if these cells aren't removed, they may develop into an invasive cancer that can spread.
- **Lobular carcinoma *in situ* (LCIS).** In this condition, the abnormal cells haven't spread beyond the lobules, and they usually don't develop into invasive cancer. For this reason, LCIS isn't considered a true cancer. However, women with LCIS are at increased risk of developing invasive breast cancer later on, in either breast. Therefore, LCIS is seen as an important marker for breast cancer risk.
- **Paget's disease.** Paget's disease is a type of breast cancer that's associated with nipple changes. The underlying cancer can be invasive or noninvasive.

More detailed information regarding breast cancer types can be found in Chapter 7.

Cancer spread

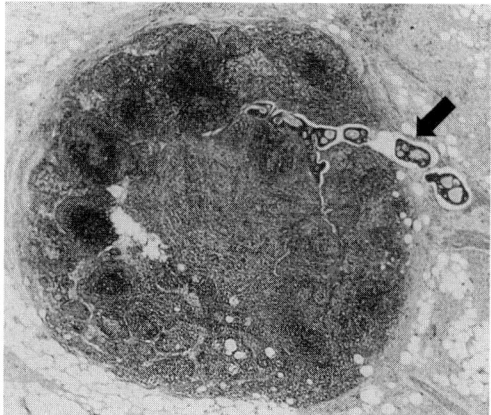

Metastatic breast cancer occurs when breast cancer cells spread to other parts of the body. The cells use lymphatic vessels and blood vessels as a means of travel to other areas. This microscopic image shows cancer cells (see arrow) entering a lymph node through a lymphatic channel.

Reprinted with permission from the *New England Journal of Medicine*

Cancer growth and spread

When cancer arises in breast tissue and spreads outside the breast, cancer cells are often found in the underarm (axillary) lymph nodes. The ability of cancer cells to spread to these nodes means that the cancer has the capacity to spread to other parts of the body as well. That's why axillary nodes are examined as part of the process of determining the extent of the disease (staging).

If breast cancer spreads to other parts of the body, it's called metastatic breast cancer. Sites for breast cancer cells to spread include the lymph nodes, skin on the chest wall, bones, liver and lungs. If, for example, breast cancer spreads to the lungs, the tumor there has the same kind of abnormal cells as the primary breast tumor. Therefore, the disease is called metastatic breast cancer, not lung cancer. It may also be referred to as distant disease.

Breast cancers grow at different rates, but some researchers estimate that the average tumor doubles in size every 100 days. Most tumors aren't large enough to feel or notice for years. It's estimated that it takes an average of at least five years for a tumor to reach a size that it can be felt. Some tumors have an even longer period in which they're undetectable (latency period). Mammography can find tumors that are too small to be felt, but most tumors have probably been growing for years before they're large enough to be visible on a mammogram. By the time most breast tumors are detected, at approximately 1 centimeter in size, they have about 1 billion cells.

For more information about how cancer develops, see Chapter 2.

What Causes Breast Cancer?

It's often impossible to explain why one woman gets breast cancer and another doesn't. Breast cancer results from a series of events that transform a normal cell to an abnormal one. Multiple factors — known and unknown — contribute to the disease. There's no single cause.

Researchers have identified a number of factors associated with an increased risk of breast cancer. These include genetic,

Features of Hereditary Breast Cancer

What if there are two or three women in your family with breast cancer? Does that mean the cancer is hereditary?

Because breast cancer is a common disease, two or more cases of breast cancer may occur in a family simply by chance. Also, family members share many things in addition to their genes, such as similar diets and environments, weight and height, patterns of childbearing, and occupations.

All of these factors can influence a woman's risk of developing breast cancer, without the presence of an inherited alteration in a specific gene.

Breast cancer that's inherited has certain hallmarks. Some indications that breast cancer cases in a family may be hereditary include the following:

- Women in each generation are affected.
- Multiple relatives are affected.
- The cancer is diagnosed at an early age — before menopause.
- Some family members also may have developed ovarian cancer.
- There's a family history of cancer in both breasts (bilateral breast cancer) or of male breast cancer.

For more information on hereditary breast cancer, see Chapter 4.

hormonal and environmental factors, as well as aging. These factors are interrelated and can all work together to contribute to cancer development.

Genetic factors

Most cancers, including breast cancer, acquire many genetic abnormalities — alterations to genes or chromosomes — as the cancer develops. In this sense, breast cancer is considered a genetic disease.

But most of the genetic problems seen in breast cancer aren't inherited. Genetic alterations may be either inherited or acquired (spontaneous). Inherited mutations are those you were born with — a defective gene that one of your parents passed on to you. Acquired alterations occur within your body's cells during your lifetime and aren't passed on. They're much more common than are inherited changes.

An acquired genetic error can happen in many ways, and the causes of most of these alterations remain unknown. Most breast cancers appear to result from a variety of spontaneous changes that ultimately lead to the development of cancer.

Alterations in two types of genes important to cell growth can turn normal cells into cancerous ones.

- **Tumor suppressor genes.** These very important regulatory genes turn off cell growth, stopping cell division and replication. Errors in these genes allow cells to grow out of control. Inherited defects in certain tumor suppressor genes, such as the breast cancer genes BRCA1 and BRCA2, result in a marked predisposition to develop breast cancer.

- **Oncogenes.** These genes turn on (promote) cell division and growth. If this type of gene is damaged or defective, cell growth runs out of control. Several oncogenes have been associated with the development of breast cancer. They include the HER-2/neu, EGFR and ras genes. Although abnormalities in these oncogenes can contribute to breast cancer, they're not inherited.

Hereditary breast cancer

An estimated 5 percent to 10 percent of breast cancers are hereditary — that is, they're caused by inherited alterations in the chemical order of a gene. Individuals from some families inherit and pass on altered genetic material that significantly increases the risk of breast cancer. If your father or mother has an altered gene, you have a 50 percent chance of inheriting that gene from him or her.

For example, inherited mutations in two tumor suppressor genes have been linked to an increased risk of breast cancer. The two most common genes associated with hereditary breast cancer are breast cancer gene 1 (BRCA1) and breast cancer gene 2 (BRCA2). People with defects in these genes have a high risk of developing breast cancer over their lifetimes. Women with an alteration in one of these genes have a 45 percent to 80 percent lifetime chance of developing breast cancer. Men also can carry a defect in BRCA1 or BRCA2, and when they do, they're at an increased risk of breast cancer. This is especially true for men who inherit a BRCA2 mutation.

The BRCA1 and BRCA2 genes are large, and many different alterations in them have been associated with an increased risk of breast cancer. Defective BRCA1 and BRCA2 genes account for about 40 percent of hereditary forms of breast cancer. Abnormalities in these genes also result in an increased risk of other cancers, especially ovarian cancer.

Several other inherited syndromes also significantly increase risk of breast cancer.

Miscarriage, Abortion and Fertility Treatments

Because hormonal and reproductive factors are known to influence breast cancer risk, a great deal of research has been conducted to determine whether having a miscarriage or abortion affects a woman's chances of developing breast cancer later. Early studies produced inconsistent results, and most of those studies were small and had scientific flaws. Since then, larger, better-designed studies have found no consistent link between miscarriage or abortion and breast cancer.

Researchers have also questioned whether treatments to boost fertility, such as those used during assistive reproductive technology procedures, can contribute to breast cancer development. Women undergoing treatment for infertility are exposed to high concentrations of estrogen and progesterone. Studies indicate that this type of ovarian stimulation doesn't appear to increase a woman's risk of breast cancer.

These include Li-Fraumeni syndrome, Cowden syndrome and Peutz-Jeghers syndrome. These conditions account for less than 1 percent of all breast cancers. Alterations in other tumor suppressor genes, including p53, PTEN and ATM, are also linked to increased breast cancer risk.

Hormonal and reproductive factors

Researchers have long observed that many of the risk factors for breast cancer relate to a woman's lifetime exposure to estrogen and other reproductive hormones. From a woman's first menstrual cycle, to the birth of a child, to the onset of menopause, the hormones estrogen and progesterone are stimulating breast cells. These hormones are essential for normal breast development and function, but they can also promote breast cancer.

Breast cancer risk is affected to some extent by several reproductive factors that increase the amount of time a woman's body produces or is exposed to estrogen. These include:

- An early age at first menstruation
- A late age at menopause
- Postmenopausal hormone therapy

Women who carry a pregnancy to term at a young age and those who breast-feed have a slightly decreased risk of getting breast cancer. On the other hand, women who don't become pregnant or who become pregnant at a later age have increased breast cancer risks.

Environmental factors

Environmental factors also play a role in the development of breast cancer. When used in reference to cancer risk, the word

Breast Cancer and Stress

Can stress cause breast cancer? The short answer is no, probably not. Most research hasn't found evidence of a direct link between stress and breast cancer. But the belief that emotional or psychological factors can cause cancer is widespread — and it's not a new idea. Almost 2,000 years ago, the Greek doctor Galen noted that melancholic women were much more susceptible to cancer than were other women. Interest in the mind-body connection and cancer has been renewed in recent decades as scientists gain a better understanding of the complex relationships among the immune system, hormones and the nervous system. Evidence suggests that stress can disturb many components of the immune system and that an impaired immune system may increase a person's risk of cancer. Stress also impacts an individual's endocrine (hormonal) system, increasing or decreasing the secretion of various hormones.

Other researchers have theorized that cancer is more likely to occur in people with certain personality traits — those who suppress their emotions, especially anger, who put others' needs ahead of their own or who have an attitude of

environment means more than just the surrounding air, water and land. Environmental factors include anything that isn't inherited or innate, including a woman's lifestyle, where she lives and works, and any exposure to carcinogens.

Research on the rates of breast cancer in different areas of the world suggests that environmental factors do affect cancer risk. For example, breast cancer rates in Asia and Africa are much lower than are those in North America. Yet, when Asians immigrate to the United States, within a couple of generations, the breast cancer rate among their descendants approaches the American rate. In addition, the rate of breast cancer in Japan has gradually increased as the Japanese lifestyle has become more westernized.

Unfortunately, determining which environmental factors contribute to breast cancer and to what extent is neither easy nor straightforward. So far, scientists haven't found many links between specific environmental factors and the risk of breast cancer.

In addition, it can be difficult or impossible to sort out environmental factors and a woman's susceptibility to such factors. For example, breast cancer rates are higher among some professional workers, but this may be because they have later pregnancies or no pregnancies, rather than because of something related to their jobs.

Nonetheless, researchers have identified some lifestyle and environmental factors that appear to affect a woman's chance of developing breast cancer. They include:

- **A sedentary lifestyle.** Some data suggest that women who are physically inactive may have a mildly increased risk of breast cancer.

helplessness or hopelessness, the so-called cancer-prone (type C) personality.

Over the years, researchers have put these theories to the test in a large number of studies investigating whether stressful life events or psychosocial factors play a role in the onset and progression of breast cancer. Results have been inconclusive and contradictory.

A few studies have shown an association between stressful life events, such as divorce, separation or the death of a spouse, close friend or relative, and the development, progression or recurrence of breast cancer. But other studies have shown just the opposite — that stressful life events are *not* associated with breast cancer risk. Similarly, most studies haven't found personality factors to be related to breast cancer risk.

In general, the evidence for a relationship among psychological and social factors and breast cancer is weak. But because of the small number of high-quality studies on the topic, some researchers say it's not possible to definitively rule out stress as a contributing factor to breast cancer.

The bottom line? If you have breast cancer, don't think that your cancer resulted or recurred because you were unable to deal with life's stresses.

- **Excessive alcohol use.** Studies show that women who drink more than one alcoholic drink a day have a greater risk of developing breast cancer than do nondrinkers or those who drink less than one drink a day.
- **Excess body weight.** Being overweight or obese has been shown to increase the risk of postmenopausal breast cancer.
- **Radiation exposure.** Women whose breasts have been exposed to significant X-ray (ionizing) radiation — such as women who received radiation to their chest lymph nodes to treat Hodgkin's disease — have an increased risk of breast cancer. The amount of radiation necessary to increase risk is much greater than that which accompanies yearly mammograms.

Researchers have also conducted studies to determine whether pesticides, pollution or on-the-job exposure to hazardous agents may contribute to breast cancer. Most of the evidence is inconclusive. For more information on breast cancer risk factors, see Chapter 4.

Aging

Increasing age is a major risk factor for breast cancer. One reason the disease is more common now than it was 100 years ago is that women are living almost twice as long (see Chapter 2). Breast cancer is uncommon among women under age 30, but your risk of getting it increases as you get older. Seventy-five percent of breast cancers occur in women older than age 50.

The National Cancer Institute estimates that about one in eight women in the United States will develop breast cancer at some point during her lifetime. But this figure is somewhat misleading because it refers to the risk a woman has during her entire life if she lived to be more than 89 years old. For a woman who lives to age 79, the chance of getting breast cancer is one in 10.

How Common Is Breast Cancer?

According to the World Health Organization, breast cancer is the most common life-threatening cancer to affect women worldwide, with more than 1 million new cases of the disease occurring each year.

Breast cancer rates are highest in developed, affluent regions, such as the United States, the United Kingdom, Northern and Western Europe, and Australia, where incidence rates are greater than 80 per 100,000 women. But even in these regions, the death rate from breast cancer has begun to decline, thanks to improvements in early detection and treatment.

Low incidence and death rates for breast cancer are found in most Asian and African countries, and intermediate rates are found in Southern European and South American countries.

In the United States, in 2004 an estimated 215,990 new cases of invasive breast cancer will be diagnosed in women, and the number of estimated deaths is 40,110.

The incidence of breast cancer has generally increased in the last 25 years. Between 1996 and 2000, among all women

A woman's chance of developing breast cancer increases with age

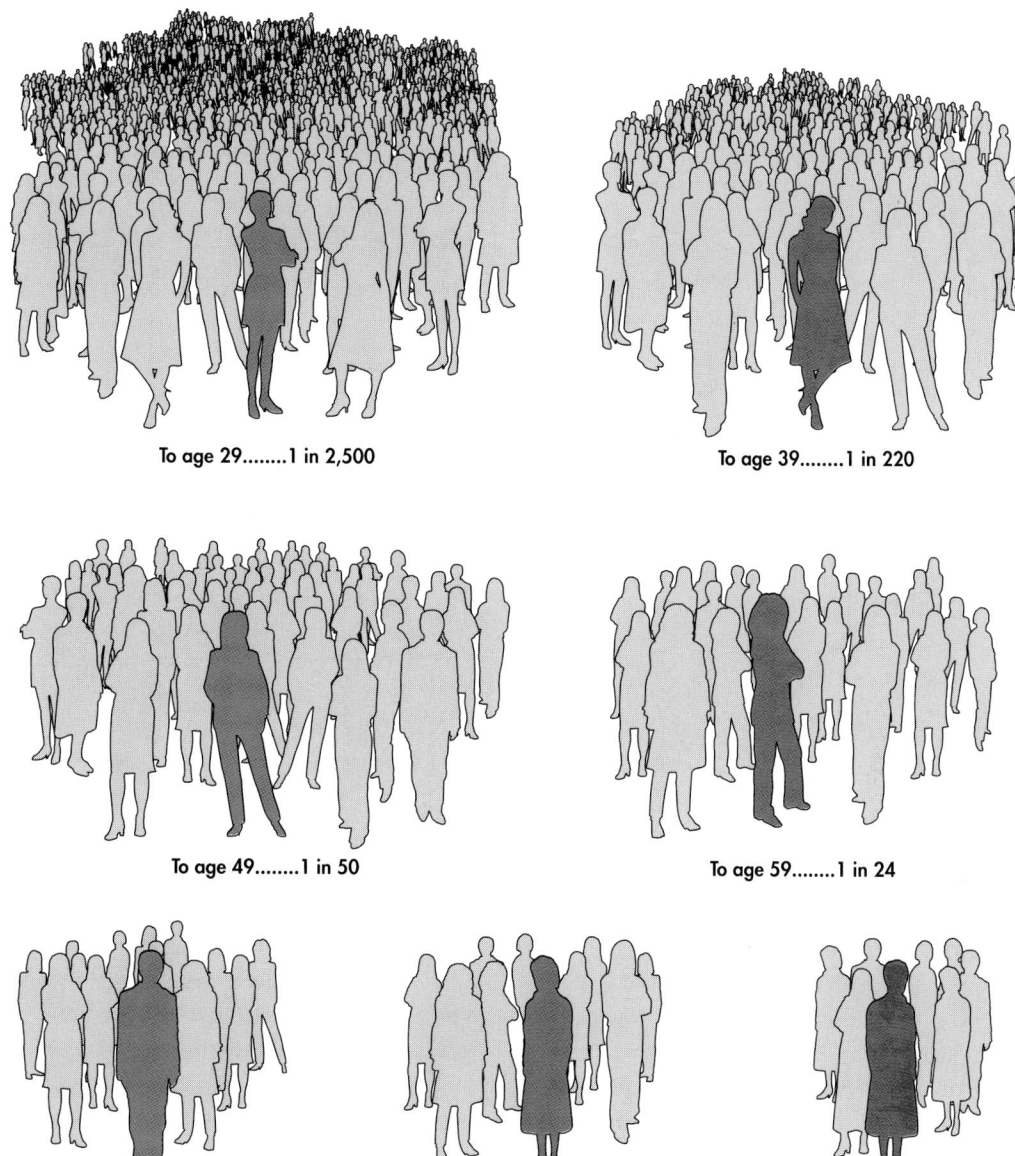

To age 29........1 in 2,500

To age 39........1 in 220

To age 49........1 in 50

To age 59........1 in 24

To age 69........1 in 14

To age 79........1 in 10

89 and older........1 in 8

Modified from Surveillance, Epidemiology, and End Results (SEER) data, National Cancer Institute, 2003

BREAST CANCER

BREAST CANCER

Incidence of breast cancer worldwide

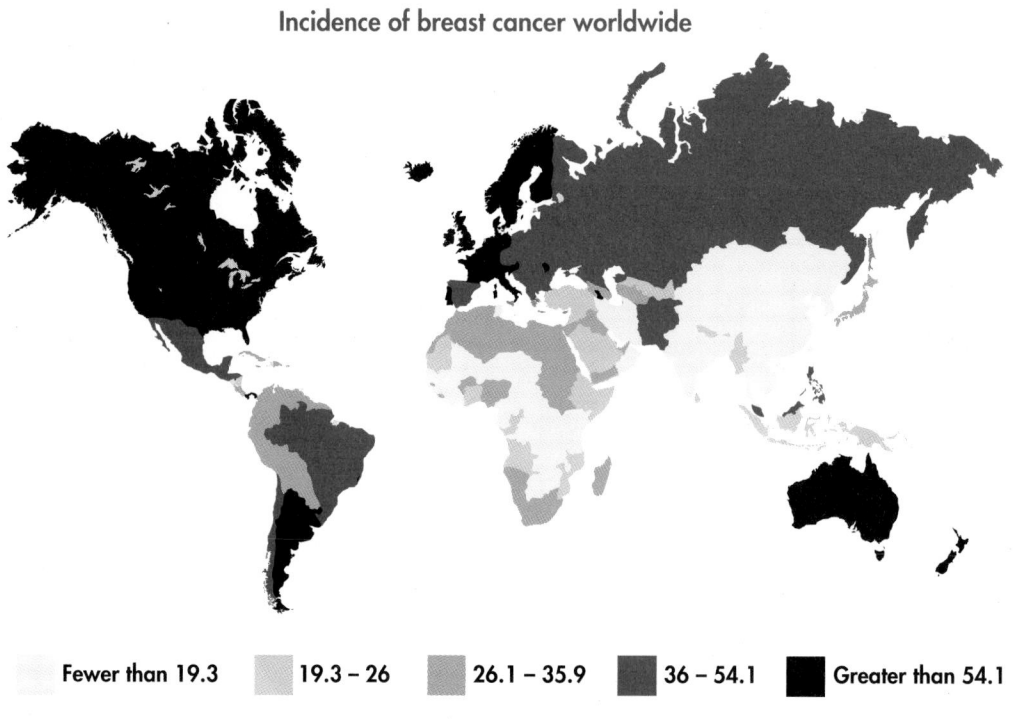

| Fewer than 19.3 | 19.3 – 26 | 26.1 – 35.9 | 36 – 54.1 | Greater than 54.1 |

Number of breast cancers per 100,000 women

Developed regions such as the United States, the United Kingdom, Northern and Western Europe, and Australia have the highest rates of breast cancer. Lifestyle is thought to be a key factor in breast cancer incidence.

Source: World Health Organization, 2003

in the United States, breast cancer incidence was 135 per 100,000 women. In recent years, there has been a slight decline in deaths from breast cancer, a decrease attributed to earlier diagnosis and more effective treatment. Among women of all races in the United States, the death rate from breast cancer between 1996 and 2000 was 28 per 100,000 people.

Breast cancer incidence also varies according to a woman's race and ethnicity. In the United States, white and black women have the highest levels of breast

cancer risk, while Hispanic and American Indian women and women of Asian and Pacific Islander groups have lower levels of risk. Some of the lowest levels of risk occur among Korean and Vietnamese women. Breast cancer is more frequent in Jewish women compared with non-Jewish women.

Racial and ethnic differences in survival rates

Studies reveal racial and ethnic disparities in survival rates among American women with breast cancer. Black, American Indian, Hispanic, Indian and Pakistani women are more likely to receive a diagnosis of advanced breast cancer than are white women, according to a study of nearly 125,000 U.S. women from 17 different races and ethnic groups.

The study also found that black, American Indian, Hawaiian, Hispanic and Vietnamese women face a greater risk of dying of breast cancer, once they develop it, than do white women, even though breast cancer isn't as common among these racial and ethnic groups as it is among white women.

Researchers speculate that some of these disparities are due to delays in diagnosis and differences in the treatment received by women of various ethnic and racial groups. Other possible explanations include socioeconomic, cultural and lifestyle factors, such as reduced access to health care and lack of health insurance, as well as underuse of mammography screening.

Advancing Science

As is true of any type of cancer, the biology of breast cancer is extraordinarily complex. Still, in the last two decades, scientists have made remarkable strides in understanding the differences between normal cells and cancer cells, and in developing new treatments to take advantage of this expanding knowledge.

Advances in technology and completion of the Human Genome Project — an effort to identify all of the genes in humans — are expected to further increase the pace of discovery, allowing researchers to better determine breast cancer risk and to further tailor therapies to target specific molecular characteristics that can cause or stimulate cancer development.

DNA

New technologies now allow scientists to probe the molecular machinery of breast cancer cells in greater detail.

BREAST CANCER

Incidence of invasive breast cancer among U.S. women

Race/ethnicity	Rate per 100,000 women (1996-2000)
All races	135.0
White	148.3
Black	121.7
Asian and Pacific Islander	97.2
Hispanic	89.8
American Indian and Native Alaskan	58.0

Source: Surveillance, Epidemiology, and End Results (SEER) data, National Cancer Institute, 2003

White women have the highest rate of invasive breast cancer among American women. Women of American Indian and Native Alaskan ancestry have the lowest rate.

For a cancerous tumor to grow, its cells must gain the ability to divide (replicate) uncontrollably. When a cell divides, its DNA is replicated so that the newly formed cells have a copy of the person's genetic material. As cells reproduce, the DNA can be damaged. Damaged DNA can lead to uncontrolled cell division and the development of cancer.

Researchers can now study the activity of many genes simultaneously, using a process called microarray technology. This technology allows scientists to compare microscopic amounts of gene products from 25,000 genes at one time. Scientists can compare genetic patterns in breast cancers with those in normal tissue, or patterns in aggressive breast cancers with those in cancers that aren't aggressive.

Proteins

Scientists are learning more about the role proteins play in the development of breast cancer. Proteins are the products of genes.

Proteomic techniques, as described in Chapter 2, allow scientists to study circulating protein patterns that occur when breast cancer begins. Identification of these protein patterns could potentially be used as a new screening tool. At the same time, the proteins provide clues regarding early changes within cells that allow for the development of breast cancer.

One protein being studied is called p53, produced by the p53 gene. This gene is an important tumor suppressor that's activated when a cell is damaged. Its job is to stop or slow further cell growth until the

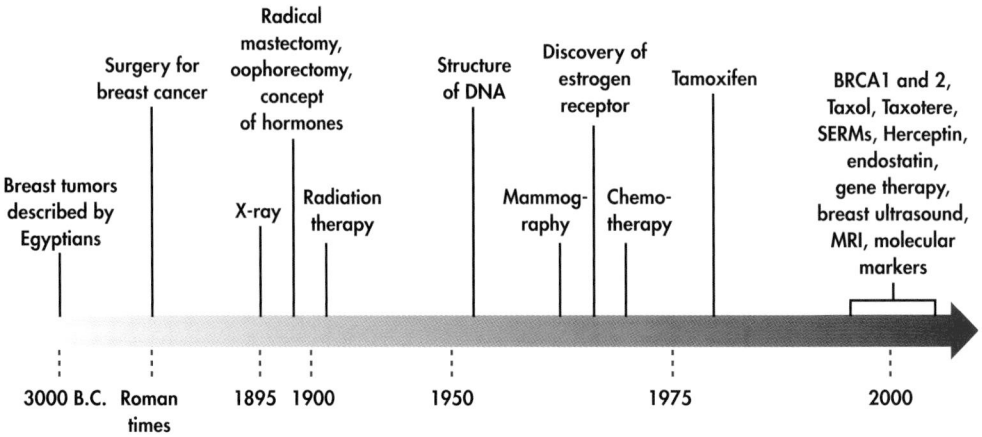

Breast cancer advances timeline

For centuries, surgery has been used to treat breast cancer. After discovery of the X-ray in 1895, radiation therapy came into use. The first use of hormone therapy was in 1896 when a young woman's ovaries were removed to treat metastatic breast cancer. But it wasn't until after discovery of the estrogen receptor and development of the drug tamoxifen that hormone therapy became a common form of treatment. Chemotherapy emerged as a standard treatment in the early 1970s. In just the last decade, the pace of discovery has accelerated dramatically. More discoveries are expected in the near future.

The Story of Herceptin

A recent success story in the development of cancer drugs is trastuzumab (Herceptin), a drug used to treat breast cancer. The story begins with the discovery of the HER-2/neu oncogene in 1987. Oncogenes — genes that can drive tumor growth — were first identified by molecular biologists in the early 1970s. Ten years later, researchers at the University of California, Los Angeles, began studying tumors to look for genetic alterations in known oncogenes.

The researchers discovered that about 25 percent to 30 percent of breast and ovarian cancers had extra copies of the HER-2/neu oncogene, causing the genes to produce too much of the growth-promoting HER-2/neu protein. This protein sends strong growth-promoting signals to cell nuclei.

The UCLA team found that the more copies of the HER-2/neu oncogene there were in a tumor, the more aggressive was the disease.

Researchers began looking for ways to block the activities of the HER-2/neu protein. They became interested in a genetically engineered antibody called Herceptin. Antibodies are part of the body's immune-system defense against foreign invaders. Genetically engineered antibodies target specific invaders that would normally escape notice by the immune system.

In the lab, Herceptin inhibited the growth of breast cancer cells that depended on excess HER-2/neu.

By 1991, the researchers began clinical trials to test Herceptin in humans. The first (phase I) trial showed it was well absorbed and produced few side effects. Phase II trials found that Herceptin was safe and effective in women with metastatic breast cancer in which HER-2/neu was overexpressed. A Phase III trial was then conducted. In this trial, women received either Herceptin and standard chemotherapy or chemotherapy alone. The women who received Herceptin and chemotherapy had slower tumor growth, greater reductions in tumor size and longer survivals, on average, than did those who received chemotherapy alone. In another study, women received Herceptin alone. In about 25 percent of these women, the tumor got smaller or disappeared.

In 1998, Herceptin was approved by the Food and Drug Administration (FDA) for the treatment of metastatic breast cancer in which HER-2/neu was overexpressed. The drug was considered a triumph because it was the first approved cancer drug directed against a specific molecular alteration. It's now being studied in earlier stage breast cancers that overexpress HER-2/neu.

Herceptin is the first in an emerging wave of new, more tailored therapies designed to fight cancer at its roots — treatments akin to a bullet rather than a sledgehammer. It's noteworthy that this whole process took over a decade of work, from the early identification of the HER-2/neu oncogene in 1987 to FDA approval in 1998.

BREAST CANCER

damage has been repaired. If the damage is too extensive to be repaired, it sends the cell into a suicide pathway.

Breast cancer, along with other cancers, often inactivates the p53 gene so that it can't perform its job. Breast cancers associated with changes to p53 tend to be highly invasive and aggressive.

Another protein important to cell growth is HER-2/neu. This protein is overexpressed — that is, too much of it is produced — in 25 percent to 30 percent of breast cancers. Scientists have developed a test to detect the presence of both the HER-2/neu protein and its gene, a type that normally promotes cell division.

Tumors that test positive for HER-2/neu generally grow faster and are more likely to spread compared with other tumors. These tumors often respond to a treatment designed to block HER-2/neu, a drug called trastuzumab (Herceptin).

Angiogenesis

To continue growing, a cancer needs nourishment. It gets the nutrients it needs by promoting the growth of new blood vessels in a process called angiogenesis. The word *angio* refers to blood or lymph vessels, and *genesis* means birth or generation. The new network of blood vessels supplies the tumor with nutrients and oxygen and takes waste products from it.

Normally, angiogenesis is a tightly regulated process that's controlled by the production of molecular chemicals known as pro-angiogenic and angi-inhibitory factors. An imbalance of these factors is seen in several conditions in which abnormal new blood vessels are formed.

Much research is being done in the area of angiogenesis. Scientists have developed methods for counting the number of blood vessels in a tumor to help predict the severity or outcome of the tumor. Researchers are also looking into ways of blocking the cellular signals that trigger angiogenesis, as well as the use of drugs that could inhibit the process.

Chapter 4: Breast Cancer

Making Sense of Risk Statistics

Most women want to know what their chances are of developing breast cancer and whether there's anything they can do to reduce their risk. Among women who've had breast cancer, one of the most common questions is, "What's my daughter's risk?" Being able to estimate a woman's risk of breast cancer is essential for making decisions about medical care.

But statistics about breast cancer risk can be confusing. It seems that practically every week headlines highlight some new medical finding on cancer risk — followed the next week or month by a study producing contradictory results. Sorting through this information and figuring out what's valid and what's not can be tricky.

The way risk statistics are presented only adds to the confusion. Maybe you read that eating a certain food increases your risk of breast cancer by 20 percent, or that a particular drug causes a threefold increase in breast cancers. Risk estimates are calculated in different ways and may be shown as percentages, ratios or plain numbers. How the information is presented can sway how you react to a finding and whether you consider changing your behaviors.

This chapter will help you make sense of information on breast cancer risk, including how risk is assessed. A risk factor is anything associated with a greater chance of getting a disease. Different cancers have different risk factors. The main risk factor for breast cancer is simply being a woman. Age also is an important risk factor. Your likelihood of getting breast cancer increases as you get older.

Understanding your risk of getting breast cancer can help you make informed decisions about your medical care and lifestyle. It can help you avoid overestimating or underestimating your risk. Having realistic information allows you to take appropriate steps to lower your risk and may ease your anxieties about breast cancer. Accurate risk assessment is especially important for women at high risk of getting breast cancer. For these women, aggressive surveillance or risk-reducing (preventive) measures may be considered.

At the same time, it's important to realize that while medical professionals know some of the risk factors that increase a woman's chance of developing breast cancer, it's uncertain exactly how, or in some cases if, all of these risk factors cause normal cells to become cancerous.

Having a risk factor, or even several risk factors, doesn't guarantee that you'll get the disease. Some women with several risk factors never get breast cancer. And some women with no known major risk factors do.

What Is Risk and How Is It Measured?

Cancer researchers use the word *risk* in different ways. For example, you may hear the terms *absolute risk, relative risk* and *lifetime risk*. When scientists talk about risk, they're referring to a probability or a ratio of probabilities — the chance that something may occur but not a guarantee that it will.

Risk estimates and risk factors for breast cancer and other diseases are determined by studying large groups of people to discover the probability that any given woman or category of women will develop the disease, and to see what characteristics or behaviors are associated with increased or decreased risk.

Absolute risk

Absolute risk refers to the actual numeric chance (probability) of developing breast cancer during a specified time — for example, in the next year, in the next five years, by age 50, by age 70 or over the course of your lifetime.

One specific type of absolute risk that you might hear about or be familiar with is lifetime risk. Lifetime risk refers to the probability that an individual will develop cancer over the course of a lifetime.

For example, the lifetime risk for an "average" American woman to develop breast cancer from birth to age 89 is about 12 percent. Another way of saying this is that the lifetime risk is one in eight, meaning that one in eight women who live to age 89 will develop breast cancer (see page 47). Lifetime risk calculated to age 79 is 10 percent, or one in 10.

In studies that test the effects of a treatment or prevention strategy, absolute risk refers to the actual number of health problems that happen or are prevented because of a specific treatment, such as a drug, or a risk-lowering strategy, such as losing weight. For example, an absolute risk might be described as "10 extra cases of breast cancer in 10,000 women who took a particular drug for five years, compared with women who didn't" or as a "1.3 percent reduction in the number of breast cancer cases in one year among women taking a certain drug, compared with women who didn't take the drug."

Relative risk

Relative risk expresses a comparison (ratio) rather than an absolute value. It shows the strength of the relationship between a risk factor and a particular type of cancer by comparing the number of cancers in a group of people with a particular exposure or trait — such as women who have a history of breast cancer — with the number in an unexposed but otherwise similar group — such as women with no history of breast cancer. Relative risk can also express the likelihood that a person who uses a certain treatment or prevention strategy will have an increased or decreased risk of breast cancer, compared with someone who used another strategy or who didn't do anything.

When the difference in risk between two groups is compared, it's often shown as a ratio. This ratio is known as the relative risk. Another way to describe relative risk is to show it as a percentage increase or decrease in risk. For example, women who go through menopause after age 55

FASTFACT

Relative risk at a glance

Relative risk	% increase	Risk factor	Type of cancer
25	2,400%	Smoking	Lung
20	1,900%	BRCA1 gene mutation	Breast
6	500%	Use of estrogen therapy, without progesterone	Endometrial
5 or greater	400% or more	Lobular carcinoma *in situ* Chest radiation therapy for Hodgkin's disease	Breast Breast
3-4	200-300%	Past history of breast cancer	Breast
2-3	100-200%	First-degree relative with premenopausal breast cancer	Breast
1.5	50%	Postmenopausal obesity	Breast
1.25	25%	Modest alcohol intake Hormone replacement therapy	Breast Breast

have a risk of developing breast cancer that's about 1.5 times the risk in women who go through menopause when they're younger than 45. A relative risk of 1.5 means that their risk of developing breast cancer is increased by 50 percent. A relative risk of 1.0 means there's no increased risk. A relative risk of 0.5 means the risk is reduced by 50 percent.

Fifty percent sounds like a very large increase in risk because many people assume when they hear a percentage that 100 percent is the highest possible increase, but that's not the case. In fact, a relative risk of 1.5 may represent a very small increase in absolute risk. Unfortunately, there isn't an easy way to translate relative risk estimates into actual numeric risks, which are usually the most understandable.

A relative risk of 1.5 is also modest in the context of all cancer risk factors. For example, smoking increases the risk of lung cancer. What is the relative risk of lung cancer in smokers compared with nonsmokers? It's 25. This means that smokers are 25 times as likely to develop lung cancer as are nonsmokers. To translate this into a percentage, subtract from the number and multiply it by 100, to result in 2,400 percent increase in risk.

The message to remember is, when you hear that a study found a risk increase of 50 percent or 100 percent, keep in mind that 100 percent is not the upper limit of the possible increase. The chart on page

Relative Risk vs. Absolute Risk

Research studies may be reported in terms of relative risk or absolute risk, and you may have a very different reaction to the two numbers, or you may be confused about how the studies are interpreted.

A relative risk often sounds more alarming than an absolute risk. For example, consider the results of a well-known clinical trial called the Women's Health Initiative (WHI). One of the goals of this study was to identify the risks and benefits of using hormone replacement therapy (HRT) — combined estrogen plus progestin — after menopause. The study monitored the development of a number of diseases, including heart disease, breast cancer and osteoporosis.

In the summer of 2002, WHI researchers stopped the estrogen plus progestin part of the study because they found that the possible risks of therapy outweighed the benefits. In a widely publicized finding, the investigators reported that combined estrogen and progestin increased the risk of breast cancer by 26 percent.

That percentage increase represented a relative risk of 1.26, comparing the chance that a woman taking estrogen plus progestin would get breast cancer with the chance that a woman taking an inactive pill (placebo) would get breast cancer. It didn't mean that 26 percent of the women taking hormone therapy got breast cancer. The absolute risk translat-

55 lists some relative risks associated with various cancer risk factors.

Putting risk into perspective

Most information about cancer risk and risk factors comes from epidemiologic studies, which are studies conducted in large, well-defined groups of people. In the last 50 years, epidemiologists have identified many of the major environmental factors that contribute to cancer, including smoking for lung cancer and sunlight for skin cancer. But uncovering more subtle cancer risks has proved more difficult.

Randomized controlled trials, such as the Women's Health Initiative (WHI), are the gold standard of research studies. But they aren't always practical for studying cancer risk factors. These types of studies can take years or decades to complete and often require the participation of thousands of people. For some risk factors, it would be unethical to subject healthy participants to possible cancer-causing agents (carcinogens). In addition, for investigations of some risk factors, a randomized trial isn't feasible.

Instead, most epidemiologic studies of cancer risk factors rely on observational approaches. In these studies, researchers keep track of a group of people for several years without trying to change their lives or provide special treatment. This can help scientists find out who develops a

ed into eight more cases of breast cancer each year among 10,000 women taking estrogen and progestin.

For any individual woman, the absolute risks of these adverse events are fairly small. However, when spread across an entire population, the risks become more significant, which is why the study was stopped.

When you're evaluating information about your risk of breast cancer, it's helpful to know the difference between relative risk and absolute risk.

Women's Health Initiative findings

Risk or benefit	Relative risk	% change	Absolute risk each year
Heart attacks	1.29	29% increase	7 more cases in 10,000 women
Breast cancer	1.26	26% increase	8 more cases in 10,000 women
Strokes	1.41	41% increase	8 more cases in 10,000 women
Blood clots	2.11	111% increase	18 more cases in 10,000 women
Hip fractures	0.66	33% decrease	5 fewer cases in 10,000 women
Colon cancer	0.63	37% decrease	6 fewer cases in 10,000 women

disease, what those people have in common and how they differ from the group that wasn't sick or didn't get sick. But observational studies are more prone to bias and are considered less reliable. Sometimes, differences between the groups are caused by something the investigators aren't aware of. An example of the limitations of epidemiologic studies is provided by data from the WHI study. This gold standard trial demonstrated that hormone replacement therapy (HRT) increased the incidence of heart disease, while multiple previous epidemiologic studies had consistently suggested that HRT would protect against heart disease.

Because of these limitations, most epidemiologists agree that one observational study by itself isn't authoritative. Only further research can better determine whether the finding is true. The media, though, often report each new study in isolation, rather than as part of an evolving picture. This can sometimes cause unnecessary alarm or confusion.

When looking at information about risk and risk factors, keep a critical perspective about the source of the information and the strength of the research.

Quantifying Risk

Estimating breast cancer risk for any individual woman is difficult, in part because most breast cancers occur in women who don't have major risk factors for the disease other than gender and age. In addition, each risk factor by itself is an isolated piece of information. In reality, many factors work together to cause breast can-

cer, and some risk factors may interact, working in a combined fashion to further increase risk.

To quantify a woman's risk of breast cancer using a combination of risk factors that may have an additive effect, researchers have developed computer-generated risk models based on data collected from many women. The information they provide can help doctors determine which women should be tested for possible inherited genetic abnormalities. The models also help women and their doctors make decisions about screening, lowering risk and treatment. Women who are at very high risk of getting breast cancer may consider options such as risk-reduction medications or surgery.

Several different risk models are available that are based on data from large epidemiologic or clinical studies.

Gail model

The most commonly used tool for general breast cancer risk assessment is the Gail model, which is based on data gathered from more than 280,000 women over a period of seven years. The model allows doctors to estimate the likelihood that a woman with certain risk factors will develop invasive breast cancer in the next five years or during her lifetime.

Risk factors used in the Gail model include:
- Current age
- Age at first period (menses)
- Age at first live birth
- Number of previous breast biopsies
- Presence of atypical hyperplasia on a breast biopsy (see page 142)

- Number of first-degree relatives (mother, sister or daughter) with breast cancer

A doctor does the assessment using a computer or a hand-held device similar to a calculator. The result is given as an absolute risk percentage.

Examples

Here are two examples of results using the Gail model:

Susan is 51 years old, going through menopause and considering estrogen for the treatment of hot flashes. She's concerned about her breast cancer risk because her mother developed breast cancer at age 60.

To calculate Susan's risk, the Gail model assessment seeks the following information regarding Susan and her personal and family health history:

- Current age: 51
- Age at first period: 13
- Age at first live birth: 28
- Number of previous breast biopsies: 0
- Number of mother + sister(s) + daughter(s) with breast cancer: 1

Putting these figures into the program, the Gail model predicts Susan has a 2 percent risk of developing breast cancer over the next five years and that her lifetime risk is 16.6 percent. Many breast cancer experts wouldn't consider Susan to be at very high risk.

Jackie also is 51. She shares many similarities with Susan but has some key differences. Jackie's mother and two sisters developed breast cancer, and Jackie has had previous breast biopsies:

- Current age: 51
- Age at first period: 13
- Age at first live birth: 28

- Number of previous breast biopsies: 2
- Number of mother + sister(s) + daughter(s) with breast cancer: 3

Jackie's predicted five year risk of breast cancer using the Gail model is 5.2 percent. Her lifetime risk is 37.8 percent. Most cancer experts would agree that Jackie is at high risk of breast cancer and that it would be beneficial for her to see a genetic counselor to further review her family history.

Other models

The Gail model, though useful for many women, doesn't take into consideration other important risk factors, including breast cancer on the father's side of the family, breast cancer in second-degree relatives (aunts, cousins, grandmothers), the age at which relatives developed breast cancer, lobular carcinoma *in situ* and a family history of ovarian cancer. To address these gaps, the Claus model may be used. The Claus model estimates the probability of developing breast cancer in women with a family history of breast cancer.

The Claus model calculates risk either as a lifetime probability or for a 10-year period. This model is appropriate only for women with at least one female relative with breast cancer. But the model doesn't take into account some other risk factors associated with breast cancer, such as age at first menstruation or first live birth.

Other risk-prediction models have been developed for use in women suspected of having an inherited susceptibility to breast cancer. These models (including Couch, Shattuck-Eidens, Frank and

BRCAPRO) estimate the probability of detecting mutations in breast cancer genes BRCA1 and BRCA2 in a given individual or family. They help doctors determine if a woman is likely to benefit from genetic testing.

Another risk-prediction approach that's sometimes used in high-risk women is to use data from studies that apply to a specific group or population. For example, regardless of family history, up to 30 percent of Jewish women of Ashkenazi (Eastern European) descent diagnosed with breast cancer before age 40 have one of the BRCA1 or BRCA2 mutations common to this population. Information such as this is summarized in "prevalence tables," which give estimates of the prevalence of a BRCA1 or BRCA2 mutation in particular population groups.

Beyond the numbers

Risk-prediction models can provide women with useful information about their risk of developing breast cancer. But these numbers are just estimates, and none of the models is perfect.

Depending on a woman's particular situation, a given model may be more relevant than another. For example, the Gail model wasn't developed based on women with a strong family history of breast cancer or among nonwhite women and may underestimate risk in these groups. That is why doctors generally don't rely solely on risk models when recommending a preventive measure or genetic testing. Doctors also take other factors into consideration that are unique to a woman's situation.

Risk Factors

Women who've been diagnosed with breast cancer often wonder, "What did I do? How did I let my body down?"

Let yourself off the hook because it's highly unlikely that anything you did caused your breast cancer. Very few strong risk factors for breast cancer have been identified. Therefore it's often impossible to say why one woman gets the disease and another doesn't. And most of the known risk factors, such as gender, age, menstrual history and family history, aren't things that you can control or change.

As mentioned earlier, simply being a woman is the main risk factor for developing breast cancer. Although men have breast tissue and can get breast cancer, the disease is 100 times more common among women. That's because women have more breast cells than men do, and their breast cells are constantly being exposed to the growth-promoting effects of female hormones.

Age also is a major risk factor. Three-fourths of women with breast cancer are older than age 50 when they receive the diagnosis.

Family history

After gender and age, a family history of breast cancer is the strongest known risk factor for breast cancer. About 15 percent to 20 percent of breast cancers occur in women with some family history of the disease. The affected family members may be on your mother's side of the family or your father's.

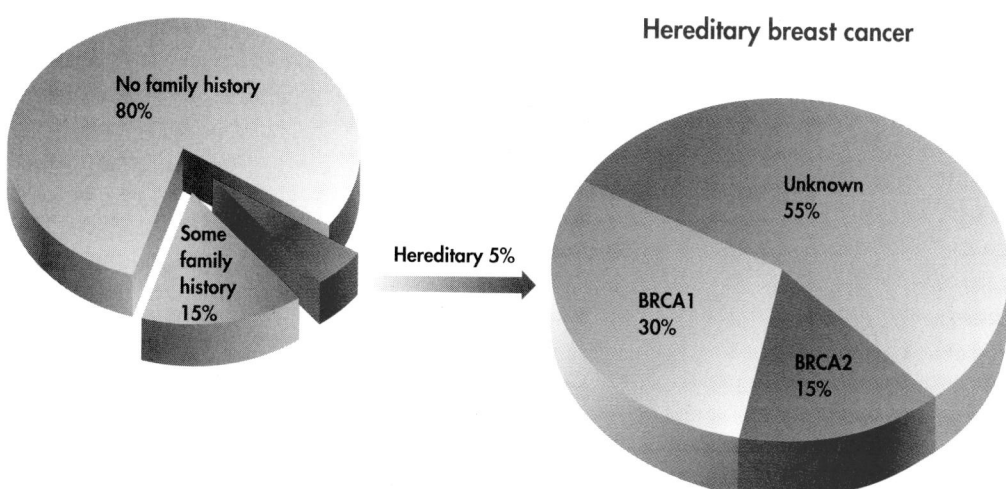

All breast cancer cases

No family history 80%

Some family history 15%

Hereditary 5%

Hereditary breast cancer

Unknown 55%

BRCA1 30%

BRCA2 15%

If you have one close or first-degree relative — a mother, sister or daughter — with breast cancer, your relative risk of getting the disease is approximately doubled, compared with that of women who have no first-degree relatives with the disease. The relative risk is 1.5 if you have one second-degree relative, such as an aunt or grandmother, with breast cancer.

A woman's risk of breast cancer is strongly related to the number and closeness of relatives with breast cancer, as well as the age at which those relatives were diagnosed.

In general, the more first-degree relatives you have with breast cancer, the greater your risk. In addition, the younger your relatives were when they were diagnosed, the greater your risk. These key factors — number of relatives and early age at diagnosis — signal the possibility of an inherited predisposition to the disease in the family.

Is it hereditary?

When a woman is diagnosed with breast cancer, one of the first things her doctor wants to determine is if she has a hereditary form of the disease. That is, is her cancer the result of an abnormal gene that's being passed on in the family?

A detailed family health history is an important first step in identifying hereditary cancer. Clues that point to inherited breast cancer include:

- A history of breast cancer on either your mother's or your father's side of the family
- Multiple women on either side of the family diagnosed with the disease
- Women diagnosed at a young age — younger than age 50
- A history of ovarian cancer on either your mother's or your father's side of the family
- Male breast cancer on either your mother's or your father's side of the family

Nonhereditary disease

Just because a woman has one or two relatives with breast cancer doesn't mean there's an inherited abnormality in the family. In most women with a family history of breast cancer, there isn't a specific inherited gene that's responsible for the cancer. Other factors that increase breast cancer risk are at play instead.

Breast cancer may occur more often in some families because of shared reproductive or environmental risk factors. In these women, their risk of breast cancer is much lower than that of women with an inherited mutation. For a woman who has a mother or sister with breast cancer and no other affected relatives and no identified genetic alteration, the probability that she will develop breast cancer by age 70 is between 7 percent and 18 percent. The risk increases as the number of relatives with breast cancer goes up but is still less than the risk for women who carry a known genetic mutation.

Hereditary disease

About 5 percent to 10 percent of all breast cancers are thought to be hereditary — caused by an inherited alteration (mutation) in a single gene. Several of these genes, known as cancer susceptibility genes, have been identified.

The first genes to be discovered were breast cancer gene 1 (BRCA1) and breast cancer gene 2 (BRCA2). Together, defects in these genes account for about 45 percent of hereditary breast cancer cases, or about 1.5 percent to 3 percent of all breast cancers (see page 61).

- **BRCA1.** Defects in this gene, located on chromosome 17, appear to be responsible for breast cancer in about 30 percent of families with multiple cases of the disease and up to 90 percent of families who have both breast and ovarian cancers. By age 70, a woman who carries a mutation in this gene has approximately a 65 percent chance of developing breast cancer and a 39 percent chance of getting ovarian cancer. Defects in the BRCA1 gene may also be associated with an increased risk of prostate and colon cancers.

- **BRCA2.** Mutations in this gene, located on chromosome 13, account for about 15 percent of multiple-case family breast cancers. By age 70, carriers of this gene mutation have about a 45 percent chance of developing breast cancer and an 11 percent chance of developing ovarian cancer. BRCA2 mutations also may be associated with an increased risk of several other cancers, including colon, prostate, pancreatic, gallbladder, stomach and melanoma. BRCA2 families also show an increased risk of male breast cancer.

BRCA1 and BRCA2 are tumor suppressor genes found in all humans. Normally, they regulate activity within a cell that helps to suppress the chance of cancer development. The BRCA genes produce proteins that help detect and repair DNA damage that can occur during normal cell division. When a BRCA gene is altered (mutated), the DNA repair process can go awry, and genetic defects can accumulate. This allows abnormal cells to multiply and cancer to develop.

BRCA1 and BRCA2 are both very large genes that contain codes for large proteins. Nearly 2,000 distinct mutations in

Gene Search

The first breast cancer susceptibility gene, BRCA1, was identified in 1994. For years, researchers had known that women with a strong family history of breast cancer were at higher risk of getting the disease than were other women. The search for a gene responsible for breast cancer began with studies of families with multiple cases of breast cancer. By studying these families, researchers were able to identify a pattern (autosomal dominant inheritance pattern) for how the disease was passed on to family members (see page 65).

With the advent of technology that made it possible to analyze DNA, researchers were able to begin searching for the actual gene that was altered in people with a family history of breast cancer. In 1990, a team of scientists narrowed the search by discovering a link between early-onset breast cancer in families and a region of chromosome 17. The researchers called the region BRCA1. Four years later, the region was narrowed to the specific gene where mutations were found to occur. This discovery enabled the development of genetic testing for mutations in BRCA1. The first commercial testing for BRCA1 mutations was performed in 1996. BRCA2 was identified on chromosome 13 in 1995.

Discovery of BRCA1

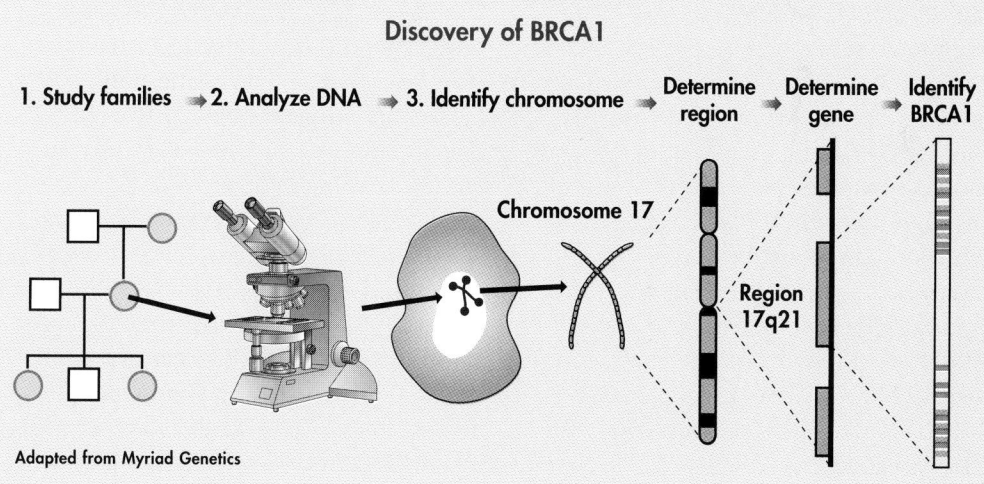

1. Study families → 2. Analyze DNA → 3. Identify chromosome → Determine region → Determine gene → Identify BRCA1

Chromosome 17

Region 17q21

Adapted from Myriad Genetics

BRCA1 and BRCA2 have been described. For example, in one mutation seen in women of Ashkenazi Jewish ancestry, just two pieces of the genetic code are missing out of a sequence of 6,000 — this one small deletion can result in an increased susceptibility to breast cancer. The mutations associated with an increased risk of cancer cause either missing or nonfunctional protein products.

Breast tumors that arise as a result of an inherited BRCA1 defect have some features of more aggressive cancers — they're higher grade, and they usually are estrogen receptor negative. These features are discussed in Chapter 7. BRCA2-related breast cancers are more likely to be estrogen receptor positive, similar to nonhereditary breast cancers.

Before BRCA1 and BRCA2 were found, women with a strong family history of breast cancer were usually assumed to be carriers of a gene mutation, but no tool was available for testing them. Some women had their breasts or ovaries removed to prevent cancer, even though there was no way to tell for sure that they carried the genetic defect. Thanks to the advances in gene mapping and genetic testing, women can now be tested before making such major decisions.

It's important to note that in families where an altered BRCA1 or BRCA2 gene is present, not all family members will inherit the gene mutation. That's why genetic testing may be especially helpful. Only family members who test positive for a known genetic mutation are at increased risk. In family members who aren't carriers, their risk isn't any greater than is the average woman's.

Meanwhile, researchers continue to work to identify other breast cancer susceptibility genes.

Inheriting a genetic mutation

Mutations in BRCA1 or BRCA2 are inherited in what's called an autosomal dominant pattern. What this means is that one parent, either the father or the mother, transmits the genetic alteration to approximately half of his or her children. Each child has a 50 percent chance of inheriting the mutation. This is because the parent has one normal copy of the gene and one abnormal copy. Either can be passed on.

Because both men and women have chromosomes 17 and 13, a mutation in one of these genes can come from either your father or your mother. Women may not realize they have a family history of breast cancer if the cancer is on their father's side of the family.

Inheriting a genetic mutation associated with the development of breast cancer greatly increases the likelihood of getting the disease, but it's not a given. A woman with a 25 percent chance of developing breast cancer may get the disease, and a woman with a 75 percent chance of getting it may not. Some women with a BRCA1 or BRCA2 mutation develop early and multiple cancers, while others develop cancer later in life or not at all.

There are several possible reasons for the individual variation in cancer susceptibility among carriers of BRCA1 or BRCA2 alterations. First, genetic mutations located at different places in these genes may lead to different levels of risk. Second, other risk factors, such as reproductive history, may influence breast cancer risk associated with these mutations. Environmental factors also interact with the genetic susceptibility, and other genes may interact with the BRCA genes to modify an individual's risk.

Genetic counseling and testing

Women who are thought to be at high risk of carrying an inherited genetic mutation are often referred to a geneticist for a

Passing on a defective gene

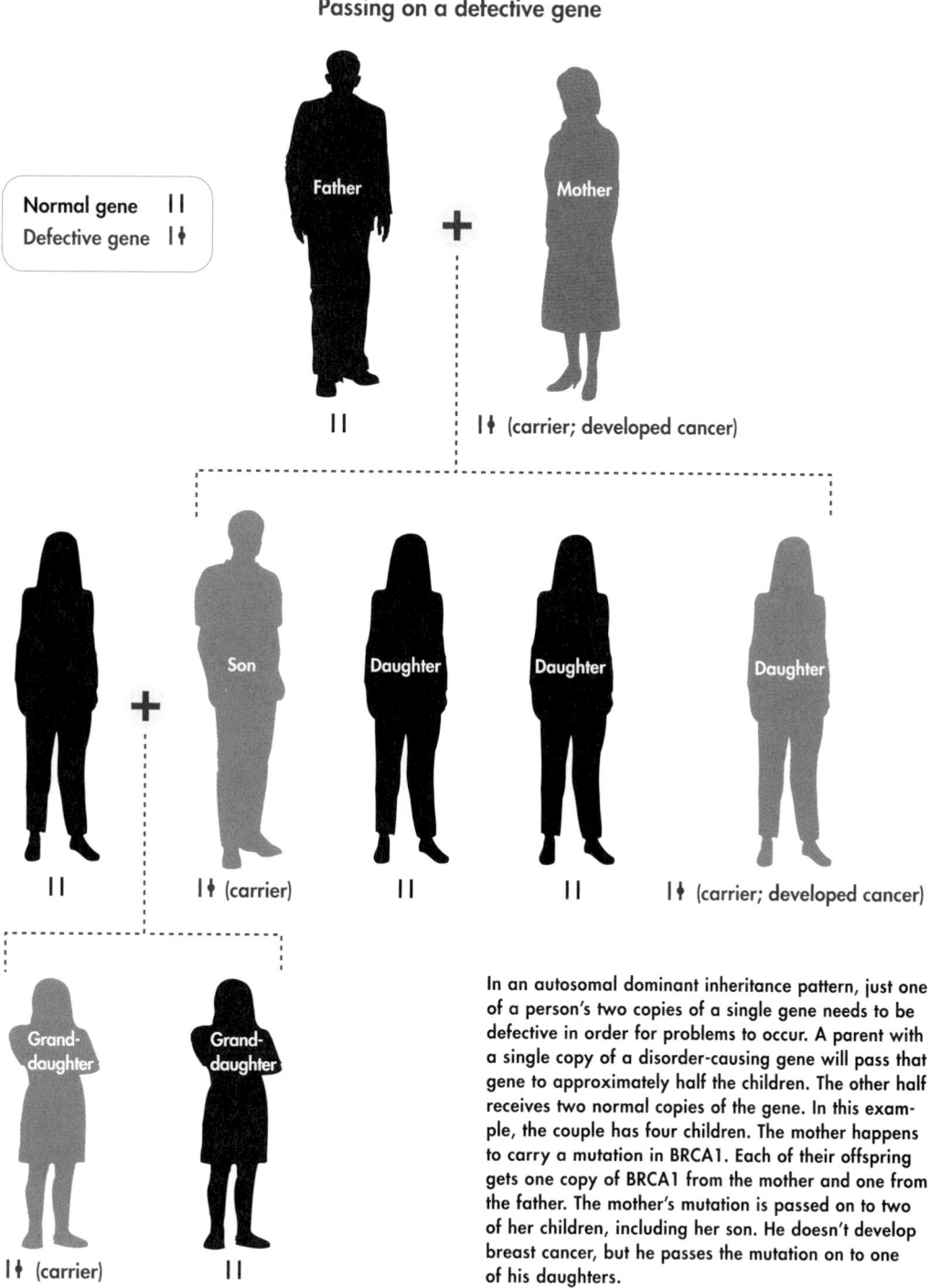

In an autosomal dominant inheritance pattern, just one of a person's two copies of a single gene needs to be defective in order for problems to occur. A parent with a single copy of a disorder-causing gene will pass that gene to approximately half the children. The other half receives two normal copies of the gene. In this example, the couple has four children. The mother happens to carry a mutation in BRCA1. Each of their offspring gets one copy of BRCA1 from the mother and one from the father. The mother's mutation is passed on to two of her children, including her son. He doesn't develop breast cancer, but he passes the mutation on to one of his daughters.

cancer risk assessment, which may include genetic counseling and testing.

For women's cancers, genetic testing analyzes one or more specific genes — usually BRCA1 and BRCA2. Genetic testing can help determine whether you carry a specific gene mutation that puts you at increased risk and what the probability is that you'll develop the disease in your lifetime. However, genetic testing is just one component of a comprehensive cancer risk assessment plan.

Who should be tested?

Doctors generally recommend genetic testing only for individuals with a family history that suggests they may be carriers of a BRCA1 or BRCA2 mutation. A genetic test can distinguish women who carry an inherited mutation from those who don't. For example, one sister in a family may test positive and have a greatly increased risk of breast cancer. Another sister may test negative, meaning she's not a carrier. Her risk of developing breast

Breast cancer incidence among BRCA mutation carriers

Age	Incidence among BRCA1 carriers	Incidence among BRCA2 carriers
20	0.0%	0.0%
25	0.1%	0.1%
30	0.6%	0.7%
35	4.3%	2.5%
40	11.6%	6.2%
45	23.7%	10.4%
50	38.4%	16.2%
55	46.0%	23.3%
60	53.5%	30.6%
65	59.2%	37.8%
70	64.7%	44.7%

This chart indicates the likelihood, by age, that a woman who carries a mutant BRCA gene will develop breast cancer. Incidence is expressed in percentages. For example, a woman who is a BRCA1 carrier has a 38.4 percent chance of developing breast cancer by age 50. As she gets older, her risk increases.

Ovarian cancer incidence among BRCA mutation carriers

Age	Incidence among BRCA1 carriers	Incidence among BRCA2 carriers
20	0.0%	0.0%
25	0.0%	0.0%
30	0.0%	0.0%
35	0.9%	0.0%
40	2.3%	0.1%
45	6.5%	0.5%
50	13.2%	1.2%
55	17.3%	4.1%
60	22.1%	7.6%
65	30.4%	9.4%
70	38.6%	11.3%

This chart indicates the likelihood, by age, that a woman who carries a mutant BRCA gene will develop ovarian cancer. Incidence is expressed in percentages. For example, a woman who is a BRCA1 carrier has a 13.2 percent chance of developing ovarian cancer by age 50. As she gets older, her risk increases.

Source: Jeffrey Slezak, Mayo Clinic, with data borrowed from A. Antoniou, et al., "Average Risks of Breast and Ovarian Cancer Associated with BRCA1 or BRCA2 Mutations," *American Journal of Human Genetics*, 72:5 (2003), pages 1117-1130

cancer is the same as that of women with-out any family history of the disease.

What's involved?

Genetic counseling is typically recom-mended to make sure you fully under-stand the risks, benefits and psychological effect of learning that you may carry a gene that puts you at increased risk of developing cancer. The counseling team may include a genetic counselor, nurse, doctor, psychologist and social worker.

Topics covered may include:

- Your risk status and family history
- Your perceptions of risk and motivation for testing
- Education about genetics, inheritance and risk
- Limitations, risks and benefits of testing
- Test procedures
- Diagnosis and treatment options
- Privacy and confidentiality issues
- Emotional and psychological conse-quences of testing

How much does it cost?

For many women, the cost of genetic test-ing is a major concern. The price varies, depending on the situation. For a woman who's the first person in her family to be tested, the test currently costs about $2,800. If she tests positive for a specific genetic mutation, then another relative in her family can be tested for that specific mutation at a lesser cost, generally about $325. This testing is much less costly because the geneticists know exactly where to look for the mutation.

For women of Ashkenazi Jewish descent, the initial test screens for the three most common genetic alterations in

Questions to Ask

During the genetic counseling process, ask any questions you may have. They may include:

- Where can I be tested?
- How much will the test cost?
- Does insurance cover it?
- Who else will know my results, and will it affect my ability to get insurance?
- Should all my family, including my children, be tested?
- How might this information affect my relationship with my family?
- When will I get my results?
- If I test positive, what are my options?

BREAST CANCER

that population. These mutations account for the majority of hereditary cases of breast and ovarian cancer in Ashkenazi Jewish women. If the result is negative, a woman may choose to have more exten-sive testing done.

Many insurance plans cover the cost of genetic testing or part of it. But some health plans don't, and some women aren't comfortable having their insurer know they're being tested. While many women are concerned that genetic testing could lead to insurance discrimination, there are few known instances in which this has occurred. To learn what your options are, talk to your doctor or insurer.

Making a decision

About half the women who are referred for genetic counseling decide not to have the test. It's a personal decision. Some women feel relieved to know their risk status, even if it's bad news, because they feel empowered. They believe that the information they've gained will help them make the right decisions. Others worry about discrimination from health insurers or employers or about the cost of testing. For most women, the issue of genetic testing is emotionally charged, which is why counseling is critical.

If you decide to be tested, the appropriate test will be selected and ordered, and your blood will be drawn. The test is a simple blood test. It generally takes about three to four weeks to get the results. The counseling team will likely discuss your results with you in person.

Mapping Your Family Health History

To help determine if you have an inherited risk of breast cancer, your doctor may construct your pedigree. A pedigree is a chart that shows your family tree and indicates which family members developed cancer, what kind of cancer they had and at what age they developed it. A pedigree, like the one illustrated below, can reveal a strong inheritance pattern for breast, ovarian and other cancers.

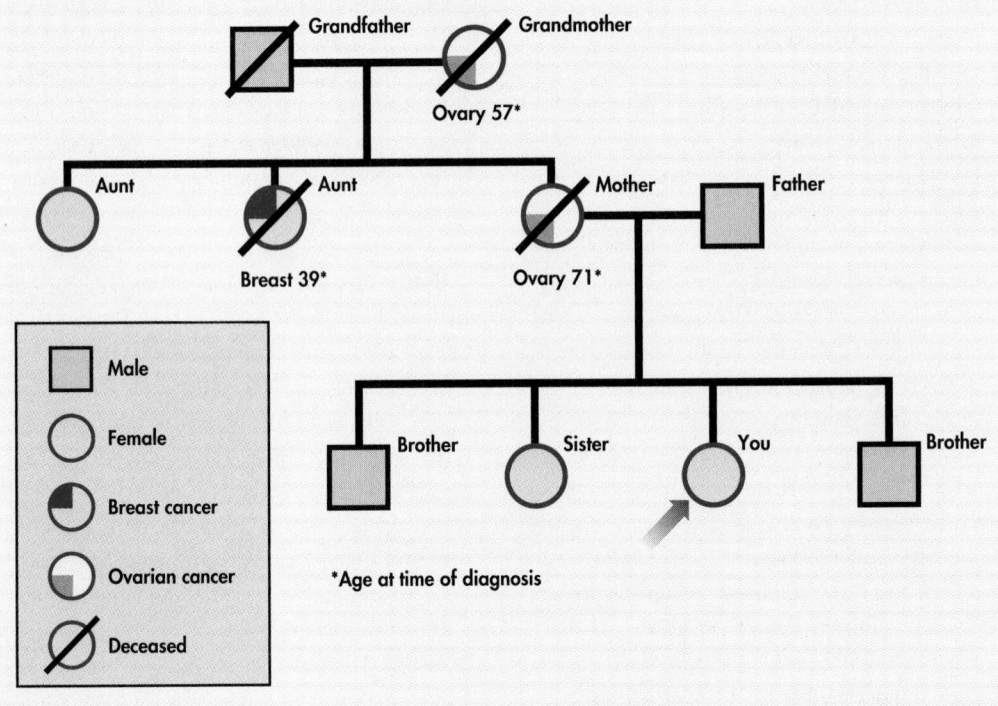

*Age at time of diagnosis

If the test is positive, your follow-up care will likely include counseling and an individualized management plan that will address screening and surveillance procedures and prevention options. You and your counseling team may also discuss whether you want to share the results of your test with other family members who also may be at increased risk.

Keep in mind that just as a positive test doesn't automatically mean you'll develop cancer, a negative test doesn't mean you're not at risk. You still have the same risk as the general population.

One Family's Story

Here is one story of a hereditary cancer that was revealed over a several-month period.

When Janet noticed a dimpling under her left breast while doing her monthly breast self-exam, she knew it was cancer, though she had no reason to suspect it. Janet was only 38 years old, a runner and in good health. She didn't smoke, didn't drink and wasn't aware of any family history of breast cancer — because Janet's mother was adopted, the health history on that side of the family was unknown.

Being a physician, Janet was only too aware that dimpling is a common sign of breast cancer. Then there was also the mild pain she had been experiencing while breast-feeding her youngest son, something she had easily dismissed to nursing — until now. What she didn't know standing in front of a mirror that November day was how her discovery would profoundly change not only her life but also the lives of four other women.

Janet immediately saw her doctor. A mammogram and additional tests confirmed her fears. It was cancer. While awaiting the final test results, Janet sat in her husband's lap and cried, agonizing over how her young sons would cope without her. "In my mind, I just went right to the worst-case scenario, that I had stage IV cancer."

Fortunately, the cancer was only at stage II. Janet had her left breast removed, followed by a regimen of chemotherapy, radiation and the hormone medication tamoxifen, which she continues to take today.

Not surprisingly, Janet's diagnosis came as a shock. She grew up in a tightknit family, and her parents and three sisters were devastated when Janet called with the news. Her younger sister, Jill, drove from Michigan to Minnesota to be with Janet and help take care of the boys during Janet's first round of chemotherapy.

At Janet's insistence, her sisters each made appointments to have mammograms. The news was good; the results came back fine. A sigh of relief, but unfortunately it would be short-lived.

It was less than six months after Janet's diagnosis when her sister Jill experienced a perplexing event. A young child jumped into Jill's arms, accidentally kicking her in the breast. The incident caused intense pain, and it bothered Jill that such a minor mishap should bring about such pain. Later, while examining her breasts at home, Jill felt a lump — the same one she first noticed before her recent mammogram. Her doctor had told her then that the lump was likely a cyst and not to worry about it. And, for a while, Jill didn't, having been reassured by the "normal" finding on her mammogram that everything was OK. But Jill didn't like that the lump hadn't gone away and that it didn't seem to move. To be safe, she made another appointment to see her doctor. Still feeling it was just a cyst, Jill's doctor ordered a biopsy to comfort Jill's concerns. The results weren't comforting. It was cancer.

In July 2002, while Janet was just beginning her radiation therapy, 31-year-old Jill underwent a mastectomy. For Jill, the diagnosis was more severe. The tumor was close to 8 centimeters, and she had several involved lymph nodes — a stage III cancer. Her treatment would be even more extensive than Janet's.

Janet made plans to travel to Michigan to be with Jill during her initial round of chemotherapy. Though tired from her radiation treatments, Janet was determined to be there for Jill, just as Jill had been there for her. Shortly before she was getting ready to leave, Janet's mother, Charlotte, called. The call didn't turn out to be the routine, "Hi, how are you doing?" Charlotte had just been in for a mammogram. She had had previous mammograms, but this was the first since her two youngest daughters had been diagnosed with breast cancer. The results showed an "axillary abnormality." She didn't know what it meant. Janet did. Her mother had an enlarged lymph node under her arm, likely due to breast cancer. For Janet, the news was almost too much to bear. "I was talking to her on the phone and I said, 'I cannot take another diagnosis of cancer right now.' This was literally weeks after Jill." Within a

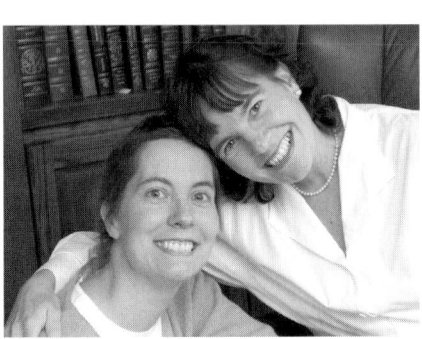

Jill, left, and Janet, right, following their cancer treatments.

few days, 71-year-old Charlotte underwent surgery to remove a small cancerous mass in her breast that had spread to lymph nodes under her arm.

For the two oldest sisters, Julann and Jean, it suddenly felt as if their breasts had turned into ticking time bombs. Julann made an appointment with a surgeon to discuss the possibility of preventive (prophylactic) mastectomy. Though genetic tests showed that the family didn't carry the BRCA1 or BRCA2 breast cancer gene, it was apparent that some genetic abnormality was at play, which current technology can't yet identify.

After a battle with her insurance company, 46-year-old Julann finally received approval for surgeons to remove and reconstruct both of her breasts. As Janet sat in the waiting room and received updates from the operating room nurse, she became worried. The general surgeon was still in the room. "He should be done by now," Janet thought. "This isn't good." The surgeon would later tell Janet what she already suspected. During the surgery, the surgical team found cancer. Fortunately, it was still in its early stages.

For the fourth time in just over a year, cancer had raised its ugly head in this family. For these women, their once-normal routines became vague recollections. Janet recalls a single week in January 2003. Her mother was in the hospital, Jill was just completing radiation treatments, Julann was starting chemotherapy, and Jean was going in for a breast biopsy because a mammogram had revealed an abnormal mass.

For Jean, finally, there would come a break. Her biopsy results came back negative. But she decided there would be no more waiting, no more gambling with time. She decided to have prophylactic surgery.

As they did during those long and often-grueling months, faith, family and a sense of humor continue to keep the women going today. "As hard as it was, sometimes you just had to step back and laugh," says Jill. "If you didn't laugh about it, you would cry all the time."

The women believe that they're free of cancer today because they were proactive. They performed self-exams, had regular mammograms and took preventive action. For Jill, it's difficult to imagine what might have happened if she hadn't gone back to her doctor to have the lump re-examined. "You think, 'Who gets breast cancer at 31?' But if I hadn't persisted and questioned the changes, who knows where I'd be right now? You might not always know what's happening (inside your body), but you know when something isn't right."

Following her diagnosis, Jill made a little booklet of the top 10 things she wants to do or see in her lifetime. She has since added to it. It's now the top 50. She figures if she does one thing each year, she'll have her list completed by age 82. "They may be dreams, but I think you have to have something to focus on."

Hormonal and reproductive factors

More than a century ago, the first effective treatment for metastatic breast cancer in premenopausal women was reported — removal of the ovaries. It wasn't until years later, though, that the underlying link between the ovaries and production of the female sex hormones estrogen and progesterone was established. In the 1960s, estrogen receptors were discovered. Estrogen receptors are proteins in breast tissue cells that interact with estrogen and allow estrogen to bind to DNA, which turns on gene and protein production. Estrogen receptors are also found in other tissues, such as the uterus, bones, brain and heart, which are "targets" for estrogen. When estrogen binds with an estrogen receptor, the hormone influences the cell's activities.

Experimental evidence suggests that estrogen plays a key role in the development of breast cancer. In animals, the hormones estrogen and progesterone stimulate the growth of breast tumors. Although a precise cause-and-effect relationship hasn't been established, it's known that the greater a woman's lifetime exposure to estrogen is, the higher her risk of breast cancer. If a premenopausal woman has her ovaries removed — reducing her exposure to sex hormones — her risk of breast cancer drops by about 50 percent.

Several risk factors for breast cancer are related to a woman's hormonal and reproductive history.

Menstrual history

Women who start menstruating before the age of 12 or who go through menopause after age 50 have a slightly higher risk of breast cancer. Compared with someone who begins menstruating after age 15, a girl who has her first period before age 12

BREAST CANCER

has a 30 percent greater risk of developing breast cancer later in life.

At the other end of the reproductive spectrum, women who don't reach menopause until age 55 or older have about a 50 percent greater chance of getting breast cancer than do women who experience menopause between the ages of 45 and 55.

Earlier menstruation and later menopause translate into more years of breast tissue exposure to higher levels of hormones, which are thought to influence breast cancer risk.

Pregnancy and breast-feeding

Women who never become pregnant or who give birth to their first child after age 30 have approximately double the risk of breast cancer compared with women who give birth when they're younger than age 20. Giving birth at a young age significantly reduces the risk of breast cancer, though if an early pregnancy isn't carried to completion, the protective effect is lost.

Some studies have shown that breast-feeding can lower breast cancer risk. Other studies, though, haven't. One study of 100,000 women concluded that for every 12 months of breast-feeding, a woman's risk is lowered by 4.3 percent. The study also reported that every birth reduced a woman's breast cancer risk by 7 percent.

One reason early pregnancy and breast-feeding may reduce breast cancer risk is that these circumstances push breast cells into their final phase of maturation. Breast cells that are fully mature (differentiated) may be less vulnerable to the influence of carcinogens later in life.

Use of oral contraceptives

Some studies suggest that women using birth control pills have a slightly increased risk of developing breast cancer. The increased risk appears to return to normal 10 years after a woman stops using oral contraceptives. A few studies have also shown that women with a strong family history of breast cancer — who are at increased risk of getting the disease — have an even higher risk if they use birth control pills.

It's important to note, though, that some studies that suggested an elevated risk of breast cancer with oral contraceptives involved earlier formulations of the pill, which contained higher concentrations of estrogen and progestin. Since the introduction of oral contraceptive pills in the early 1960s, the dose of hormones in them has continued to decrease, so today's pills contain much lower doses. Many other studies of oral contraceptive use and breast cancer risk have not found evidence of increased risk.

Although the relationship between oral contraceptives and breast cancer risk remains somewhat controversial, most experts think that current versions of the pill don't increase breast cancer risk.

Hormone replacement therapy

Use of the female hormones estrogen and progesterone (progestin) to help ease menopausal symptoms was first recommended in the early 1970s. Twenty years later, nearly 40 percent of postmenopausal women in the United States were using hormone replacement therapy (HRT) to control symptoms of menopause and prevent osteoporosis. By this time, though, reports began to appear linking hormone use with a slightly increased incidence of breast cancer.

The most conclusive evidence about HRT and breast cancer risk stems from the Women's Health Initiative (WHI), a clinical trial involving thousands of postmenopausal women. Participants in the study were selected at random to receive either an inactive pill (placebo) or HRT. If a woman had had a hysterectomy, she received estrogen alone. If she still had her uterus, she received estrogen plus progestin. (Use of estrogen alone in a woman who still has her uterus has been linked to increased risk of uterine cancer.) The WHI was designed to gather information on ways to prevent and reduce heart disease, osteoporosis and colorectal cancer, while monitoring the effect of hormones on breast cancer.

In July 2002, researchers prematurely stopped the part of the study evaluating the use of combined estrogen and progestin because they found possible risks of the therapy exceeded the safety limits established at the beginning of the study. There was a 26 percent increase in the risk of invasive breast cancer over a five-year period. This confirmed the increased risk reported in previous epidemiologic studies. When the relative risk estimate is translated into an actual number, it equals eight additional breast cancers among 10,000 women who take estrogen and progestin for one year.

A more recent analysis of the WHI data has raised additional concerns about HRT and breast cancer risk. The new study provides more detailed information about characteristics of the cancers that occurred

in the women taking estrogen and progestin. Compared with the breast cancers that occurred in women who took placebos, the cancers that developed in women taking estrogen and progestin had higher risk features — on average, the tumors were slightly larger and the cancer was more likely to have spread to the lymph nodes. It should be noted that larger studies have not shown such a trend. Some have shown just the opposite — that breast cancers in women taking hormones had better risk features.

The WHI also found that women taking the combined hormones were more likely to have abnormal mammograms, perhaps related to increased breast density from the hormones, requiring additional follow-up and evaluation. These WHI results come from women taking both estrogen and progestin.

What about use of estrogen alone after menopause? Estrogen taken by itself has some risks. In women who haven't had a hysterectomy, estrogen taken alone can increase their risk of endometrial cancer. A recent large study showed no increase in breast cancer risk with estrogen alone, even in women who had taken it for more than 20 years. However, other studies have shown a slight increased risk of breast cancer with longer-term use (five years or longer) of estrogen alone. Among participants in the WHI who took estrogen alone, the results didn't show any increase in risk of breast cancer.

Environmental factors

Over the years, much attention has been given to environmental and lifestyle risk factors — from a high-fat diet, to pesticides to power lines — as possible risks for breast cancer. But unlike the clear connection between cigarette smoking and lung cancer, there's little strong evidence to link environmental factors and breast cancer development.

Diet

Several aspects of diet have been studied in relation to breast cancer risk. Researchers have long observed that breast cancer rates are much lower in most Asian and developing countries than in affluent Western countries, and dietary factors have been suggested as one reason for the variation. What's more, women who migrate from a country with a lower incidence of breast cancer to a country with a higher incidence over time acquire the same level of risk as women in the new country. Despite these intriguing hints, there isn't a clear-cut relationship between diet and breast cancer risk. Research has produced conflicting results and uncertainty.

One aspect of diet that has received a lot of hype is fat intake. Common thinking used to be that high-fat diets increased breast cancer risk. This belief was largely based on observations that breast cancer rates are highest in countries where consumption of dietary fat is highest. But well-controlled studies comparing intake of dietary fat and development of breast cancer have not been able to establish a clear link between the two. Some scientists, though, believe that the range of fat intake being studied isn't large enough to detect possible differences in risk.

Weight

Being overweight or obese increases risk of breast cancer in postmenopausal women by about 50 percent — roughly twice the increase than that resulting from use of hormone replacement therapy. This is especially true if the extra weight is gained during adulthood. Risk doesn't seem to be increased among women who have been overweight since childhood. Obesity in premenopausal women is actually associated with a modest reduction in breast cancer risk, but since obesity before menopause usually leads to obesity after menopause, excess weight at any age is seen as a risk factor for breast cancer.

Although your ovaries produce most of your estrogen, fat tissue can convert other hormones, such as those made by your adrenal glands, into estrogen. Thus, having more fat tissue increases your estrogen levels and may increase your breast cancer risk. Obesity also contributes to increased levels of insulin and insulin-like growth factors, which are associated with a higher breast cancer risk.

Exercise

How exercise may affect breast cancer is a fairly new area of research. Many studies indicate that low levels of physical exercise — a sedentary lifestyle — may increase breast cancer risk. Some evidence indicates that strenuous exercise in youth might provide lifelong protection against breast cancer and that moderate to vigorous physical activity as an adult could lower your risk.

Exercise may influence levels of the hormones estrogen and progesterone. It may also promote a healthy weight

---

MYTH vs. FACT

Myth: **Most cancers are caused by environmental pollution or chemicals.**

Fact: Although it's a common belief that exposure to occupational and industrial hazards and environmental pollution or chemicals causes most cancers, research doesn't support this idea. Pollutants and environmental exposures are thought to account for fewer than 10 percent of all cancer cases.

Rather than environmental pollutants, many cancer deaths in the United States are thought to be related to unhealthy lifestyle behaviors, such as tobacco use, diet and obesity, physical inactivity and excessive use of alcohol. Practicing healthy behaviors such as not smoking, maintaining a healthy weight, being physically active, eating a diet rich in fruits and vegetables, and avoiding too much alcohol should reduce your cancer risk.

---

and healthy lifestyle habits. In post-menopausal women, less body fat translates to lower estrogen levels. Exercise is also thought to boost your body's natural immune function, which could help protect against cancer.

Alcohol consumption

Dozens of studies around the world have consistently and clearly shown that drinking alcoholic beverages increases a woman's risk of developing breast cancer and that the more a woman drinks, the higher her risk.

Compared with nondrinkers, women who consume one alcoholic drink a day have a very small increase in risk, while women who consume more than three drinks a day have about 1.5 times the risk. Compared with women who don't consume alcohol, the relative risk of breast cancer increases 7 percent to 9 percent with each extra drink of alcohol consumed daily. The risk is the same whether you drink wine, beer or hard liquor.

Light to moderate consumption of alcoholic beverages — one drink a day or less — is unlikely to significantly affect your risk of breast cancer. If you do drink, do so in moderation. Limit yourself to one drink a day or less.

Radiation exposure

Women who've had radiation therapy to the chest wall area, especially as a child or young adult, have an increased risk of breast cancer later in life. For example, for a woman who's had radiation to lymph nodes in the chest to treat Hodgkin's disease, especially if she was treated before age 30, her risk of breast cancer is five times or more than that of a woman who didn't receive the treatment. Radiation exposure can damage cells, and extensive radiation can cause enough cell damage to contribute to cancer development. The small amount of radiation exposure you receive from ordinary diagnostic exams, such as mammograms and chest X-rays, doesn't appear to pose a significant risk.

Pesticides and environmental pollution

Many people are concerned about the potential cancer-causing effects of pesticides, hazardous chemicals and pollutants in food, drinking water and the air.

Like the general public, cancer scientists also have been very interested in uncovering possible environmental factors that may influence breast cancer development. A great deal of research has been done — and more is being conducted — in this area. However, no environmental agents aside from radiation exposure have been consistently linked to breast cancer development in humans.

Occupational exposures

On-the-job exposure to hazardous materials is thought to contribute to a small percentage of all cancers. Direct, frequent and high-level exposure to materials such as benzene, styrene, solvents, dyes, radioisotopes, fertilizers and pesticides may increase cancer risk.

Most of the evidence related to occupational exposures and breast cancer risk, though, is inconclusive. Although breast cancer rates are higher among some workers, the increase may be related to reproductive factors such as later pregnancies or no pregnancies rather than to something associated with their jobs.

Prior breast cancer

Having had breast cancer indicates that a woman is at increased risk of developing a second breast cancer. Women who have had breast cancer have a threefold to fourfold increase in risk of developing a new cancer in the other breast. This is a second cancer. It's not a recurrence of the first cancer.

This increased risk is higher for women with a family history of breast cancer, for those whose first cancer was lobular in origin and for women who were young — less than age 40 — when first diagnosed.

Benign breast disease

Certain changes seen on a breast biopsy are associated with an increased risk of later breast cancer. Your risk is increased if a biopsy shows an overgrowth of cells that line the breast ducts or lobules (epithelial hyperplasia), especially if the cells appear abnormal (atypical). See Chapter 8 for more information on these conditions.

Hyperplasia

Epithelial hyperplasia may involve an overgrowth of cells that line the breast ducts (ductal hyperplasia) or lobules (lobular hyperplasia). Based on how the cells appear under a microscope, hyperplasia is classified as usual (typical) or atypical. In typical hyperplasia, there's an increased number of normal cells in a normal arrangement. In atypical hyperplasia, the cells have not only increased in number, but have also taken on some abnormal characteristics (see page 20).

Women with typical hyperplasia have a slightly increased risk of breast cancer — up to two times greater than that of women without the condition. Among those with atypical hyperplasia, the increase in risk is more significant — four to five times as great. Women with atypical hyperplasia who have a family history

5 Things That *Don't* Increase Your Risk

Many misconceptions, rumors and unproven theories about breast cancer risk factors have made the rounds. The following factors have not been demonstrated to have any significant effect on breast cancer risk:

1. Antiperspirants

People have suggested that chemicals in underarm antiperspirants interfere with lymph circulation and cause toxins to build up in the breast, leading to breast cancer. Several thorough studies haven't found antiperspirant use to increase the risk of breast cancer.

2. Underwire bras

Similar to the claim that antiperspirants cause breast cancer, individuals have suggested that bras cause cancer by blocking lymph flow. There's no scientific basis for such a claim.

3. Coffee

Following a report that women with benign breast disease experienced relief from symptoms after eliminating caffeine from their diet, researchers speculated that caffeine may be a risk factor for breast cancer. But studies have shown no increase in breast cancer risk associated with drinking coffee or tea.

4. Large breasts

Large-breasted women have the same risk of developing breast cancer as small-breasted women do. They're not more or less likely to get the disease.

5. Breast implants

Several studies have concluded that breast implants don't increase breast cancer risk.

of breast cancer are at even higher risk, about 11 times that of other women.

Lobular carcinoma *in situ*

Lobular carcinoma *in situ* (LCIS) refers to the presence of abnormal-appearing cells in the lobules of the breast. Because the cells are still confined within the membranes of the lobules and haven't spread to adjacent breast tissue, the condition is termed *in situ*. LCIS is uncommon and is often discovered unexpectedly in tissue that's removed from the breast for another reason.

Studies indicate that women with LCIS are more than five times as likely to develop invasive breast cancer later on. The invasive cancer can occur in either breast but, according to at least one recent study, is more likely to occur in the same breast in which the LCIS was found.

Increased breast cancer risk associated with LCIS is higher for women who are diagnosed with the condition at a younger age and for those with a family history of breast cancer. See Chapter 8 for more information on LCIS.

Breast density

Breasts appear dense on a mammogram if they contain more glands and connective tissue (dense tissue) and less fat. Because breast cancers nearly always develop in the dense tissue of the breast, women who have mostly dense tissue on a mammogram are at increased risk of breast cancer. Abnormalities in dense breasts can also be more difficult to detect on a mammogram.

Chapter 5: Breast Cancer

Preventing Breast Cancer

What can you do to make sure you don't get breast cancer? Unfortunately, there are no clear answers to that question. Research holds promise for developing better risk-reduction strategies, but there's no guaranteed way to prevent the disease.

What is possible? For all women, it's important to follow screening guidelines. Although screening won't prevent breast cancer, it can lead to early detection, which increases the likelihood of successful treatment. For more information about screening and detection, see Chapter 6.

It's also important that you understand your risk of getting the disease, as discussed in Chapter 4, so that you can decide what steps to take, if any, to reduce your risk. For women at average risk, a change in certain lifestyle habits, such as limiting alcohol use and maintaining a healthy weight, may lower their risk to some degree. For women at high risk, options include medications (chemoprevention) or surgery to remove the breasts or ovaries. Because these are major, difficult decisions, high-risk women are urged to learn all they can about their specific risks and the available strategies for reducing those risks.

This chapter looks at lifestyle factors that may play a role in your risk of breast cancer and discusses prevention options if you're at high risk of getting the disease.

Lifestyle Factors

If you're like most women hoping to avoid breast cancer, you're looking for something you can do — some change you can make in your life — that will steer you away from the disease. Despite a great deal of research, though, few lifestyle factors have been strongly linked with breast cancer.

Most lifestyle changes result in only a modest reduction in cancer risk, if any. Among those that have received the most attention are factors related to diet, alcohol consumption and physical activity.

Diet

Researchers began investigating the role of diet in the development of breast cancer after noticing striking variations in breast cancer rates in different populations. Breast cancer is less common in countries where people eat less fat and in countries where people eat a lot of soy foods.

Researchers are also exploring the interactions between diet and genetic factors. For example, nutrients in the diet can protect deoxyribonucleic acid (DNA) from being damaged and thus may help prevent the development of abnormal (mutated) genes related to cancer. In addition, dietary factors combined with physical activity and weight control might delay or prevent the development of breast cancer in people with an increased genetic susceptibility to the disease.

Research on diet and breast cancer risk is often widely publicized, but no single study has been able to produce the definitive word on the subject. Although several dietary factors are believed to influence cancer risk, most studies haven't found a clear-cut relationship between consumption of particular foods or beverages and breast cancer prevention. With that in mind, consider new findings in the context of continuing research.

Fats

Probably no other aspect of diet has received more attention with regard to cancer than has fat. Early studies suggested that high intake of dietary fat was associated with a higher incidence of breast cancer. And in the 1980s, public health organizations recommended that people eat less fat to reduce their risk of cancer. Since then, however, most studies have found no correlation between higher dietary fat consumption and an increased incidence of breast cancer.

One group of researchers looked at the combined results of seven different studies that examined dietary fat and breast cancer risk. The seven studies collected information on the dietary habits of more than 350,000 women. The investigators found no association between fat in the diet and breast cancer — the risk of breast cancer was the same for women who had a high intake of fat and for those who ate a low-fat diet. The study concluded that there's no evidence that even diets very low in fat protect against breast cancer.

The Skinny on Fat

Fats are classified according to the type of fatty acids — the molecular building blocks of fats — they contain. Saturated fatty acids are found in higher concentrations in animal foods such as meats and dairy products. Saturated fats, such as butter, whole milk, lard and shortening, are solid at room temperature. Polyunsaturated fatty acids are found in foods of plant origin. They include safflower, corn and sunflower oils. Polyunsaturated fats are liquid at room temperature. Monounsaturated fatty acids are found in highest concentrations in olive oil, canola oil, peanut oil, avocados and most nuts. These fats are liquid at room temperature but begin to solidify when chilled.

The mixed results in studies of breast cancer and dietary fat may be due to several reasons:

- Studies that show different breast cancer rates in different countries can't easily separate diet from other risk factors.
- It's difficult to study the effects of an individual nutrient, such as fat, because foods contain multiple nutrients.
- Diets high in fat are also high in calories and can contribute to obesity, which is a risk factor for breast cancer among postmenopausal women. Obesity is also known to increase levels of estrogen and other hormones that may influence breast cancer development.
- It's possible that the effect of diet on breast cancer risk is time-dependent — that aspects of diet during childhood and adolescence, when breasts are developing, affect breast cancer risk decades later.
- The effect of dietary fats on breast cancer may depend on the type of fat that's consumed. Several studies have tried to determine if saturated, monounsaturated and polyunsaturated fats have differ-

ent effects on the development of breast cancer. Some preliminary studies have shown a modest protective benefit from olive oil, which is high in monounsaturated fat. But studies of other types of monounsaturated fat haven't found the same association, suggesting that the benefits of olive oil may come from other nutrients in the oil besides its fat.

- At this time, experts recommend replacing saturated fats with olive oil or other monounsaturated fats to reduce the risk of heart disease. Doing so may also have a slight effect on breast cancer risk.

Omega-3 and omega-6 fatty acids

Two types of polyunsaturated fat that have been studied in relation to breast cancer are omega-3 and omega-6 fatty acids. Omega-3 fatty acids are found in fatty, cold-water fish, such as salmon, mackerel, sardines, herring, bass, shark, swordfish and tuna, and in flaxseed, walnuts and canola oil. In animal studies, a high intake of omega-3 fatty acids from fish oils has been shown to slow the development and growth of breast

Weight Control and Breast Cancer Prevention

Studies have consistently shown that weight gain between early adulthood and midlife increases the risk of breast cancer in postmenopausal women. During late teen years or early adult life, being overweight is actually associated with a lower incidence of breast cancer. Premenopausal women who are overweight have a slightly reduced risk. But weight gain after age 18 substantially increases the risk in postmenopausal women. Excess body fat can lead to higher levels of estrogen and other hormones, which are associated with increased breast cancer risk.

Excess weight has also been reported to increase the risk of developing cancers of the colon, uterine lining (endometrium), gallbladder, esophagus, pancreas and kidney. For this reason, the American Cancer Society recommends maintaining a healthy weight throughout life.

Experts recommend that postmenopausal women who are overweight and sedentary lose weight and become more physically active, both for the possible benefits in preventing cancer and to improve overall health. A weight-loss program may include dietary changes, exercise, behavior modification and ongoing medical supervision.

tumors. But most human studies have found little evidence to support the idea that high consumption of fish reduces breast cancer risk.

Omega-6 fatty acids are plentiful in vegetable oils. Some studies suggest that the ratio of omega-3 fatty acids to omega-6 fatty acids in the diet is important in reducing breast cancer risk. In animal studies, a high omega-3 to omega-6 ratio has been shown to decrease the number, size and growth of breast tumors. A few preliminary human studies have found that a high omega-3 to omega-6 ratio is associated with a lower breast cancer risk in premenopausal women.

Despite the controversy about the link between dietary fat and breast cancer, scientists agree that the issue warrants further study. Results from several large, randomized trials are expected to shed further light on the subject. For example, the ongoing Women's Healthy Eating and Living (WHEL) study is looking at the effect on breast cancer survivors of eating a low-fat diet that's high in vegetables and fruits. Another ongoing study, the Women's Intervention Nutrition Study (WINS), also is studying the effect of a low-fat diet on breast cancer recurrence in postmenopausal women. The Women's Health Initiative is testing whether a low-fat diet that's rich in vegetables, fruits and grains can help prevent breast cancer.

Vitamins and minerals

Several vitamins and minerals have been studied for their possible role in preventing breast cancer. These include vitamins A, C and E, folate (a B vitamin) and the mineral selenium. Of these, only vitamins

QUESTION & ANSWER

Q: **Will eating fruits and vegetables help prevent breast cancer?**

A: Although eating a diet rich in fruits and vegetables provides a host of health benefits, these foods don't appear to offer particular protection against breast cancer.

Studies that have looked at consumption of fruits and vegetables and breast cancer risk have produced inconsistent results. One analysis of 26 studies did report a reduction in breast cancer risk with high vegetable consumption, and a modest reduction with high fruit intake.

However, another analysis of eight previously published studies including more than 350,000 women did not find an association between fruit and vegetable consumption and breast cancer risk.

But eating fruits and vegetables brings many other health benefits, including a reduced risk of diabetes, obesity, heart disease and other cancers, such as lung and colon cancers. The American Cancer Society recommends eating five or more servings of vegetables and fruit each day.

A and folate appear to be related to a slightly lower breast cancer risk.

Vitamin A is found in animal foods such as milk, eggs and liver. Carotenoids, plant chemicals found primarily in fruits and vegetables, are another source of vitamin A. Some carotenoids are converted to vitamin A in the body. The evidence of vitamin A's protective effect is strongest for carotenoid sources of the vitamin. These include yellow and orange vegetables and fruits, such as cantaloupe, carrots and sweet potatoes. It's possible, though, that other compounds in these foods provide cancer-fighting benefits. Therefore, at this point, it's not recommended that women take vitamin A specifically for breast cancer prevention.

Several studies suggest that an adequate intake of folate may be important in preventing breast cancer, particularly among women who drink alcohol regular-

ly. Folate occurs naturally in food, and folic acid is the synthetic form of the vitamin that's found in supplements and fortified foods. The recommended daily intake of folate is 400 micrograms a day. Alcohol interferes with the body's absorption of folate and increases the excretion of the vitamin by the kidneys.

Soy and phytoestrogens

Reports of the potential health benefits from soy have made soy foods increasingly popular. You may have heard that eating soy foods helps prevent breast cancer. Some studies, though, have suggested just the opposite — that soy is harmful for women with a high risk or history of breast cancer. The real story on soy remains uncertain, with more questions than answers.

Soybeans are a source of isoflavones, a type of phytoestrogen. Phytoestrogens are plant chemicals that behave like estrogen in your body but are less potent than your natural estrogen. Similar to estrogen, phytoestrogens bind to estrogen receptors in the body's cells. The effect of a phytoestrogen may differ depending on the level of natural estrogen in the body. For example, when natural estrogen is abundant in the body, phytoestrogens may reduce estrogen's effects by displacing it from cells. But when little natural estrogen is present, such as after menopause, phytoestrogens may act like estrogen.

Much of the basis for the suggestion that soy foods protect against breast cancer comes from studies that show lower breast cancer rates in many Asian countries, where soybean products are a food staple. Studies also show that when Asian women move to the United States and adopt a Western lifestyle, their risk of breast cancer rises. But it's clear that many differences could explain these patterns. Soy consumption is just one factor.

Hundreds of studies have attempted to determine if eating soy does indeed help prevent breast cancer. The results have been contradictory. Most studies haven't found that high soy intake cuts breast cancer risk. A few studies have raised concerns that increasing your soy intake at midlife could have adverse effects. Common sources of soy protein in the American diet are tofu, soy milk, energy bars, soy protein powder and soy nuts.

Right now, it's impossible to define soy's role. The bottom line? As with most things, moderation is key. If you enjoy soy foods, it's reasonable to use soy products in your diet in moderation, whether or not you're at risk of breast cancer or have had the disease. But experts don't recommend taking soy for the sole purpose of trying to lower your breast cancer risk.

Antioxidants and Cancer Prevention

Carotenoids, selenium, vitamin C and vitamin E are all antioxidants — substances that bind to and protect the body's cells from the damaging effects of free radicals, which are highly reactive and potentially toxic oxygen metabolites within cells. Free radicals are created as a byproduct of normal metabolism, the biochemical process by which the body uses oxygen and nutrients to produce energy. The natural aging process and chronic diseases also produce free radicals. In small amounts, some of these oxygen metabolites help the immune system do its job, but as production of free radicals increases, they can damage cells.

Free radicals are neutralized by antioxidants. These substances are found in food — derived from vitamins, minerals and plant chemicals in fruits and vegetables — or taken as supplements. Because damage from free radicals is associated with increased cancer risk, antioxidant nutrients are thought to possibly protect against cancer by decreasing the adverse effects of free radicals. But studies haven't found a specific benefit of

Lignans

Lignans are another naturally occurring compound found in plants. Like isoflavones, several lignans are phytoestrogens. The richest source of lignans is flaxseed, sometimes called linseed. Flaxseed oil, however, doesn't contain a significant amount of lignans. Other sources of lignans include whole grains, soybeans, cranberries, some vegetables — broccoli, carrots, cauliflower and spinach — and black and green teas.

Like isoflavones, lignans are being studied for possible use in breast cancer prevention. But, as with isoflavones, the evidence isn't strong enough to make the case for their preventive benefits. Some studies have shown a lower incidence of breast cancer among people who eat more lignan-containing foods, and in animal studies, lignans inhibited the growth of breast tumors. But researchers have some of the same concerns about lignans as they have about soy products — that a high intake might promote breast cancer.

More studies are needed about the potential benefits of flaxseed and other lignan-containing foods.

Alcohol

Drinking alcohol is associated with a higher risk of developing breast cancer. Having two drinks a day of beer, wine or liquor increases your risk of breast cancer by about 20 percent. The risk goes up with each drink consumed in a day.

Excessive use of alcohol is also associated with a number of other health problems. Moderation, again, is key. Moderate drinking is defined as no more than one drink a day for women and for small-framed men and men older than age 65, and two drinks a day for larger men

antioxidants — whether from food sources or supplements — in protecting against breast cancer.

Despite the popular belief that antioxidants in the diet can fight disease, many questions remain unanswered about their health benefits. For example, it's possible that taking antioxidant supplements may disturb the body's normal balance of free radicals and antioxidants, increasing the risk of disease or interfering with treatment. Clinical studies of antioxidant supplements, which contain a number of antioxidant vitamins, are under way but haven't yet been shown to reduce cancer risk. In one study of 90 women with breast cancer, those who took high-dose combinations of vitamins and minerals in addition to standard treatments fared worse in terms of survival time than did women who didn't take the supplements. In another large study involving smokers, participants who took supplemental vitamins developed more lung cancers than did participants who took inactive pills (placebos).

Because of the uncertainty surrounding supplements, the best advice is to get your antioxidants by way of food sources rather than in the form of supplements.

Diet and breast cancer

Many questions still remain regarding the relationship among food, alcohol and breast cancer prevention. Here's a summary of what's currently known about various foods and alcohol:

Dietary factor	Effect on breast cancer	Recommendation
High-fat diet	Doesn't directly increase risk, but contributes to obesity, which is associated with increased risk.	Aim for a total fat intake of no more than 30 percent of calories, with 10 percent or less from saturated fat. Minimize animal sources of fat, such as meats and high-fat dairy products.
Olive oil	May have protective effect. Further research is needed.	Replace saturated fat with olive oil or other monounsaturated fats.
Fruits and vegetables	Limited.	To reap other health benefits, eat five or more servings daily.
Vitamin A	May reduce risk modestly.	Good sources of vitamin A are yellow fruits and vegetables, such as carrots, cantaloupe and sweet potatoes.
Soy products	Unknown. Studies show contradictory results.	Eat dietary soy in moderation. Soy supplements aren't recommended.
Folate or folic acid	Decreases risk, especially in women who drink alcohol.	Consume recommended daily intake of 400 micrograms.
Fish and fish oils	Reduce breast cancer development in animals. No strong effect has been shown in humans.	Eat as part of a healthy diet.
Flaxseed	Unknown.	Eat in moderation.
Alcohol	Increases risk.	If you drink, do so in moderation.

under the age of 65. One drink is defined as 12 ounces of beer, 5 ounces of wine or 1.5 ounces of 80-proof distilled spirits.

Physical activity

Physical activity, ranging from yardwork to intensive exercise sessions, pays off with a number of health benefits. Among them are cardiovascular fitness, which can help protect against heart disease, and a reduced risk of diabetes. Exercise may also decrease the risk of certain cancers, such as colon and breast cancers.

Researchers have found consistent evidence that regular physical activity lowers

FASTFACT

**Too much weight
and too little exercise**

The International Agency for Research on Cancer estimates that between one-fourth and one-third of cancers of all types could be attributed to the combined effects of being overweight and physically inactive.

the risk of breast cancer. Of 44 studies that investigated the association between breast cancer and physical activity, 32 of the studies found a reduced breast cancer risk in women who were most physically active. The average reduction in risk was 30 percent to 40 percent.

The relationship between exercise and breast cancer risk is complex, and several underlying biological factors may account for the reduction in risk that comes with physical activity. Regular exercise helps prevent obesity and weight gain, which are associated with breast cancer risk. Both physical inactivity and obesity affect normal metabolism of insulin. Regular exercise may reduce levels of insulin and insulin-like growth factors — high levels of which have been associated with an increased risk of breast cancer. Exercise may also lower levels of sex hormones, including estrogen. Estrogen is thought to act as the fuel that promotes the growth of some breast cancers.

Not every study has shown that exercise helps lower breast cancer risk. Some studies found no protective effect of physical activity. This may be because of differ-

ences in the way researchers measured exercise. In addition, the relationship between physical activity and breast cancer risk may differ depending on a woman's age, the amount of exercise she gets and at what period in her life she was most physically active. For example, some studies have found that exercise had the strongest protective effects among postmenopausal women, and other research has shown a stronger effect in premenopausal women.

Experts recommend engaging in at least 30 minutes of moderate activity five or more days of the week to reduce your risk of breast cancer. Moderate or vigorous activity is any physical activity that raises your heart rate or causes you to sweat. Examples of such activities include biking, brisk walking, jogging, swimming, recreational sports as well as heavy housework or yardwork.

Surgery and Chemoprevention

For women identified as having a high risk of developing breast cancer, prevention becomes even more critical. Knowing that you have a 40 percent to 60 percent chance of getting breast cancer can be a source of intense anxiety. Women at high risk face a number of difficult issues:

- Understanding and coming to terms with the meaning of their risk status
- Dealing with fear of harm, disfigurement, pain or death
- Coping with guilt about passing on a hereditary risk

- Managing stress, worries and intrusive thoughts
- Making decisions about preventive therapy

Women at high risk of breast cancer include those with a strong family history of the disease and those who test positive for a genetic alteration known to cause breast cancer, such as a BRCA1 or BRCA2 mutation. Other reasons a woman may be considered high risk include a personal history of breast cancer or a history of lobular carcinoma *in situ*. (See Chapter 4 for more information about breast cancer risk factors.)

Before you pursue any type of treatment aimed at reducing risk, it's essential that you have an accurate estimate of your breast cancer risk. Make an appointment with your doctor or a breast specialist to determine your risk status.

Doctors don't always agree on the most effective way to manage the care of high-risk women. Some focus on close surveillance and early detection of the disease, while others focus on risk reduction.

The goal of screening and surveillance, sometimes referred to as secondary prevention, is early detection of breast cancer. Screening in high-risk women typically involves annual mammograms beginning five to 10 years before the age of the youngest affected relative, clinical breast examinations twice a year and monthly breast self-examinations. The role of magnetic resonance imaging (MRI) in screening women at high risk of breast cancer is being studied. These procedures are discussed in Chapter 6.

Some women at high risk of breast cancer prefer to take steps to reduce their risk. They may consider surgery to remove their breasts (preventive, or prophylactic, mastectomy) or surgery to remove their ovaries (preventive, or prophylactic, oophorectomy). In premenopausal women, removing the ovaries significantly reduces the amount of estrogen their bodies produce. This can halt or slow breast cancers that depend on estrogen to grow. Another option is the use of medications to reduce cancer risk (chemoprevention). These strategies are sometimes referred to as primary prevention.

Each of these options has benefits and risks. Deciding what course to take is a highly personal decision. There's no one right answer for all high-risk women. Risk-reduction counseling can help you evaluate your options and make the decision that's right for you. With any primary preventive strategy, there's always the chance that some women who pursue it would not have developed breast cancer at all. For this reason, it's important to have a thorough understanding of your individual risk and your options for reducing that risk.

Prophylactic mastectomy

Risk-reducing mastectomy, also known as prophylactic mastectomy, is the surgical removal of one or both breasts to reduce the risk of breast cancer. Although prophylactic mastectomy was discussed as early as the 1920s, the operation wasn't commonly performed until the 1960s and 1970s, when breast implants became available for breast reconstruction and the medical community gained a greater awareness of increased breast cancer risk in some families.

Studies have shown that mastectomy of both breasts (bilateral mastectomy) is very effective in reducing the risk of breast cancer. However, the surgery doesn't completely eliminate breast cancer risk or prevent all cases of breast cancer. That's because breast tissue is widely distributed on the chest wall, extending into the armpit, and even to the collarbone, in most women. Therefore, it's impossible for a surgeon to remove all breast tissue, and breast cancer can potentially develop in the small amount of remaining tissue.

Researchers at Mayo Clinic reviewed the experience of 639 women with a family history of breast cancer who had prophylactic bilateral mastectomies between 1960 and 1993. The investigators compared the total number of breast cancers expected among these high-risk women with the number of cancers that actually occurred. Among 214 women at high risk, it was predicted that without prophylactic mastectomy, 14 years later 30 women would develop breast cancer, but only three cases occurred. Thus, prophylactic mastectomy reduced the risk of getting breast cancer by about 90 percent, and the surgery also resulted in a significant reduction in the number of deaths from breast cancer. Instead of an expected 19 deaths, there were two.

In addition, prophylactic mastectomy has been shown to decrease the risk of breast cancer in women with BRCA1 or BRCA2 mutations. In a study from the Netherlands involving 139 women who had BRCA mutations, 63 chose surveillance and 76 chose prophylactic bilateral

mastectomy. At a median follow-up of three years, there were eight cancers in the surveillance group and none in the surgery group.

Other studies have found that an opposite-breast (contralateral) prophylactic mastectomy significantly reduces the risk of a second breast cancer in women who've had cancer in one breast and are at high risk of developing it in the other.

Who's a candidate?

Prophylactic mastectomy is an elective procedure, and there aren't precise guidelines defining who should have the surgery. A number of factors are taken into consideration. The surgery may be appropriate for women who:

- Carry a BRCA mutation
- Have a strong family history of breast cancer without a known genetic mutation
- Have already had one breast removed due to cancer and have a family history of the disease
- Have had lobular carcinoma *in situ*

To make the best individual decision about whether prophylactic mastectomy is appropriate, it's crucial that you understand your true risk of breast cancer. Many women overestimate their individual risk.

It's often recommended that women considering prophylactic mastectomy talk with a genetic counselor before making this decision. Meeting with a breast surgeon beforehand to discuss the potential risks and benefits of the surgery also is beneficial. Women interested in breast reconstruction — plastic surgery to restore the shape of a breast mound — typically meet with a plastic surgeon to discuss options available. A woman may also meet with a psychologist or other mental health professional to discuss potential issues related to body image and other concerns.

How it's done

The recommended procedure for prophylactic mastectomy is a simple (total) mastectomy, an operation to remove the entire breast and nipple. Subcutaneous mastectomy, an operation that removes breast tissue but spares the nipple, isn't the preferred procedure because it leaves substantial breast tissue behind.

After a mastectomy, most women choose to have breast reconstruction. Researchers are exploring the use of skin-sparing mastectomy. This procedure may offer cosmetic advantages. Mastectomy and breast reconstruction are discussed in detail in Chapters 9 and 10.

Risks

Like any major surgery, prophylactic mastectomy may result in some physical complications either immediately after the operation or months or years later. Problems with breast implants are among the most common concerns.

One study evaluated 592 women who had both breasts removed and implant reconstruction. Almost all these women had subcutaneous mastectomies. During the next 14 years, about half the women required a second operation. The most common reason for re-operation was a problem with implants, often the development of a tight, firm capsule around the implant.

In addition to possible physical complications, prophylactic mastectomy can have psychological and social effects. Limited research has been done regarding the emotional and psychological effects of prophylactic mastectomy. In one study at Mayo Clinic, researchers interviewed women who had had prophylactic mastectomy, asking several questions about the psychological and social consequences of the surgery. About 15 years after the surgery, 70 percent of the women were either satisfied or very satisfied with their surgery. Seventy-four percent of the women said they had a lower level of emotional concern about developing breast cancer. The majority of women also reported either favorable effects or no change in emotional stability, stress, self-esteem, sexual relationships and feelings of femininity. When asked whether they would choose to have the surgery again, two-thirds said they definitely or probably would.

Women who felt they had the surgery mainly on the basis of a doctor's advice were more likely to be dissatisfied. Women who had strong support from family and friends were most satisfied with their decisions.

In smaller studies, women who had had prophylactic mastectomies reported significantly lower levels of anxiety after the surgery, but some women experienced difficulties with body image, sexual interest and functioning, and self-esteem.

The procedure has been controversial because of the lack of clearly defined criteria for who should have the surgery and because it doesn't completely eliminate the risk of breast cancer. In addition, information about the emotional and social ramifications of the procedure is limited. Some women and doctors consider removing the breasts an unacceptably extreme way to reduce risk.

Because of the potential physical and psychological effects, the decision to have prophylactic mastectomy must be made on an individual basis after carefully weighing the risks and benefits. It's important to fully consider all of your options before making a decision. You and your partner also need to understand the procedure and the effect it will have on body image and sexuality. Some women find it helpful to talk with others who have had the surgery.

Lisa's Story

After watching her mother die of breast cancer at the age of 49, Lisa, a nurse, developed cancerphobia.

Lisa's fear of cancer grew as she took stock of her family history and learned that many of her relatives had been diagnosed with either breast or ovarian cancer: her maternal grandmother, four of seven maternal aunts and two paternal aunts. "I always thought that I would die of breast cancer. So many of my family members did. I vowed to try to detect it early."

Lisa's insurance company wouldn't pay for a mammogram before age 40, so she and her husband decided to bear the cost. Doctors detected a lump when Lisa had her first mammogram. After a biopsy revealed that the lump was benign, Lisa's surgeon ordered yearly mammograms and checkups every six months, and the insurance company began to pay for the screenings.

Over the course of five years, mammography identified four lumps in Lisa's breasts. She underwent a biopsy each time — all of the lumps were benign.

But Lisa, her husband, Todd, and their two daughters began to dread the routine screenings — and the possibility that results would reveal an aggressive cancer. Noting her family history and level of distress, Lisa's surgeon asked Lisa if she had ever considered prophylactic mastectomy.

After thinking about it, Lisa decided that she was interested in learning more about the surgery. She conducted extensive Internet research on prophylactic mastectomy and weighed its pros and cons.

In January 2002, Lisa decided to go ahead with a complete genetic evaluation and risk assessment. After three days of undergoing diagnostic tests, genetic tests and genetic counseling, as well as consulting with a breast surgeon, Lisa and Todd had all of the information they needed to make a decision. Genetic modeling, genetic counseling and Lisa's history of previous breast biopsies all added up to a very high risk.

"The decision to proceed with prophylactic mastectomy became a no-brainer after we saw all those black circles indicating breast cancer on Lisa's family history pedigree," says Todd. "I was going to love her whether she had breasts or not. It didn't matter."

The procedure took about two hours. Immediately following that surgery, a plastic surgeon began an intricate reconstruction procedure that took 14 hours to complete.

Lisa required 16 weeks of rest to fully recover, but said that she's pleased with the results. She has continued finalizing her reconstruction — returning for nipple and areola reconstruction.

"Never once did we doubt our decision," Lisa points out. "Never once did we have second thoughts. I've felt the world lifted off my shoulders. My life has started all over."

Prophylactic oophorectomy

Another surgical option available to women at high risk of breast cancer is preventive (prophylactic) oophorectomy — removal of the ovaries. Removing the ovaries in premenopausal women greatly decreases the amount of estrogen a woman's body produces and may halt or slow breast cancers dependent on estrogen to grow.

Oophorectomy is usually motivated by the need to reduce ovarian cancer risk. However, if the procedure is performed before a woman reaches menopause, it also reduces breast cancer risk.

Prophylactic oophorectomy reduces the risk of breast cancer by about 50 percent in premenopausal women. It reduces the risk of ovarian cancer and peritoneal cancer by up to 95 percent in both pre- and postmenopausal women. Peritoneal cancer arises from the same cell type as ovarian cancer but develops in cells lining the abdominal cavity.

Oophorectomy is usually recommended for women who are at increased risk of both breast cancer and ovarian cancer due to an inherited mutation in the BRCA1 or BRCA2 gene. Even though the risk of ovarian cancer may be lower than the risk of breast cancer (see the tables on page 66), ovarian cancer is much more difficult to detect at an early stage. For this reason,

it's also more likely to be deadly. For BRCA1 carriers, oophorectomy is usually done between ages 35 and 40. For BRCA2 carriers, ovarian cancer risk is less than 1 percent until age 45, so the procedure may be somewhat delayed. Prophylactic oophorectomy may also be recommended for women with a strong family history of breast and ovarian cancers but no known genetic alteration.

Some women at high risk choose prophylactic oophorectomy instead of mastectomy because of concerns about body image and because breast cancer is more likely to be detected at an earlier stage than is ovarian cancer.

When oophorectomy is performed, the fallopian tubes are removed as well (this procedure is known as salpingo-oophorectomy) to avoid the possibility of tumors developing in the tubes. In addition, the fallopian tubes aren't needed if the ovaries are removed.

Although oophorectomy can greatly reduce the risk of ovarian and peritoneal cancers, the surgery doesn't eliminate all cancer risk. Women who undergo the procedure still have a slight risk (less than 5 percent) of getting peritoneal cancer.

Risks
Removal of the ovaries brings some negative consequences that need consideration. In premenopausal women, oophorectomy causes premature menopause. This can increase the risk of osteoporosis. Signs and symptoms of menopause, which include hot flashes, vaginal dryness, sexual problems, sleep disturbances and, possibly, cognitive changes, may affect quality of life. Some

women who have such surgery experience emotional and sexual effects, though there's insufficient research in this area.

Using hormone replacement therapy (HRT) after prophylactic oophorectomy is an option, especially for women who have the procedure at a young age. The effect of such hormones on breast cancer risk isn't entirely clear, but the amount of hormone given is less than what your ovaries are making.

If you're considering prophylactic oophorectomy, make sure you understand the risks and benefits of the procedure. Genetic counseling is generally recommended before oophorectomy. The timing of the procedure depends on the age at which a woman is considered at greater risk of ovarian and breast cancers. (As mentioned earlier, BRCA1 carriers are at risk of getting ovarian cancer at an earlier age than are BRCA2 carriers.) After having an oophorectomy, some women undergo other preventive strategies for breast cancer, such as chemoprevention or mastectomy. Prophylactic oophorectomy is discussed in more detail in Chapter 15.

Janice's Story

In 1994, Janice's sister was diagnosed with breast cancer. The cancer had gone undetected for some time and had spread beyond the breast. Her sister died in 1996 at the age of 43. Five years later, Janice's mother received a diagnosis of inflammatory breast cancer that had spread to her lymph nodes. Her mother's diagnosis triggered a warning for Janice — maybe these cancers weren't unfortunate coincidences, maybe they had some sort of genetic link.

To get more information, Janice called a local breast clinic. From there, she was referred for genetic counseling. During genetic counseling, Janice filled out a questionnaire about her family history of cancer. The results revealed not only a few cases of breast cancer on her mother's side but also a strong history of colon cancer on her father's side. For Janice, the results of the evaluation indicated that she was at increased cancer risk.

The next step was deciding what to do about it — if anything. Janice learned that she had a number of options to reduce her risk. Because she didn't feel there was one clear-cut preventive strategy that would be best for her, Janice decided to take her time and keep her options open.

For the time being Janice, who is 48, has a mammogram regularly to check for any breast changes. She also decided to have her uterus and ovaries removed (hysterectomy and oophorectomy). The purpose of this surgery was twofold: Removing her uterus would reduce her risk of uterine cancer, which is greater in families with a strong history of colon cancer. And removing her ovaries would decrease the amount of estrogen produced in her body, helping reduce her risk of breast cancer.

While Janice had initially been reluctant to have genetic testing, she later decided to proceed and is awaiting the results.

For Janice, one of the hardest parts is keeping the situation in perspective. "You kind of live in this worst-case scenario world," she says. At times, it's been difficult for Janice to not get wrapped up in the uncertainty of her future — to not feel like the cancer risk is a life sentence. "You need to try to separate yourself from what's going on around you." Janice's advice to others is to try not to dwell on the what-ifs.

The results of her genetic tests may also benefit more than just Janice. Janice is concerned that her daughter and niece may be at increased cancer risk, and the results of her tests may help them with their health decisions.

Janice has also decided to turn this time of struggle into an opportunity to pursue her dream. She has always wanted to be a writer and loves learning, so she has returned to school to work toward a master's degree in health journalism. She's enjoying school, feels well and so far is happy with the decisions she's made.

Medication

Using medications to prevent the development of cancer is called chemoprevention. Currently, only one drug, tamoxifen (Nolvadex), is approved by the Food and Drug Administration (FDA) for reduction of breast cancer risk in women at high risk of getting the disease. Other drugs are being investigated for their potential to reduce the risk of breast cancer. These include raloxifene (Evista), a drug that's currently used to prevent osteoporosis in postmenopausal women, as well as a group of drugs called aromatase inhibitors and yet another group of medications called nonsteroidal anti-inflammatory drugs.

Tamoxifen and raloxifene both belong to a class of drugs called selective estrogen receptor modulators (SERMs). These drugs bind to the same protein partner that the hormone estrogen needs to exert its effects — the estrogen receptor (ER).

Estrogen is thought to act as a fuel that promotes the growth of breast cancer cells. But SERMs are different from estrogen. In some tissues they mimic the effect of estrogen, and in others — such as in breast tissue — they block or work against estrogen. The pattern of activity varies with each SERM.

In the following pages, tamoxifen, raloxifene, aromatase inhibitors and nonsteroidal anti-inflammatory drugs are discussed in more detail.

Tamoxifen

Tamoxifen has been used to treat breast cancer for more than 25 years. It's used to treat advanced cancer and, for women with early-stage, estrogen receptor positive breast cancer, it's used as an additional (adjuvant) treatment to reduce their risk of recurrent cancer. In addition, the drug is approved for women who haven't been diagnosed with breast cancer but who are considered to be at high risk of the disease.

Four large clinical trials have examined whether tamoxifen reduces the risk of breast cancer in women who don't have the disease but are at high risk of developing it. One of these studies, the Breast Cancer Prevention Trial, began in 1992. More than 13,000 women in the United States were enrolled in this randomized controlled study, which was sponsored by the National Cancer Institute. The results, released in 1998, showed that compared with an inactive pill (placebo), tamoxifen reduced the short-term (five year) risk of invasive breast cancer by 49 percent. The risk of noninvasive breast cancers was reduced by 50 percent.

The 50 percent risk reduction refers to relative risk. What does this mean in absolute terms? Say that a woman has a 4 percent actual risk of developing breast cancer in the next five years if she doesn't take tamoxifen. By taking the drug, she reduces the risk to 2 percent. In other words, out of 100 similar-risk women, four would develop the disease over five years if they didn't take tamoxifen. If they did, two would develop the disease.

Another large clinical trial, the International Breast Cancer Intervention Study, found a 32 percent relative reduction in risk with use of tamoxifen. But two European trials found no reduction in risk. In early 2003, an overview of the combined results of four breast cancer prevention trials was published. Altogether, the studies involved more than 25,000 women. The analysis showed that use of tamoxifen resulted in a 38 percent reduction in the incidence of breast cancer overall and a 48 percent reduction in the incidence of ER positive cancers — tumors that have receptors for estrogen and are sensitive to the hormone. But tamoxifen was ineffective in preventing ER negative breast cancers.

Based on the results of the initial Breast Cancer Prevention Trial, in 1998 the FDA approved the use of tamoxifen for breast cancer risk reduction for women who are at least 35 years old and have a five-year breast cancer risk greater than 1.66 percent. When used, tamoxifen is generally prescribed for a period of five years.

Side effects and risks

The most common side effects of tamoxifen are hot flashes and vaginal discharge. Some women also experience menstrual irregularities.

Women who take tamoxifen are at increased risk of developing blood clots, although this is uncommon, occurring in less than 1 percent of women who take the drug. Tamoxifen also increases the risk of two types of cancer that can develop in the uterus — endometrial cancer, which begins in the lining of the uterus, and uterine sarcoma, which arises in the muscular wall of the uterus.

In the Breast Cancer Prevention Trial, women who took tamoxifen had about two and a half times the chance of developing endometrial cancer, as did women who took a placebo. The absolute risk is small — about two additional cases of endometrial cancer among 1,000 women taking tamoxifen each year. The increased risk was seen only among women who were age 50 or older. Women under 50 who took tamoxifen had no increased risk of endometrial cancer.

Tamoxifen isn't effective against breast cancer that doesn't express the estrogen receptor. This raises questions about the benefits of tamoxifen for women with an inherited gene mutation, because BRCA1 carriers are more likely to have ER negative tumors. For BRCA2 carriers, however, a greater proportion develop ER positive breast cancer, so in this group, tamoxifen may be more beneficial. How much women who carry a genetic mutation can lower their breast cancer risk by taking tamoxifen isn't yet known.

In addition, none of the clinical trials found that tamoxifen improves overall survival. In fact, in the International Breast Cancer Intervention Study, there were slightly more deaths among women taking tamoxifen, due to an increase in blood clots.

If you're considering taking tamoxifen to reduce your risk of breast cancer, you need to weigh the potential benefits and risks in light of your individual risk profile. Unless you're at high risk of developing breast cancer, the potential risks of tamoxifen may outweigh any benefits. The decision will depend on your age, risk status, family history, medical history, lifestyle, personal values and preferences. For example, if you have a history of blood clots, your doctor may well advise you not to take tamoxifen.

In general, tamoxifen provides the greatest benefit with the fewest side effects in:

- Women at highest risk of developing breast cancer, such as women with a personal or family history of breast cancer or those with ductal or lobular carcinoma *in situ*
- Premenopausal women who are less likely to develop blood clots or uterine cancer
- Women who've had a hysterectomy and no longer have a uterus

A number of questions remain to be answered about the use of tamoxifen to reduce the risk of breast cancer. For example, it's not known how long the risk reduction will last or whether the drug will eventually result in fewer deaths from breast cancer.

Raloxifene

Like tamoxifen, raloxifene binds to estrogen receptors in breast tissue and blocks estrogen's effects in the breasts. On bone tissue, on the other hand, the drug behaves like estrogen, stopping bone loss.

Currently, raloxifene is approved only for use in preventing and treating the bone-thinning disease osteoporosis. But research is under way to investigate whether it also may be of benefit as a therapy to reduce breast cancer risk.

A large clinical trial, the Multiple Outcomes of Raloxifene Evaluation (MORE), was conducted to determine if raloxifene treatment could reduce the risk of bone fractures in postmenopausal women with osteoporosis. It did. In this trial, researchers also monitored breast cancer outcomes, although the participants weren't selected because of breast cancer risk. The trial showed that, compared with a placebo, raloxifene reduced the risk of estrogen receptor positive breast cancers by 76 percent . The drug didn't affect breast cancers that were estrogen receptor negative. Other studies comparing raloxifene with a placebo reported a somewhat smaller reduction in breast cancer risk, about 54 percent.

Based on the findings from the MORE trial, the National Cancer Institute launched the Study of Tamoxifen and Raloxifene (STAR) trial, which began in 1999. This ongoing study is designed to see whether raloxifene is more or less effective than tamoxifen is in reducing breast cancer occurrence in postmenopausal women at increased risk of getting the disease. The STAR trial will involve about 19,000 women, and results are expected in 2007. Another ongoing clinical trial, Raloxifene Use for the Heart (RUTH), will study the effects of raloxifene compared with those of a placebo in preventing both heart disease and breast cancer in postmenopausal women.

Raloxifene hasn't been studied in premenopausal women. Because its safety in younger women is unknown, the drug isn't recommended for these women.

Similar to tamoxifen, raloxifene increases the risk of blood clots slightly, but unlike tamoxifen, it doesn't appear to increase the risk of endometrial cancer.

Aromatase inhibitors

Aromatase inhibitors are drugs that reduce estrogen levels in a woman's body by blocking an enzyme called aromatase, which is involved in converting other hormones to estrogen. These medications present an alternative hormonal approach to breast cancer treatment. Three aromatase inhibitors, anastrozole (Arimidex), exemestane (Aromasin) and letrozole (Femara), are currently used to treat breast cancer in postmenopausal women.

One large clinical study, the Arimidex, Tamoxifen, Alone or in Combination (ATAC) trial, evaluated anastrozole as an additional (adjuvant) treatment for breast cancer. The study found that anastrozole was slightly better than tamoxifen in reducing the risk of breast cancer recurrence in women with estrogen receptor positive tumors. The ATAC trial also found that anastrozole reduced the risk of developing a new cancer in the other breast by 58 percent.

These promising results have led researchers to embark on a number of studies to evaluate the effectiveness of aromatase inhibitors in preventing breast cancer. A large-scale international clinical trial called the International Breast Cancer Intervention Study will compare anastrozole with a placebo in postmenopausal women at high risk of breast cancer. Another study will evaluate exemestane taken with or without a nonsteroidal anti-inflammatory drug (NSAID).

Researchers are excited about the potential of aromatase inhibitors because they appear to be at least as effective and possibly better than tamoxifen, with fewer side effects. Serious adverse effects such as blood clots and endometrial cancer are less of a concern with aromatase inhibitors. Some aromatase inhibitors may contribute to bone loss, but the extent of this potential side effect has not yet been fully determined. Further studies in women are planned to gain more information.

Nonsteroidal anti-inflammatory drugs

Several studies have tried to determine if aspirin and other NSAIDs have an effect on breast cancer risk. NSAIDs include many common over-the-counter painkillers, such as ibuprofen and naproxen sodium. All the studies to date have been observational studies, which don't provide the strongest level of evidence.

Some research has found that people who regularly take aspirin or other NSAIDs have a slightly decreased risk of breast cancer. But other studies have not shown a significant association between breast cancer risk and NSAID use. In studies involving animals, NSAIDs inhibit the development of breast tumors.

A recent analysis of data from the Women's Health Initiative study found that postmenopausal women who took two or more NSAID tablets (aspirin,

Options for women at high risk of breast cancer

Option	Advantages	Disadvantages
Surveillance	• Preserves breasts. • Allows for other options. • Requires no treatment for women who don't develop breast cancer.	• Doesn't prevent disease. • Mammography has a high rate of false-negatives in younger women. • Effectiveness unknown in younger, high-risk women.
Chemoprevention*	• Tamoxifen reduces risk of breast cancer up to 50 percent. • Preserves breasts. • Allows for other options.	• Effective only for estrogen receptor positive breast cancer. • Has side effects (hot flashes, vaginal discharge, others) and increases risk of endometrial cancer and blood clots. • Effectiveness for BRCA1 and BRCA2 carriers uncertain. • Optimal length and timing of treatment uncertain. • No improvement in overall survival has been shown. • Duration of benefits unknown.
Prophylactic mastectomy	• Reduces risk of breast cancer by up to 90 percent. • Has a long-term effect.	• Requires major surgery that results in loss of breasts. • Is an irreversible decision. • Has potential psychological and physical effects — body image issues, numbness in chest, and so on. • Has a high rate of re-operation with implant reconstruction.
Prophylactic oophorectomy	• Reduces risk of breast cancer by 50 percent in premenopausal women. • Reduces risk of ovarian cancer by up to 90 percent. • Preserves breasts.	• Results in premature menopause, causing short-term side effects (hot flashes, vaginal dryness, others) and long-term effects, including increased risk of osteoporosis. • Results in loss of fertility. • Is an irreversible decision.

*Raloxifene, aromatase inhibitors and nonsteroidal anti-inflammatory drugs had not been established as chemopreventive agents at the time this book was published. Ask your doctor about updated information on these drugs.

ibuprofen or related drugs) a week for five to nine years cut their risk of breast cancer by 21 percent. Regular use for 10 years or more was associated with a 28 percent reduction in risk. In that study, use of ibuprofen was associated with greater protection. Other studies have found greater risk reduction with use of aspirin.

The benefits of NSAIDs in lowering breast cancer risk were seen only with standard doses, not low (baby aspirin) doses. Acetaminophen, which isn't an NSAID and has a different mechanism of action, is the active ingredient in pain relievers such as Tylenol. It wasn't associated with a lower breast cancer risk.

It's not known for certain how aspirin and other NSAIDs may help protect against breast cancer. In animals, these drugs are capable of triggering cell death in abnormal breast cells. The medications work by blocking cyclooxygenase (COX) enzymes, which are involved in many important body processes, including inflammation and cancer development.

Priscilla's Story

Although she has never had cancer, Priscilla has seen and experienced its effects. Her sister, Hope, was 63 when she received a diagnosis of breast cancer in 2000. During the course of her cancer treatment, Hope underwent eight sessions of chemotherapy and six sessions of radiation treatment. Because Hope lived about 80 miles from where she received her treatments, Priscilla would drive her to the appointments and stay with her afterward.

In May of 2002, Priscilla felt some lumps in her breasts that were painful and made an appointment for a mammogram. Her mammogram results were inconclusive, so her doctor ordered an ultrasound. Priscilla's lumps turned out to be benign cysts, but the experience increased her fear of developing breast cancer, like her sister.

During one of Priscilla's appointments, she talked with a nurse practitioner about her sister's experience with breast cancer. The nurse practitioner mentioned a clinical trial called the STAR trial, in which researchers are testing two drugs — raloxifene and tamoxifen — to see if one drug is more beneficial than the other in preventing breast cancer in women at increased risk of the disease. After talking with the trial coordinator, Priscilla decided she wanted to participate in the STAR trial.

The first step in enrolling in the trial was to see if she qualified to be a participant. Priscilla filled out a form indicating her family's history of cancer. Her sister and two of her maternal cousins had breast cancer, and one maternal cousin had ovarian cancer. In addition, her maternal grandmother had died of breast cancer at age 56. Priscilla also had some blood tests and an additional mammogram. When the results came back, Priscilla learned that she qualified for the trial and she enrolled.

Each day, Priscilla takes two pills and will continue to do so for five years. Because the medications are randomly assigned, she doesn't know whether she's receiving tamoxifen or raloxifene. Every six months, Priscilla has a physical, including a clinical breast exam, and once a year she receives a mammogram, Pap test and blood tests. STAR trial results are expected in 2007.

After a year in the trial, Priscilla is happy with her decision and has yet to experience any side effects from the treatment. Her sister, Hope, also is cancer-free. Both Priscilla and Hope closely monitor their health and lead active lives. Priscilla's advice to other women is to not be afraid to ask about preventive therapy. She urges women to do whatever they can to try to prevent cancer or detect it as early as possible.

Future Directions

It would be great if doctors knew just what to do to prevent breast cancer, but in reality few factors are known to provide strong protection against the disease. The options for women at high risk are fairly limited and far from ideal. But breast cancer prevention is the focus of a wide range of ongoing research. Advances in the understanding of cancer are providing more targets and tools to achieve the ultimate goal of preventing breast cancer.

Chapter 6: Breast Cancer

The Latest on Screening

Until scientists find a way to prevent breast cancer, the best strategy for fighting the disease remains the same — to find it as early as possible. You've likely heard or read this many times, but it bears repeating: The earlier cancer is detected, the better the chance for successful treatment and long-term survival. That's why screening is so important.

The purpose of screening for a particular disease is to identify the condition before it starts producing signs and symptoms and while it's the most receptive to treatment. The makeup of most cancers is such that if a mass of cancerous (malignant) cells is caught early enough, the need for aggressive treatment is reduced and the chance for a cure is increased.

Screening for breast cancer has traditionally been accomplished with three methods:

- Mammography, a procedure in which X-rays are taken of your breasts to detect masses too small to be felt
- Clinical breast examination (CBE), a procedure in which your doctor examines your breasts for lumps or changes
- Breast self-examination (BSE), a procedure in which you examine your own breasts for lumps or changes

Many experts believe that increased awareness and the use of breast cancer screening, particularly mammography, has played an important role in the decrease in deaths caused by breast cancer. Breast cancer death (mortality) rates have been declining every year in the United States since 1989. Between 1995 and 1998, age-adjusted rates decreased more than 3 percent annually.

Current Controversy

Despite a steady decrease in deaths, many details regarding breast cancer screening remain controversial. Largely because of conflicting studies, not all doctors and medical organizations agree on the benefits of today's screening methods, the age at which women should begin screening and how often they should be screened (screening intervals). As a result, there are differences of opinion on when or how often screening should be done, or even if it should be done at all. Much of the controversy centers on mammography screening, although both clinical breast examinations and breast self-examinations have come under scrutiny as well.

Studies to better determine the value of breast cancer screening methods are ongoing, but it may be some time until the results of these studies are known. In the meantime, it's helpful to understand the benefits and limitations of today's screening methods. By being aware of these issues, you may be less anxious when you have your annual physical examination, which often includes a mammogram. In addition, you may be better able to evaluate the significance of various breast cancer studies reported by the media.

A bit of background

For years, conventional thinking has been that postmenopausal women who receive regular mammography screening are less likely to die of breast cancer, because screening helps to detect cancer while it's still in an early stage and more responsive to treatment. But several studies, particularly a Danish study published in 2000, have questioned this. The Danish study evaluated eight previously published mammography trials, which included more than half a million women in the United States and Europe. The researchers claimed that six of the eight studies had serious flaws in their design and execution, and their results couldn't be trusted. The remaining two studies found that mammography screening had no effect on the reduction of breast cancer deaths.

The resulting outcry from the medical community — from men and women who have spent years trying to convince women of the value of regular mammograms — was understandable. The following year, the Danish team did a reanalysis of its controversial study, again coming up with the same conclusions. As a result, the U.S. Preventive Services Task Force (USPSTF), a group of health experts who review published literature and make recommendations about preventive health care, commissioned a review of the mammography studies.

In its review, the task force concluded that the studies in question did have limitations (as all studies do). But, despite these weaknesses, the task force concluded that the studies' results were still valid and that they constituted fair enough evidence that mammography screening reduces breast cancer deaths among women ages 40 to 74.

More recent studies indicate that regular mammography screening does save lives. The results of a large Swedish trial of 210,000 women, published in early 2003, found that regular mammography screening reduced breast cancer deaths in women ages 40 to 69 years by about 45 percent. However, although a 45 percent reduction sounds like a large decline in deaths, the number of lives saved may not be as large as you might think. For example, among women ages 40 to 49, for every 10,000 women screened, only six breast cancer deaths are prevented. The benefit is greater among women ages 50 to 69. In this age group, 40 breast cancer deaths are prevented for every 10,000 women screened.

In addition to mammography, the value of clinical and self breast examination are being questioned. The USPSTF reviewed the latest data regarding the two exams. The task force found no evidence that clinical breast examination (CBE) provides additional benefits to mammography screening. It also found no role for breast self-exams (BSEs) in reducing breast cancer deaths. A large study conducted in Shanghai, China, also failed to show any differences in death rates among women who did breast self-exams versus those who didn't do the exams. The women involved in the Chinese study weren't receiving mammograms or clinical breast exams.

Screening risks

Adding to the controversy, investigators point out that screening has some risks. It's possible that a tumor may be missed during screening — what's known as a false-negative result — leading to a false sense of security. If a woman notices a lump in her breast and a mammogram isn't able to detect the tumor, resulting in a negative or "normal" finding, the woman may be inclined to think "It's nothing," when it may be cancer. On the other hand, screening may detect an abnormality when no cancer is present — a false-positive result — resulting in unnecessary anxiety and testing.

In addition, some cancers detectable with mammography may grow so slowly that they may never pose a threat to life. This can lead to unnecessary tests and procedures, as well as needless fear and anxiety. Follow-up tests and procedures may pose some risk of side effects and can be expensive and time-consuming. Unfortunately, it's not possible to judge which cancers might fit into this category.

Making sense of it all

Breast cancer is a well-publicized disease, and with the media attention given to one study and then to another, it's easy to feel lost in a sea of statistics and opinions. You may find yourself asking, "If these exams aren't that useful, then why do them?"

The truth is, despite their limitations, they do appear to be useful. Current screening methods may not be as good as once thought, but that doesn't mean they aren't beneficial. Many women have

BREAST CANCER

found their cancers by doing self-exams or incidentally while dressing or after being bumped. It's also a fact that doctors do detect breast changes during clinical breast exams. And most research shows that breast cancers found in women who have regular mammograms are more likely to be smaller than those found in women who don't get mammograms.

Screening Recommendations

So, when should you be screened and how often? Most health organizations still support regular breast cancer screening, particularly mammography, and most recommend that women at average risk of breast cancer have their first mammogram at age 40. If you're at high risk of breast cancer, you and your doctor may decide to begin screening tests at an earlier age.

The benefit of mammography increases with age, with the strongest benefit coming after age 50. This occurs partly because your chances of developing breast cancer increase as you get older. In addition, normal breast tissue is generally less dense in postmenopausal women, making cancers easier to detect. However, when breast cancer occurs in younger women, it tends to grow more rapidly. For this reason, most organizations advocate that women between the ages of 40 and 49 also be screened frequently.

The U.S. Preventive Services Task Force recommends mammograms every one to two years for women age 40 and older, as does the Department of Health and Human Services and the National Cancer Institute. The American Cancer Society (ACS) has different recommendations. In May 2003, the ACS released new screening guidelines based on its interpretation of the latest research.

The ACS recommends:
- All women in their 20s and 30s should have a clinical breast exam every three years as part of a general physical examination. Women age 40 and older should have such an exam annually.
- All women age 40 and older should have an annual mammogram for as long as they're in good health.

Are You at High Risk?

Factors that have the most significant effect on breast cancer risk include:
- Older age — beyond 65
- A personal history of breast cancer
- Two or more first-degree relatives — such as your mother or sister — who had breast cancer diagnosed at an early age
- Inherited genetic mutations for breast cancer — such as the BRCA1 and BRCA2 genes

For more information on breast cancer risk factors, see Chapter 4.

Screening guide

The following chart offers an overview of the latest recommendations and where most organizations stand on screening:

Age	Consensus	Recommendation
Women in their 20s and 30s, average risk	General agreement	• Breast self-exam optional. • Clinical breast exam every three years, as part of general physical. • No mammogram.
Women ages 40 to 49, average risk	Some disagreement	• Breast self-exam optional. • Clinical breast exam annually, as part of general physical. • Mammogram every one to two years.
Women ages 50 to 74, average risk	Some disagreement	• Breast self-exam optional. • Clinical breast exam annually, as part of general physical. • Mammogram every one to two years.
Women age 75 and older, average risk	General agreement	• Regular screening as long as an individual is in good health.
Women of all ages, high risk	General agreement	• Breast self-exam recommended. • Clinical breast exam every 6-12 months, as part of general physical. • Mammogram annually. • Talk to your doctor for an individualized program. You may benefit from shorter screening intervals and use of other screening tools, such as ultrasound or MRI.

BREAST CANCER

• Optional use of breast self-exams. It's OK to do them irregularly or not at all.
• Women at high risk of breast cancer consider earlier and more frequent screening and use of other screening tools, such as ultrasound and magnetic resonance imaging (MRI).

These are guidelines. Ultimately, your screening schedule should be determined by you and your doctor, based on evaluation of your personal risk factors.

Breast Self-Examination

For years, doctors and women's health advocacy groups have emphasized the need for regular breast self-examination (BSE) to promote early detection of tumors. However, because recent research has failed to show that regular breast self-examination reduces the number of deaths caused by breast cancer, there's less emphasis on this screening method. Doctors are increasingly taking the stance that if breast self-examination causes you more anxiety than it's worth, it's OK not to do it or to do it only on occasion.

This doesn't mean, though, that self-exams aren't useful. Over the years, many women have detected breast tumors through self-examination or incidentally. This examination method can help identify breast cancer in its earlier stages, before signs and symptoms develop. Because of

this, some organizations continue to support self-exams as part of a comprehensive screening program.

Perhaps more important than adhering to a strict monthly schedule is simply increasing your awareness of your breasts — what they look like and how they feel. If you make a habit of examining them every so often, you'll find it easier over time to notice what's normal for you and what's not. When a new change is detected, seek prompt medical attention.

Fibrocystic Breasts

Many women have lumpy breasts, a condition called fibrocystic breasts or fibrocystic changes. This condition occurs when growth or proliferation of fibrous connective tissue and ducts — in combination with cyst development — causes breasts to feel lumpy. The lumpiness is typically more prominent in the upper-outer region of your breasts.

Fibrocystic breasts may also be associated with variations in hormone levels during your menstrual cycle, sometimes causing painful breasts. Caffeine also can contribute to breast tenderness. Your doctor may recommend that you eliminate caffeine from your diet to relieve breast discomfort. There's no evidence, though, that caffeine increases the risk of breast cancer.

Fibrocystic breasts may be found in approximately half the women in the United States. The condition is more common in women in their 20s and 30s. Having fibrocystic breasts doesn't mean that you're more likely to develop breast cancer, but if your breasts are lumpy, performing breast self-exams can be more challenging. Try to become familiar with what's normal for your breasts. This will help make the detection of new lumps or changes easier.

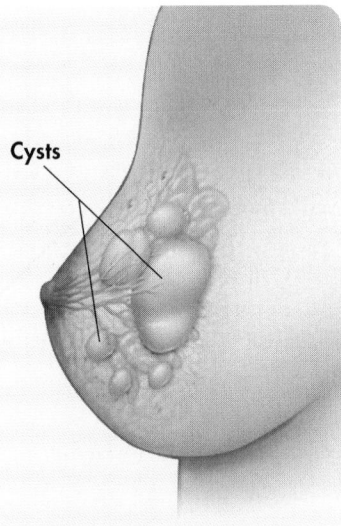

Cysts

Many women have lumpy (fibrocystic) breasts. The condition is most often associated with changes in hormone levels that occur with menstruation.

How to do a breast self-exam

A breast self-exam includes three basic steps:

1. Visual examination in front of a mirror
2. Examination while standing in the shower
3. Examination while lying down

The following tips can help you get the most out of a breast self-exam, but don't obsess so much with technique that you avoid doing it for fear of doing it wrong.

It's also important for premenopausal women to remember that breast tissue changes throughout the month. It responds to changes in hormone levels that occur during the menstrual cycle, causing swelling and engorging of the breasts due to increased blood flow. With your menstrual flow (menses), your breasts return to normal size.

If you're premenopausal, the best time to examine your breasts is about one week after the start of your period. That's when breasts are less likely to be tender or swollen. Women who are pregnant or breast-feeding also should be aware that during these times their breasts are likely to feel more lumpy than normal.

Visual examination

Here are some suggestions to help you view your breasts from different angles. You might want to do a visual exam right before you get in the shower.

- Stand in front of a mirror with arms at your sides, inspecting both breasts carefully. Turn from side to side to view the outer portions of your breasts. If this is your first time, get a good look at them and try to familiarize yourself with their

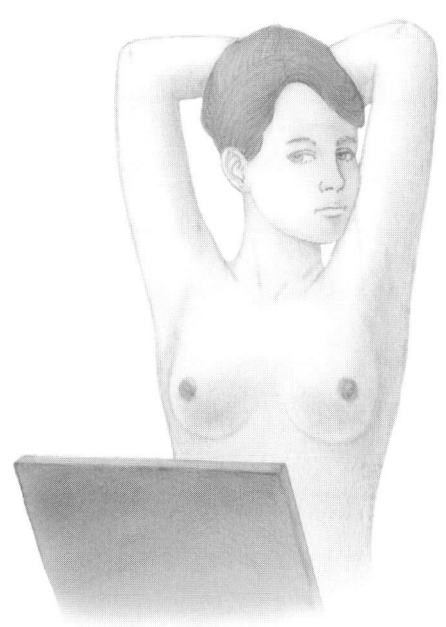

In front of a mirror, visually inspect your breasts for changes in shape and size, dimpling, nipple changes and skin changes, such as discoloration or scaling.

size and shape. During subsequent self-exams, look for changes since the last time you inspected them.

- Rest your palms on your hips. Press down firmly on your hips to flex chest muscles and firm your breasts, and again, turn from side to side.
- Raise both arms above your head and press your palms together to flex your chest muscles and firm your breasts. Again, turn from side to side.

Standing in the shower

It's usually easier to feel (palpate) your breasts for changes when your skin is wet and soapy.

- Use your right hand to examine your left breast. Raise your left arm overhead to allow your breast to lie flat against

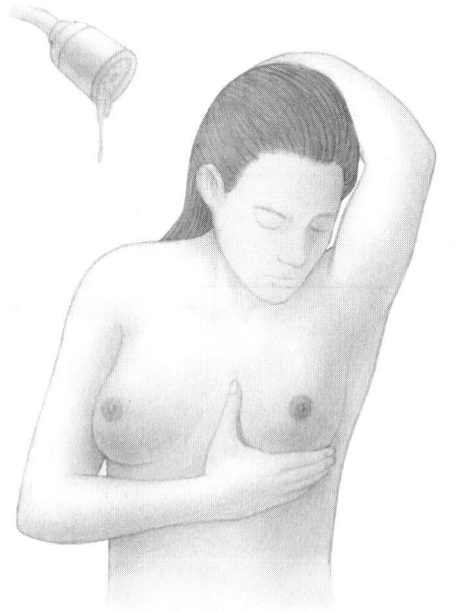

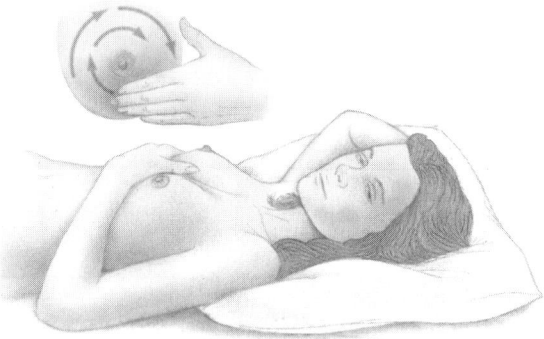

While lying on a flat surface and using the pads of your fingers, move your fingers in a circular fashion around each breast, beginning at the nipple and moving outward.

In the shower, use the pads of your fingers to feel for lumps or thickened tissue in your breasts or under your arms.

your chest, or if you have larger breasts, support your breast with your left hand.

- Use the pads of your fingers instead of your fingertips to examine your breast.
- Move your fingers systematically all over your breast. This can be in a circular, up-and-down line or wedge pattern. Just be sure to feel all your breast tissue. Remember that breast tissue extends up toward the collarbone and under your arm, where lymph nodes are located. Lymph nodes are small nodules that filter foreign substances from your system. A ridge of firm tissue in the lower curve of each breast is normal.
- Check the tissue under the nipple and look for discharge from the nipple.
- Perform a similar exam of your right breast.

- Do this exam the same way every time so that you can notice any changes.

Lying down

Lie down on a flat surface and use the same procedure that you used in the shower, plus these additional guidelines:

- To examine your right breast, place a folded towel under your right shoulder blade. Place your right hand behind your head to distribute the breast tissue more evenly on your chest.
- Repeat the exam on your left breast with the folded towel under your left shoulder blade and your left hand behind your head.
- You may want to use lotion or powder on the pads of your fingers to make the motion easier.

Possible signs of cancer

Some changes to watch for when examining your breasts include lumps, dimpling or thickening in a breast or under the arm; a nipple that's not pointing straight ahead (retracted); redness of breast skin, flaking or redness around a nipple; nipple discharge that's clear or bloody; and breast skin that takes on the appearance of an orange peel (peau d'orange changes). If you notice any changes, bring them to your doctor's attention, even if your mammograms have been normal.

Dimpling

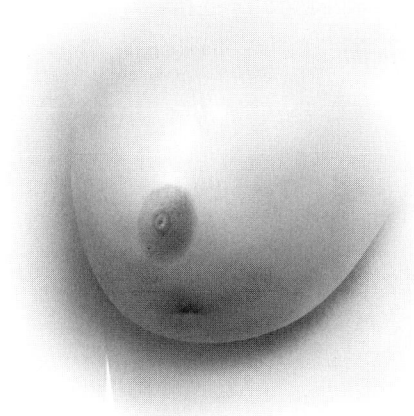

Nipple retraction

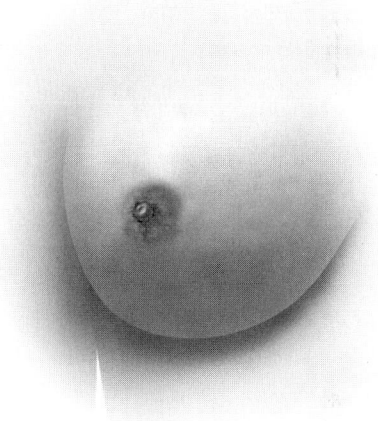

Inflammation

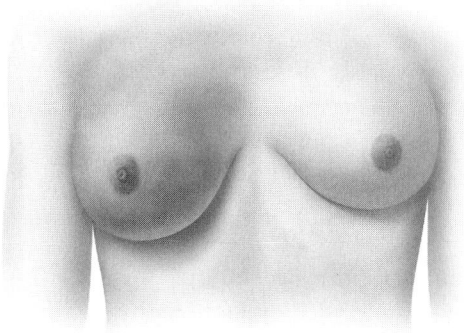

Peau d'orange changes

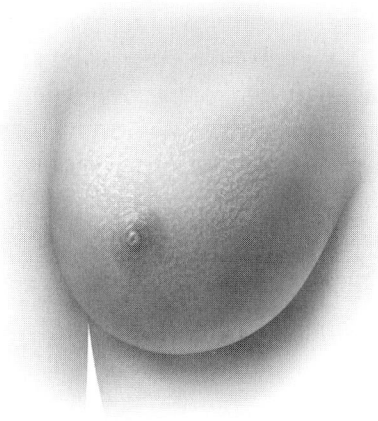

Clinical Breast Examination

A clinical breast examination (CBE) is an inexpensive and noninvasive screening test performed by a health care provider, typically a doctor. During this exam, your doctor visually inspects your breasts for changes in shape, size and appearance and then feels your breasts for lumps or other abnormalities. Your doctor may also examine your armpits (axillae) for enlarged lymph nodes, another indication of possible breast cancer. A clinical breast exam is often performed in conjunction with mammography or as part of an annual physical examination.

In light of recent studies suggesting that clinical breast exams don't reduce breast cancer deaths, some organizations no longer recommend them, though many doctors continue to do them. The American Cancer Society continues to advocate the test, suggesting that women in their 20s and 30s have such an exam every three years and women age 40 and older have the exam annually.

If a clinical breast exam is done shortly before your mammogram, areas within your breasts that feel suspicious during the exam can be targeted for special attention during mammography. If you or your doctor find a suspicious lump, it should be investigated further, even if the mammogram comes back normal. At times, a clinical breast exam can find a cancer that mammography doesn't.

The presence of a lump, however, doesn't mean cancer. The lump may be noncancerous (benign). In addition, normal

Not all lumps can be felt

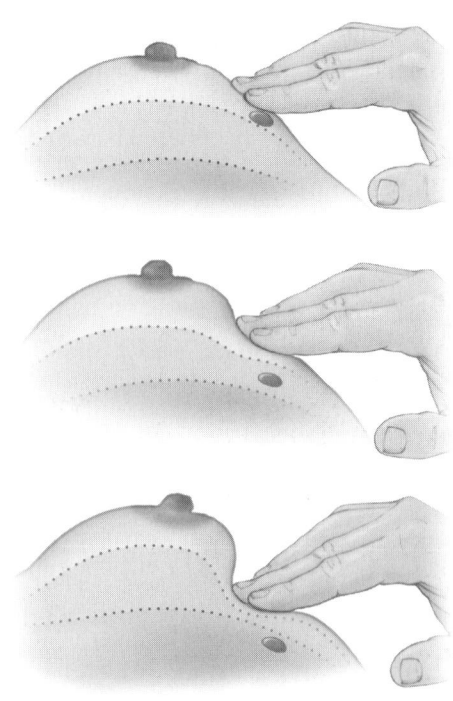

The illustrations above point out how some lumps — those closer to the surface of the breast — can be felt during a self or clinical breast exam, while others — deeper lumps closer to the chest wall — can't be.

breast tissue can feel lumpy. Of lumps that appear to be benign, less than 1 percent actually turn out to be a cancer. Therefore, close observation of such a lump is reasonable.

Mammography

Mammography is generally performed in two situations. It's used to screen for breast cancer and to help make a diagnosis if breast cancer is suspected.

Two mammography views

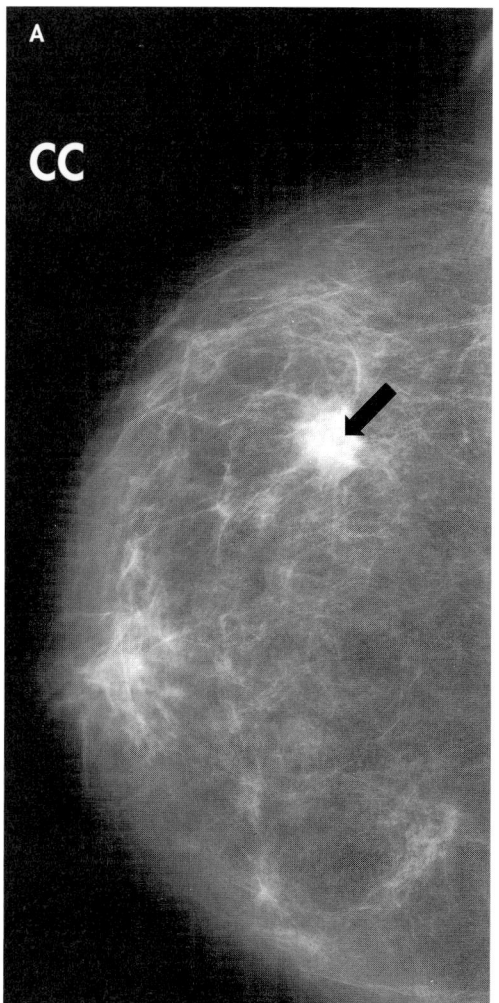

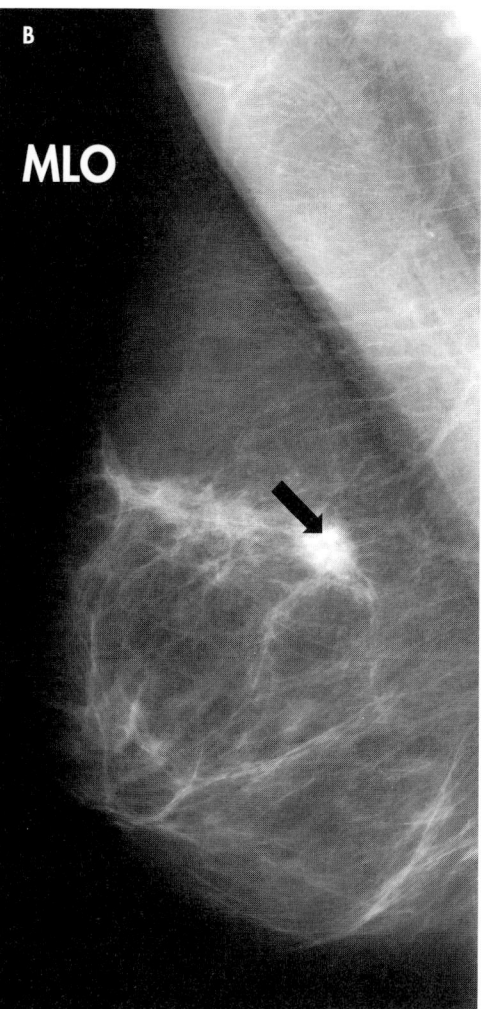

Image A shows an X-ray of the breast taken from above the breast, looking down. This is known as a cranial-caudal (CC) view. Image B shows a side-view X-ray of the breast, taken from the middle of the chest, looking toward the armpit. This is known as a mediolateral-oblique (MLO) view. By putting the two images together, radiologists can determine the location of a tumor. In this case, it's located in the upper-outer portion of the breast.

Screening mammograms

A screening mammogram is a breast X-ray that's taken to look for suspicious masses or breast tissue changes in women who have no signs or symptoms of breast cancer. It usually requires two views of each breast — one from above (cranial-caudal view) and one from an inside angle of the breast (mediolateral-oblique view). For a cranial-caudal view, the X-ray film is placed below the breast, and the X-ray beam is aimed from above the breast down through the breast (see image A on page 111). A mediolateral-oblique view is obtained by having the X-ray film placed to the side, basically under the armpit (see image B). If a tumor or suspicious area is identified, a radiologist can put these two images together to determine its approximate location.

Your first screening mammogram is typically called your baseline mammogram. Radiologists — doctors who specialize in interpreting X-ray images — will compare it with future mammograms to look for changes.

Diagnostic mammograms

A diagnostic mammogram is a breast X-ray used to further investigate breast changes such as a lump, nipple thickening, nipple discharge, and a difference in breast size, shape or overlying skin. It's also used to evaluate abnormal findings on a screening mammogram or to evaluate the breasts of women who have implants, which can obscure signs of disease. A diagnostic mammogram is usually more complex and takes longer than does a screening mammogram. For more information on diagnostic mammograms, see Chapter 7.

Preparing for your mammogram

When scheduling your first screening mammogram, or if you're switching to a new doctor, gather information about your personal and family history of breast

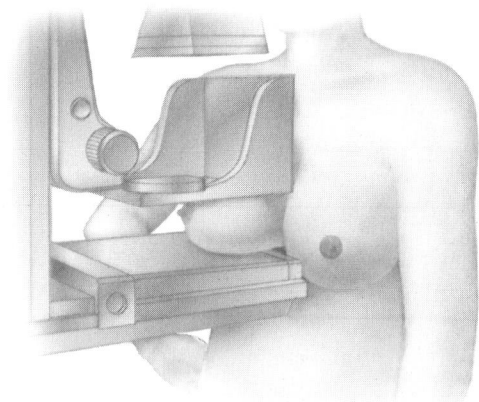

During mammography, your breast is pressed against the X-ray platform by a clear, plastic plate used to spread out the breast tissue. The breast is compressed to even out its thickness and allow X-rays to penetrate and distinguish tissues.

disease. In addition, be prepared to discuss the following:

- Any problems with your breasts
- Past breast biopsies or surgeries
- Whether you have breast implants
- Whether you're pregnant or nursing
- Whether you're taking hormone replacement therapy (HRT) or hormone treatments for a breast disorder
- The timing of your menstrual cycle or when you started menopause

If you've moved or changed doctors and this is the first time you're having a mammogram at a particular facility, bring with you prior mammograms for comparison. Bring the original mammogram films, not copies, plus accompanying reports. This allows the radiologist to make the best possible interpretation.

Because your breasts will be compressed during mammography, avoid testing at times when they may be most tender. This often includes the weeks before and during your period. Usually, your breasts are least tender the week after your period. If you have a history of breast pain (mastalgia) or tenderness, you might consider taking an over-the-counter pain medication about an hour before your mammogram.

You'll likely be given instructions before you come in for the test. Don't apply deodorants, antiperspirants, powders, lotions, creams or perfumes under your arms or on your breasts. Metallic particles in powders and deodorants could be visible on your mammogram and make interpretation difficult.

The day of the test

At the screening facility, you're typically given a gown and asked to remove neck jewelry and clothing from the waist up. For the mammogram itself, you stand in front of an X-ray machine designed for mammography. This machine delivers a lower dose of radiation than do many standard X-ray devices. The technician places one of your breasts on a platform that holds the X-ray film and raises or lowers the platform to match your height. The technician also helps you position your head, arms and torso to allow an unobstructed view of your breast.

Your breast is then gradually pressed against the platform by a clear, plastic plate. Pressure is applied for a few seconds to spread out the breast tissue. The pressure isn't harmful, but it may be uncomfortable, and some women find it painful. If you experience too much discomfort, tell the technician.

Because of the low dose of radiation administered, your breast must be compressed to even out its thickness and permit X-rays to penetrate and distinguish tissues that might hide an abnormality. The pressure also holds your breast still, decreasing the chance of blurring from movement. You'll be asked to stand still and hold your breath during the X-ray exposure.

After the technician has taken pictures of both breasts, you may be asked to wait while the quality of the film is checked. If the views are inadequate for technical reasons, you may have to repeat part of the test. The entire procedure usually takes less than 30 minutes.

A radiologist interprets these images and sends a written report of the findings to your doctor.

Understanding the results

Most women who have a mammogram receive normal results. According to the American Cancer Society, about 10 percent of women who are screened receive results that show an abnormality that requires further testing. Out of these women, only 8 percent to 10 percent end up needing a biopsy, and 70 percent of those biopsies test negative for cancer. In short, only about one or two mammograms out of every 1,000 lead to a diagnosis of cancer.

Abnormalities that may prompt additional tests include:
• Calcium deposits (calcifications) in ducts and other tissues
• Masses
• Distorted tissues

- Dense areas that appear in only one breast
- Dense areas not seen on your last mammogram

Calcifications may be the result of cell secretions, cell debris, inflammation, trauma to the breast, previous radiation therapy or foreign bodies. They're not related to calcium in your diet or calcium from supplements.

There are two types of calcifications. Tiny, irregular deposits called microcalcifications may be associated with cancer. Larger, coarser deposits called macrocalcifications tend to result from benign conditions such as aging, injury and common noncancerous tumors of the female breast (fibroadenomas).

Breast calcifications are common. Many women have at least one breast calcification that can be seen on a mammogram. Most calcifications are benign, but if they appear worrisome, a radiologist may order a diagnostic mammogram that provides magnified views of the suspicious area. If the pattern or appearance of the calcifications remains suspicious after further testing, your doctor may recommend a biopsy.

Dense areas seen on a mammogram may indicate tissue with many glands that make calcifications and masses more difficult to identify, or they may represent cancer. Distorted areas on a mammogram may suggest tumors that have invaded neighboring tissues.

A mammogram alone generally can't prove that an abnormal mass is breast cancer. To determine the cause of an abnormality, additional diagnostic tests are usually necessary.

Limitations of mammography

Mammography isn't foolproof. The accuracy of the procedure depends in part on the quality of the X-rays taken and the experience and skill of the radiologist. If these are inadequate, cancerous growths may be missed. However, even with the best techniques and radiologists, some breast cancers aren't detectable with mammography. The breasts of some women contain more glands and fibrous tissue than those of other women. These features can hide tumors and make interpretation of a mammogram more difficult.

In general, younger women and post-menopausal women taking estrogen have denser breasts than do older women. However, some older women have breasts that appear dense on mammography even without the use of estrogen.

Drawbacks associated with screening mammography include:

- **False-negatives.** *False-negative* is the term for a test result that comes back normal when cancer is actually present. According to the National Cancer Institute, 10 percent to 20 percent of breast cancers are missed during mammography screening. False-negatives are more common in younger women because of higher breast density.
- **False-positives.** A false-positive is an indication that cancer is present when it's not. False-positives are more common in younger women, women who've had previous breast biopsies, women with a family history of breast cancer and women who are taking the hormone estrogen, such as that used in hormone replacement therapy.

Detection can be difficult

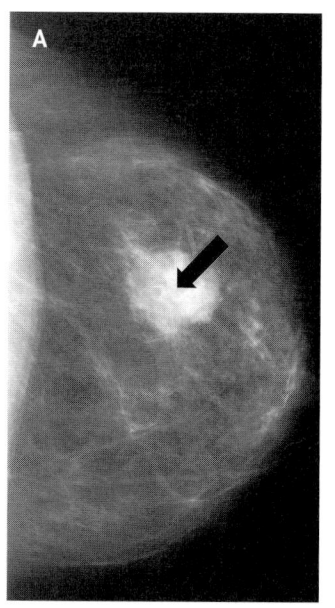

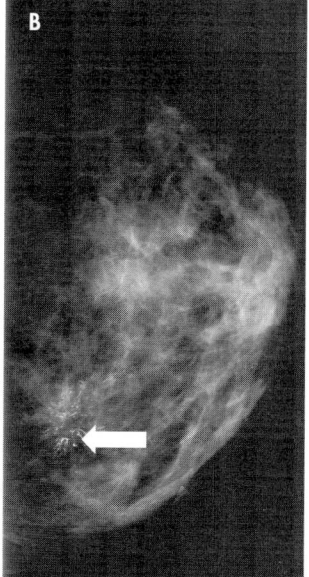

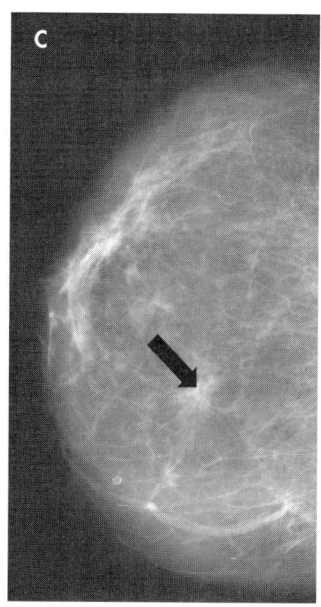

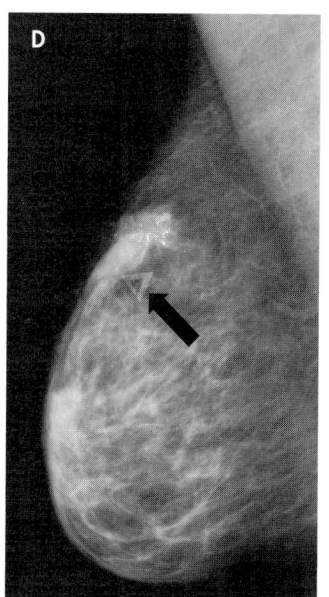

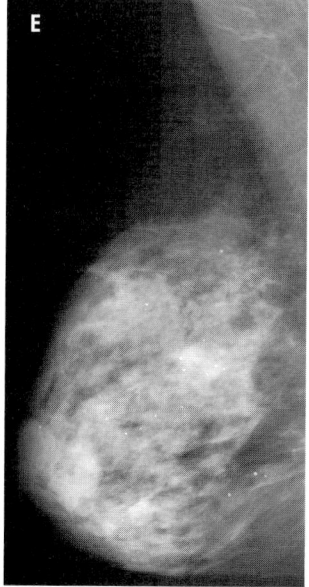

Image A shows a large tumor in a woman with less dense breasts. The tumor is clearly visible. But not all tumors or potentially cancerous lesions are that easy to identify. Image B shows tiny, irregular deposits (microcalcifications) that may be associated with cancer. Image C shows an area of more subtle tissue distortion that may be associated with cancer. Image D comes from a woman with more dense breasts. The triangle is a marker put on the woman's skin, indicating an area where a doctor felt a lump. On the mammogram, the lump isn't easily identifiable. Image E comes from a woman with very dense breasts. In women with dense breasts — typically younger women — tumors and microcalcifications may be difficult to see on mammography.

- **Limited benefit.** Even if a tumor is discovered through mammography, the discovery doesn't always mean that survival is guaranteed. Mammography can detect most tumors that are 5 to 10 millimeters (mm) — about $\frac{1}{4}$ inch — and some as small as 1 mm. But certain types of breast cancer grow very rapidly and are more aggressive in spreading to other parts of the body. Such a cancer may grow and become apparent, in the form of a lump, in between scheduled mammography visits.

Where to get a mammogram

Mammograms may be performed at your doctor's office, in a hospital or in a clinic. Or your doctor may refer you to a mammography facility or an X-ray or imaging center. Mobile units may offer screening even at shopping malls, community centers and offices.

All mammography facilities are required to have Food and Drug Administration (FDA) certification. To be certified by the FDA, a facility must meet strict quality standards set up by the Mammography Quality Standards Act, a federal law designed to ensure the safety and reliability of mammograms. A certificate with an expiration date should be displayed.

To get the best quality mammogram, look for a medical facility that regularly performs mammograms and that has a radiologist dedicated to interpreting them. Experienced technicians and radiologists have been shown to substantially increase the accuracy of mammography results.

New Screening Approaches

Although mammography is currently the best-accepted tool for finding breast cancer in its early stages, experts agree that it's not perfect. An ideal screening tool would be accurate, reliable, inexpensive and readily available to the public.

Alternative breast cancer screening methods being investigated by researchers include:

Ultrasound

Ultrasound is an imaging procedure that uses high-frequency sound waves to display images of the inside of the human body on a screen. To produce the images, sound waves are bounced off body tissues, and the returning waves are measured and recorded. By analyzing a computer image of breast tissue, a doctor may be able to tell if a lump detected on a mammogram or a physical exam is a cyst or solid mass. Cysts, which are sacs of fluid, aren't cancerous, but a solid mass may be.

Ultrasound is most often used to help determine if a lump or suspicious area on a mammogram or clinical exam is solid or fluid-filled. Some researchers suggest that ultrasound may also be helpful in screening women with dense breast tissue, a characteristic that makes abnormalities difficult to see on a mammogram.

But ultrasound isn't a good method for detecting small calcium deposits, which often precede cancer. That's why it's not recommended as a substitute for mammography.

Computer-aided detection

Computer-aided detection (CAD) is a computer technique that gives radiologists an additional tool for interpreting questionable areas found on standard mammograms. After a radiologist reviews a standard mammogram, the film is scanned into a computer. A software program analyzes the image and flags any suspicious-looking lesions. The radiologist then compares the original mammogram with the scanned one to make sure no areas of concern were missed in the initial review.

The Food and Drug Administration approved the first CAD device in 1998. Research indicates that CAD may increase the rate of breast cancer detection by nearly 20 percent, without greatly increasing the number of women called back for more tests. However, not all cancers are detected by CAD.

Magnetic resonance imaging

Magnetic resonance imaging (MRI) uses a magnetic field and radio waves to create a detailed, two-dimensional representation of your body.

Most recently, MRI has been used in breast imaging in conjunction with a contrast material that's injected into a vein just before or during the procedure. The contrast material enhances areas with abnormal blood vessels, like cancers. MRI may also be used to further assess suspicious areas found on a mammogram or to determine cancer spread (staging).

Given its powerful imaging abilities, MRI is being studied as a potential tool for routine breast cancer screening. But there are several obstacles. Although MRI detects some abnormalities that mammography doesn't, it's uncertain how well it distinguishes between what's cancerous and what's not. The procedure picks up some abnormalities that aren't cancerous. MRI is also expensive. Still, preliminary studies indicate that MRI in conjunction with mammography may be useful in screening women at high risk of breast cancer or with very dense breast tissue.

Nuclear medicine studies

Nuclear medicine studies of the breast use tiny amounts of radioactive tracers that are injected into your body, usually by way of a vein in your arm. A special camera detects the tracers in your body and produces images in areas where they've accumulated.

The tracers can help detect cancer because tumors tend to attract more of certain radioactive materials than does normal tissue. Side effects from the procedure are minimal because the radiation dose is very low, and the tracers usually leave your body within a few hours. Two procedures being studied are the technetium sestamibi (Miraluma) scan and positron emission tomography (PET).

Technetium sestamibi scan

During this test, the radioactive agent technetium sestamibi is injected into a vein in your arm. After a few minutes — giving the tracers time to flow through your bloodstream — a special camera records areas of higher absorption in your breasts.

This test may be used to help diagnose breast cancer if your doctor still has questions about an abnormality after diagnostic mammography has been performed. But the procedure isn't very accurate in finding very small abnormalities — less than 1 centimeter (cm) — which makes it less sensitive than mammography for breast cancer screening.

Positron emission tomography

During a positron emission tomography (PET) scan, your doctor injects a small amount of a radioactive tracer, typically a form of blood sugar (glucose), into your body. Most tissues in your body absorb some of this tracer, but tissues that are using more energy — those exhibiting increased metabolic activity — absorb greater amounts. Tumors are often more metabolically active than is healthy tissue and may absorb more of the tracer, which allows the tumors to appear on the scan.

PET scanning might enable doctors to detect cancer in a lymph node before enlargement occurs, allowing for earlier detection and treatment. But like the technetium sestamibi scan, a PET scan isn't considered a reliable tool in the detection of tumors smaller than 1 cm or of slow-growing tumors. Researchers are working to improve the accuracy of this procedure.

Ductoscopy and ductal lavage

Because most breast cancers develop from cells in the milk ducts, researchers are looking for ways to screen the ducts for precancerous or cancerous cells that may not be visible with mammography.

Ductoscopy involves use of an endoscope, a slender tube with a microscopic video camera at its tip. The endoscope is inserted into very small ducts on the nipple, allowing a doctor to see the lining of

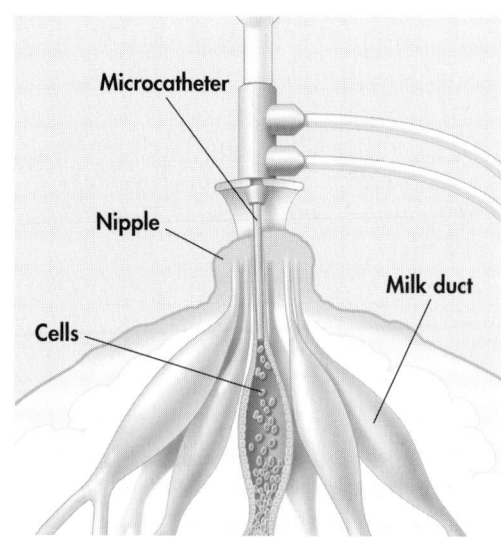

Ductal lavage can detect the presence of abnormal cells in the milk ducts of the breast, the place where most breast cancers begin.

the ducts and to look for precancerous cellular changes.

Ductal lavage is a procedure by which sterile salt water (saline) is injected into a breast duct on a woman's nipple and then withdrawn. The fluid and cells that are withdrawn are examined under a microscope for abnormalities that may indicate cancer.

Both ductal lavage and ductoscopy are still being evaluated as potential screening tools for high-risk women.

Chapter 7: Breast Cancer

Diagnosing Breast Cancer

What happens if you find a lump in your breast or if a mammogram or another test shows an abnormality? Although this may suggest the possibility of cancer, it doesn't automatically mean that you have cancer. It does indicate, though, the need for further tests to determine what the lump or abnormality is. This is called the diagnostic process.

A breast cancer diagnosis is based on a number of factors, including your signs and symptoms, if you have any; examination of your breasts; the results of imaging tests; and, ultimately, the removal and examination of a sample of cells from the abnormal area (biopsy). If cancer is present, other tests are typically done to determine whether the cancer has spread to other parts of your body and to identify certain characteristics of the tumor that may help you and your doctor decide on the type of treatment you should receive.

The diagnostic process may take several days. This is often a time of great uncertainty and emotional stress. Not knowing whether you have cancer can sometimes be worse than knowing that you do. Knowledge allows for action, but uncertainty frequently hinders your ability to formulate a plan, causing anxiety from a fear of the unknown. This is precisely why diagnosis is so important. An accurate diagnosis is key to your plan of action, and getting the diagnosis right often takes more than one test. Waiting for the results can be difficult. It might help to use this time to learn more about breast cancer and how it's treated. This way, if the tests reveal cancer, you have a leg up on what comes next. At the same time, remember that noncancerous (benign) breast conditions are far more common than cancerous (malignant) ones.

Signs and Symptoms

The most common sign of breast cancer is a lump (mass) or thickening in one breast that can be felt (palpated). Often, the lump is painless, but occasionally a tumor may cause pain or tenderness. A lump that's cancerous is usually firm to hard and may have irregular borders, although some cancerous lumps are more soft and rounded. Most tumors develop in the upper-outer portion of your breast, close to your armpit.

A tumor that can be felt (a palpable mass) is most often discovered by a woman herself, either by accident or through breast self-examination (BSE). Sometimes a feeling of discomfort or a blow to a breast may draw attention to a lump. Less often, a lump is discovered by a partner during lovemaking or by a doctor during a routine physical exam.

Typically, signs and symptoms of breast cancer occur in one breast only. In addition to a lump, other signs and symptoms may include:

- Differences in the size and shape of one breast compared with the other.
- A generalized swelling of part of your breast.
- A spontaneous nipple discharge from one breast that's not breast milk. Usually, the discharge is bloody or clear leaning to yellow or green.
- A recent inversion of one of your nipples that can't be turned outward again.
- Thickening or irritation of a nipple that may be accompanied by an itching, burning or sharp, sticking sensation (Paget's disease of the nipple).
- Dimpling, thickening or puckering of the skin of one of your breasts.
- A change in the skin of the breast where it takes on the consistency of an orange peel. You may occasionally hear this referred to by its French name, which is peau d'orange.
- Enlarged lymph nodes in your armpit area, or less commonly, above your collarbone.

In the earliest stages of breast cancer, and even in some of the later stages, there are no signs or symptoms. This is where screening mammography becomes helpful. A mammogram may reveal a lump or abnormality that can't otherwise be visually or palpably detected.

Medical History

If there's any suspicion of breast cancer, the first thing your doctor likely will want to do is get your complete medical history, if he or she doesn't already have it.

Although most women who develop breast cancer don't have a high number of risk factors for the disease, information about your particular risks will help your doctor assess your situation.

Your doctor may wish to gather information regarding:

- Recent changes in your breast or new signs and symptoms
- Previous breast problems or biopsies
- Previous breast cancer diagnosis and the test results that led to it
- Previous hysterectomy, including why you had it done and whether your ovaries were removed
- Your family history of breast and ovarian cancer
- Use of hormone replacement therapy (HRT)
- Use of oral contraceptives
- Your reproductive history, including your age at your first period; age at menopause, if applicable; number of pregnancies and age at first pregnancy; and breast-feeding history

Your doctor may use the Gail model risk assessment described in Chapter 4 or another method for evaluating your risk. He or she may also want to see previous mammograms and ultrasound examinations of your breasts. This may help provide a frame of reference for the current evaluation.

Physical Examination

After gathering as much information as possible about your personal and family medical history, an examination of both of your breasts usually follows. The exam is very similar to your routine clinical breast examination. While you're seated facing your doctor, he or she may visually inspect your breasts, making note of any differences between the two, any scars, skin irritations or other characteristics. Some lumps aren't immediately apparent in a normal seated position, so you may be asked to place your hands on your hips and then raise your arms above your head so that your doctor can see your breasts from different angles. Your doctor may also feel (palpate) your armpits and the area around your collarbone to check for enlarged lymph nodes.

Next, you may be asked to lie down while your doctor feels your breasts, using a similar technique to that used for breast self-examination (see page 108). This way, your doctor can evaluate the size, shape and firmness of any noticeable lumps or masses. Your nipples may also be examined for asymmetry, inversion, irritation and discharge.

If your signs and symptoms are suggestive of cancer — even if prior mammograms have been normal — it's likely your doctor will recommend additional tests. For women age 30 and older, this may be a diagnostic mammogram.

Further testing is often based on the results of the mammogram. If you're under age 30, your doctor may recommend an ultrasound because at a young age the high density of your breasts may prevent a mass from being seen on a mammogram. An ultrasound helps to determine whether a mass is solid or fluid-filled (cystic). If the mass is solid, a biopsy procedure — a fine-needle aspiration or core needle biopsy — may be performed. Breast cancer is rare in younger, average-risk women, so your doctor may also recommend waiting and watching for one or two menstrual cycles to see if the lump persists.

If you don't have any signs or symptoms but your screening mammogram suggests a suspicious abnormality, further testing is typically recommended, usually in the form of a diagnostic mammogram, an ultrasound or a biopsy.

Imaging Tests

The obvious advantage of imaging tests is that they may be able to locate tumors deep within breast tissue that can't be felt. They can also show whether there's more than one suspicious area. Imaging tests may also be used to guide a needle biopsy procedure.

The most common imaging tests used in the diagnosis of breast cancer are diagnostic mammography and ultrasound. Other tests, including magnetic resonance imaging (MRI), positron emission tomography (PET) scans and other radioactive tracer tests, are being investigated for possible use. Presently, these tests are used mainly to check for the spread of cancer to other parts of the body. However, results of various studies suggest that MRI may soon play a greater role in the screening and diagnosis of breast cancer.

Diagnostic mammography

Diagnostic mammography may be used for several purposes — to assess signs and symptoms of breast cancer, to precise-ly locate or further evaluate an abnormality visible on a screening mammogram, and to follow up on women who've had lumpectomies for previous breast cancer.

Like screening mammography, diagnostic mammography consists of X-raying your breast. The test is similar to screening mammography (see Chapter 6), but it may include more views than the standard two done during routine screening. For example, during a diagnostic mammogram, a spot compression view can focus pressure on the breast at the site of the abnormal tissue area (lesion). This spreads out the breast tissue and allows for a better view of the lesion. A magnification view may zoom in on an area to bring out the details of a small mass or clusters of tiny, irregular calcium deposits (microcalcifications).

When you have a diagnostic mammogram, your doctor may mark the site of the lesion on your breast so that the radiologist will know where to focus attention. Your radiologist may also ask you to point out where you've experienced any signs or symptoms. Often, both breasts are X-rayed so that they can be compared for symmetry. Ideally, current mammograms are compared with previous images to look for small changes in breast tissue that may not be apparent on a single mammogram.

Ultrasound imaging is often used to further evaluate a finding, such as a mass, and to determine its characteristics. Benign masses, such as cysts and fibroadenomas, often have a characteristic appearance with ultrasound, and therefore a biopsy may not be needed. Ultrasound is less invasive than is a biopsy.

Interpreting mammography results

The American College of Radiology has developed a system for interpreting mammograms that standardizes the results and provides doctors with consistent terminology with which to write their reports and make uniform recommendations to women. This reduces differences in interpretation and decreases the margin of error. The system is called the Breast Imaging Reporting and Data System (BI-RADS) and is widely used.

The BI-RADS system divides results into the categories listed below:

Category	Description
Category 0: Needs additional imaging evaluation	Category 0 is usually used to describe a screening mammogram in which a possible abnormality has been found. The evaluation is considered incomplete, and more testing is necessary to arrive at a definitive category (1, 2, 3, 4 or 5). Additional testing might include mammography with spot compression, magnification or special views, or ultrasound or another test.
Category 1: Negative	The findings don't appear worrisome. The breasts are symmetrical, and no suspicious abnormalities are present.
Category 2: Noncancerous (benign) finding	This also is a negative mammogram in that no cancer has been found, but your radiologist may wish to describe a cyst, fibroadenoma or other benign characteristic present in the breast.
Category 3: Probably benign finding; short interval follow-up suggested	A finding in this category generally has a high probability of being benign, but your radiologist may feel that it's better to be safe than sorry and recommend a follow-up mammography exam after a specified period of time. This may be four to six months.
Category 4: Suspicious abnormality; biopsy should be considered	A lesion in this category doesn't have the exact characteristics of cancer but has a definite probability of being malignant and, therefore, a biopsy is often recommended.
Category 5: Highly suggestive of being cancerous (malignant); appropriate action should be taken	The lesion that appears on the mammogram has a high probability of being cancerous, and it should be biopsied.

Adapted from the American College of Radiology (ACR) Breast Imaging Reporting and Data System (BI-RADS), third edition, 1998

Signs of cancer on a mammogram include dense masses with irregular borders, suspicious microcalcifications, tissue distortions and asymmetrical breasts. Typically, when a finding falls into category 4 or 5 (see page 123), a biopsy is done.

Ultrasound

Ultrasound technology, also referred to as ultrasonography or sonography, uses sound waves to create images of unseen areas. Ultrasound is used aboard ships to determine ocean depths and aboard fishing vessels to find fish. In the medical field, it's used to create images of structures within your body.

A breast ultrasound works by directing very high-pitched (high-frequency) sound waves at the tissues in your breast. These sound waves bounce off the curves and variations of breast tissue and are visually translated into a pattern of light and dark areas on a screen. The patterns form a visual image of the tissue inside your breast.

During an ultrasound exam, a gel-like substance is applied to the skin over your breast. The gel acts as a conductor for sound waves and helps to eliminate air bubbles between your skin and the transducer. A transducer is a small plastic device that sends out the sound waves and records them as they bounce back. The person performing the exam (ultrasonographer) moves the transducer back and forth over your breast, directing the sound waves into the tissue and capturing the waves' echoes. The returning echoes are digitally converted into black-and-white images on a screen.

A disadvantage of ultrasound is that it can't reliably detect microcalcifications, which commonly accompany cancer. This is one of the main reasons this procedure isn't used for screening. But ultrasound has several important uses in the diagnosis of breast cancer. They include:

- **Evaluating a questionable mammographic finding.** Ultrasound may be used to further evaluate a suspicious abnormality on a mammogram.
- **Distinguishing a cyst from a solid mass.** Cysts are benign sacs filled with fluid. Sound waves pass through fluid more easily than through a solid mass. A cyst, which isn't malignant, generally has a different appearance on an ultrasound image than does a solid mass, which may or may not be malignant. If a definitive diagnosis of a simple cyst is made using ultrasound, usually no further testing is required. If the mass has a complex structure, a fine-needle aspiration may be recommended. If the mass is solid, a biopsy is generally done.
- **Evaluating dense breast tissue.** In younger women, especially women under age 30, breast tissue can be dense. Breast density can obscure masses or abnormalities on a mammogram. In such cases, an ultrasound may provide a clearer image. That's why it's often the tool of choice for evaluating a younger woman with a mass that can be felt. If the mass turns out to be a simple cyst, no further testing is needed. If the mass is solid, a mammogram may be recommended to determine the presence of any calcifications, or a biopsy may be done to determine whether the mass is benign or malignant.

- **Evaluating breasts with implants.** Ultrasound can distinguish between the materials used in implants and breast tissue, making it useful in evaluating women with breast implants who have implant complications or masses that can be felt.
- **Guiding needle biopsy procedures.** Ultrasound may also be used to help guide a needle biopsy procedure by providing an image of the needle as it's being inserted into the breast tissue. The image can help your doctor direct the needle to the appropriate area.

Biopsy Procedures

A biopsy involves removal of a small sample of tissue for analysis in the laboratory. It's generally the only way of knowing for certain that a suspicious lesion is cancer. It's most often recommended after a physical examination and an imaging test have raised the possibility of cancer. Besides identifying cancerous cells, a biopsy can provide important information about the type of cancer you may have and whether it might respond to a form of treatment known as anti-estrogen therapy.

Currently, the three common types of biopsy procedures are fine-needle aspiration biopsy, core needle biopsy and surgical biopsy. Each has its own advantages and disadvantages, and in a given situation, one may be more appropriate than another. The following section describes each one. If you don't understand why you're having one type of biopsy instead of another, ask your doctor to explain his or her recommendation in greater detail.

Fine-needle aspiration biopsy

This is the simplest type of biopsy and is most often used for lumps that can be felt. For the procedure, you lie on a table. A local anesthetic might be used. Sometimes an anesthetic isn't used, though, because it may cause more discomfort than the procedure. While steadying the lump with one hand, a doctor uses the other hand to direct a very fine needle — one more slender than that used to obtain a blood sample — into the lump. The needle is attached to a hollow syringe. Once in place, a sample of cells is collected.

Your doctor may use this type of biopsy as a quick-and-easy method to distinguish between a cyst and a solid mass, and avoid a more invasive biopsy.

- **Cyst.** A cyst typically yields fluid, and your doctor may drain all the fluid. If the fluid is clear and the mass disappears, this is usually a sign of a simple cyst. If cancer is present, which isn't very common when fluid can be withdrawn, the fluid is usually bloody and part of the mass remains. In this case, the fluid is typically sent to a laboratory for examination.
- **Solid mass.** If the mass is solid, your doctor may feel resistance to the needle and no fluid will be retrieved. A sample of cells is then obtained by passing the needle through the mass several times while maintaining suction. The cells collected in the syringe are spread onto one or more slides and sent to a laboratory. A pathologist — an individual who studies tissue samples for signs of disease — will inspect the specimen for the presence of cancer cells. In some cases, a

Needle biopsy

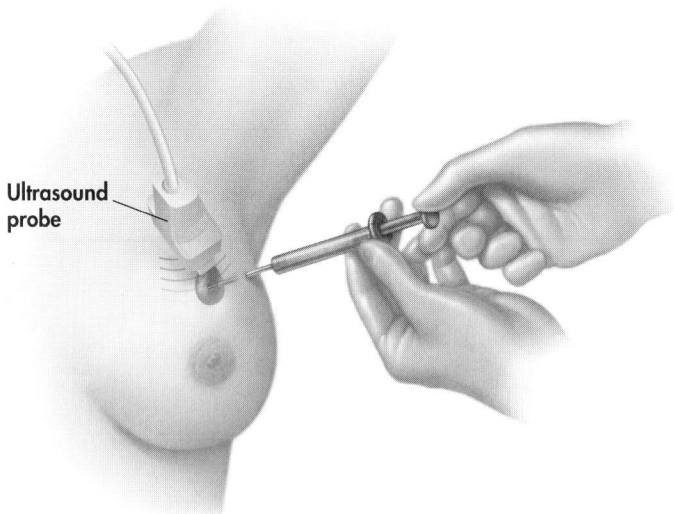

Ultrasound probe

During fine-needle aspiration and core needle biopsy, a needle is inserted into the suspicious mass and tissue is removed for examination. A larger needle is used in core needle biopsy than is used in fine-needle aspiration. In both procedures, ultrasound may be used to guide the needle to the correct location.

pathologist can determine right away whether enough cells have been collected. If not, a repeat biopsy may be performed so that an adequate sample can be collected.

Image guidance

If the mass is hard to feel, your doctor may use ultrasound or mammography imaging to guide the needle to the correct site. With ultrasound, your doctor can watch movement of the needle on the ultrasound monitor. In case of mammography, the procedure is called stereotactic core needle biopsy. Stereotactic methods are usually used with a larger needle biopsy (core needle biopsy), but on occasion they're used with fine-needle aspiration biopsy. Two mammograms are taken

from different angles, and the mass is mapped out by a computer, which then guides the needle to the precise location. This procedure is described in more detail later in this chapter.

Pros and cons

The advantages of fine-needle aspiration biopsy are that it's quick, relatively inexpensive and fairly painless. It can be done in your doctor's office, and you can obtain an immediate report.

One of the biggest potential advantages, or disadvantages, relates to the experience of the person performing the procedure. Studies have shown that experienced staff can produce very accurate results. Fine-needle aspiration biopsies performed by inexperienced staff, though, aren't as reliable. Interpretation of the sample also requires special expertise.

A disadvantage of the procedure is that it may not be able to distinguish between noninvasive (*in situ*) and invasive cancer. As a result, many medical facilities in the United States prefer to use a core needle biopsy, which often can provide more definitive results.

Core needle biopsy

A core needle biopsy may be used on a mass that can't be felt but is visible on a mammogram or ultrasound. A core needle biopsy involves a larger needle than does a fine-needle aspiration, and a small cylinder of tissue (core) rather than just cells is withdrawn from the mass, giving the pathologist more tissue to examine. In most cases, the procedure is performed under the guidance of a radiologist and with imaging equipment. For a lump that can be felt, it may be performed by a surgeon.

A core needle biopsy can provide a definitive diagnosis about 90 percent of the time, thus eliminating the need for a surgical biopsy. A core needle biopsy carries a small risk of infection and bleeding.

Preparation
Before the procedure, tell your doctor if you've been taking aspirin or any blood-thinning medications. These can keep your blood from clotting properly during the procedure and may cause more bleeding. You may be asked to temporarily stop taking the medication. In addition, don't wear deodorant, talcum powder, lotion or perfume the day of the test because they

may interfere with imaging used during the procedure. You may also be asked not to eat for a certain amount of time before the test. Some facilities may request that you wear a bra, to hold an ice pack against your breast after the procedure. An ice pack generally helps to ease pain and swelling.

During the procedure
The process varies depending on the type of procedure you have.

Stereotactic core needle biopsy
With this procedure, you generally lie facedown on a padded biopsy table with one of your breasts positioned in a hole in the table. The table is usually raised several feet, and the radiologist sits below the table. Some facilities use a standing procedure similar to a screening mammogram. Your breast is then firmly compressed between two plates while mammograms are taken to determine the exact location of the lesion for the biopsy. However, it's very important to keep still once your breast has been positioned so that the correct spot is biopsied.

Ultrasound-guided core needle biopsy
During this procedure, you lie on your back on an ultrasound table. You may be asked to raise your arm over your head on the side of the breast to be biopsied. This allows stretching of the soft tissue so that the radiologist can get a better image of the abnormality. The radiologist then locates the mass with an ultrasound probe. Ultrasound guidance may be used if the abnormality can be clearly seen on an ultrasound image.

Needle Biopsy and Magnetic Resonance Imaging

Radiologists at Mayo Clinic and other institutions are studying the ability of magnetic resonance imaging (MRI) to guide needle biopsies. Previously, image guidance of needle biopsies had been limited to mammography and ultrasound. If a tumor was detected on an MRI scan, it would have to be found again on a mammogram or ultrasound before a needle biopsy could be done. In some women, particularly those with dense breast tissue, a lesion found on an MRI might not show up on mammography or ultrasound, leaving surgery (surgical biopsy) as the only option to evaluate the area in question. Use of MRI to guide a needle biopsy streamlines the diagnostic process for many women who otherwise might not be eligible for a needle biopsy.

With both procedures, the site of the needle puncture is usually numbed with a local anesthetic. A small incision, approximately $1/8$ inch to $1/4$ inch, may be made to allow the biopsy needle to be inserted more easily. When the biopsy is taken, you might hear a quick popping sound as the device removes a tissue sample. Several cores of tissue are removed to ensure adequate sampling. Generally, people don't experience too much discomfort with this type of biopsy.

The tissue that's removed is sent to a pathologist for examination. Although the biopsy takes only about 15 minutes, the whole process may take up to 90 minutes.

Occasionally, a tiny, stainless steel clip is inserted in the biopsy site within the breast to mark the spot of the biopsy, in case the area needs to be checked again later. The clip can only be removed surgically and is only visible with special equipment. It can't be felt.

Pros and cons

The advantages of core needle biopsy over fine-needle aspiration biopsy include the ability to distinguish noninvasive (*in situ*) cancer from invasive cancer, greater accuracy in diagnosis and better identification of breast calcifications in the tissue removed. Occasionally, a core needle biopsy may miss a cancer (false-negative result) or, very rarely, lead to a false diagnosis of cancer when, in fact, no cancer is present (false-positive result). The procedure is also more expensive than is fine-needle aspiration. Nonetheless, core needle biopsy has become relatively standard. Individuals — both women and their doctors — like to know if cancer is present before surgery. It allows for better surgical planning, among other reasons.

Surgical biopsy

In some instances, the amount of tissue obtained with a needle biopsy isn't enough, and a surgical biopsy must be performed. Or the suspicious mass is small and palpable, and your doctor may recommend both diagnosing and removing the mass in one procedure. In other situations, it may be determined that a relatively prominent lesion needs to be surgically removed, regardless of the needle biopsy results.

As its name implies, surgical biopsy involves minor surgery, and you likely will be able to leave the hospital on the same day. Surgical biopsy remains the most accurate way of determining if a breast lump is cancerous.

The two types of surgical biopsies are incisional and excisional:

- An incisional biopsy removes a portion of the mass for examination.
- An excisional biopsy removes the whole mass and, if all the cancer cells have been removed, may serve as treatment as well as a diagnostic procedure. A lumpectomy falls into this category.

Preparation

The procedure is usually performed in an operating room with sedation and a local anesthetic or, in some cases, under general anesthesia. Tell your doctor if you're taking blood-thinning medications, including aspirin or other nonsteroidal anti-inflammatory drugs (NSAIDs) or any other medicines or herbal products that affect blood clotting. You may also be asked to not eat for a certain amount of time before the procedure. You'll also want to arrange for someone to drive you home.

Wire localization

If the mass can't be felt (it's nonpalpable), your radiologist may use a technique called wire localization to map the route

Wire localization

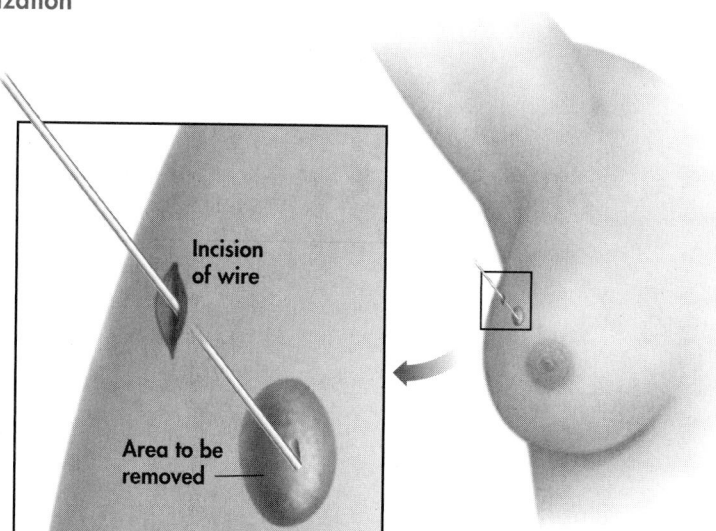

Incision of wire

Area to be removed

In case of a lesion that can't be felt, a tiny wire may be inserted in the breast through a small incision in the skin. With the aid of mammography, the wire is guided through breast tissue until its tip reaches the area in question. The surgeon then has good guidance as to where to remove tissue.

From identification to removal

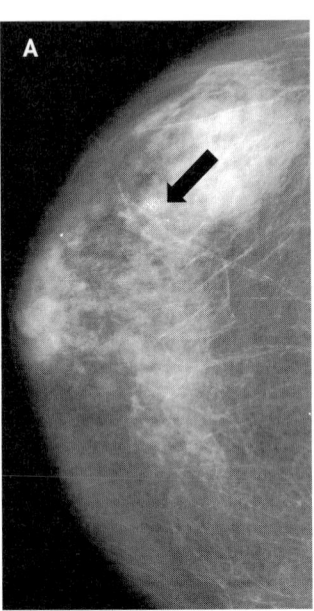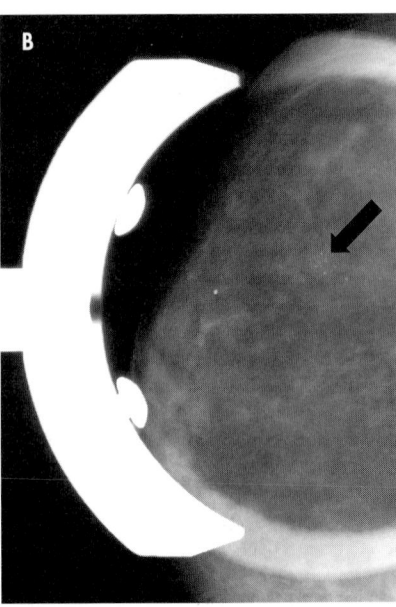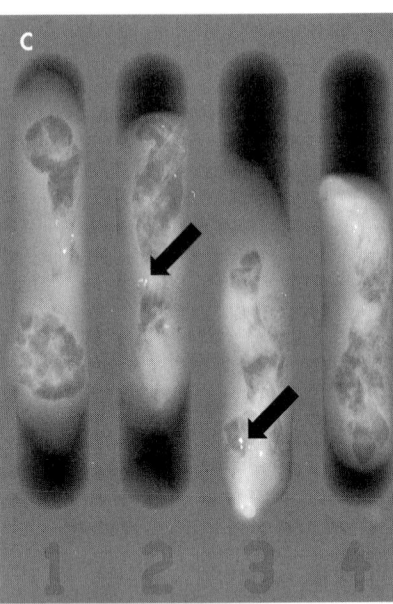

Image A is a screening mammogram indicating possible tiny, irregular deposits, called microcalcifications. Because the microcalcifications aren't easily identified, a magnification view of the area is taken, as illustrated in image B. Here the microcalcifications can be seen more easily. A needle biopsy is then performed (see the illustration on page 126). Tissue samples taken from the area in question may be X-rayed to see if microcalcifications are present

to the mass for the surgeon. This is usually done immediately before surgery. For the procedure, you're positioned for a mammogram, which locates the mass in question on a grid. Then a needle with an attached wire is inserted into your breast at a depth corresponding to the coordinates on the grid. You may be given a local anesthetic beforehand, but sometimes the anesthetic can be more uncomfortable than can insertion of the needle.

The tip of the wire is positioned within the mass or just through it. Two more mammographic views are taken to check the position of the wire. If necessary, the wire can be adjusted. After the correct positioning is obtained, the needle is

removed and the wire is left in place. A hook at the tip of the wire keeps its position secure. Another mammogram is taken of the wire and sent to the operating room. Sometimes, if the lesion is better viewed with ultrasound, the radiologist will use ultrasound instead of mammography to guide insertion of the wire.

The biopsy

Once all preliminary steps are complete, your surgeon carefully examines the diagnostic images to decide on the best surgical approach. During surgery, he or she will attempt to remove the entire mass, along with the wire. The surgeon may

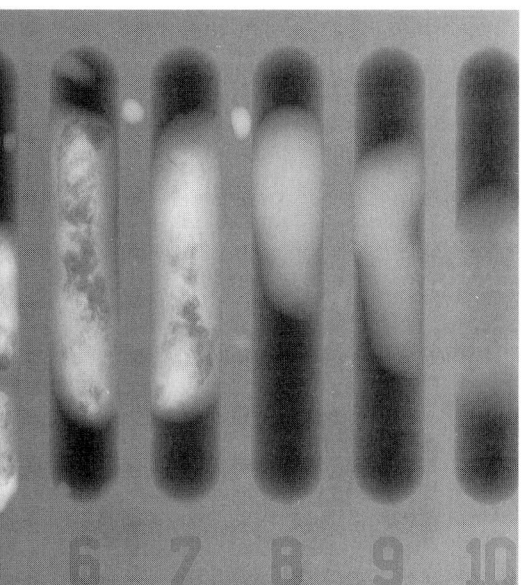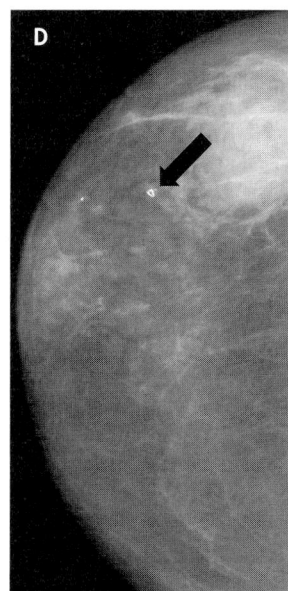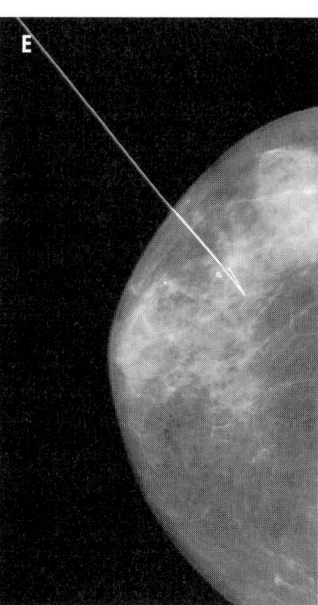

in the samples, as shown in image C. During the biopsy procedure, a small clip is placed in the location where the samples were taken, as shown in image D. Using the clip as a guide, a wire is then placed in the area to direct the surgeon where to remove additional tissue to help make sure all of the microcalcifications have been removed. This is shown in image E.

mark the edges (margins) of the removed tissue (specimen) with sutures to orient the specimen for the pathologist. The specimen's margins may also be marked with ink so that when it's cut open, the pathologist may determine whether cancer cells are at the margins.

The surgeon may have the tissue X-rayed before it goes to the pathologist to help determine if all of the calcifications are included in the sample. If the margins have cancer cells (positive margins), this means that some cancer may still be in the breast and more tissue needs to be removed. If the margins are clear (negative margins), it's more likely that all the cancer has been removed.

Occasionally, only by removing the breast (mastectomy) can the entire area of abnormal tissue be removed.

Risks and aftercare

The risks of surgical biopsy are similar to those of any minor surgery, including bleeding, infection and bruising around the site. You may find it best to take the rest of the day off and relax. For the next five to six days, avoid activities that may cause you discomfort. You may shower or take a bath after the dressing is removed. The dressing is usually removed during a return appointment. If not, you may be able to remove it a day or two after surgery. Minimal drainage is expected the

Q: **Why do I have to have the same test twice?**

A: Findings from different diagnostic tests, such as your physical exam, mammogram and biopsy, may at times disagree. In some of these situations, one or more of the tests may need to be done again, or additional tests may be needed.

For example, if your physical exam reveals a mass that can be felt but a mammogram shows nothing, the mammogram may need to be repeated or another imaging test may be selected. Or if a mammogram indicates suspicious microcalcifications but your biopsy shows no abnormalities, your doctor may recommend a second biopsy to make sure the tissue area in question was actually sampled.

first few days. A small gauze pad inside your bra may help absorb the drainage. A bra also provides support to the incision. Call your doctor if you develop symptoms of infection, such as foul-smelling drainage, increased swelling, redness or tenderness at the incision, or a fever.

Pathology Report

After a pathologist has studied the tissue that was removed, he or she writes up a detailed pathology report containing information about the specimen.

In addition to personal information, the report may list relevant parts of your medical history and any special requests to medical personnel. It also explains the site from where the specimen was taken and gives a description of what the specimen looks like to the naked eye. Its size, color and consistency may be noted. The pathologist should indicate whether cancer cells were present at the edges of the specimen (positive or negative margins) and what the noncancerous tissue looks

like. He or she may also detail how many tissue sections of the specimen were taken for examination.

If cancer is present, a pathologist will outline a number of details about the cancer to help you and your doctor decide on the best type of treatment. These details include the type of cancer present (invasive or noninvasive), histologic type (ductal or lobular), how abnormal the cancer cells appear (tumor grade), whether the tumor cells contain certain proteins called hormone receptors (estrogen and progesterone receptor status), and whether the tumor cells have a surface protein receptor called HER-2/neu.

Type of cancer

By looking at the distribution of cancer cells in the specimen, a pathologist is able to tell if the cancer is invasive (infiltrating) or noninvasive *(in situ)*. Invasive cancer spreads beyond the membrane that lines a breast duct or lobule, into surrounding connective tissue (see page 39). From there it's able to travel (metastasize) to other parts of the body. Noninvasive cancer usually stays in one location, although it can become invasive. Noninvasive cancer has a better projected outcome (prognosis) than does invasive cancer.

Invasive

The most common type of invasive cancer, which accounts for about 75 percent of all invasive breast cancers, is invasive ductal carcinoma. Invasive lobular carcinoma makes up about 15 percent of invasive breast cancers. The remaining 10 percent of invasive cancers are rare types.

Invasive lobular cancers can be particularly hard to detect with mammograms, so they're generally not detected until they're quite large and can be felt.

Some of the rare types of invasive breast cancer include medullary, tubular and mucinous breast cancers. These invasive cancers tend to have a better prognosis than does invasive ductal or lobular carcinoma and may be treated differently from the more common invasive cancers. Another rare cancer called metaplastic cancer can behave more aggressively than invasive ductal cancer.

Noninvasive

Noninvasive cancer (carcinoma *in situ*) is less common than is invasive breast cancer. Ductal carcinoma *in situ* (DCIS), the most common type of noninvasive breast cancer, appears to be confined to the breast's duct system, and it doesn't invade the breast's connective tissue. Lobular carcinoma *in situ* (LCIS) begins in the lobules instead of the ducts. Most breast cancer specialists don't consider LCIS to be a true breast cancer. But

women with this diagnosis have an increased risk of developing future invasive cancer in either breast, not just the breast containing the LCIS.

With appropriate treatment and follow-up, both of these noninvasive conditions carry an excellent prognosis.

Tumor grade

In addition to determining what type of cancer is present, a pathologist also assigns a grade to the cancer. The grade is based on how normal or abnormal the cells appear when examined under a microscope. Generally, the lower the grade, the fewer the abnormalities and the better the prognosis.

Pathologists often use a grading system called the Scarff-Bloom-Richardson system, or some variation of this system, for grading invasive breast cancers. One variation that may be used is called the Elston-Ellis modification.

In medical terms, the grade refers to the appearance of the cancer. The grade a cancer receives is based on three features of the tumor: tubule formation, nuclear grade and mitotic activity. Each of these features is given a score of 1 to 3.

- **Tubule formation.** Normal breast ducts are shaped like small tubes (tubules). Cancer cells tend to become more and more distorted as the cancer progresses. A specimen that contains more than 75 percent normal cellular tubular structures is given a score of 1. A tubular composition of 10 percent to 75 percent represents a score of 2. If less than 10 percent of cells have a tubular form, the score is 3.

- **Nuclear grade.** The nuclear grade reflects how the nucleus of each cell appears. The nucleus of a normal cell has a regular structure, and the cells are small and uniform (well-differentiated). The more aggressive a cancer is, the greater the variation in size and structure of the cancer cells' nuclei (poorly differentiated). A score of 1 for nuclear grade implies a close resemblance to a normal nucleus, 2 represents a moderate increase in size and variability, and 3 represents marked variation between normal and cancerous cells.
- **Mitotic activity.** Mitosis is the process of cell division. The score for mitotic activity indicates how many of the cancer cells are dividing. To obtain this score, a pathologist counts the number of cells undergoing mitosis compared with the number of cells observed. A score of 1 implies slow growth, a score of 2 implies intermediate growth and a score of 3 implies fast growth.

The scores of each of the three measurements are added together to obtain an overall tumor grade, giving a possible total of 3 to 9 points. A total score of 3, 4 or 5 is classified as grade 1 (low-grade or well-differentiated), a total score of 6 or 7 is grade 2 (intermediate-grade or moderately differentiated), and a total score of 8 or 9 is grade 3 (high-grade or poorly differentiated). Grade 1 implies the cells still look fairly normal, and the mass doesn't appear to be growing too fast. If the specimen is a grade 3, the cells have lost their proper structure and function, or they're dividing rapidly, or both. Grade 2 cancers aren't as normal in appearance as grade 1, but they aren't as abnormal as grade 3.

Hormone receptor status

Scientists have discovered that two female hormones, estrogen and progesterone, affect the growth of most breast cancers. One of the tests that's often performed on a biopsy specimen is a hormone receptor test. A receptor is a cell protein that binds to specific chemicals, drugs or hormones traveling through the bloodstream.

Normal breast cells have receptors that bind with estrogen and progesterone. When bound to the receptors, the hormones interact with appropriate genes, helping to promote breast development during puberty and prepare breasts during pregnancy. Some breast cancer cells also have these hormone receptors.

If a pathologist detects estrogen receptors (ER) or progesterone receptors (PR) on the cancer cells, he or she will report the tumor cells as ER positive or PR positive, respectively, or both. If no ER or PR receptors are detected, the tumor is reported as ER negative or PR negative, respectively, or both.

The good news about being ER positive or PR positive is that you may benefit from hormone therapy, which consists of medications designed to interfere with the growth of these cancers. Hormone receptor positive cancers typically grow more slowly than do hormone receptor negative cancers.

HER-2/neu status

Human epidermal growth factor receptor 2 (HER-2/neu) is a protein receptor that's produced by the HER-2/neu gene. Normally, substances that attach to this receptor stimulate cell growth. When too many of these receptors are present, they can cause cell growth that becomes out of control. About 20 percent to 25 percent of breast cancers have an excess of the HER-2/neu protein.

There are two ways to test for HER-2/neu receptors: One is by a technique called immunohistochemistry (protein overexpression) and the other is by a method called fluorescent *in situ* hybridization (FISH), also known as gene amplification.

- **Immunohistochemistry tests.** These tests, which were developed first and are less expensive than are FISH tests, are generally done first. They use certain easily identifiable antibodies that bind to HER-2/neu to measure the number of receptors on a cancer cell surface. Scores range from 0 to 3+. A score of 0 or 1+ is considered negative, which means the tumor cells don't have an excess of HER-2/neu receptors. A score of 3+ indicates the tumor cells are overexpressing HER-2/neu protein, and is considered positive. A 2+ score is considered borderline.
- **FISH test.** For 2+ immunohistochemistry results, a doctor may recommend a FISH test to confirm whether the HER-2/neu gene is overamplified (positive). FISH uses fluorescent DNA markers to find extra copies of the HER-2/neu gene. The results are generally reported as being either positive or negative. Some facilities are now using FISH testing first and eliminating the use of immunohistochemistry tests.

In some situations, knowing that your cancer cells contain too much HER-2/neu

can be important information that can help determine the treatment you receive. The drug trastuzumab (Herceptin), for example, is a specific antibody that binds to HER-2/neu, shutting it down and, thereby, reducing the growth rate of the cancer (see Chapter 3).

Staging

Once a doctor knows cancer is present, he or she also wants to know if the cancer is confined to the breast or has spread to other areas. This knowledge is obtained through a process called staging. Staging is another aspect of diagnosis that's essential to determining the best form of treatment. It's also the most significant factor in predicting your prognosis.

Staging tests

Several additional tests may be needed as your doctor determines the stage of your cancer, including blood tests, a chest X-ray, bone scan, magnetic resonance image (MRI), computerized tomography (CT) scan and positron emission tomography (PET) scan. It's important to note, though, that most women receiving a diagnosis of breast cancer don't need all of these tests. This is partly because the tests have limited usefulness and partly because the chances that the cancer has spread beyond the breast and lymph nodes are low.

Blood tests

A complete blood count (CBC) can help your doctor assess your general health. A CBC measures:

- Red blood cells, which carry oxygen
- White blood cells, which help fight infections
- Platelets, cells that help your blood to clot when you bleed

A blood chemistry test measures the level of substances that indicate whether your organs, such as your kidneys and liver, are functioning correctly.

Abnormal levels of certain substances in your blood, called tumor markers, might suggest the presence of cancer. But unless other evidence suggests your cancer has spread to distant parts of your body — which occurs in only 5 percent to 10 percent of women when they're initially diagnosed — tests for these markers generally aren't used because they don't provide much useful information at this point. In addition, no one tumor marker is specific for breast cancer.

Chest X-ray

Your doctor may recommend a chest X-ray to check for any evidence that the cancer has spread to your lungs. If your tumor is very small and the cancer cells haven't spread to your lymph nodes, a chest X-ray may not be necessary.

Bone scan

A bone scan is used to check for spread of the cancer to your bones. The test usually isn't done unless other evidence indicates possible spread, such as pain in your bones or abnormal blood tests.

During the test, you receive an injection that contains a tiny amount of a radioactive tracer. The tracer is drawn to cells involved in bone remodeling. Throughout a person's lifetime, bone tissue is continu-

Diagnostic Basics

Most women with a new diagnosis of breast cancer don't need to undergo all the diagnostic tests available. The following examinations and tests — in addition to a biopsy of the tumor or suspicious area — are often all that's necessary to determine the stage of the cancer:
- Medical history
- Physical examination
- Mammogram
- Chest X-ray
- Blood tests

ously removed and replaced by new bone tissue, a process called remodeling. When cancer cells spread to bone, remodeling typically increases. A special camera scans your body and records whether the tracer has accumulated in certain areas (hot spots). A hot spot may indicate that cancer has spread to your bones, but it could also indicate infection or arthritis, another cause of increased bone remodeling.

Computerized tomography scan

Computerized tomography (CT) is an X-ray technique that produces more-detailed images of your internal organs than do conventional X-ray studies.

The procedure involves an X-ray tube that rotates around your body and a large computer to create cross-sectional, two-dimensional images (slices) of the inside of your body. When these images are combined, a doctor may be able to see tumors, measure them and later biopsy them if necessary. This test is generally only used if your doctor suspects the cancer has spread.

Magnetic resonance image

Like computerized tomography, a magnetic resonance image (MRI) also views the inside of your body in cross-sectional slices, but it uses an extremely strong magnet instead of X-rays. The magnet manipulates water molecules in your body so that they tumble, which produces a faint signal. A sensitive receiver — similar to a radio antenna — picks up those signals. A computer used to generate the pictures manipulates the resulting signal.

Depending on their chemical makeup, different tissues produce stronger or weaker signals. This allows a doctor to differentiate a tumor from normal tissue. In some cases, MRI can be a more sensitive test than can a CT scan. Typically, though, this test isn't necessary to stage breast cancer.

Positron emission tomography scan

Positron emission tomography (PET) is different from a CT or MRI scan in that it records tissue activity rather than tissue structure. As opposed to normal cells, cancer cells often exhibit increased metabolic activity. During a PET scan, your doctor injects a small amount of a radioactive tracer — typically a form of blood sugar (glucose) — into your body. Most tissues in your body absorb some of this tracer, but tissues that are using more energy — exhibiting increased metabolic activity — absorb greater amounts. Tumors are usually more metabolically active and tend to absorb more of the

sugar tracer, which allows the tumors to light up on the scan.

Your doctor may recommend a PET scan if he or she suspects the cancer has spread but is uncertain of the location to which it has spread.

Staging classification

After the biopsy and any additional tests are complete, your doctor or team of doctors gathers all the information provided to determine the stage of your cancer. The most commonly used method of doing this is the TNM staging system created by the American Joint Committee on Cancer. This system addresses three key issues:

- **T (tumor).** How big is the tumor, and has it spread to the skin or to chest wall muscle?
- **N (node).** Have cancer cells spread to nearby lymph nodes?
- **M (metastasis).** Has the cancer spread to other, distant areas of the body?

Numbers are assigned to each of these categories, indicating the degree to which the tumor has grown or spread. *T* receives a number from 0 to 4, indicating the size of the tumor and if it has spread to the skin or chest wall. *N* receives a number from 0 to 3, indicating the degree of spread to the lymph nodes and how many lymph nodes are involved. *M* is rated either 0 or 1, indicating no spread or spread, respectively, to distant parts of the body.

A higher number indicates a larger tumor or more advanced spread of the cancer. More detailed notations also may be assigned to these categories, such as to indicate whether the cancer is *in situ*

Summary of Staging Definitions*

Primary tumor status

Tis: Carcinoma *in situ*

T0: No primary tumor evidence

T1: ≤ 2 cm of invasive cancer

T2: 2.1-5 cm of invasive cancer

T3: > 5 cm of invasive cancer

T4: Direct extension to the chest wall, or skin ulceration, or skin nodules, or inflammatory breast cancer

Regional lymph node status

N0: None involved

N1: 1-3 involved axillary nodes, or microscopically involved internal mammary node detected by sentinel node biopsy procedure

N2: 4-9 involved axillary nodes *or* clinically apparent internal mammary nodes

N3: ≥ 10 involved axillary nodes, or infraclavicular node, or supraclavicular node, or axillary nodes *and* internal mammary nodes

Metastasis

M0: No distant metastasis

M1: Distant metastasis

*More detailed definitions can be found at S.E. Singletary, et al., "Revision of the American Committee on Cancer Staging System for Breast Cancer," *Journal of Clinical Oncology*, 20:17 (2002), pages 3628-3636

(as opposed to invasive), or a lowercase letter after the number to signify a subcategory. For example, a T1c, N0, M0 classification means that the tumor is more than 1 centimeter (cm) in size but less than 2 cm, it hasn't spread to the lymph nodes, and it hasn't metastasized. These classifications may be modified after surgery when the pathologic data are complete.

Once the TNM classification is made, your doctor can determine the stage of your cancer, which usually is labeled as a Roman numeral. A lower number indicates that the cancer is still in its early stages, and a higher number means a more advanced, serious cancer. The T1c, N0, M0 tumor described above would be a stage I tumor.

Stages 0 to IV

Breast cancer staging is complicated and constantly changing as doctors learn more about breast cancer, its spread and how it responds to treatment.

The accompanying chart lists the latest stage groupings for breast cancer. Your doctor can identify for you which designation describes your cancer. Following is some general information about the stages of breast cancer.

Stage 0

This is very early *(in situ)* breast cancer that hasn't spread within the breast or to other parts of the body.

Stage I

This stage refers to breast cancer that's 2 centimeters (cm) or less — smaller than an inch — in size with no lymph node involvement.

Stage II

Stage II is subdivided into IIA and IIB. Stage II cancer is more extensive than stage I, but not as extensive as stage III. A cancer 5 cm or less — about 2 inches or less — that has spread to the lymph nodes would fall into this category.

Stage III

Stage III breast cancers are subdivided into three classifications: IIIA, IIIB and IIIC. Stage III cancers include a number of criteria that make this a broad category. Stage III cancers are sometimes referred to as local-regionally advanced cancers. One of the main criteria with stage III cancers is that there's no evidence the cancer has spread (metastasized) to distant sites.

Stage IV

In stage IV, the cancer has spread to other, distant parts of the body, such as the lungs, liver, bones or brain.

Ideally, staging is done after examination of tissue specimens (pathologic material) obtained during surgery. This is called pathologic staging. Staging can be attempted before pathologic examination.

Breast cancer stage grouping

Stage	T	N	M
Stage 0	Tis	N0	M0
Stage I	T1	N0	M0
Stage IIA	T0	N1	M0
	T1	N1	M0
	T2	N0	M0
Stage IIB	T2	N1	M0
	T3	N0	M0
Stage IIIA	T0	N2	M0
	T1	N2	M0
	T2	N2	M0
	T3	N1	M0
	T3	N2	M0
Stage IIIB	T4	N0	M0
	T4	N1	M0
	T4	N2	M0
Stage IIIC	Any T	N3	M0
Stage IV	Any T	Any N	M1

Source: American Joint Committee on Cancer, 2002

Tis: Indicates noninvasive *(in situ)* cancer
T 0-4: Refers to tumor size and spread
N 0-3: Indicates degree of spread to the lymph nodes
M 0-1: Indicates spread to distant parts of the body

This method, termed clinical staging, is less accurate.

Estimating survival

Based on statistics assembled from other women's experiences, scientists are able to estimate how many women might survive for at least five years after a diagnosis of breast cancer. This is commonly known as the five-year survival rate. Specifically, it refers to the percentage of women who are still alive five years after their cancers were diagnosed.

This doesn't mean that survivors live for only five years after being diagnosed with cancer. In fact, most cancer survivors live much longer. On the other hand, it doesn't mean that women living for five years after breast cancer are cured. Of all women who experience a breast cancer recurrence, less than half of the time does the recurrence happen in the first five years.

Advances in early detection and treatment have increased survival periods, and today women diagnosed with breast cancer are living longer than did women diagnosed 20 or 30 years ago.

A study published in 2002 concluded that standard long-term survival rates for most cancers were overly pessimistic. It also estimated that, in more recent years, these rates have improved substantially. For example, the standard 20-year survival rate generally quoted for breast cancer is just over 51 percent. According to the study's authors, the 20-year survival rate is now more likely to be 65 percent.

Finally, remember that statistics don't tell the whole story. They only serve to give a general picture and a standard format for doctors to discuss prognosis. Every woman's situation is unique. If you have questions about your own prognosis, discuss them with your doctor or cancer care team. They will help you find out how these statistics relate, or don't relate, to you.

More information on breast cancer prognosis is provided in later chapters.

Chapter 8: Breast Cancer

Precancerous Conditions & Noninvasive Cancer

Sometimes, when doctors look for cancer, they don't find it, but they find a condition that may lead to cancer. For example, when a pathologist examines breast tissue removed during a biopsy, he or she may find abnormalities that don't meet the criteria for invasive cancer but that signal an increased risk of developing invasive breast cancer in the future.

One such breast abnormality is a condition called hyperplasia, in which too many cells line the wall of a milk duct or lobule. If the extra cells begin to take on a strange-looking appearance, the condition is known as atypical hyperplasia. Atypical hyperplasia is generally thought of as a precancerous condition — it isn't cancer but it can be a forerunner to its development.

As the cells keep multiplying and become more abnormal, the condition becomes known as carcinoma *in situ* or noninvasive cancer (see the illustration on page 20). The abnormal cells have reached the point where they're now considered cancerous, but they remain confined within the duct. They haven't broken through the duct wall to invade connective tissue within the breast, which contains blood vessels and lymph channels. Another commonly used term for carcinoma *in situ* is *stage 0 cancer*. Approximately 20 percent to 30 percent of breast cancers diagnosed in the United States each year are noninvasive.

The two main noninvasive breast cancers are lobular carcinoma *in situ* (LCIS), which occurs in the milk-producing glands (lobules), and ductal carcinoma *in situ* (DCIS), which occurs in the breast ducts. It's important to note that while LCIS is called a carcinoma, which means cancer, the exact nature of this condition is still being determined. Presently, most doctors don't consider it a true cancer.

Researchers still have many unanswered questions about these conditions. For instance, it's not clear if some precancerous conditions are actual precursors to cancer or if they're just cancer markers, indicating an increased risk — but not the certainty — of future breast cancer. And studies have yet to confirm which women with DCIS may be at greatest risk of invasive cancer or recurrent DCIS and benefit from more aggressive treatment.

In general, precancerous conditions and noninvasive cancer aren't life-threatening. With appropriate therapy and monitoring they have a very good outcome. Treatment for these conditions varies a bit from that of invasive breast cancers, although many of the same procedures are used.

Atypical Hyperplasia

Atypical hyperplasia of the breast may be diagnosed after a biopsy to evaluate a suspicious spot on a mammogram. It can take two forms — atypical ductal hyperplasia and atypical lobular hyperplasia — depending on the location of the abnormal cells. These conditions aren't considered cancerous, but they do represent an increased risk of breast cancer, and they may be associated with the presence of a cancerous growth elsewhere in the breast. A woman with either atypical ductal hyperplasia or atypical lobular hyperplasia has about a fourfold increased risk of eventually developing breast cancer, compared with a woman who doesn't have either condition.

Atypical hyperplasia of the breast is generally treated with surgery to remove the abnormal cells to prevent them from turning cancerous. After surgery, your doctor may want to talk with you about other ways of trying to lower your risk of cancer developing. Chapter 5 has more information on these methods for women considered at high risk of the disease.

Lobular Carcinoma *In Situ*

Lobular carcinoma *in situ* (LCIS) occurs within the lobules located at the end of the breast ducts. It's most often diagnosed in premenopausal women and found incidentally as a result of biopsies done for other reasons. LCIS is less likely than is DCIS to show up on mammograms.

Over the years, most cancer experts haven't considered LCIS to be cancer in and of itself. Rather, they've viewed it as an area of abnormal tissue growth that signals an increased risk of developing invasive breast cancer later on. The increased risk applies not just to the breast where the LCIS occurred but to both breasts.

Investigators continue to explore whether in some situations LCIS may actually be a preinvasive cancer, just like ductal carcinoma *in situ*. At this time, though, LCIS is still most often viewed as a marker that predicts an increased risk of breast cancer in both breasts, as opposed to a preinvasive cancer.

Statistics suggest that women with LCIS have a 25 percent lifetime risk of developing invasive breast cancer in either breast.

Treatment options

A number of factors are weighed in the treatment decision-making process, one of the most important being personal choice.

Given the relatively low likelihood of developing invasive breast cancer in the first five years after receiving a diagnosis, some women with LCIS choose not to do anything other than closely monitoring their breasts with yearly screening mammograms, monthly breast self-examinations and regular clinical breast exams.

This approach works best in women who have breasts that are relatively easy to examine by clinical examination and mammography, as opposed to women who have lumpy breasts or women whose breast tissue appears very dense on mammograms.

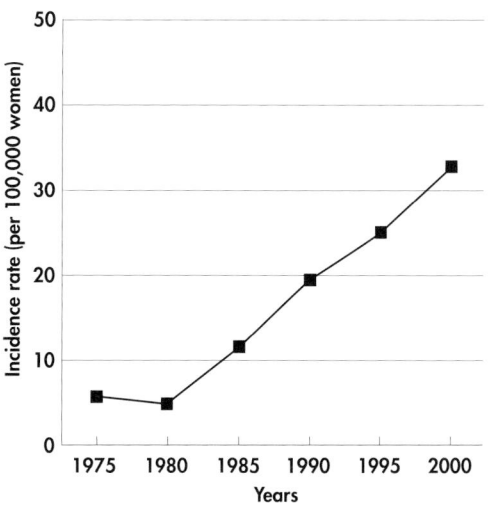

Increased diagnoses of noninvasive cancer over the years

The rate at which noninvasive (carcinoma *in situ*) breast cancers are diagnosed has increased sharply in the last two decades, due to increased use of screening mammography.

Source: "SEER Cancer Statistics Review, 1975-2000," National Cancer Institute, 2003

Cancer prevention strategies

Because of the increased risk of developing invasive breast cancer, it's also reasonable for women diagnosed with LCIS to consider cancer risk reduction (prevention) strategies.

Options include surgically removing both breasts (bilateral prophylactic mastectomy) or cancer-preventing (chemoprevention) medications, such as tamoxifen (Nolvadex). A large study evaluating the chemoprevention properties of tamoxifen found that the drug can help reduce a woman's risk of invasive breast cancer. Among both pre- and postmenopausal

BREAST CANCER

women with LCIS who took tamoxifen, their risk of invasive breast cancer was reduced by 56 percent over five years.

To learn more about breast cancer prevention strategies, see Chapter 5.

Ductal Carcinoma In Situ

Ductal carcinoma *in situ* (DCIS) is the most common type of noninvasive breast cancer, accounting for approximately 85 percent of all diagnoses of carcinoma *in situ* of the breast. In the United States in 2003, about 55,000 women were diagnosed with DCIS.

Other terms used to describe this condition include *intraductal carcinoma* or *noninfiltrating carcinoma*. Unlike lobular carcinoma *in situ* (LCIS), this noninvasive cancer is more likely to develop into invasive cancer if left untreated.

Ductal carcinoma *in situ* is usually found during mammogram screenings, but it can be difficult to detect. On mammograms, DCIS is often characterized by the presence of tiny groups of calcium deposits called microcalcifications. Because of increased mammography screening, the rate at which DCIS is diagnosed has increased dramatically in recent years. In some cases, a mass can actually be felt (palpated).

DCIS is typically diagnosed either with a core needle biopsy, a procedure that uses a needle to remove a small sample of tissue for examination, or by way of an open excisional biopsy, which involves a small surgical incision to remove a tissue

Ductal carcinoma *in situ*

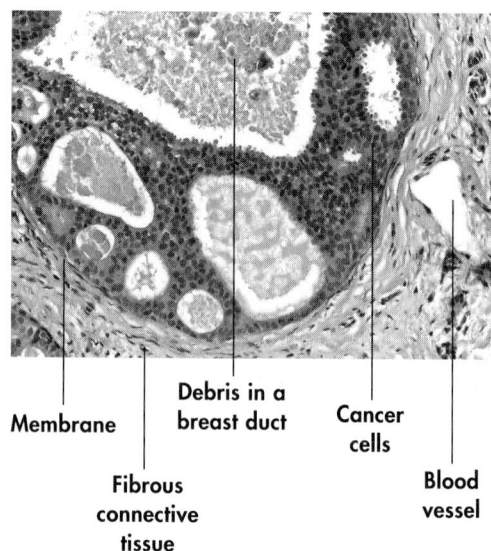

Membrane · Debris in a breast duct · Cancer cells · Fibrous connective tissue · Blood vessel

This slide shows a large duct in the center that's expanded by layers of cancer cells. Debris from dying cells is present in the duct. Most importantly, the membrane around the duct is intact — there's no invasion into surrounding tissue.

sample. These biopsy procedures are discussed in more detail in Chapter 7.

Fortunately, treatment of DCIS results in a high survival rate, approaching 100 percent in most reports in medical journals. Different treatment options are available. Ideally, the therapy chosen should be one that neither overtreats nor undertreats the condition.

Factors that influence treatment

Several factors may influence the behavior or aggressiveness of DCIS, although the precise effect of each factor is still being studied. Researchers are attempting to identify women at high risk of recurrence and those at low risk, to help determine the best treatment for each group, based on the following factors:

- **Pathologic margins.** If cancer cells extend close to the edge of the tissue samples removed during a biopsy, there's a higher likelihood that some cancer cells have been left behind. In such a situation, wide excision lumpectomy or a mastectomy may be necessary.
- **Tumor size.** A small tumor has a better chance of being adequately removed with lumpectomy than does a larger tumor.
- **Grade.** In DCIS, grade refers to the appearance of the control centers (nuclei) of the cells. If, when examined under a microscope, the nuclei of the cells still appear fairly similar to the nuclei of normal cells and very few cells are dividing, the tumor is low grade. If the nuclei are markedly different from the nuclei of normal cells, the tumor is high grade, or the cells are dividing rapidly, or both. High-grade tumors have a higher rate of recurrence than do low-grade tumors.
- **Cell structure.** Two major subtypes of DCIS are distinguished by the structure of their cells. One type is characterized by large, atypical cells with a central area of dead or degenerating cells (comedo necrosis). The other type is characterized by the lack of these qualities. The presence of comedo necrosis generally signifies a more aggressive cancer. Tumors with comedo necrosis have a higher rate of recurrence than do DCIS tumors without comedo necrosis.

Women who have high-grade DCIS with comedo necrosis may be advised to have a procedure called sentinel node biopsy (see Chapter 9). In this procedure, the lymph nodes to which the cancer would most likely spread first are examined for the presence of cancer cells. Because DCIS with comedo necrosis has a higher risk of invasion than do other types of DCIS, studying the sentinel lymph nodes is a way to double-check for any cancer spread to the lymph nodes. If no cancer is found, chances are the cancer is still confined to the breast.

- **Age.** Women with DCIS younger than age 40 may be at higher risk of recurrence than women age 40 and older.

Treatment options

Three treatment options are generally considered in women with ductal carcinoma *in situ* (DCIS):

- Surgery (lumpectomy or mastectomy)
- Radiation therapy (a consideration in women who choose lumpectomy)
- The drug tamoxifen

Surgery

When a woman is diagnosed with DCIS, generally one of the first decisions she has to make is whether to treat the condition with a mastectomy or lumpectomy.

Mastectomy

Mastectomy is the medical term for surgical removal of the entire breast. For the treatment of DCIS, a simple (total) mastectomy is performed rather than a modified radical mastectomy. A modified

A Gray Zone

Exactly when does ductal carcinoma *in situ* become invasive cancer? Sometimes, it can be hard to tell. There's a continuum of change that occurs at the cellular level between DCIS and a diagnosis of invasive cancer. At times it can be difficult for a pathologist to determine whether a particular breast tumor is a noninvasive cancer or an invasive one.

Some breast tumors are still labeled DCIS even though they show some evidence of microinvasion — the beginnings of invasive cancer. In these situations, a surgeon might recommend a sentinel node biopsy to provide better assurance that the cancer hasn't spread to the lymph nodes under the arm.

radical mastectomy is commonly used for invasive breast cancer, particularly cancers that have spread to the lymph nodes. A simple mastectomy removes the breast tissue, skin, areola and nipple, but not underarm lymph nodes. A modified radical mastectomy removes all these components, including underarm lymph nodes.

Before widespread use of mammography, the DCIS mass was often large and a simple mastectomy was the standard treatment. With regular mammography screening, DCIS was detected earlier. When lumpectomy combined with radiation became an accepted treatment for invasive breast cancer, doctors questioned the use a more extensive surgical procedure (mastectomy) for a less aggressive condition (DCIS). Researchers studied lumpectomy as a potential treatment for DCIS, leading to its widespread use today.

In some situations, though, mastectomy may still be preferable to a lumpectomy:

- The DCIS area is large compared with the size of your breast. If the area is large, a lumpectomy may not produce acceptable cosmetic results.

- There's more than one DCIS area, and it would be difficult to remove all the areas with a lumpectomy.
- Examination of tissue samples removed from the breast shows cancer cells at or near the edge of the tissue specimens. This may mean that there's more DCIS than originally thought, and a lumpectomy may not be adequate.
- You're not a candidate for radiation therapy, which commonly follows a lumpectomy. You may not be a candidate for radiation if you're pregnant, you've already received radiation to your chest area or you have a condition that makes you more sensitive to the side effects of radiation therapy.
- You have extremely dense breast tissue, which may make it difficult to detect a recurrence on a mammogram.
- You're a BRCA gene carrier and you and your doctor are concerned about an increased risk of new breast cancers.
- You prefer to have a mastectomy rather than a lumpectomy for any of a number of reasons, including a desire not to undergo radiation therapy.

Breast reconstruction is almost always a possibility after a mastectomy. It can be done during the same surgery to remove the breast or at a later time. See Chapter 10 to find out more about breast reconstruction.

Lumpectomy

Lumpectomy, also known as breast-conserving therapy, removes only a portion of tissue from your breast. The procedure allows you to keep as much of your breast as possible and, depending on the amount of tissue removed, usually eliminates the need for reconstructive surgery.

Lumpectomy followed by radiation therapy is the most common treatment for DCIS. Although no study has officially compared lumpectomy with removal of the entire breast (mastectomy) for the treatment of DCIS, research suggests that lumpectomy combined with radiation produces survival rates similar to those of mastectomy. Most women with DCIS are candidates for lumpectomy, although in some situations mastectomy may be necessary.

For DCIS, lumpectomy generally doesn't involve removal of lymph nodes from under the arm because this is a noninvasive cancer and the chance of finding can-

cer in the lymph nodes is exceedingly small. If tissue obtained during surgery leads a doctor to think the cancer may have spread outside the breast duct, he or she may recommend a sentinel node biopsy or removal of some lymph nodes. Chapter 9 discusses lumpectomy and lymph node removal in more detail.

Radiation therapy

Radiation therapy after lumpectomy reduces the chance that DCIS will come back or that it'll progress to invasive cancer. This was illustrated by a study that randomly assigned women with DCIS to receive either lumpectomy alone or lumpectomy with radiation. After an average follow-up of seven and a half years, researchers found that women who underwent radiation had less risk of recurrent DCIS and invasive breast cancer in the affected breast (see the table below).

Some doctors have suggested that in the study just mentioned, the amount of normal breast tissue around the DCIS tissue may not have been as large as is desirable to assure that all the DCIS was removed. They contend that if larger areas of normal tissue are removed, radiation therapy might not be needed. Nonetheless, this study forms the basis for why radiation

BREAST CANCER

Risk of recurrent DCIS and invasive cancer in the same breast

	Lumpectomy alone	Lumpectomy plus radiation
Recurrent DCIS	13%	8%
Invasive breast cancer	13%	4%

Source: B. Fisher et al., "Lumpectomy and Radiation Therapy for the Treatment of Intraductal Breast Cancer: Findings from the National Surgical Adjuvant Breast and Bowel Project B-17," *Journal of Clinical Oncology*, 16:2 (1998), pages 441-452

therapy is recommended for most women with DCIS who have a lumpectomy.

Radiation therapy uses high-energy X-rays to kill cancer cells or damage them to the point where they lose their ability to grow and divide. Cells that grow out of control, such as cancer cells, are more vulnerable to the effects of radiation than are normal cells and thus are more likely to be damaged.

The two basic types of radiation therapy are external and internal. External beam radiation therapy is most commonly used for treatment of DCIS. See Chapter 9 for more information on radiation therapy.

Tamoxifen

Tamoxifen (Nolvadex) is a synthetic anti-estrogen hormone that has been shown to be beneficial in the treatment of invasive breast cancer. It's also used as a cancer prevention agent for women at high risk of breast cancer.

Due to this drug's success in treating invasive breast cancer, doctors wanted to know if it might benefit women with ductal carcinoma *in situ* (DCIS). That question was addressed in a study called the National Surgical Adjuvant Breast and Bowel Project (NSABP) B-24 trial. It involved approximately 1,800 women with DCIS who had undergone lumpectomies and radiation therapy. These women were randomly assigned to receive either tamoxifen or an inactive pill (placebo) for five years.

Researchers wanted to know if women taking tamoxifen experienced reduced rates of recurrent DCIS and invasive breast cancer, compared with women taking a placebo. The results are shown in the table below.

As the table indicates, 7 percent of the women who took a placebo developed invasive breast cancer, compared with 4 percent of the women who took tamox-

---

Tamoxifen vs. a placebo

Cancer-related events	Placebo group	Tamoxifen group
All types of breast cancer	13%	8%
Invasive	7%	4%
Noninvasive (DCIS)	6%	4%
Cancer in the same breast as the original tumor		
All cancers	9%	6%
Invasive	4%	2%
Noninvasive	5%	4%
Cancer in the opposite breast		
All cancers	3%	2%
Invasive	2%	2%
Noninvasive	1%	0%

Source: B. Fisher, J. Dignam, N. Wolmark, et al., "Tamoxifen in Treatment of Intraductal Breast Cancer: National Surgical Adjuvant Breast and Bowel Project B-24, Randomized Controlled Trial," *The Lancet* 353 (9169) pages 1993-2000, 1999

ifen. The results of this study led to the Food and Drug Administration's approval of tamoxifen as a treatment for women with DCIS.

What this study didn't address, though, was whether hormone receptor status was an important factor in the study's results. (See Chapters 7 and 9 for more on hormone receptor status.) A group of researchers went back and addressed this issue. They found that women with estrogen positive receptors in their biopsy specimens benefited from taking tamoxifen, whereas women with estrogen negative receptors didn't. As a result, hormone receptor status is typically determined in DCIS tissue specimens.

For women who choose to have a mastectomy, there's less reason to use tamoxifen. With a mastectomy, the risk of invasive breast cancer or DCIS in the small amount of remaining breast tissue is almost zero. Any potential benefit from tamoxifen would apply only to the opposite breast.

The bottom line is that tamoxifen is a treatment option to be considered among women with DCIS. However, for some women, it may not provide much benefit. Discuss the pros and cons of tamoxifen with your doctor. For more information on tamoxifen, see Chapter 9.

Making the Decision

If you've been diagnosed with ductal carcinoma *in situ* (DCIS), you may wonder what would be best for you. Not all DCIS is the same, so it's important to consider treatment options in the context of your own situation and to make a decision with which you feel comfortable.

If you're trying to decide whether to have a lumpectomy or a mastectomy, Chapter 9 contains a list of several questions to ask yourself that may help you. If you're deciding whether to have radiation therapy after a lumpectomy, discuss the benefits and risks with your doctor.

The stories of three women with DCIS follow. Each of the women made a different choice regarding her treatment.

Geraldine's Story

Geraldine was 68 years old when she received a diagnosis of DCIS. The diagnosis came at the same time she learned that she had some abnormal cells in her cervix. After a biopsy of her right breast, where a mammogram detected a small abnormality, she had a double surgery. Doctors removed abnormal tissue in her right breast with a lumpectomy, followed by removal of abnormal cells in her cervix.

After the surgery, Geraldine knew she had some decisions to make. One of them was whether to undergo radiation therapy to the remaining tissue in her right breast. Geraldine wanted to thoroughly study the matter before making a decision. After reviewing the medical literature, Geraldine decided that radiation therapy wasn't for her. She decided to undergo monitoring every six months with mammography. She also has a Pap test regularly to monitor the health of her cervix.

Geraldine's decision not to have radiation was based on several factors:
- The DCIS was very small, about half a centimeter.

- One of the side effects of radiation therapy was possible damage to her lungs.
- The amount of time and travel involved in receiving radiation every day for six weeks was fairly extensive.

On weighing the risks versus the benefits, Geraldine felt, with the support of her doctors, that radiation therapy posed more disadvantages than it was worth to her. Her children worried about her decision but were supportive. As Geraldine likes to point out, it's her life and she's the one who has to live with her decisions.

Geraldine is quick to emphasize the need to make your own decision and to not let others control your life. She sums up, "Do research, put your life in God's hands and make a choice that's good for you."

Cathy's Story

Like Geraldine's, Cathy's DCIS was first detected on a routine mammogram. Cathy was 42 years old at the time. She had had a baseline mammogram at age 38 and thought it would be a good time to have another mammogram. A practicing radiologist, Cathy had ready access to the mammography suite and had her examination while a friend was working in the area. Before long, they were getting extra views of the affected breast. Cathy recognized new clusters of microcalcifications that didn't appear either obviously benign or definitely malignant, but worrisome enough to warrant a biopsy.

A biopsy revealed DCIS with at least three areas of calcifications. Because of this, Cathy opted for a mastectomy. A sentinel node biopsy performed at the same time confirmed that the cancer hadn't spread to the lymph system. This gave Cathy assurance that all the DCIS areas had been removed and that there was no cancer spread to the lymph nodes. After a six-month follow-up mammogram and clinical exam of her other breast, she has returned to annual screening of her remaining breast.

Cathy decided against immediate reconstructive surgery so she could deal with additional treatment that might be necessary after surgery. She wears a prosthesis and is keeping reconstruction as a future option when her children are older.

Her advice to other women is to regularly perform breast self-examinations and to have clinical examinations and mammograms on a regular basis.

Agnes' Story

At the age of 72, Agnes was diagnosed with DCIS. She was given the treatment option of a lumpectomy with radiation or a mastectomy. Agnes decided on a lumpectomy with radiation, and she also had a sentinel node biopsy to provide some assurance that the cancer hadn't spread. Agnes' surgery went smoothly, as did the follow-up radiation therapy. She had almost no side effects from her daily radiation sessions.

Standing by to offer Agnes support were two close friends and a sister-in-law with similar experiences. One friend had been disease-free for eight years following a lumpectomy and radiation, a factor that helped Agnes make her decision.

Agnes has been satisfied with her decision. She hopes that the future will confirm that her decision was the right one.

Chapter 9: Breast Cancer

Treating Invasive Breast Cancer

A
fter coming to grips with a breast cancer diagnosis, the next questions are often, "What now?" and, "How do I deal with this cancer?" The good news is that breast cancer is highly treatable. Survival rates are continuously increasing, and much research is being done to develop better treatment options. But as options increase, so does the information needed to make appropriate treatment decisions. The goal of the next few chapters is to help you become more informed about what's available to treat breast cancer.

This chapter focuses on treating invasive cancer that hasn't spread to other parts of your body, what's known as localized breast cancer (stages I and II). Chapter 11 includes information on treatment of locally advanced breast cancer (stage III). Treatment for recurrent cancer — cancer that returns after initial treatment — is covered in Chapter 13. Chapter 14, meanwhile, focuses on breast cancer that has spread (metastasized) to distant parts of the body (stage IV).

If you're still grappling with your diagnosis, it's OK to wait awhile before delving into your treatment options. Take the time you need to understand and absorb your situation. This is a life-changing event for many women, and it frequently leads to a time of re-evaluating priorities and life goals. It's also a time to strengthen your connections with family and friends and to gather the support you need for the days ahead.

When you're ready, find a quiet spot to read the following information. Remember that taking a bit of time — up to a couple of weeks — to carefully weigh your options isn't likely to alter the outcome. Thorough consideration of your values, lifestyle and personal priorities will make all the difference in how satisfied you are with the choices you make. Even if you decide you're more comfortable asking your doctor to decide on your treatment, the knowledge you've acquired may make the process a little less scary.

Treatment Options

The primary goal of treatment for localized breast cancer is to get rid of all cancerous (malignant) cells that are in your body. In general, the two ways of accomplishing this are with locoregional therapy and systemic therapy:

- **Locoregional therapy.** Locoregional therapy is targeted directly at the tumor and the nearby tissue. Locoregional therapy includes surgery and radiation therapy.
- **Systemic therapy.** Systemic therapy is aimed at treating cancer cells through-

out your body. It involves medication that's usually given by mouth or injected into your bloodstream. Systemic therapy includes chemotherapy and hormone therapy.

If you have localized invasive cancer, locoregional therapy is usually the first line of treatment. It may be followed by systemic therapy to get rid of any cells that may have split off from the primary tumor and traveled to other parts of your body. This type of additional therapy is called adjuvant systemic therapy. The goal of both locoregional therapy and adjuvant systemic therapy is to cure your cancer.

Surgery

Surgery to remove the tumor is usually the first form of treatment for localized breast cancer. In addition to removing the cancerous mass, surgery provides additional information about the type and extent of the cancer that's present. This information can help guide further treatment decisions.

For some women, the most difficult part of surgery is deciding which type of breast surgery to have. In general, two options are available: removal of the tumor only (lumpectomy) and removal of the whole breast (mastectomy). Lumpectomy combined with radiation therapy is known as breast-conserving therapy because it allows a woman to receive effective breast cancer treatment and still keep the breast. Making a choice between mastectomy and lumpectomy can be difficult. It's hoped that the following information will be helpful to you in this process. It describes the possible surgical procedures and outlines the pros and cons of each option.

Lumpectomy

With a lumpectomy (breast-conserving surgery), only the part of your breast that contains the tumor is removed. This allows as much of your breast to be saved as possible. Because tumors are now detected at an earlier stage and often are smaller in size, and because of the procedure's proven success in research studies, lumpectomy is much more common today than it was in the past.

During a lumpectomy, a surgeon makes an incision in the breast large enough to allow removal of both the tumor and a margin of healthy tissue surrounding the tumor. The margin is taken to help ensure that all the cancer cells are removed.

As noted in Chapter 7, a lumpectomy can perform dual roles. If you didn't have a biopsy previously, tissue from the lumpectomy may be used to confirm a diagnosis of breast cancer. In addition, a lumpectomy can serve as a first line of treatment.

Lumpectomy is usually followed by radiation therapy to try to eliminate any cancer cells that may not have been removed during surgery.

Because breast tissue remains after a lumpectomy, with this procedure there's a slightly higher chance that the cancer could return, compared with a mastectomy. This is particularly true if a lumpectomy isn't followed with radiation treatment. Lumpectomy without radiation isn't a commonly accepted treatment

When Lumpectomy May Not Be the Right Choice

Most women with stage I or II breast cancer are eligible for a lumpectomy (breast-conserving surgery). But in some situations, a lumpectomy may not be recommended. For example:

- You have a tumor larger than 5 centimeters (about 2 inches) in diameter.
- You have a large tumor relative to the overall size of your breast. You may not have enough breast tissue left after a lumpectomy to achieve an acceptable cosmetic result.
- The tumor is located beneath the nipple, and a lumpectomy would require removing the nipple. For some women, removal of the nipple may not leave an acceptable cosmetic result.
- You have multiple tumors in different areas of your breast.
- You have widespread malignant-appearing microcalcifications on your mammogram.
- You're unable to receive radiation therapy because you're pregnant, you've had previous radiation to your chest area or you have a connective tissue disease, such as systemic lupus erythematosus (SLE) or scleroderma.
- You're at high risk of developing another new breast cancer, and you're considering prophylactic surgery to remove both breasts.

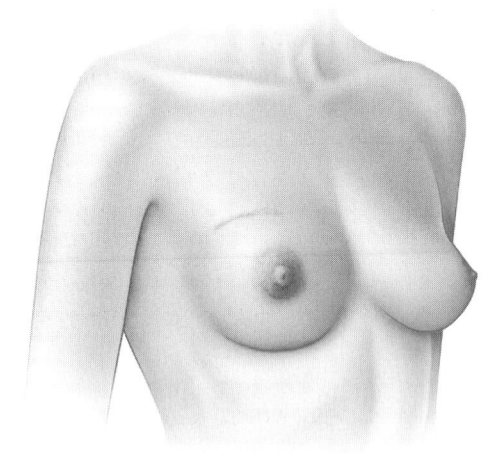

During a lumpectomy, the tumor is removed along with some healthy tissue around the tumor.

option for invasive breast cancer because the risk of a cancer recurrence in the breast — 35 percent to 40 percent — is unacceptably high.

If cancer does return in a breast after a lumpectomy, then a mastectomy is almost always necessary. However, most women treated with a lumpectomy don't have a local cancer recurrence.

A breast-conserving procedure similar to lumpectomy is a partial mastectomy (quadrantectomy or segmental mastectomy), which removes significantly more tissue than does a lumpectomy. It generally isn't performed in the United States.

Mastectomy

Mastectomy is a general term for removal of a breast. A mastectomy may be performed when a lumpectomy isn't possible or when a woman prefers it.

Up until the 1980s, mastectomy was almost always recommended for the treatment of breast cancer. Researchers then learned that smaller operations combined with radiation could successfully treat the disease as well. The most important finding of their studies was that survival — the length of time lived after diagnosis — was the same, regardless of the type of surgery chosen: either a lumpectomy with radiation or a mastectomy. In other words, for most breast cancers, it's not necessary to have a mastectomy in order for the treatment to be successful.

During a mastectomy, the surgeon usually makes a single incision across half the chest that allows for removal of the breast and, if necessary, adjacent underarm (axillary) lymph nodes. Several types of mastectomies may be performed: radical, modified radical and simple (total).

Radical mastectomy

A radical mastectomy is a procedure that requires removal of the largest amount of tissue, including the breast, some of the chest wall muscles, all the lymph nodes under the arm, and some additional fat and skin. From the early 1900s through the 1970s, this was the standard treatment for women with breast cancer. Today it's used only in cases of locally advanced cancer that's spread to chest wall muscles.

Modified radical mastectomy

During the last three decades of the 20th century, the most common mastectomy used to treat invasive breast cancer was modified radical mastectomy. It involves removing the entire breast, including the skin, areola and nipple, as well as some of

and nipple, but not the lymph nodes. This procedure is generally used when the axillary lymph nodes don't need to be removed, for example, when a sentinel node was examined and showed no sign of cancer cells (see "Sentinel node biopsy," page 156). A simple mastectomy is also an option for the treatment of noninvasive breast cancer, such as ductal carcinoma *in situ*, and it's used to prevent breast cancer in women at high risk of the disease (see Chapter 5).

Lymph node removal

Lymph nodes are small, compact structures where cells of your immune system congregate. They're linked by tiny vessels along the lymphatic system. They're generally clustered in certain areas of your body, such as your neck, armpits and groin. The job of lymph vessels is to drain excess fluid that's not absorbed by blood vessels. Lymph nodes filter out foreign substances, such as bacteria and cancer cells. As a cancerous tumor grows, cancer cells may spread to nearby lymph nodes.

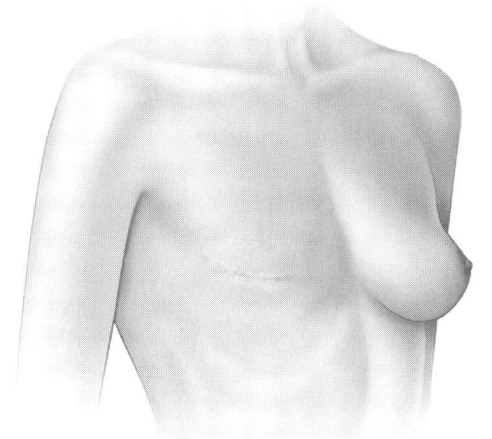

During a modified radical mastectomy, the breast is removed as well as some underarm lymph nodes. Chest muscles are left intact.

the lymph nodes under the arm. It spares the chest wall muscles, thereby leaving a more normal chest wall contour than does radical mastectomy.

Simple mastectomy

A simple (total) mastectomy involves removal of the breast tissue, skin, areola

---

QUESTION & ANSWER

Q: **What are positive margins?**

A: When your surgeon removes a cancerous (malignant) tumor, he or she tries to make sure that all the cancer has been removed. The edges of the removed tissue are called the margins. In a laboratory, these margins are examined to see if any cancer cells are at the margin or close to it. If cancer cells have spread to the edges of the tissue sample, the sample is said to have positive margins. This means there's a high probability that cancer cells still remain in the area from where the tumor was taken. Additional tissue is usually removed in this situation until cancer-free (negative) margins are obtained.

Some may get past the lymph nodes and travel to other parts of the body.

An early location for breast cancer to spread is the lymph nodes under the arm, called the axillary lymph nodes. That's why women with invasive cancer generally have these nodes surgically evaluated. If your surgeon doesn't plan to do this, be sure that you understand why. One reason may be that you have a noninvasive cancer, so there's no reason to believe cancer cells have spread to the lymph nodes.

Surgeons use two methods to examine underarm lymph nodes for cancer cells: axillary lymph node dissection and sentinel node biopsy.

Axillary lymph node dissection

In an axillary lymph node dissection, a surgeon removes multiple lymph nodes under the arm in an attempt to detect any cancer cells that may have traveled away from the primary tumor. These nodes, along with tissue samples from your cancer, are examined under a microscope. If the lymph nodes contain cancer, the chances are higher that the cancer has escaped and traveled to other parts of the body. Your doctors may recommend other treatments that would attempt to destroy these traveling cells. You'll read more about this later in the chapter.

One of the potential side effects of removing multiple underarm lymph nodes is that the surgery disrupts the lymphatic channels that drain fluid from your arm to the rest of your body. The result can be a buildup of fluid in your arm and hand, causing swelling (lymphedema). The swelling may be mild or quite extensive.

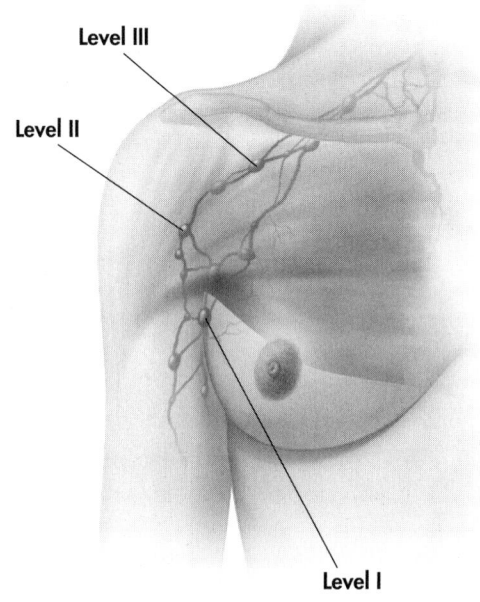

The three major levels of axillary lymph nodes are as follows: Level I nodes are located below the lower edge of the major chest muscle. Level II nodes are underneath the chest muscle. Level III nodes are above the upper edge of the chest muscle. During a conventional axillary lymph node dissection, levels I and II nodes are usually removed as a triangular piece of fatty tissue, and the lymph nodes are later extracted from that tissue and examined for cancer.

Other uncommon side effects include recurrent skin infections of that arm, numbness, pain and a reduced range of motion in the upper arm and chest. These side effects may be temporary or permanent. For more information on lymphedema and other potential side effects, see Chapters 35 and 36.

Sentinel node biopsy

Sentinel node biopsy is a procedure designed primarily to reduce the risk of lymphedema associated with axillary lymph node dissection. This procedure has become increasingly popular in the past few years. It focuses on finding those lymph nodes that are the first to receive drainage from breast tumors (sentinel nodes) and, therefore, the first to collect cancer cells. If these nodes test negative for cancer cells, it's not necessary to proceed with axillary lymph node dissection.

Surgeons typically use two methods to find sentinel nodes. One is to inject blue dye in the area of the tumor within the breast. The dye is absorbed in lymphatic channels and travels to a sentinel node or sometimes up to a few sentinel nodes (see the color illustration on page 261). In the early days of the procedure, the dye was injected around the area of the cancer. But later tests showed that no matter where the dye is injected into the breast, it still tends to travel to the same sentinel lymph nodes.

The other frequently used method is to inject a small amount of radioactive solution into the breast and use a special gamma detector to see in which lymph nodes the radioactive solution accumulates. At times, both methods are used to better ensure that the appropriate sentinel nodes are removed.

Identification and removal of the sentinel nodes are often combined with lumpectomy or mastectomy surgery. To remove sentinel lymph nodes during a lumpectomy, the surgeon makes a separate incision under your arm. During a mastectomy, removal of the breast and sentinel nodes is usually done with a single incision.

Axillary procedures and breast procedures can be paired in any combination. In other words, the type of breast surgery you choose doesn't affect whether a sentinel node biopsy can be done. In addition, even if cancer is found in the sentinel nodes, a lumpectomy can still be done. You don't have to have a mastectomy.

If the sentinel nodes are found to be free of cancer cells, the chances of finding cancer in any of the remaining axillary lymph nodes are very small, and no other nodes need to be removed. This spares many women the need for a more extensive

When Sentinel Node Biopsy Isn't Appropriate

Sentinel node biopsy isn't appropriate for all women. Axillary lymph node dissection may be performed instead of sentinel node biopsy in the following situations:
- There's not an experienced team to do it.
- The tumor is larger than 5 centimeters (about 2 inches) in diameter.
- You've had previous chemotherapy or hormone therapy. It's still controversial whether the sentinel node procedure is accurate in these situations.
- Your underarm lymph nodes feel enlarged. It may be that the sentinel lymph node is so full of cancer that it can't take up the blue dye or radioactive tracer.
- A fine-needle aspiration biopsy of an enlarged lymph node is positive for cancer.

operation and greatly decreases their risk of complications such as lymphedema. If cancer is found in the sentinel node, a conventional axillary lymph node dissection is usually done.

In some larger medical institutions, tissue removed during surgery (surgical specimen) is examined while surgery is still taking place. This is done with a technique called frozen section analysis (see "Frozen section for quick analysis," page 160). With this type of immediate analysis, the surgeon is notified right away whether additional lymph nodes need to be removed.

Although the frozen section technique can be helpful in avoiding additional surgery, it doesn't always provide all the necessary information. So the pathologist chemically preserves the tissue specimen overnight and re-examines it the following day. A small percentage of the time, he or she finds some cancer the next day, when the lymph node is examined more extensively. This may mean further surgery to remove additional lymph nodes.

Sentinel Node Biopsy Controversies

With any new procedure, questions are raised about its effectiveness, its limitations and how it should be used in actual (clinical) practice. This is true of the sentinel node biopsy procedure.

Sentinel node biopsy rapidly became commonplace in clinical practice. To many surgeons, the procedure made a lot of sense and seemed to offer an improved alternative to standard axillary lymph node dissection. But some surgeons say that the new procedure became established too rapidly, before information from large research studies was available with which to compare the two methods. These physicians argue that it may still be too early to tell whether sentinel node biopsy is appropriate for use in general practice.

A number of ongoing research studies are seeking to address some of the unanswered questions regarding sentinel node biopsy:

- One trial asks, "Is it appropriate to do a more sensitive analysis called immunohistochemical staining of the removed sentinel lymph nodes?" The goal is to see whether this method can improve care, compared with more traditional pathologic staining methods.
- Another trial asks, "When a sentinel lymph node is positive for cancer, is it necessary to go back and surgically remove all the other lymph nodes?" Would subsequent radiation therapy to the breast, systemic drug therapy or both be enough to effectively eliminate any cancer in the other lymph nodes, thus sparing women the risks associated with a standard lymph node dissection?

Better answers to these questions should be available in the next few years.

Some common side effects of a sentinel node biopsy include bruising or bleeding near the incision, blue-stained breast skin that may persist for weeks or months, blue-stained urine for a couple of days, and pain or tenderness where the dye was injected that may last one or two weeks.

What to expect

Regardless of whether you've had surgery before, the idea of having an operation can be stressful. The information that follows is intended to give you a general idea of what to expect during breast cancer surgery. If you have any questions, be sure to ask your doctor, surgeon or other health care professional. In addition, read any materials that your surgeon or hospital provides on how the procedure you're having is performed.

Before surgery

Before your surgery, you'll likely meet with your surgeon and perhaps an anesthesiologist to discuss your operation, review your medical history and determine the plan for your anesthesia — whether you'll receive local, regional or general anesthesia. Local and regional anesthesia don't put you to sleep but rather numb only the area where the surgery is to be performed. You may also receive a mild sedative. In other words, you're conscious for the surgery, but you don't feel any discomfort. With general anesthesia, you're given drugs that make you unconscious and block the memory of the surgery. When you receive this type of anesthesia, people commonly say that you're being put under or put to sleep.

Before your surgery, you may be asked to sign a consent form to allow the surgeon to perform the operation. And you may be asked to sign an informed consent document allowing researchers to use for research purposes some of your tissue and blood that's not used for diagnosis.

You'll likely be asked a number of questions about allergies or other chronic problems you may have, medications you're taking and whether you smoke or drink alcohol daily. Some medications — such as aspirin and other nonsteroidal anti-inflammatory drugs (NSAIDs) and blood-thinning medications (anticoagulants) — can cause excessive bleeding during surgery. Other medications and herbal supplements may interact with the anesthetics and cause problems. Your doctor may ask you to stop using these medications and supplements for a period of time before and after your surgery.

In addition, you may need to have blood tests and perhaps an assessment of your heart function with an electrocardiogram (ECG). Just before surgery, you'll likely be asked to fast for six to 12 hours.

The day of your surgery or the night before, you'll be admitted to the hospital. A nurse will talk with you and prepare you for the operation. Your family and friends will be told where they can wait for you.

During surgery

After you receive an anesthetic and enough time has passed for it to take effect, your surgeon will make an incision in the area of the tumor to remove it and some of the surrounding tissue. The amount of tissue removed depends on whether you've decided to have a lumpectomy or a mastectomy. Following removal of the tissue, the surgeon may also insert one or two plastic drains, which are the thickness of a pen, where your breast tissue was removed or under your arm to draw off fluids from the wound and reduce swelling. The tubes are sewn into place, and the ends are attached to a small drainage bag.

A lumpectomy usually takes less than two hours. Sometimes, lymph node removal is done as a separate procedure.

A mastectomy that doesn't include breast reconstruction takes one to four hours. If you're having breast reconstruction done at the same time, the surgery is generally longer.

After surgery

After your surgery, you'll go to a recovery room where a nurse checks your vital signs and makes sure you're recovering from anesthesia. You may have an intravenous (IV) catheter in one of your arms to provide access for medications. You'll have a bandage on your incision. If drainage tubes were inserted, a nurse will check that they're draining properly and begin teaching you how to take care of them. This typically involves emptying and measuring fluid and letting your doctor or nurse know of any problems. When drainage slows to less than an ounce of fluid a day — usually after one or two weeks — the tubes are removed.

If lymph nodes were removed, in most cases hospital staff will try to have you move the affected arm as soon as possible so that it doesn't get stiff. In addition to pain in the breast area, you may experience sensations of numbness and tingling in your underarm. This is because sensory nerves are cut during the surgery, though

Frozen Section for Quick Analysis

Around the early 1900s, Mayo Clinic surgeons weren't satisfied with having to wait overnight or even several days to process tissue for pathologic analysis. The surgeons felt that important microscopic information, obtained while a patient was still under anesthesia, could help guide surgical planning. In response to this, Mayo Clinic pathologist Louis Wilson, M.D., decided to test a rather controversial new idea — frozen tissue examination.

It's said that on a cold winter day in Minnesota, Dr. Wilson set a tissue specimen on an outside windowsill. After the specimen froze, he cut it and examined it under a microscope. The microscopic image of the frozen specimen provided sufficient information to help direct the surgical team. This was the start of Mayo Clinic's practice of obtaining frozen sections of surgical specimens.

The advantage of a frozen section is that it allows the pathologist to examine the tissue immediately. To perform a frozen section, the specimen is quickly frozen with a freezing coolant and cut into thin sections. The sections are

the nerves to the muscles are preserved. Over time, usually several months, these nerves typically grow back, restoring sensation to the area. In some cases, a woman may experience decreased sensation that's permanent.

Your surgeon or nurse will give you instructions about how to care for yourself at home, including how to care for your incision and drains, how to recognize problems such as an infection, when to resume wearing a bra or start wearing a breast prosthesis, which activities you may need to restrict and how to take your medications. While you're in the hospital, someone also may talk with you or give you information regarding some of the psychological and emotional factors associated with the surgery.

You'll probably meet with an oncologist after surgery to discuss your laboratory results and whether you may need further treatment. You may see your oncologist while you're hospitalized or after you're released from the hospital.

If you've had a lumpectomy, you may need to stay in the hospital overnight, depending on whether you had lymph nodes removed at the same time. Some lumpectomies are performed on an outpatient basis, allowing you to go home the same day. In case of a mastectomy, you may need to stay in the hospital one or two days.

Radiation Therapy

Radiation therapy uses high-energy X-rays to kill cancer cells or to cause them to lose their ability to grow and divide. Rapidly growing cells, such as cancer cells, are more susceptible to the effects of radiation therapy than are normal cells.

stained with a colored dye so that the cells can be easily seen. Then they're mounted onto glass slides. A pathologist examines them under the microscope and, within minutes of receiving the specimen, reports the findings to the surgeon.

A surgeon may request a frozen section analysis to determine if a sentinel node is positive for cancer or if the tissue margins of a lumpectomy contain cancer cells. If the lymph node or the lumpectomy margins are positive, the surgeon may remove additional nodes or take out more tissue to ensure that the margins are clear. In difficult cases, a pathologist may defer the final diagnosis until conventional tissue processing is complete, typically the next day. In some cases, cancer cells aren't detectable on a frozen section and analysis of a preserved section the following day reveals that cancer cells are indeed present. In these cases, another surgery may be needed to achieve negative margins or to perform an axillary lymph node dissection.

Although frozen tissue examinations are routine at some medical institutions, it requires a particular expertise to do them well. That's why they're not routinely done at all institutions.

Radiation therapy may be used to treat breast cancer at almost every stage. For primary breast cancer in stages I and II, radiation therapy is used along with lumpectomy as part of locoregional therapy. In some instances, radiation is also used after a mastectomy.

This section discusses radiation therapy as a treatment for early-stage breast cancer. Radiation therapy is also used to treat locally advanced breast cancer (stage III). In certain situations it's also used to control breast cancer that has spread (metastasized) to distant parts of the body (stage IV). Radiation treatment for stages III and IV breast cancer is described in Chapters 11 and 14, respectively.

Radiation after lumpectomy

Radiation therapy is usually recommended after a lumpectomy because with lumpectomy alone there's a relatively high chance of cancer recurrence in the affected breast months to years later. This is called in-breast recurrence.

Without radiation therapy, the risk of in-breast recurrence over a 10-year period after a lumpectomy ranges from 20 percent to 35 percent, depending on disease characteristics. When radiation therapy is added after surgery, the rate generally decreases to 5 percent to 10 percent.

In a few situations, though, radiation may not be appropriate and mastectomy may be needed. This may be the case if:
• You're pregnant.
• You have a connective tissue disease, such as lupus or scleroderma.
• You've previously had radiation to the involved breast.

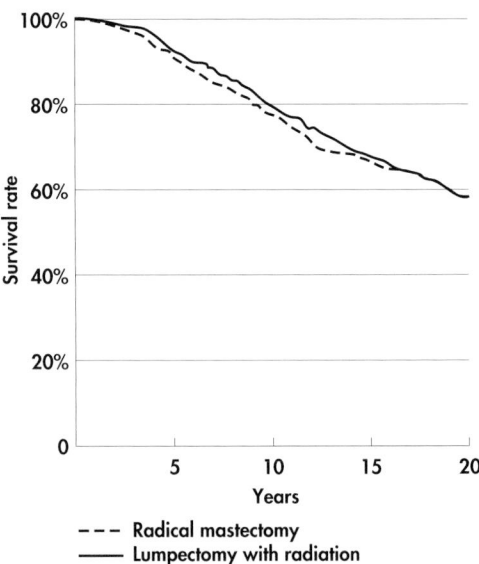

Survival by treatment option

- - - Radical mastectomy
—— Lumpectomy with radiation

Both mastectomy and lumpectomy with radiation have proved to be equally effective in terms of survival. In a number of clinical trials, women with invasive breast cancer were treated with either mastectomy or lumpectomy with radiation, and the outcomes of their surgeries were compared. After follow-up periods of up to 20 years, survival rates for both groups were found to be virtually identical. The above graph is from one such trial.

Source: The *New England Journal of Medicine*, October 17, 2002

Radiation after mastectomy

If you've had a mastectomy and you're at high risk of a recurrence of the cancer on the chest wall, your doctor may recommend radiation therapy to reduce your risk. Factors that may put you at high risk of chest wall recurrence include:
• Underarm (axillary) lymph nodes that test positive for cancer cells
• A tumor greater than 5 centimeters (about 2 inches) in diameter

- Very narrow margins or margins that test positive for cancer cells in the removed (excised) tissue

The value of radiation therapy for women with just a few positive lymph nodes is controversial. Some studies have shown that radiation after a mastectomy decreases breast cancer deaths but increases deaths from other causes, such as heart-related problems, because radiation can damage the coronary arteries. Researchers speculate the deaths were related to use of older radiation techniques and this may no longer be a significant issue. Another study of women who received radiation therapy in the 1970s and 1980s after a mastectomy found that the women were at increased risk of lung cancer. A recent report indicates risk of lung cancer after radiation is higher in smokers than in nonsmokers.

Today, with newer planning and delivery techniques, radiation exposure to the heart and lungs is more limited. Recent studies show an increase in survival of women with any number of positive lymph nodes who receive radiation after a mastectomy. Data suggest that radiation therapy after a mastectomy may increase 10-year survival by 5 percent to 10 percent. Further study is still needed to more accurately determine radiation therapy benefits after a mastectomy.

If your biopsy shows cancer spread to the lymph nodes, discuss the potential benefits of radiation with your doctor.

How radiation works

Radiation therapy for breast cancer may be delivered in a couple of ways.

Radiation that comes from an external source and is directed to the whole breast and to some surrounding areas containing lymph nodes is the most commonly used method. This is known as external beam radiation therapy.

Another way of delivering radiation is internal radiation therapy (brachytherapy). In this procedure, small amounts of radioactive material contained in tubes or catheters are placed directly in your breast tissue and allowed to stay there for a period of time. This allows only the localized area to receive radiation. External beam radiation and brachytherapy may be used together, with one method following the other, but this is less commonly done.

External beam radiation therapy

External beam radiation therapy generally begins a few weeks after surgery. If you're also planning on receiving chemotherapy, radiation therapy is typically given three to four weeks after you've completed your chemotherapy treatment. External beam radiation treatment is usually given daily, Monday through Friday, for approximately five to six weeks.

During each visit, you lie flat on a table while a machine moves around you, directing the radiation toward your breast from different angles (see the color illustration on page 271). The procedure is similar to getting an X-ray, but the radiation is more intense. Sometimes, the lymph nodes above your collarbone (supraclavicular lymph nodes) or near your sternum (internal mammary lymph nodes) also are targeted.

Each treatment is painless and takes just a few minutes. In many treatment centers, you can set up an appointment at the same time each day so that your treatment becomes part of your daily routine. Generally, several health care professionals work together in providing your radiation treatment. Team members usually include:

- **A radiation oncologist.** This person is a doctor who specializes in treatments using radiation. He or she determines the appropriate therapy for you, follows your progress and adjusts your treatment if necessary.
- **A radiation physicist and dosimetrist.** These two people make special calculations and measurements regarding your radiation dosage and its delivery.
- **A radiation therapist.** This individual actually delivers your daily treatments.

Before treatment

Before your first treatment session, you'll go through a simulation process in which a radiation oncologist carefully maps your breast to pinpoint the precise location of your cancer. During the simulation, a radiation therapist helps you into a position best suited to locating the affected area. Sometimes, pads or other devices are used to help you maintain the position.

Using a special X-ray machine or computerized tomography (CT) scanner, the radiation oncologist locates the area that needs to be treated. You'll hear noise from the X-ray or CT equipment as it moves around you. Sometimes, this can be unnerving, but try to relax and remain still during the simulation because this will help ensure consistent, accurate treatments.

After the area to be treated is located, ink marks or tiny permanent tattoo dots are placed on your skin to provide a reference point for the radiation therapist when administering the radiation. Be sure not to wash the ink marks off until you're allowed to do so. If the marks can't be seen, you may need to go through the mapping process again.

The dosimetrist, radiation physicist and radiation oncologist then use a computer to plan the dosage of radiation you'll receive and how long the beam must be applied to deliver the right amount.

During treatment

After the simulation and planning are complete, you can begin treatment. When you arrive at the hospital or treatment facility, you'll be taken to a special room that's used specifically for radiation therapy. You may need to remove your clothes and put on a hospital gown for the session. The radiation therapist carefully helps you into the exact position that you were in during the simulation. The therapist then leaves the room and turns on the machine, called a linear accelerator, that's used for delivering the radiation. Although the therapist isn't in the room, he or she can see you on a television monitor, and usually you and the therapist can talk with each other through an intercom.

The treatment itself lasts only a few minutes, but the whole process may take 10 to 30 minutes each visit. The customary schedule for radiation treatments is therapy five days a week for five to six weeks. Occasionally, a boost treatment to the location where the tumor was removed (tumor bed) may be recommended. This typically involves an additional five therapy sessions. Boost treatments are used to further reduce the chances of recurrence in women with stage I or II cancer who are at higher risk. This may include younger women, those in whom cancer cells were found in the tissue (margins) around the tumor that was removed, and those with associated ductal carcinoma *in situ*, which is discussed in Chapter 8.

After treatment

After the radiation session is over, you're free to go about your regular activities. Generally, no special precautions are necessary.

Internal radiation therapy

Internal radiation therapy (brachytherapy) uses implants of radioactive substances, sealed up in thin wires, catheters or tubes, to deliver a high dose of radiation to a small area of your body, such as a section of your breast.

The objective of internal radiation is to place the radiation as close as possible to the site where the cancer was removed (see the color illustration on page 271). This method concentrates the radiation to the site at highest risk of a cancer recurrence and attempts to reduce damage to nearby normal tissue, such as your lungs, heart and normal breast tissue. Internal radiation can be done in a much shorter time than can external therapy — usually three to five days.

During lumpectomy, or later as a separate procedure, a catheter or another holder for the radioactive material is implanted in the area from where the tumor was taken (tumor bed). The holder is then

RESEARCH UPDATE

Improved radiation delivery

Doctors continue to study alternative ways to deliver radiation that may result in fewer side effects and more effective and convenient treatments.

- For women with early-stage breast cancer, researchers are studying use of external beam radiation to only part of the breast, instead of the entire breast.
- Researchers are experimenting with dividing up a daily dose of radiation into smaller doses given twice a day (hyperfractionated therapy) in the hope that it may be more effective than is standard dosing.
- For individuals who live a long distance from a medical center and need to be away from home while receiving treatment, doctors are investigating giving a larger daily dose of radiation to shorten the time required to complete the treatments.
- Scientists are investigating whether internal radiation may be used as an alternative to external beam radiation. Because of the brief treatment period, it may be an option for women who aren't able to receive daily treatments for several weeks.
- Researchers are studying whether a large, single external beam radiation treatment could be safely and effectively given during a lumpectomy when the incision is still open, to decrease the amount of radiation needed after surgery.

loaded with seeds of radioactive substances that radiate nearby cancer cells.

In general, internal radiation may be given as low-dose rate (LDR), in which the implants stay in place for several days, or high-dose rate (HDR), in which the radiation is delivered for a short period twice a day for fewer days. High-dose radiation is more common, but either method may be used.

What to expect

Low-dose internal radiation usually requires a few days' hospital stay. If the radiation holder wasn't implanted during your cancer surgery, a doctor may insert it in a separate procedure under local, regional or general anesthesia. After the holder is in place, the radioactive seeds are loaded into the holder.

Because other people can be exposed to the radioactive materials inside you, you'll stay in a private room and visitors will be limited. Children and pregnant women probably should wait to see you until you're out of the hospital to avoid risk of unnecessary exposure. Hospital staff will work quickly with you to avoid exposure themselves. This is to limit unnecessary radiation exposure, even at low levels, to individuals other than the person being treated. Don't be afraid to ask for help, though, if you need it, and don't feel offended. Remember, the radiation is performing a therapeutic function.

After the scheduled amount of time, the implants are removed. Once the implants are taken out, your body no longer contains any radioactivity, and you're free to spend as much time with others as you wish.

Side effects

Radiation is a cumulative process. With daily external beam radiation therapy, side effects tend to become more of an issue as treatment continues. Fatigue is the most common side effect. It's a good idea to plan for this possibility so that you can rest whenever you feel the need. Sometimes, putting your feet up for 15 to 20 minutes is enough.

Other side effects include skin irritation, such as itchiness, redness, shininess, soreness, peeling, blistering, swelling and decreased sensation or hypersensation. Many of these signs and symptoms may be similar to those you've experienced with a sunburn. They gradually go away after treatment ends. To reduce skin irritation, take precautions to avoid exposing the radiated area to direct sun.

A small percentage of women experience more serious problems that may be temporary or chronic, such as swelling in the arm, lung damage, nerve damage and increased susceptibility to broken ribs.

Some changes to the breast may be permanent after radiation. These include a difference in skin color, a feeling of heaviness in the breast, changes in the texture of the breast and even changes in breast size.

Internal radiation therapy usually produces fewer skin reactions. However, this form of radiation may cause swelling of your breast and possibly infection at the site of the implant.

If you develop any bothersome signs and symptoms during or after radiation treatment, make sure to discuss them with your doctor.

Decision Guide: Lumpectomy vs. Mastectomy

Deciding between a lumpectomy and a mastectomy isn't always easy. A number of issues need to be considered, including the stage of your cancer, your risk of recurrence, how you feel about having a breast removed and how convenient it is for you to receive follow-up radiation therapy after a lumpectomy.

Many women prefer to keep their affected breast, despite a slightly higher chance of in-breast (local) recurrence. Others prefer mastectomy. Women who feel anxious about the possibility that the cancer might return may be willing to sacrifice their breast for a lower risk of a local recurrence. Neither option is right, and neither is wrong. It's a personal choice.

The table on page 169 lists some of the pros and cons of removing just a portion of your breast (lumpectomy) or all of it (mastectomy). In addition, following is a list of frequently asked questions and answers that may help address some of your questions. Finally, we've included the stories of three women who've undergone breast surgery. They talk about how they decided on their treatments and how they feel about their decisions now.

It's hoped that this information will help you in making your decision. But it's also important that you talk with your doctor about your situation. If you have questions about your diagnosis, treatment or prognosis, be sure to have your doctor explain things to you in detail and make

sure that you understand what he or she is saying.

Factors to consider

As you make decisions on the best way to treat your breast cancer, you'll want to weigh each choice against your personal values and with your lifestyle in mind. The following questions may help you work through this process:

How do you generally approach health care?

Think about how you approach other health care issues. Are you the type of person who needs to feel that she has done everything medically possible to fight this disease? If so, you may be more comfortable if you're more aggressive in your treatment. If you're more conservative when it comes to medical intervention, you might prefer to avoid the risks and inconveniences of more aggressive treatment.

Once treatment ends, how much do you think you'll continue to worry?

If you choose lumpectomy and radiation, how will you feel living each day with a breast that once harbored cancer? Despite the scientific evidence that the long-term outcomes of mastectomy and lumpectomy with radiation are virtually the same, some women discover that they worry more about recurrence when breast tissue remains. If you still have part of your breast after treatment, will that increase your worry? If so, would removal of the entire breast significantly reduce that worry? These are clearly psychological

BREAST CANCER

questions rather than medical ones, but they're worth asking yourself.

How do you feel about losing a breast?

For some women, the loss of a breast is not significant when weighed against their fear of dying of cancer. For others, breasts are closely connected to their self-image. They feel that removing a breast is too great a sacrifice when it doesn't improve overall survival.

How will your choice affect your partner?

Ultimately, the decision is yours to make. But if you're married or in a relationship, you may want to think about how your choice will affect your partner. This is a difficult area for many couples. But a frank and open discussion before any surgery will help to avoid problems afterward. Whether you choose mastectomy or lumpectomy with radiation, your partner's sexual attitude toward you may be affected. With some couples, the loss of a breast might leave a permanent, daily reminder of the cancer to both partners. On the other hand, during radiation treatment many women experience fatigue, and some women experience hypersensitivity in their breasts and don't want to be touched. If you opt for breast reconstruction, the resulting change in sensation may alter your sexual practices. Information from your medical team or a breast cancer support group may help you consider all these possibilities.

Can your lifestyle accommodate the daily routine of radiation therapy?

Making the decision to have radiation can be different from living with that decision.

Look closely at your support system. Can you meet the Monday through Friday commitment for the five to six weeks needed for radiation treatment? Are you physically able to drive to the treatment center each day? Is public transportation an option? Some women need someone to accompany them. Others need help with child care. Some take their children along and couple the outing with an activity of interest to the children.

How will your treatment choices affect your family?

Again, the decision is yours to make, not your family's. But you may want to consider the time that your treatment will involve and how that will affect your family.

- You'll need time to recuperate from your surgery.
- If you choose radiation, you'll need to commit to appointments each weekday for five to six weeks.

The type of treatment you decide on will affect how much you can do. Will your family be able to adapt to your treatment demands? It's a good idea to talk through these issues with all members of your family in advance so that they'll know what to expect and so that all of you, as a family, can plan how best to meet each person's needs while you're being treated for your cancer.

How will your treatment choices affect your work?

If you work outside the home, can your job accommodate your treatment schedule? Radiation requires a daily weekday commitment for five to six weeks. Ask if

Lumpectomy vs. mastectomy: The pros and cons

The following table lists some of the advantages and disadvantages of a lumpectomy with radiation and a mastectomy. For more information on the risk of cancer recurrence and the different types of recurrence, see Chapter 13.

Procedure	Pros	Cons
Lumpectomy with radiation	**Keeping your breast.** This can be of great psychological value for some women. **Near-normal appearance.** Your breast may appear much the same as before surgery.	**Risk of cancer recurrence.** Carries a slightly greater risk of an in-breast (local) recurrence than does a mastectomy. Younger women have higher risk. **Need for a second operation.** If all the cancer isn't removed during the first surgery, you may need a second lumpectomy or a mastectomy. **Unsatisfactory cosmetic results.** This may happen if you have a large amount of tissue removed. **Need for radiation.** Radiation requires regular appointments for about five to six weeks. Side effects of radiation therapy may include swelling and pain in your breast, fatigue, and temporary skin reaction similar to a sunburn, as well as long-term skin and tissue changes.
Mastectomy	**Radiation may not be needed.** After a mastectomy, many women don't need radiation therapy. **No need for a second operation.** Because the entire breast has been removed, there's rarely a need for additional surgery, other than reconstruction, if you so desire. **Reduced risk of cancer recurrence.** Usually has less risk of a local recurrence than does a lumpectomy. However, cancer can still recur in the mastectomy scar. The chance of developing a new tumor in remaining chest wall tissue years later is low.	**Loss of a breast.** There's often a certain amount of grieving after losing a breast. The surgery may leave a daily physical reminder of your disease, which can be difficult. **Sexual self-image.** Sometimes, the absence of a breast raises issues regarding sexual self-image and feminine identity. However, these often pass with time and support. **Feeling lopsided.** Some women, particularly those with large breasts, feel lopsided. Most get accustomed to the feeling over time. For others, the issue may be resolved with breast reconstruction. **Unusual sensations.** Infrequently, some women experience chronic tenderness or soreness around the scar.

you can schedule a regular appointment outside working hours, perhaps on your way to work or just after. Talk with your employer about taking time off during the workday. Think about the proximity of your workplace to your treatment location and how long you'll need to get there and back. Will your co-workers be able to accommodate if you require additional time off?

Meet other women

Each woman is unique. And so is her decision-making process. Sometimes, though, it's helpful to hear about someone else's experience. It may offer reassurance regarding the decision you make.

Below you'll find the stories of three women. Each made different treatment choices, and each is happy with the choices she made. These women don't necessarily represent the most typical treatment decisions, and the three stories together shouldn't be considered the three most common treatment paths. They're simply three people sharing their personal stories.

Jan's Story

Jan received a diagnosis of breast cancer at age 29. She chose to have both breasts removed (bilateral mastectomy), along with reconstruction, chemotherapy and radiation. This was considered unusually aggressive treatment at the time.

I'm the type of person who wants all the information, and I don't want it sugarcoated. I want members of my health care team to talk to me openly and honestly. Otherwise, you just don't have what you need to make the right decisions.

In 1987, when I was 29, my husband and I had been trying to have a child for some years. On a Friday morning, I went to an infertility clinic for an evaluation. During my basic physical, my doctor found a lump in my right breast. She assured me it was probably nothing but ordered a mammogram just to be sure. The right breast turned out to be fine, but my left breast had some calcifications that concerned the doctors.

Within an hour I saw a surgeon to talk over treatment options, and I saw a plastic surgeon to discuss reconstruction. The surgeon told me that at my age (if cancer was found in one breast) the risk of developing cancer in the other breast in my lifetime was 25 percent to 30 percent. That seemed pretty high to me.

When the biopsy determined it was cancer, I decided to have a double mastectomy. One factor in my decision was knowing that it's easier to get reconstructed breasts to match if you do the same thing to both breasts. A nurse showed me implants and talked about how I would look, which was very helpful. They were using silicone implants then, saline implants were just getting started. This was still Friday. The surgery was scheduled for Monday.

I was actually eager to go to surgery. I could've taken more time to decide, but I understood from the X-ray that it was likely to be cancer. At the same time, I knew this meant at least a delay, if not a change, in my plans to have a child.

On Monday they found a cancer measuring 4 centimeters. All my lymph nodes were benign. Thursday, I was home recuperating.

Shortly thereafter, I saw an oncologist. He reviewed my situation, went over all the test results, talked about where medical science was, discussed ongoing chemotherapy trials and told me there might be some benefit in having radiation or chemotherapy or both. I decided to go for both.

After six weeks of surgical leave, I returned to work from 8 a.m. to 3 p.m. and after work headed for chemotherapy. I had no severe side effects. I tried to remain really upbeat. I thought of therapy as my ally, something that would help me live longer.

Within a few weeks after finishing chemotherapy I started radiation. I went for five or six weeks, every day. I always made it a point to come out of the radiation with a big smile on my face to show other people that it was OK.

I kept a journal throughout the experience, which was really helpful because it gave me a place to record my feelings and let me go back and see where I had been. Occasionally, I still look at it, and it brings back some nice memories. It wasn't all bad. In a way, it was a gift to get this at age 29, because it let me know what was important to me and who was important to me. It brought up spirituality issues and a lot of other things that often don't occur to some people until much later in life.

The decisions I made were the right ones for me, and I'm very comfortable with them. I'm extremely glad that I saw different oncology doctors beforehand. The information I got from them really helped me make intelligent decisions.

Since my diagnosis, I've had three children, so now most of my focus is on being a mom to an eight-year-old girl and to five-year-old twin boys.

Colleen's Story

Colleen was 45 when she found out she had breast cancer. After weighing her treatment options, she chose a mastectomy.

In 1993, a close friend of mine was diagnosed with breast cancer, so I decided I should get myself checked, too. I had a history of fibrocystic disease, so I was accustomed to finding cysts when I checked my breasts. So when I felt a lump in my right breast, I thought it was probably a cyst. A cyst was confirmed by a mammogram and ultrasound. And I was told to watch it and check back again in a year.

More than a year passed. Then, early one morning while I was still in bed, I had this feeling someone was near the bed nudging me to get this lump checked again. When I opened my eyes, no one was there. But I mentioned it to my doctor that day, and that I thought the cyst was bigger. He scheduled me for a diagnostic mammogram and an ultrasound. That was in July 1994.

An ultrasound showed that the cyst had changed and was growing. The doctor offered me a choice of a needle biopsy immediately or surgery a week or so later. I opted for the needle biopsy because I could get the results sooner. When they called the next day, they told me I needed another appointment. I had cancer. I met with the surgeon on Monday, and that Wednesday I was in surgery.

The surgeon gave me the option of lumpectomy with radiation or a mastectomy. My husband and I talked. It turned out we felt the same way. I decided I would rather have the mastectomy and not have to deal with any other treatment.

I was OK about making decisions quickly, but I don't think it really hit me until I was waiting to be rolled into surgery. I wound up lying on the gurney with tears rolling down my face. The nurses were very comforting.

They found a stage II cancer, but no lymph nodes were involved. Because the tumor was deeper than they expected, my doctor told me afterward that mastectomy was probably the best call.

My family handled it well. My daughter in college was initially upset but felt better once she learned that lymph nodes weren't involved. One son had just entered Marine boot camp, and we weren't even able to reach him until it was all over. My older son was very involved in supporting me. And my husband was very understanding. Also, my sisters are close and were supportive.

I didn't have a lot of pain waking up. That came later because a rather large nerve was cut. I still have a lot of numbness under my arm. I wasn't really prepared for that. And it probably took three years for my hand to get its full strength back. That surprised me the most.

I just finished a five-year course of tamoxifen. I still go for a follow-up every four to six months because my oncologist wants me checked that often. I'd like to say it doesn't bother me but it does. You want to go because you want to hear it's OK. But you don't want to go because you're afraid they're going to find something.

Once you've had a close call with cancer, you always have to be prepared for the worst. I know I may develop cancer one day, but I also know I'm watched carefully, which means it's more likely to be caught early. I try to enjoy each day because I never know what's ahead.

Rosemarie's Story

Rosemarie was 48 when she noticed a lump. She decided to have a lumpectomy followed by chemotherapy and radiation.

In October 1995, I was standing, talking with someone, and I crossed my arms and felt this pecan-sized lump in my breast. I wasn't really worried because everyone told me that if it was cancer, it wouldn't hurt, and this lump felt sore. I called my gynecologist who sent me for a mammogram, and while I was there, they did an ultrasound, too. The radiologist thought I might have a cyst, but when she tried to drain it with a needle, the lump appeared to be solid. Then she told me I needed a biopsy. I was scheduled to take a trip and decided I wanted to do that first, so I didn't have the biopsy until late November 1995 when they removed a small section of tissue.

My gynecologist called a week later and asked me to come to his office on a Saturday morning and suggested I bring a friend. That's when he told me I had cancer. The section of breast that was removed during the biopsy didn't leave clean margins, so my doctor told me I needed a mastectomy. Mine wasn't an aggressive cancer, so I took some time to think about it.

I wound up seeing a breast specialist on Dec. 18, my 49th birthday. He told me I could have a lumpectomy if I chose. That's what I decided to do. I had the surgery on Dec. 26. This time, they removed a bigger section of tissue and 21 lymph nodes, which all turned out to be negative. I wish I had known beforehand about a sentinel node biopsy, because then I wouldn't have had to have so many nodes removed.

The only unexpected part of the surgery was managing the drains. That felt kind of overwhelming, but fortunately my mother came to stay with me and helped.

My oncologist told me that if I had chemotherapy, it would increase my survival chances 20 percent, and radiation would increase those chances another 10 percent. I decided to do both.

I had the chemotherapy first, four treatments, 21 days apart. My biggest fear about chemotherapy was losing my hair, and I did. About 14 days after the first treatment, nearly all of it came off one day in the shower. The few clumps that were left, I just pulled out. For about a week, I wore a wig that I hated. Then I tried new and different ways to wrap scarves around my head. And some days, I just went out without anything. I was more bothered by the loss of my eyelashes and eyebrows than the hair on my head because that's what really makes you look like a cancer patient.

The first seven days after each treatment was really the worst time for me. I felt weak. I didn't really want to get out of bed, and I did feel nauseated, although I never actually threw up. But I kept going to work. For me, being with people helped me deal with having cancer.

Once the chemo ended, I went for radiation. The treatments weren't too bad. I went on my lunch hour. Midafternoon I'd get a little tired. About midway through treatment I did develop a radiation burn on the underside of my breast. That was uncomfortable, and they finally put a bandage on it to block it from rubbing against my bra.

Since my treatment, I've had some problems with lymphedema. I try not to use that arm for lifting, and when I travel, I wear a

pressurized sleeve. That part has been frustrating. I also developed costochondritis, a kind of arthritis between the chest and rib bone that my internist told me is a result of radiation. Some days I can't touch my chest because of pain, and then other days I don't feel a thing.

Being in a support group has helped a lot. You get so much information and so many helpful hints. And when I get an ache or pain, chances are when I check with the group, someone else has had the same thing. So then I don't have to worry.

Now that I've passed the five-year mark, I only see my oncologist once a year. I haven't forgotten I had cancer. I know it can always come back, but I don't let things bother me. It took me awhile to get there, but I'm appreciating life more. I look at all the little things that make me happy, and whatever makes me happy, I do.

Adjuvant Systemic Therapy

Surgery and radiation are referred to as locoregional therapy because they target cancer cells in one specific area. However, doctors can't be certain that all the cancer cells were removed during surgery or destroyed with radiation. There's always the possibility that some cells have been left behind. Or, some may have broken off from the primary tumor and traveled to other parts of your body through the bloodstream or the lymph system. These cells may hide, growing until they reach a size in which they can be seen on an X-ray or felt during examination.

To try to eradicate any microscopic cancer cells, your doctor may suggest additional (adjuvant) whole-body (systemic) therapy in addition to local therapy. The goal of adjuvant systemic therapy is to destroy any remaining cancer cells throughout your body to help you remain cancer-free and live longer. Most women with invasive breast cancer are candidates for some form of additional therapy.

Might you benefit?

Several key pieces of information need to be taken into account when considering adjuvant systemic therapy. The first of these are called prognostic factors, factors that are based on characteristics of your tumor and on your own personal characteristics. Prognostic factors, such as the degree of cancer spread to the lymph nodes, the tumor size, your age and the tumor grade, can help predict the outcome of your cancer (prognosis). Using this information, along with other factors, and keeping in mind the benefits and risks of each type of therapy, you and your doctor can decide on the best plan for you.

You may benefit from additional (adjuvant) therapy if:

The cancer has spread to lymph nodes

The degree of cancer spread to underarm (axillary) lymph nodes (nodal status) is the prognostic factor that typically provides the most information about your chances of being cured. As discussed previously in this chapter, during surgery the surgeon usually does a sentinel node biopsy or removes some of the lymph nodes in your axillary nodes to look for cancer cells that may have spread from your breast. If cancer is found in any of the nodes, there's a greater chance that cancer cells may have spread to other parts of your body.

The tumor is larger in size

Tumor size is the second most important prognostic factor. Women with smaller tumors usually have better outcomes than do women with larger tumors, especially tumors larger than 5 centimeters (about 2 inches) in diameter.

You're younger

Younger women, especially those 35 and younger, sometimes have a more aggressive type of breast cancer and a poorer prognosis than do older women with otherwise similar tumor characteristics.

The tumor is high grade

The grade of a tumor refers to how it looks under a microscope. Tumor cells that resemble normal breast cells are called well differentiated or low grade (grade 1). Those that look very abnormal are referred to as poorly differentiated, or high grade (grade 3). Moderately differentiated (grade 2) cells fall somewhere in between. Well differentiated cancers usually have the best prognosis.

Other factors

Scientists are exploring additional factors that may help predict who will benefit from adjuvant systemic therapy. Some factors under investigation include:

- **Cell proliferation.** This test measures the percentage of tumor cells that are

QUESTION & ANSWER

Q: What's adjuvant therapy?

A: Adjuvant therapy is another name for additional treatment. Adjuvant therapy is given to a person who has no visible evidence of any leftover cancer after the first (primary) treatment — usually surgery — has been completed and who may be cured of his or her cancer.

Because there's a risk that an individual may still have some cancer cells in his or her body that weren't detected during primary treatment, additional treatment is given to decrease the chance that the cancer will come back.

dividing (proliferating). A higher rate of cell proliferation may indicate a more aggressive cancer and thus a greater need for additional therapy.

- **Oncogene activation.** An oncogene is an altered gene that causes uncontrolled cell growth. In their normal states, these genes have useful functions, such as regulating cell division and tissue repair. When they become damaged (mutated), they're labeled as oncogenes, and the proteins they produce can turn normal cells into cancer cells. HER-2/neu is an oncogene associated with breast cancer. Its presence usually signals a more aggressive breast cancer, and it may predict an increased risk of resistance to some anti-cancer drugs.

Therapy options

Adjuvant systemic therapy may consist of hormone therapy, chemotherapy or a combination of the two. Many women with hormone receptor positive cancer cells receive both chemotherapy and hormone therapy, as these two different types of therapy can complement each other.

Hormone therapy is usually given after chemotherapy.

Chemotherapy

Chemotherapy is the term for a group of medications that are toxic to cancer cells. The drugs interfere with uncontrolled cell growth, a common characteristic of cancer cells. Unfortunately, chemotherapy drugs can also affect rapidly dividing normal, healthy cells, leading to a number of adverse side effects. However, the drugs don't affect healthy cells as much as they do cancer cells. Most of your normal, healthy cells aren't dividing and, therefore, they aren't as susceptible to the effects of chemotherapy medications as are cancer cells.

Chemotherapy is usually given over a period of three to six months in one- to four-week cycles. The medications are most often given intravenously, but some types can be taken orally. At times, two or three different chemotherapy drugs are given at the same time, to attack tumors in a variety of ways. Each treatment session is followed by a period of recovery

Making a Decision

To help you make an intelligent choice regarding the use of adjuvant systemic therapy, consider the following steps:

1. Find out and understand what your chances are of being cured without adjuvant systemic therapy.
2. Find out and understand the benefits of adjuvant systemic therapy in terms of increasing your chances of a cure.
3. Find out and understand the risks (side effects) associated with different adjuvant systemic therapy options.
4. Weigh the benefits against the risks.
5. Make an informed personal decision with your health care team.

before the next session. For instance, if you received a round of chemotherapy today, you might receive the next treatment in one to four weeks. You can usually go to an outpatient clinic to receive your treatment, which doesn't require a hospital stay.

Some commonly used chemotherapy drugs and drug combinations include:

Cyclophosphamide

Cyclophosphamide (Cytoxan, Neosar) was one of the earliest chemotherapy agents used as adjuvant systemic therapy. This drug interferes with the growth of cancer cells by blocking the ability of cancer cells to copy their genetic material (DNA). Common side effects include nausea, vomiting, hair loss, lowered blood counts, fatigue, fever, chills and drug-induced menopause.

Doxorubicin

Doxorubicin (Adriamycin) belongs to the general group of medicines known as anthracyclines. Chemotherapy regimens containing anthracyclines have been found to have a slight advantage over many that don't. Common side effects include nausea, vomiting, hair loss, lowered blood counts and fatigue. Very rarely, doxorubicin can cause leukemia or heart damage. With correct dosing, these long-term risks are minimal but they should be taken into account when considering use of doxorubicin.

5-fluorouracil

5-fluorouracil, which is also called 5-FU (Adrucil), is an antimetabolite. It interferes with the growth of cancer cells by blocking enzymes necessary for DNA synthesis. Side effects of fluorouracil include mouth sores and diarrhea.

Methotrexate

Methotrexate also belongs to the group of medicines known as antimetabolites. It works by blocking an enzyme needed by cells to make DNA. Common side effects of methotrexate include lowered blood counts and mouth sores.

Taxanes

Paclitaxel (Onxol, Taxol) and docetaxel (Taxotere) come from the group of drugs called taxanes. These are relatively new adjuvant therapy agents. They disrupt cell division by interfering with the cellular machinery that separates a dividing cell into two new cells.

Because these drugs have been used with success in treating metastatic breast cancer, scientists began evaluating their use in adjuvant systemic therapy. Relatively new data show that these drugs — in addition to the medications doxorubicin (Adriamycin) and cyclophosphamide (Cytoxan, Neosar) — may further improve survival. Common side effects include muscle aches, hair loss, numbness or tingling in fingers or toes, and lowered blood counts. Allergic reactions also can occur.

Side effects

Chemotherapy can cause both short-term and long-term side effects that may affect your quality of life.

Hormone Receptor Status

Estrogen, the principal female hormone, is known to influence the growth and development of certain breast tumors. Normal breast tissue cells contain receptors for estrogen and progesterone, another female hormone. Receptors are cell proteins that bind to specific substances in your bloodstream, such as hormones. You might think of receptors and hormones as a lock and key. If the hormone fits with the receptor, it opens the door for the cell to grow (see page 182).

Many breast cancer cells have hormone receptors for estrogen, progesterone or both. These cancers are called hormone (estrogen or progesterone) receptor positive. Breast cancer cells are analyzed in the lab to see if they have hormone receptors. Hormone receptor positive cancers may shrink with hormone therapy. Hormone receptor negative cancers usually don't.

Although the hormone receptor status of your cancer doesn't say much about your chances of a long-term cure — that is, it's not a good prognostic factor — it can tell your doctor whether hormone therapy treatment is likely to help. The hormone receptor status is called a predictive factor, a factor that helps predict what treatment might be useful.

Whether you've entered menopause also is a predictive factor in your treatment decision. During menopause, your ovaries make less estrogen and progesterone until eventually they stop producing them altogether. This may make a difference in the type of therapy you receive. For example, if you've already entered menopause, shutting down your ovaries (ovarian ablation) wouldn't be of much benefit to you, but a fairly new class of drugs called aromatase inhibitors may be, as you'll find out later in the chapter.

Chemotherapy Combinations

Over the years, evidence has suggested that combining chemotherapy drugs decreases the chance that resistance will develop and thereby increases the chance of a cure. Often, women receiving additional therapy are given two or more chemotherapy drugs at once.

Drug combinations often are abbreviated using the first letter of each drug. Those combinations frequently used in adjuvant systemic treatment of breast cancer are:

- **AC:** Doxorubicin (*A* is for Adriamycin, a brand name) and cyclophosphamide
- **AC + paclitaxel:** Doxorubicin (Adriamycin), cyclophosphamide and paclitaxel (Taxol)
- **CAF:** Cyclophosphamide, doxorubicin (Adriamycin) and fluorouracil
- **CEF:** Cyclophosphamide, epirubicin (similar to doxorubicin) and fluorouracil
- **CMF:** Cyclophosphamide, methotrexate and fluorouracil
- **TAC:*** Docetaxel (Taxotere), doxorubicin (Adriamycin) and cyclophosphamide
- **TC:*** Paclitaxel (Taxol) and cyclophosphamide
  These combinations are relatively new.

To determine the best combination for you, your doctor looks at a number of factors, including any pre-existing conditions you might have and how well the two of you think that you can manage the side effects of different drugs.

Short-term side effects

Normal, healthy cells located in your blood, hair follicles and digestive tract are some of the most rapidly dividing cells in your body. Many anti-cancer drugs have been designed to target rapidly dividing cancer cells. But they may also damage rapidly dividing normal cells, such as those in the hair follicles, bone marrow and digestive tract. The result may be a number of side effects.

Different chemotherapy drugs given at different dosages cause different side effects in each woman. Some women lose their hair and their appetite, and others may experience increased appetite, nausea, vomiting, diarrhea, lowered blood counts or mouth sores. The effect of chemotherapy on blood cells may make you more prone to infection, bruising and bleeding. In addition, you may have less energy during and after treatment. It's not possible to know ahead of time all of the side effects you may experience. Most short-term side effects go away when treatment ends. For example, your hair will grow back, although it may return with a different color or texture or both.

Medications are available that help block nausea and vomiting caused by chemotherapy. Sometimes, changing the dose of chemotherapy you receive or adjusting your chemotherapy schedule will help counter side effects. If chemotherapy caused your infection-fighting (white) blood cells to drop too low, your doctor may recommend that you avoid people who are sick or give you a medication with the next chemotherapy cycle to stimulate your bone marrow to make blood cells faster. For more information on managing short-term side effects of chemotherapy, see Chapter 35.

Long-term side effects

A possible long-term side effect of chemotherapy in premenopausal women is ovarian dysfunction. This may cause menstruation to stop (amenorrhea), sometimes permanently. When permanent, this condition is often called chemotherapy-induced menopause. How often this occurs varies with different types of chemotherapy drugs and the age of the woman receiving the medication. Cyclophosphamide tends to produce a higher rate of amenorrhea than do some of the other chemotherapy drugs.

The chances of chemotherapy-induced menopause are much higher for women over age 40. In younger women, menstruation may return after chemotherapy is completed, although in some cases many months later. For the majority of women over age 40 — especially those over 45 —

chemotherapy will cause menstruation to permanently stop.

Loss of ovarian function may cause several side effects, including menopausal symptoms such as hot flashes, insomnia, mood swings and vaginal dryness. In addition, similar to what occurs in menopause, you may experience a reduction in bone mineralization, leading to osteoporosis and an increased risk of bone fractures. You may wish to have periodic bone density tests and consider treatments to prevent bone loss.

Some medications, such as paclitaxel (Taxol), can also cause damage to nerve endings in your fingers and toes. This can result in numbness, tingling or both. In rare cases, chemotherapy with anthracyclines has resulted in heart damage (congestive heart failure) and secondary cancers, such as cancer of the blood cells (leukemia). However, with the dosages of chemotherapy most commonly given for adjuvant chemotherapy, the chance of

Chemotherapy Before Surgery

In some cases, a doctor may recommend that a woman receive chemotherapy before surgery in order to shrink a large tumor and perhaps make it possible to have a lumpectomy instead of a mastectomy. Chemotherapy before surgery is called preoperative (neoadjuvant) therapy.

Chemotherapy has also been studied as an initial form of treatment for women with relatively small breast cancers. A large clinical trial randomly assigned women with stage II breast cancer to receive either neoadjuvant chemotherapy or standard postoperative adjuvant chemotherapy. No differences in survival or recurrence rates were noted in the two groups. However, there was a higher probability that women who received neoadjuvant chemotherapy were able to have a lumpectomy rather than a mastectomy because of a reduction in the size of the tumor, caused by the chemotherapy.

BREAST CANCER

each of these conditions occurring is generally less than 1 percent.

Hormone therapy

Hormone therapy is possibly the most important form of adjuvant systemic therapy for breast cancer when a tumor is estrogen or progesterone receptor positive, or both. The goal of hormone therapy is to block the effects of the female hormone estrogen, which is known to fuel a majority of breast cancers. Another female hormone, progesterone, also may play a role. Normally, estrogen and progesterone circulate through your bloodstream and latch on (bind) to certain cell proteins called receptors. Most breast cancer cells still make these receptors, and estrogen is believed to help these cancer cells grow and develop.

In one of the laboratory tests done on your breast tumor after it's removed from your breast, a pathologist — a specialist in diagnosing disease in tissue samples — checks to see if the tumor's cells are hormone receptive positive. He or she checks for both estrogen receptors and progesterone receptors.

If the cancer cells are hormone receptor positive, you may benefit from hormone therapy to control tumor growth. If your cancer cells are hormone receptor negative, hormone therapy isn't beneficial.

Adjuvant hormone therapy may take one of three different approaches:
- Use of anti-estrogen drugs, such as tamoxifen
- In premenopausal women, procedures to shut down the ovaries (ovarian ablation)
- In postmenopausal women, use of aromatase inhibitors

Tamoxifen

Anti-estrogen drugs work by attaching to estrogen receptors in estrogen receptor positive cancer cells and preventing them from binding with estrogen, thereby inhibiting growth of the cancer cells (see the illustration on page 182).

The most common anti-estrogen drug for the treatment of breast cancer is the synthetic anti-estrogen pill tamoxifen (Nolvadex). Tamoxifen is probably the most widely studied and — over the past couple of decades — the most widely used anti-cancer medication in the world. It has been credited with playing an important role in the reduction in breast cancer deaths.

Tamoxifen was first used to treat advanced breast cancer that had spread to other parts of the body (metastatic cancer). Subsequent studies have repeatedly shown that adjuvant tamoxifen can also reduce risk of cancer recurrence and death in women with early-stage breast cancer.

In recent years, the Early Breast Cancer Trialists' Collaborative Group published its third review of all the randomized clinical trial data pertaining to tamoxifen used as adjuvant therapy. Data from 37,000 women in 55 clinical trials showed that adjuvant tamoxifen treatment substantially lowered the rates of cancer recurrence and it improved 10-year survival in both premenopausal and postmenopausal women with estrogen receptor positive tumors.

Typically, the drug has been taken every day for five years. Research shows that

QUESTION & ANSWER

Q: **I've heard some women talk about chemo brain. What is it?**

A: *Chemo brain* (cognitive dysfunction) is a term often used to describe a poorly understood phenomenon that appears to occur in some women during or after chemotherapy. These women experience short-term memory and concentration problems. It's not known whether chemotherapy or something else causes this, how long it lasts or what can be done about it. This is a subject of active clinical research. Ongoing trials are addressing the potential causes of this phenomenon. Other trials are designed to test whether some substances, such as the herb ginkgo, might lessen the severity of the problem.

five years of tamoxifen use is better than short-term use in helping women live longer and cancer-free. But the bulk of available evidence suggests that using tamoxifen for more than five years, compared with stopping at five years, doesn't provide any greater benefit and it might actually be related to increased cancer recurrences and side effects. This may be because with longer-term exposure to tamoxifen, this drug may begin to act more like estrogen on breast cancer cells (see "Tamoxifen's dual role" on page 183).

New evidence now suggests that in women past menopause, a type of medication called aromatase inhibitors might be added to, or even replace, tamoxifen. A discussion of aromatase inhibitors begins on page 183.

Side effects

Tamoxifen's most common side effects are hot flashes and vaginal discharge. Tamoxifen is also associated with an increased risk of cancer of the uterus (endometrial cancer or uterine sarcoma).

In women who haven't had a hysterectomy, it can increase the rate of uterine cancer threefold. Although this sounds like a pretty big increase, it means that it can increase a postmenopausal woman's chance of developing uterine cancer from a one in 1,000 chance a year to a three in 1,000 chance a year. About 80 percent of tamoxifen-induced uterine cancers can be cured by removal of the uterus (hysterectomy), with or without the use of additional radiation therapy.

The most common sign of uterine cancer in postmenopausal women is vaginal bleeding, which in this case is actually uterine bleeding passing through the vagina. If this occurs, a gynecologic evaluation along with a sampling of uterine (endometrial) tissue should be done. But don't panic if you experience vaginal bleeding while taking tamoxifen. Vaginal bleeding isn't always related to uterine cancer. Rather, it may stem from a noncancerous (benign) cause.

Tamoxifen also affects bone density. In postmenopausal women, tamoxifen helps to preserve bone density because it appears that bones react to tamoxifen as an estrogen-like agent. In a pre-menopausal woman, though, tamoxifen may actually compete with estrogen in binding with estrogen receptors in bone cells. Because tamoxifen is not as strong of a bone-growth stimulator as estrogen is, it can cause bone thinning in pre-menopausal women.

Tamoxifen can also increase the risk of blood clots. When a blood clot travels to your lungs, it's called a pulmonary embolism. In one study, .9 percent of tamoxifen users developed a blood clot over a five-year period, compared with .15 percent of nonusers. Tamoxifen is also associated with increased cataract problems and, rarely, retinal problems.

Ovarian ablation

Ovarian ablation is the oldest form of systemic therapy for premenopausal women with early-stage breast cancer. It consists of shutting down your ovaries to reduce

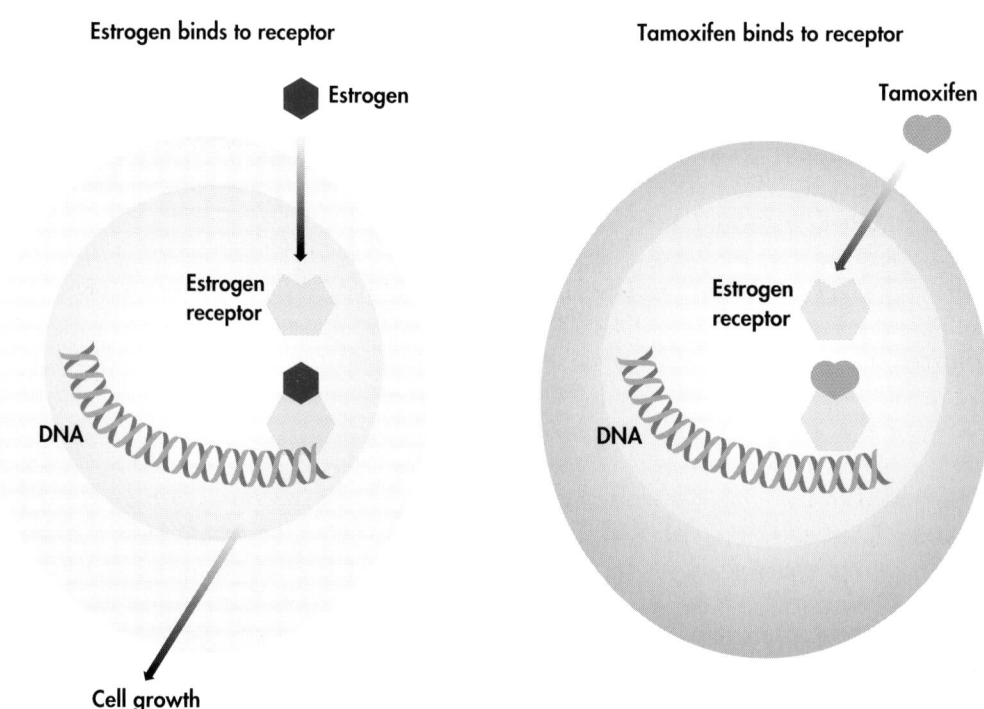

Estrogen receptor positive cell

Estrogen binds to receptor

Estrogen

Estrogen receptor

DNA

Cell growth

Tamoxifen binds to receptor

Tamoxifen

Estrogen receptor

DNA

The illustration on the left shows how the hormone estrogen attaches to estrogen receptors within cells, stimulating cell growth. The drug tamoxifen (right) also attaches to estrogen receptors. It prevents estrogen from binding to the receptors, inhibiting the growth of cancer cells.

Tamoxifen's Dual Role

Tamoxifen (Nolvadex) is used to treat breast cancer because of its anti-estrogen properties. But in some body tissues, it actually behaves like estrogen. Therefore, it's said to be both an estrogen agonist and estrogen antagonist.

What does that mean? It means that tamoxifen works in different ways in different parts of your body. In some breast cells, such as those found in women with estrogen receptor positive breast cancer, it attaches to the receptors in cancer cells and blocks estrogen binding and activity, which means it's functioning as an antagonist. In other tissues, such as in the uterus and bones, tamoxifen attaches to estrogen receptors and promotes cell growth and activity in a way similar to estrogen, meaning it's functioning as an agonist. Because of tamoxifen's estrogen-like effects on the uterus, it increases the chance of uterine cancer. At the same time, it's thought to help maintain bone strength in postmenopausal women.

the production of female hormones in your body. This may be done with surgery, with radiation or with the use of hormones — luteinizing hormone-releasing hormone (LH-RH) agonists, also known as gonadotropin-releasing hormone (Gn-RH) agonists.

A review of 12 trials of ovarian ablation by surgery or radiation revealed that it improved the 15-year survival rate in premenopausal women. Ovarian ablation wasn't beneficial, though, for postmenopausal women. This, most likely, is because their ovaries had already naturally stopped producing hormones.

During the past few decades, adjuvant ovarian ablation therapy has fallen out of favor, especially in North America, with more interest being given to chemotherapy. However, European oncologists have compared ovarian ablation and chemotherapy, concluding that ovarian ablation may be as good as some types of chemotherapy. This issue continues to be one of much study and debate. Trials are under way to see if ovarian ablation may provide additional benefit when combined with chemotherapy, tamoxifen or both.

Side effects

The side effects of ovarian ablation are the same as those of menopause, including halting of menstruation, infertility, vaginal dryness, hot flashes, osteoporosis and mood swings.

Aromatase inhibitors

Although your ovaries are the main source of estrogen, your body can produce the hormone in other ways, even after menopause. Your adrenal glands, located above your kidneys, produce several hormones, including androgens. An enzyme called aromatase that's predominant in tissues such as fat, liver, muscle and brain — as well as in normal breast tissue and breast cancer tissue — converts androgens into estrogens.

Q: **If I'm taking tamoxifen but haven't gone through menopause yet, will I still continue to get my period?**

A: Probably. Among premenopausal women taking tamoxifen, the ovaries usually continue to function, although among some women their periods may stop or become irregular. In fact, tamoxifen may cause premenopausal women to produce more estrogen. It's essential that you avoid getting pregnant while taking tamoxifen because it could harm the fetus.

Medications called aromatase inhibitors work by keeping aromatases from creating estrogen. So far, the drugs appear useful only in postmenopausal women. In premenopausal women, aromatase inhibitors aren't able to decrease total estrogen production by a significant amount, and therefore aren't effective. That's because the ovaries are still producing estrogen.

Aromatase inhibitors include the drugs anastrozole (Arimidex), letrozole (Femara) and exemestane (Aromasin).

Aromatase inhibitors vs. tamoxifen

The aromatase inhibitor anastrozole was studied in one of the largest breast cancer drug trials ever, with more than 9,000 women participating. In this study, postmenopausal women with recently diagnosed, early-stage breast cancer were given anastrozole, tamoxifen or both, to be taken for five years.

Early results indicate that anastrozole is better than is tamoxifen in improving disease-free survival — but only by about 1 percent to 2 percent. Anastrozole also produced fewer short-term side effects than did tamoxifen.

Although the findings of this study are promising for the use of anastrozole — particularly because tamoxifen carries an increased risk of blood clots and uterine cancer — more research is still needed. Among other things, anastrozole was associated with a higher rate of some side effects, such as musculoskeletal pain, than was tamoxifen. There's also some suggestion — but no proof — that the drug may increase risk of osteoporosis.

Additional studies

Two other studies have added to the aromatase inhibitor vs. tamoxifen debate. The first involved 5,000 women who had completed five years of tamoxifen therapy. The women were given either the aromatase inhibitor letrozole (Femara) or an inactive pill (placebo), which they took for another five years. Early study results, published in October 2003, showed a significant reduction in new breast cancer problems among women receiving letrozole, compared with those taking a placebo. Ninety-three percent of the women who took letrozole had no breast cancer-related troubles, compared with 87 percent of women taking a placebo.

Overall, the medication was well tolerated. Some participants experienced muscle aches and pains, but these were generally mild. Women taking letrozole tended to report more trouble with osteoporosis and bone fractures. But so far, there hasn't been definitive proof of significant differences between the letrozole and placebo groups with regard to bone problems.

Further analyses of the data from this study — and that of similar clinical trials involving use of aromatase inhibitors — will provide more helpful information regarding which women might benefit from the medication, and by how much. But based on what's known now, women who've taken tamoxifen for five years might want to consider additional treatment with letrozole.

The other study involved more than 5,000 women who had taken tamoxifen for only two to three years. The women were divided into two groups. One group continued to take tamoxifen for a total of five years. Women in the other group switched to the aromatase inhibitor exemestane (Aromasin), which they took for two to three years, for a total of five years of hormone treatment.

Early results of this study, reported in March 2004, favored the tamoxifen plus exemestane group, indicating a 5 percent reduction in breast cancer recurrences.

Exemestane was generally well tolerated with a slight increase in the incidence of joint pain and osteoporosis, compared with the tamoxifen only group. However, women in the exemestane group had a lower incidence of gynecologic symptoms, including muscle cramps and blood clots.

What next?

The studies conducted so far demonstrate that aromatase inhibitors appear to play an important role in treatment of postmenopausal women whose breast cancer is hormone receptor positive. However, it's still too early to clearly define exactly how these medications should be used. Many questions remain: Should aromatase inhibitors be used instead of tamoxifen, or should they be started after two to five years of tamoxifen use? How long should they be used? What are their long-term side effects?

Until researchers learn more about aromatase inhibitors, some doctors continue to recommend tamoxifen as the medication of first choice. Others are comfortable recommending an aromatase inhibitor instead of tamoxifen. Newer data will continue to influence these opinions.

Most doctors agree, though, that for women who can't take tamoxifen because of the risk of blood clots, an aromatase inhibitor should be recommended.

Watchful waiting

For women with small, node-negative cancers, local treatment alone may provide an excellent prognosis, and additional (adjuvant) therapy may not be needed. Watchful waiting can be a reasonable choice depending on a woman's particular situation. Some women feel there's not enough potential long-term benefit from adjuvant therapy, compared with its potential risks and side effects. Some women live long, healthy lives after breast cancer surgery without receiving any additional type of systemic treatment.

Herceptin

Trastuzumab (Herceptin) is a medication that has been found to be helpful in some women whose breast cancer has spread (metastasized) to distant areas of the body and who have specific receptors (HER-2/neu) on their cancer cells. You can read more about this drug in Chapter 3.

Because this drug is beneficial for some women with metastatic breast cancer, the question arises whether it might be helpful for women with HER-2/neu positive early-stage breast cancer. Women are participating in large clinical trials to address this question, but at present the actual advantages and disadvantages of taking this drug for early-stage breast cancer haven't been determined. If laboratory results of tissue cells taken from your tumor indicate the presence of HER-2/neu receptors, you may want to ask your doctor about the current status of Herceptin as adjuvant treatment for early-stage cancer.

Watchful waiting isn't the same as doing nothing. If you decline additional therapy, or it's not recommended, your doctor will encourage you to be vigilant with breast self-exams and mammograms. It's also important to have regular follow-up clinical examinations.

Watchful waiting has its own risks, mainly, an increased risk of cancer spread. However, for women with cancers that have a good prognosis, this increased risk may be very low.

Decision Guide: Adjuvant Systemic Therapy

Whether to receive adjuvant therapy isn't always a simple decision. A number of issues need to be considered in determining if it's the best choice for you.

Factors to consider

Following are some frequently asked questions and answers about adjuvant therapy. You'll also find stories of two women who talk about the decisions they made regarding adjuvant therapy and how they feel about it today. It's hoped that this information will help you in making your decision. If you have questions about your diagnosis, treatment or prognosis, discuss them with your doctor.

Do you want to do everything possible to prevent cancer from coming back?

If so, you may be more comfortable in the long run if you're more aggressive in your treatment choices. If, on the other hand, you generally prefer a more conservative approach when it comes to medical intervention, you might prefer to avoid the risks and side effects of more aggressive treatment.

Is there evidence that adjuvant systemic therapy helps a woman with cancer like yours live longer?

Adjuvant systemic therapy can help many women, but the benefit gained is different for each woman depending on a number of factors such as her age, the size of her primary tumor, her lymph node status and her hormone receptor status. With mathematical models of statistical averages, your doctor can help you figure out an estimate of the specific benefits to be gained in your situation.

For example, one such tool is called the Numeracy program (see "Calculating your own odds"). Its survival estimates are based on the results of multiple clinical trials and the opinions and experience of 11 practicing breast cancer oncologists from around the United States.

Consider the case of a woman less than 50 years of age with a hormone receptor positive tumor that's 1.5 centimeters in diameter. During surgery, the surgeon also found two lymph nodes that were positive for cancer. Using the Numeracy program, this woman has an estimated 56 percent chance of living without a cancer recurrence (disease-free survival) for 10 years with locoregional therapy alone. By taking tamoxifen, her chances of living disease-free for 10 years are calculated to increase to 65 percent. A combination of four cycles of standard chemotherapy and tamoxifen increases her chances of surviving 10 years without a recurrence of breast cancer to 73 percent.

If four more cycles of a different type of chemotherapy (paclitaxel) are added, the prognosis increases to 77 percent. And if eight cycles of chemotherapy are given every two weeks instead of every three, it's estimated her chance of living disease-free for 10 years would increase to 83 percent. In this situation, an additional medication called colony stimulating factor

Calculating Your Own Odds

You can access an easy-to-use Internet tool to help you calculate your chance of being cured by logging on to *www.MayoClinic.com* and searching under the term *Adjuvant Therapy for Breast Cancer*. Click on "Your Own Chances."

To use the calculator, you'll need to know:
• The size of your breast tumor in centimeters
• The grade of your tumor (grade 1, 2 or 3)
• Whether you had lymph nodes that contained cancer cells and, if so, how many
• Whether your cancer cells were found to be hormone receptor positive

Keep in mind, this tool isn't a substitute for an individual treatment plan. Be sure to ask your doctor to help you interpret the statistics to see how they may apply to you. It's also important to remember that such calculators generate only statistical averages, and their purpose is primarily to show how much you might benefit from adjuvant therapy, *not* to predict exactly how long you have to live.

needs to be given to stimulate your bone marrow to make white blood cells faster, so that the interval between chemotherapy treatments can be shortened.

It's important to understand that estimates are based on the most reliable assumptions available and that they're not perfect. However, understanding these numbers can help a woman and her doctor can make an informed decision.

Do the benefits of adjuvant systemic therapy appear to outweigh the risks?

Adjuvant chemotherapy and hormone therapy can improve cancer-free survival in many women. But there's a price to pay in the side effects that these drugs may cause. Have you weighed the pros and cons? How much importance do you place on the possibility of benefit from these drugs, compared with the potential side effects of the therapy?

Are you still hoping to have children?

Adjuvant systemic therapy can cause your ovaries to stop producing female hormones and may cause infertility.

Meet other women

Here are the stories of two women, Nancy and Jane, who made two different choices about adjuvant systemic therapy.

Although they're more than 20 years apart in age, they were both in their 30s (ages 30 and 36) when they received a diagnosis of breast cancer. Their therapy choices were different, but each choice made sense in each woman's case. Remember you, too, have choices. There's no one right answer for all women.

Nancy's Story

Nancy was 30 years old when she found a lump in her breast. Tests showed that she had a second lump that couldn't be felt. The larger lump was about 2 to 3 centimeters (cm), which is about 1 inch, in diameter, and one sentinel lymph node tested positive for cancer. Nancy looked for the best information she could find about the outcomes of women her age in her situation. She decided to have the AC chemotherapy combination — the A stands for Adriamycin, a brand name of the generic drug doxorubicin, and the C stands for cyclophosphamide. Her chemotherapy was followed by tamoxifen hormone therapy. She shared her story four months after she had completed chemotherapy and two months after returning to work. At this time, she had already begun taking tamoxifen.

Before she found the lump, Nancy was, in her words, "At the top of my game ... trucking along, doing what I do." She was 30, married, had a healthy baby daughter and had just stopped breast-feeding. She was also a busy doctor-in-training — a surgical resident. Then she stopped trucking. "I feel like my life was sort of derailed."

She found a lump in her breast through some unusual circumstances. She had recently had some fevers and wondered if she had a viral illness. Because she had just finished breast-feeding her daughter, her doctor had her check for signs of a breast infection, which may occur after breast-feeding. When she went home and did a breast self-exam, she found the lump. She remembers feeling something solid — thicker than other breast tissue — that was about a half-inch to three-quarters of an inch in diameter.

Nancy felt no pain, and nothing else seemed different.

A mammogram showed nothing abnormal. So an ultrasound test was done. It showed two lumps, one of which Nancy had not felt. Biopsies were done, and both lumps were shown to be invasive cancer.

Nancy chose to have a mastectomy on both breasts — even though nothing had been found in the other breast. Her age, the unreliability of the mammogram in her case and the fact that two lumps had been found — one of which no one could feel — all factored in her decision.

She was devastated by news that the cancer had spread to a lymph node. She remembers questioning herself. "I thought I had caught it relatively early. How could it have spread already?" Nancy had always thought that if you had cancer and it had spread, you wouldn't feel good. She felt great.

She already knew that adjuvant systemic therapy would be something to consider because of her relatively young age and the size of the cancer. That the cancer had spread to her lymph nodes pushed the decision even more. "Having the ability to do something more than just the surgery was sort of reassuring to me."

Nancy used statistics to help guide her decision. Her oncologist considered her age, tumor size, lymph node status, and that her tumor cells were hormone receptor positive. These factors helped Nancy and her doctor look at the best estimates of what happens to women like her over time when they choose adjuvant systemic therapy and when they don't. She also carefully analyzed the risks of adjuvant systemic therapy. In the end, she thought she had more to

gain than to lose by having both chemotherapy and tamoxifen.

During chemotherapy Nancy endured nausea, anemia, fatigue, hair loss and the knowledge that she may not be able to have more children. Energy was a major issue for her. She returned to a demanding job, on call every other night. At home were her 2-year-old daughter and her husband. Tamoxifen gave her hot flashes at first, but eventually they stopped.

If she had not had her young daughter, she might have made a different choice about adjuvant systemic therapy. "Absolutely, I'd hoped to have more children and again that jury's still out, but, you know, I have a healthy daughter now."

Jane's Story

Jane has had plenty of time to reflect calmly on a health history that could have been devastating. At the time she shared her story, it had been 17 years since she received her first breast cancer diagnosis and 14 years since she received a second diagnosis.

Jane wasn't always so cool about her experiences with breast cancer: "I was in my 30s, and the only thing I thought of was death sentence." She says that once you have cancer, you're always a little paranoid about your health. "In your first year (after the first diagnosis), you worry about every ache and pain. And then in your second year, it has to be more significant to get your attention," she recalls. "Well, the third year I was feeling pretty confident, and then all of a sudden I get another diagnosis. But I did get through that one too, and now it's 14 years later."

BREAST CANCER

Both times Jane had a lumpectomy and radiation. Both times she declined any adjuvant systemic therapy. Jane says she wasn't convinced about two things. She wasn't convinced that the benefits of adjuvant systemic therapy were proved in people like her with very small tumors and no cancer in the lymph nodes. And, she wasn't convinced that the benefits would outweigh the harms — especially in the long term. She says she wasn't very worried about hair loss or nausea or fatigue. It was the possibility that the therapy itself could cause other cancers that gave her the most concern.

A former vice president of an international technical education company, Jane has been comfortable analyzing numbers for years. She once taught a course in statistics. So she wasn't intimidated by statistics when it was time to make this important health care decision. The numbers just didn't stack up in favor of accepting adjuvant systemic therapy, so she declined with confidence. And she was determined to make a decision and never look back.

But Jane has also been vigilant. For the first year after her second lumpectomy and radiation, she saw a surgeon and radiation oncologist every three months. Then she slowly reduced the frequency of those visits. She continues to have annual mammograms. Her doctors carefully compare them with films from past years to scrutinize what might be scarring and what might be something else.

It's not just her breast health that her doctor checks. Jane has had colonoscopy procedures because of her family colon cancer history and her own cancer history.

"I view myself as cured of cancer, but at a higher than average risk of additional problems," she explains. "I'm quite optimistic about my battle with cancer, and I'm really excited and optimistic about what's happening in medical science."

She has become active in breast cancer advocacy work and gets satisfaction from conveying to women that "you can make good decisions, and you can survive."

Clinical Trials

A number of new approaches to breast cancer treatment and, in particular, adjuvant therapy, are being studied. The emphasis of breast cancer research is to find new or improved methods that can successfully treat women or extend their survival with the fewest side effects.

Much of what's practiced today in breast cancer treatment is the result of prior clinical trials in which thousands of women participated. Many previous clinical trials have led the way for treatments used today in clinical practice.

If you have breast cancer, you may wish to consider participating in a clinical trial. By taking part, you may be the first in line to receive the potential benefits of cutting edge breast cancer treatment. It's important to discuss the benefits and disadvantages of participation in a clinical trial with your doctor. For more information on clinical trials, see Chapter 2.

Chapter 10: Breast Cancer

Breast Reconstruction

A common concern of many women when deciding on surgical treatment for breast cancer is their appearance after surgery. This is especially true of women considering a mastectomy. While you're gathering information about your treatment options, you may also want to gather information on breast reconstruction.

Some women choose not to have any reconstructive surgery after mastectomy. That's OK. Such a decision is perfectly acceptable. In addition, some women decide not to wear a prosthesis, an artificial breast. Many women who take this route are content with this choice.

For women who do choose reconstructive surgery, there are several options available to consider. Breast reconstruction is a surgical procedure designed to restore a more naturally shaped breast mound after mastectomy. Reconstructive surgery, which is generally performed by a plastic surgeon, is complicated, and it can require a longer recovery than does mastectomy alone. At the same time, some women find reconstructive surgery easier to tolerate than a mastectomy because they perceive it as part of their emotional recovery.

Immediate vs. Delayed

Reconstruction may be performed at the same time as a mastectomy (immediate reconstruction), or it can be done later (delayed reconstruction). In general, immediate reconstruction brings the most favorable cosmetic results. In addition, some women feel much better when they wake up from a mastectomy with a reconstructed breast. With immediate reconstruction, a plastic surgeon typically works in tandem with the surgical oncologist who performs the mastectomy.

An important consideration in deciding whether to have immediate or delayed reconstruction is that radiation therapy can cause problems to a newly reconstructed breast. So, if you need radiation therapy, you may want to delay reconstruction. Among women with large tumors and those whose cancer has spread to the underarm (axillary) lymph nodes, radiation therapy is often recommended after mastectomy. Because it can take a day or two after a mastectomy before doctors have a definitive answer as to whether the cancer has spread to the lymph nodes, you may not know before your surgery whether you'll need radiation. For this reason, immediate reconstruction has become less popular.

As for chemotherapy, you can receive it after immediate breast reconstruction, but you'll need to wait about two to three weeks after your surgery before you can begin treatments. A complication from the surgery, such as an infection, could further delay the start of chemotherapy.

With delayed breast reconstruction, surgeons generally recommend that you wait until you've completed radiation therapy and chemotherapy before having reconstructive surgery. Some plastic surgeons think that the results are better when a woman waits until she's healed thoroughly from cancer treatment.

Types

If you want to reconstruct a breast that's removed during mastectomy, basically you have three options to consider:
- Breast reconstruction with implants or tissue expanders

QUESTION & ANSWER

Q: **Does breast reconstruction make it more difficult to detect a cancer recurrence?**

A: With very rare exceptions, the answer to this question is a strong *no*. This is because the most likely site for recurrence is in the tissue located just underneath the skin (subcutaneous tissue). During reconstruction, the artificial breast mound is placed deep below the subcutaneous tissue, which pushes the subcutaneous tissue forward. Therefore, recurrent tumors can still be felt during a self-examination or clinical breast examination.

- Breast reconstruction with your own tissue, which is called flap (autologous) surgery
- No reconstruction, but use of an external prosthesis

Keep in mind that reconstruction may require multiple surgical procedures. Usually, at least two surgeries are required to achieve a correctly positioned and symmetrical breast mound. Some women also wish to undergo additional areola and nipple reconstruction, or they may have surgery on the opposite healthy breast so that it more closely matches the shape and size of the reconstructed breast.

A nonsurgical option to replace a breast that's removed during mastectomy is a prosthesis. A prosthesis is an artificial breast that's worn externally.

Implants

If you decide you would like breast reconstruction, one option is reconstruction with a breast implant. An implant is a breast-shaped device that's placed under the pectoral muscles of the chest. This technique may be performed in slender, smaller-breasted women who don't have a lot of excess tissue in their abdomens or other parts of their bodies that could be used for autologous breast reconstruction.

The two kinds of implants are saline and silicone. Implants filled with salt water (saline) are more common today. The Food and Drug Administration has limited the use of implants filled with silicone gel because of some concern that these implants could cause health problems. The limitations may eventually be lifted because many of the concerns about silicone implants appear to have been unfounded.

An implant may be placed at the time of the mastectomy or during a later surgery. Implants may cause pain, swelling, bruising, tenderness or infection. There's also a long-term possibility of rupture, deflation and shifting. Another complication of implants is capsular contracture, a condition in which tight scar tissue forms around the implant. This causes the breast

BREAST CANCER

Tissue expansion before an implant

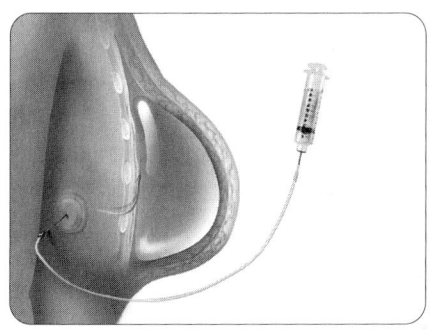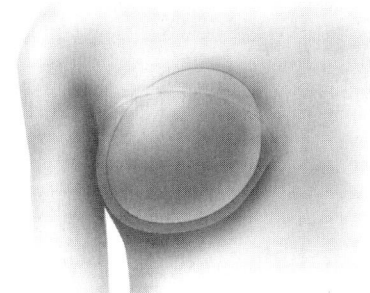

During a process called tissue expansion, a balloon is placed under the chest muscle and gradually filled with saline to stretch the chest skin to accommodate an implant.

mound to become excessively firm so that it no longer has the feel of breast tissue. Sometimes, a capsular contracture can cause discomfort. Whether to surgically correct a contracture is an individual decision, often based on the severity of the symptoms.

If you've had radiation therapy or complications such as a blood clot or infection, you may be at a higher risk of capsular contraction. Your plastic surgeon may recommend that you consider another reconstructive option.

Tissue expanders

Most women aren't able to simply have an implant placed in their breasts at the time of a mastectomy. First, they need to undergo a process called tissue expansion to stretch the remaining chest skin to accommodate the implant. This usually takes place over several months.

To begin the process, a balloon is surgically placed under the chest muscle with a small valve that can be accessed by a needle puncturing the skin. During a series of regular office visits over the next few months, this balloon is gradually expanded with saline by injecting the saline into the valve. The filling is done gradually to give the skin covering the balloon a chance to stretch between visits. The balloon is pumped up much bigger than is wanted for the end result.

This hyperexpanded state is maintained for a few months. Then some of the fluid is removed so that the eventual result

TRAM flap surgery

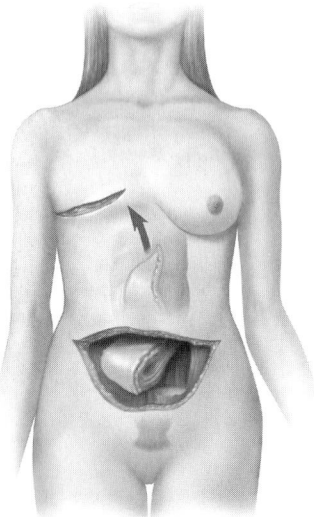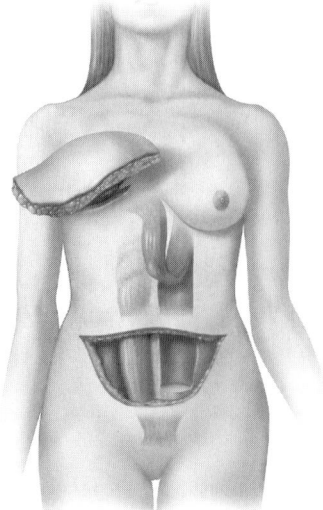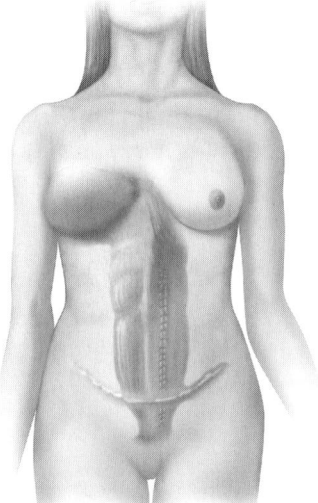

With **TRAM** flap surgery, a section of skin, muscle, fat and blood vessels is taken from a woman's abdomen and used to create a new breast mound.

BREAST CANCER

allows the breast mound to sag a bit, as happens with a normal breast. When the tissue expansion is complete, the balloon may be replaced with a permanent implant, requiring additional surgery. In some cases, a permanent expander is used that serves as both expander and implant, and then only the inflation valve needs to be removed. A nipple also can be reconstructed using skin from the new breast mound. This is generally done after the reconstructed breast has time to heal and settle. Later, a tattoo may be applied to color the nipple and create an areola.

The entire process — using an expander and an implant — takes about nine to 12 months. If the implant ruptures or capsular contraction occurs, additional surgery may be required.

Breast flap

The most complex reconstructive procedure with the longest initial recovery period is breast reconstruction using a woman's own tissue. During this surgery, a section of skin, muscle, fat and blood vessels is taken from one part of your body and is used to fashion a new breast mound. Incisions are made in the area where the tissue is removed, and the surgical wounds can be large.

Most often, the tissue is taken from the lower abdomen. This is called a TRAM flap. The term *TRAM* stands for transverse rectus abdominal muscle. The flap of tissue isn't completely removed from the body. Its blood supply remains attached. During the procedure, the flap

Latissimus flap surgery

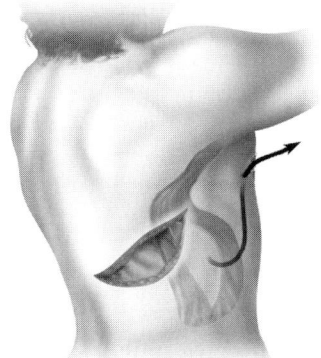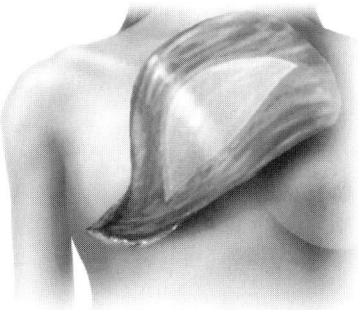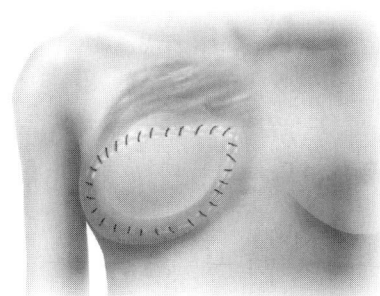

Latissimus flap surgery is performed much the same way as is TRAM flap surgery, but the section of tissue used to create a new breast mound comes from the back instead of the abdomen.

Nipple reconstruction

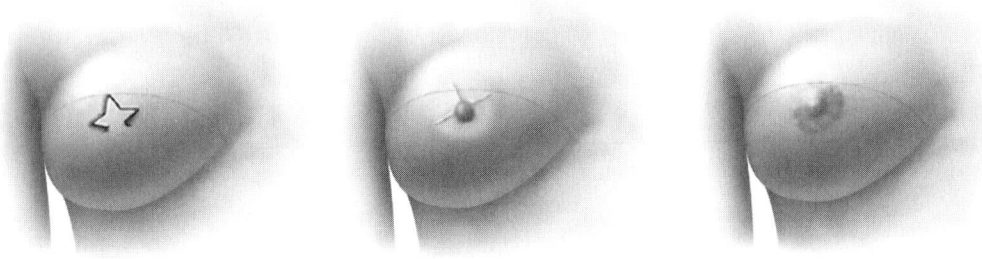

After a reconstructed breast has healed, a plastic surgeon can reconstruct a new nipple and areola.

is tunneled under the skin to the chest area, where it's brought through the mastectomy incision.

For women who don't have enough tissue available on the abdomen for this procedure, the tissue can instead be taken from the back. This is called a latissimus flap, from the Latin word for the muscle involved in the procedure. The flap is moved to the chest site in the same manner as is done with the TRAM flap.

In some instances, neither the abdomen nor the back is suitable for taking a tissue flap. In this case, the tissue is generally taken from the buttocks. This is a more complex procedure because the blood vessels must be detached from the flap and then reattached at the breast site.

The main advantage of flap reconstruction is that the reconstructed breast is made from your own body tissue. The mound remains quite soft and, unlike with an implant, contracture isn't a possibility. In addition, if the tissue is taken from the abdomen, you get a tummy tuck. However, because the flap is human tissue, it requires an adequate blood supply.

If blood supply to the flap is poor, the tissue may not survive. This may lead to significant complications and an unsatisfactory result.

Once the reconstructed breast has healed, a nipple may be formed using skin from the new breast mound, and a tattoo may be applied to color the nipple and create an areola.

If you smoke, your doctor may recommend against breast flap reconstruction because smoking can impair your circulation. In addition, an abdominal flap may not be an option if you've had previous abdominal surgery.

Prosthetics

Some women choose a prosthesis over reconstructive surgery. A prosthesis is shaped like a breast, but it remains outside your body. It's usually made from nylon, rubber, silicone or Dacron fiberfill, and you slip it into your bra. Immediately after your surgery, you may select from prostheses in a range of shapes and sizes that can be used temporarily. For long-

The Do's and Don'ts of Reconstruction

People have many misconceptions about breast reconstruction after cancer surgery. It's important to approach the procedure with realistic expectations.

What breast reconstruction can do:
- Give you a permanent breast contour
- Provide symmetry to your breasts so that they look similar under clothing or a bathing suit
- Help you avoid the need for an external prosthesis

What breast reconstruction may do:
- Improve your self-esteem and body image
- Partially erase physical reminders of your disease
- Require additional surgery to correct reconstructive problems

What breast reconstruction doesn't do:
- Make you look exactly the same as before
- Give your reconstructed breast the same sensations as your normal breast

term use, you may want to consider getting a more customized, permanent prosthesis.

Check with your insurance company to see what kind of coverage you have. Sometimes, a prescription for a prosthesis from your doctor helps with insurance coverage. Some companies cover either a prosthesis or reconstruction but not both.

Issues to Consider

In making your decision on whether to have reconstruction, or what type of reconstruction to have, consider these issues:
- Will you be able to cope with complications of reconstruction if they occur,

such as implant deflation or the need for multiple surgeries to achieve breast symmetry?
- If you choose immediate reconstruction, would a complication such as an infection compromise the start of your chemotherapy or radiation therapy?
- How soon does your surgeon need to know your preferences regarding reconstruction? Occasionally, during surgery to remove the cancer, additional masses or tumors are discovered that may necessitate an unplanned mastectomy. In other cases, your surgeon likes to know if you may want breast reconstruction — whether now or later — so that he or she can perform the proper surgery. During what's known as a skin-sparing mastectomy, a surgeon

Decision Tips

As you think about reconstruction, here are some suggestions to help you in the decision-making process:

- Gather reputable information on breast reconstruction after a mastectomy. Some organizations you might contact include the American Cancer Society and the National Cancer Institute (see page 601 for more information on these organizations). Your doctor's office may have pertinent brochures from organizations such as the American Society of Plastic Surgeons.
- Talk with your surgeon before you make your decision and make sure all of your questions are answered. Jot down questions as you think of them so that you can make the most of your visit with the surgeon. Try to establish a relationship with your surgeon that's open, clear and honest.
- Ask to see pictures of the results of different procedures. Keep in mind that doctors tend to keep pictures of their best outcomes.
- Talk to women who have gone through the various reconstructive procedures. They can give you the personal details that you might want.

removes most of the breast tissue, including the nipple and areola, but leaves the surrounding skin and natural breast landmarks to allow for better reconstruction.

- Are you doing this for yourself or because of pressure from others? Although you may wish to please your partner or family, you don't want to resent them later on for pressuring you into a procedure that you didn't really want to have.
- Are you having reconstruction to make yourself forget you ever had cancer? Unfortunately, this usually isn't possible. Even if, physically, you look closer to the way you did before, emotional and psychological aspects of your condition still need to be addressed.
- Have you given yourself enough time to make a decision you're comfortable

with? Women are often so overwhelmed and in such a state of shock after receiving a diagnosis of breast cancer that they just want to have the surgery, get the cancer out and be done with it. This is understandable, but it's usually OK to take a few days to a couple of weeks to sort things out and think through your decision. The primary goal of breast surgery is to treat the cancer. Sometimes, a plastic surgeon will recommend delaying reconstructive surgery so that the reconstruction doesn't interfere with your cancer treatment regimen.

If you have any questions regarding reconstruction, be sure to consult your doctor, your oncologist or a plastic surgeon. He or she can usually help clarify the issues for you.

Chapter 11: Breast Cancer

Special Situations

Most women diagnosed with breast cancer have a common type of breast cancer that's still in its earlier stages. Some women, though, develop less common forms of breast cancer. Signs and symptoms of the cancer may not be the same, and — depending on the type of cancer or the situation in which it was diagnosed — the treatment may be different.

Some women also are at higher risk of breast cancer than is the general population, and because their risk is increased, their treatment may be different as well. Breast cancer during pregnancy poses yet another unique situation in which treatment may be altered because of the circumstances.

If you are diagnosed with an uncommon type of breast cancer, are at high risk or are facing unique circumstances, it's important that you see an experienced breast cancer specialist. Talking with someone who's familiar with your condition helps to ensure that you receive an accurate diagnosis and appropriate treatment.

This chapter discusses special breast situations, outlining differences in treatment approaches, compared with those for more common forms of breast cancer.

Locally Advanced Breast Cancer

About 5 percent to 10 percent of breast cancers are diagnosed as locally advanced breast cancers. Locally advanced breast cancer, which generally falls under the category of stage III breast cancer, refers to larger breast tumors with one or more of the following characteristics:

- Greater than 5 centimeters (about 2 inches) in diameter
- Extensive cancer spread to regional lymph nodes
- Cancer spread to the chest wall or skin, sometimes causing open sores (ulcerations)

However, with stage III breast cancer, there's no evidence that the cancer has spread (metastasized) to other parts of the body.

Locally advanced breast cancers sometimes occur in women who fail to get medical attention when they first notice a breast lump. Often, this is because they fear receiving a diagnosis of cancer. Locally advanced breast tumors can also occur because mammography isn't always able to detect breast tumors, and the cancer may not produce easily identifiable signs and symptoms. This is most often the case with a type of breast cancer known as invasive lobular breast cancer. These breast tumors can be very large but not apparent by breast self-exams, clinical

Inflammatory Breast Cancer

Inflammatory breast cancer is a type of locally advanced cancer that occurs in a very small percentage of women with breast cancer. In addition to spreading to fibrous connective tissue inside your breast, the cancer spreads to lymphatic vessels located in breast skin, causing noticeable skin changes.

Typically, a lump in your breast is the classic sign of breast cancer, but with inflammatory breast cancer, the lump or mass may not be apparent. Common signs and symptoms of inflammatory breast cancer include:

- A breast that appears red, purple, pink or bruised

- Swelling that makes your breast feel and appear larger than usual
- A warm feeling in the breast
- Itching
- Ridged or dimpled skin texture, similar to an orange peel — often referred to by the French term *peau d'orange*
- Swelling of lymph nodes in one or more of the following locations: under the arm, above the collarbone, below the collarbone

In spite of its name, inflammatory breast cancer isn't caused by an inflammation or infection. It occurs as a result of lymphatic drainage channels in breast skin becoming plugged by cancer cells. Inflammatory breast cancer usually grows rapidly, and skin changes can become apparent in a matter of days to weeks.

examination or mammography. This may be because they occur in very large breasts or because they infiltrate into normal breast tissue not by forming a large mass but rather in a diffuse pattern that can feel like normal breast tissue.

Treatment

Prognosis is generally less favorable for a stage III breast cancer than it is for a stage I or II breast cancer. However, there's still hope for a cure. Treatment regimens generally include drug treatments (chemotherapy, hormone therapy or both), surgery and radiation.

Instead of performing surgery first, as is usually the case with stage I and II breast cancers, for stage III breast cancer, chemotherapy to shrink the tumor is often the first course of action. Usually, an anthracycline medication is recommended, such as doxorubicin (Adriamycin) or epirubicin (Ellence), and a taxane medication, such as paclitaxel (Taxol) or docetaxel (Taxotere). Chemotherapy is usually given for four to eight cycles over a period of three to six months.

The next step typically is surgery. A mastectomy is most often required to remove the tumor in the breast and lymph nodes under the arm. In some instances of locally advanced cancer, a lumpectomy (breast-conserving surgery) and a lymph node dissection may be performed instead of a mastectomy.

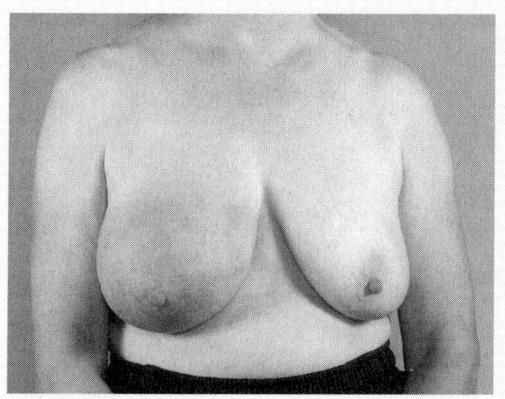

Inflammatory breast cancer is generally characterized by redness of the breast skin and swelling. In this photo, inflammatory breast cancer is present in the woman's right breast. The skin is red, and the breast is swollen (see the color illustration on page 262).

Although it's not an infection, inflammatory breast cancer can easily be confused with a breast infection (acute mastitis). Breast infections tend to occur in women who are breast-feeding. They cause a fever, and they're easily treated with antibiotics. Inflammatory breast cancers don't cause a fever, and they don't respond to antibiotics.

If you have signs and symptoms associated with inflammatory breast cancer, your doctor will likely want to evaluate the breast, which may involve a biopsy. A biopsy can confirm the presence or absence of cancer. In some cases, redness, warmth and swelling of the breast are caused not by an infection or cancer but rather a previous surgery or radiation therapy that involved the outer breast or underarm. These procedures can cause partial blockage of lymphatic channels, producing breast edema and redness.

Lumpectomy isn't an option, though, for inflammatory breast cancer.

After surgery — depending on how much chemotherapy was given before surgery and the response of the cancer to the medication — more chemotherapy may be recommended. Radiation therapy also is typically recommended to destroy any remaining cancer cells in the chest wall area. If laboratory reports indicate that you have a hormone receptor positive cancer, your doctor may also recommend hormone therapy.

For more information on these types of treatment, and how they're performed, see Chapter 9.

Women at High Risk

Some women have a higher risk than do others of developing breast cancer. Two such groups include:

- Women who carry an alteration in the breast cancer genes BRCA1 or BRCA2
- Women who received radiation therapy before the age of 30 for treatment of Hodgkin's disease

In situations where breast cancer is identified in a woman at high risk of the disease, treatment decisions tend to be more complex than for a woman at normal risk. That's because women at high risk of breast cancer are also at greater future risk of new cancers in the same breast or in the other breast.

However, there's no evidence a woman at high risk of developing breast cancer is at a higher risk of a cancer recurrence, than is a woman at normal risk with similar cancer characteristics.

BRCA carriers

If you've been diagnosed with breast cancer and genetic tests indicate that you carry a mutation in BRCA1 or BRCA2, you may want to consider surgical removal (mastectomy) of the affected breast, or perhaps both breasts, to decrease your risk of developing new cancers in the same or opposite breast. If you're diagnosed with breast cancer and your doctor suspects but doesn't yet know if you carry an altered BRCA1 or BRCA2 gene, decisions regarding your treatment are more complicated. This is because a formal evaluation of your genetic risk, which typically includes examination of your family history, genetic counseling and possible genetic testing, may take several weeks.

Some women undergoing genetic testing choose to proceed with a breast lumpectomy to remove the tumor, along with sampling of the underarm (axillary) lymph nodes to check for cancer spread. They hold off on having more extensive surgery until they've received the results of the genetic tests. Other women choose to proceed with more extensive surgery, such as mastectomy, rather than being faced with the possibility of further surgery in the future.

Once genetic test results are available, you and your doctor can make decisions regarding other possible treatments to help prevent the development of new breast tumors. Because the BRCA1 and BRCA2 genes also increase your risk of ovarian cancer, you and your doctor may also discuss strategies to prevent development of ovarian cancer.

BREAST CANCER

For more information on the BRCA genes, see Chapter 4. For more information on cancer prevention strategies, including preventive (prophylactic) mastectomy, see Chapter 5.

Hodgkin's disease survivors

Women who've had Hodgkin's disease and received radiation therapy to lymph nodes in their chest as part of their treatment are at increased risk of developing breast cancer. This is especially true among women who received such treatment during adolescence.

Factors that play key roles in determining a woman's risk of breast cancer after treatment for Hodgkin's disease include:

- **Age.** If a female is experiencing puberty when she receives treatment for Hodgkin's disease, her risk of breast cancer is greater because her breasts are exposed to radiation during the time when radiation has the greatest effect on growing breast cells. As a woman matures, risk decreases. Women who are age 30 or older when they receive radiation therapy to the chest area to treat Hodgkin's disease generally have a breast cancer risk similar to that of the general population.
- **Time.** Breast cancer usually develops approximately 15 years after radiation treatment for Hodgkin's disease. Therefore, a woman treated for Hodgkin's disease should begin breast cancer screening about 10 years after her radiation treatments, or even earlier. Some researchers believe screening should begin as early as five years after receiving radiation therapy.

- **Radiation dose.** Older methods of radiation therapy involved high doses of radiation and wider exposure of the breasts to radiation. The higher the dose of radiation received, the greater the subsequent risk of breast cancer. In recent years, treatment regimens for Hodgkin's disease have greatly improved. Now, lower doses of radiation are used that more effectively target lymph node areas, reducing exposure to surrounding breast tissue.

Treatment

For Hodgkin's disease survivors who later develop breast cancer, a mastectomy has been the standard treatment. Additional radiation often isn't possible because normal tissues typically won't tolerate further radiation therapy. However, because lower doses of radiation are now used to treat Hodgkin's disease, it may be possible for some women to have a lumpectomy followed by breast radiation therapy, as long as the total amount of radiation they receive is within acceptable limits.

Because there's an increased risk that cancer may also develop in the other breast, some women choose to have prophylactic mastectomy of the other breast.

Bilateral Breast Cancer

Only a small percentage of women with newly diagnosed breast cancer have cancer in both breasts at the time of their diagnoses. This is called synchronous bilateral breast cancer. Because breast cancer rarely spreads from one breast to the other in its early stages, the two tumors — one in each breast — are almost always two different breast cancers.

Bilateral breast cancers tend to be more common in women with a strong family history of breast cancer. Having bilateral breast cancer doesn't mean your prognosis is doubly worse. Similar to breast cancer that's confined to one breast, the prognosis for women with bilateral breast cancer depends on the characteristics of the individual tumors, including their size and whether the cancer has spread to the lymph nodes under the arm. In this situation, prognosis is generally based on the least favorable of the tumors.

Treatment

Treatment of synchronous bilateral breast cancer depends on the size, grade and lymph node status of each tumor. Options include a bilateral lumpectomy and radiation or a bilateral mastectomy. Sometimes, based on the results of a sentinel node biopsy of each breast, the lymph nodes under one of the arms need to be removed but those under the other arm don't.

If you choose to have a lumpectomy, radiation therapy usually follows. Decisions regarding additional (adjuvant) therapy, such as chemotherapy or hormone therapy, are based on the characteristics of the tumors and whether one or both carries a high risk of recurrence.

See Chapter 9 for more information on the sentinel node biopsy procedure and adjuvant therapy.

Bilateral breast cancer also refers to primary cancers that develop in both breasts but at different times. These are known as metachronous bilateral breast cancers.

Treatment for metachronous bilateral breast cancer also is based on the characteristics of the tumor being treated. When treating the second breast cancer, your doctor likely will take into account the type of therapy you received for your first breast cancer, as well as other factors, such as your family history.

Unknown Primary Cancers

Occasionally, a woman may develop an enlarged lymph node under her arm yet not have a detectable tumor in her breast. If a biopsy of the lymph node reveals cancer, the tissue sample is studied closely under a microscope to determine if the cancer looks like breast cancer. The pathologist needs to make sure — as much as is possible — that the cancer in the lymph node isn't a different cancer, such as melanoma or lymphoma. Unless a different cancer can be identified, the cancer is considered to be breast cancer and treated as such.

The breast located next to the affected lymph nodes is carefully examined to try to find a hidden tumor. This usually includes a complete physical examination, a mammogram and an ultrasound exam. If these aren't helpful, other tests may be used, such as magnetic resonance imaging (MRI) or a positron emission tomography (PET) scan.

If a tumor is found in the breast, a treatment regimen is developed, based on the size and grade of the tumor and number of lymph nodes involved. If no tumor is found and the cancer cells in the lymph nodes appear to be breast cancer cells, both the lymph nodes and the adjacent breast are treated.

In the past, treatment usually consisted of a mastectomy. In approximately half the cases in which a tumor couldn't be identified on diagnostic imaging tests, the pathologist was able to locate cancer cells in breast tissue removed during surgery. However, even in women in whom no cancerous cells were found in the breast, their cancers generally behaved similarly to breast cancer.

Today, an alternative to mastectomy is radiation therapy to the breast with close follow-up screening of the breast for any developing tumors. In virtually all cases, the lymph nodes in the affected underarm area also are removed (axillary lymph node dissection). Typically, the recommended treatment for such cancers is chemotherapy, hormone therapy or both.

Prognosis for women with an unknown primary tumor is similar to that of other women with stage II breast cancer that has spread to the underarm lymph nodes.

Metaplastic Breast Cancer

Most breast cancers are classified as adenocarcinomas — a subset of carcinomas arising from glands or glandular tissue, such as that in your breasts.

Metaplastic breast cancer is a rare type of breast cancer that undergoes a process of transformation called metaplasia. The cells start out looking similar to adenocarcinomas and then they transform into cells that take on a nonglandular growth pattern. This transformation may affect all of the cells within a tumor or only a small portion of them. When viewed under a microscope, metaplastic tumors typically display a mixture of adenocarcinoma-type cells and nonadenocarcinoma-type cells.

As in other breast cancers, the predominant indication of cancer is a lump in the breast. Metaplastic breast cancer is most often seen in women who are older than age 50, although it can occur at a younger age. Generally, this type of breast cancer doesn't spread to the lymph nodes under the arm, and its cells are hormone receptor negative.

In spite of the fact that the cancer generally doesn't spread to the lymph nodes, metaplastic breast cancer is often more aggressive than are adenocarcinomas, and it carries a higher risk of recurrence than do adenocarcinomas.

This type of cancer is generally treated with a lumpectomy or mastectomy. Your doctor may also recommend radiation therapy. Because metaplastic breast cancer is often hormone receptor negative, hormone therapy isn't effective. Chemotherapy to help prevent a recurrence would seem to be a logical choice, but experience has shown that this type of cancer often doesn't respond well to chemotherapy. Presently, there's no drug therapy regimen that's been shown to be beneficial against this particular type of breast cancer.

BREAST CANCER

Lymphomas and Sarcomas

As just mentioned, most breast cancers start in the glandular tissue of the breast, such as the ducts and lobules. A very few breast tumors — about 1 percent — develop in the lymphatic or connective tissues of the breast.

Tumors that originate in the lymphatic tissue are called lymphomas. Those that develop in the connective tissue are called sarcomas. Lymphomas and sarcomas are more likely to develop in other parts of the body than in the breast.

Breast lymphoma

Lymphoma accounts for one in 1,000 breast cancers. Like carcinomas of the breast, breast lymphoma typically develops into a mass, but its growth is usually more rapid than that of carcinomas of the breast. The cancer may also develop into multiple masses or occur in both breasts. Occasionally, this type of cancer is accompanied by night sweats, fever and weight loss. A biopsy is needed to confirm the diagnosis.

In general, breast lymphoma is treated with chemotherapy and radiation therapy. A combination chemotherapy regimen called CHOP (cyclophosphamide, hydroxydaunomycin, Oncovin and prednisone) is often used. A review of breast lymphoma cases at one medical institution found that 11 out of 20 women treated with CHOP were still disease-free an average of 80 months (just under seven years) after their diagnoses.

Breast sarcoma

The most common type of breast sarcoma is called a phyllodes tumor. Phyllodes tumors are usually noncancerous (benign), but they can be cancerous. On a mammogram, the tumors appear similar to benign masses called fibroadenomas.

Phyllodes tumors tend to occur in women around age 45 — about 20 years later than the average age at which fibroadenomas are diagnosed, but earlier than the age at which most breast cancers tend to occur.

To make an accurate diagnosis, a biopsy of the tumor is required. Prognosis for this type of breast cancer is generally dependent on factors such as the grade and size of the tumor.

Treatment

The primary treatment for a breast sarcoma is to surgically remove the tumor along with a wide margin of healthy tissue. Depending on the size of the tumor and its relation to your breast size, your doctor may recommend either a lumpectomy or a mastectomy.

Because phyllodes tumors — if they do spread — tend to spread through the bloodstream, there's generally no need to examine lymph nodes under the arm. Phyllodes tumors, if they recur, tend to do so locally in the breast or spread to the lungs.

In addition to surgery, chemotherapy and radiation therapy are sometimes considered. However, unlike for treatment of typical breast cancer, there's much less proof that these therapies are effective in treating breast sarcomas.

Radiation Therapy and Sarcoma Risk

Studies and reports of individual cases suggest that radiation therapy to treat breast adenocarcinomas, the most common type of breast cancer, carries an increased risk of development of subsequent sarcomas in the bone or tissue of the irradiated area.

To further investigate this issue, two groups of researchers reviewed data from the National Cancer Institute's Surveillance, Epidemiology, and End Results (SEER) program. SEER is a database that collects cancer-related information from nine areas in the United States. These areas collectively represent almost 10 percent of the population.

The investigators found that radiation therapy does increase a woman's risk of developing a sarcoma. But the increase in risk is extremely small, and it doesn't outweigh the benefits that radiation therapy generally provides in treating breast adenocarcinomas.

Paget's Disease

Paget's disease of the breast is a rare form of breast cancer that starts in the breast ducts and spreads to the skin of the nipple and the areola, the dark circle of skin around the nipple. Paget's disease of the breast isn't related to Paget's disease of the bone, a metabolic bone disease.

Paget's disease of the breast is most common in middle-aged women. Signs and symptoms may include:

- Crusted, scaly, red skin of the nipple and areola
- Nipple discharge, such as bleeding or oozing
- A burning or itching sensation in the nipple area
- A lump in the nipple area

Early detection of Paget's disease is important. If you have a lump or skin irritation in the nipple area that persists for more than one or two months, see your doctor.

A doctor may be able to diagnose the cancer by inspecting discharge from the affected nipple for cancer cells or by biopsying the involved area.

Because of the underlying breast cancer associated with Paget's disease, a mammogram should be performed to check for any masses or abnormalities in the breast. Paget's disease can be associated with both noninvasive and invasive breast cancer.

Treatment for Paget's disease depends on the size of the tumor and whether the cancer has penetrated surrounding tissues or spread to nearby lymph nodes. A small, noninvasive tumor may require removal of just the nipple area plus a surrounding margin of healthy tissue, followed by radiation therapy. A larger, more aggressive tumor may require a mastectomy.

Prognosis is often dependent on the size of the tumor. Generally, the smaller the tumor, the better the prognosis.

Breast Cancer and Pregnancy

It's very difficult and emotionally trying when a woman is pregnant and is diagnosed with breast cancer. Fortunately, this is uncommon, ranging from one in 3,000 to one in 10,000 deliveries. Women in this situation are usually in their 30s.

During pregnancy, the ducts and lobules in a woman's breasts multiply, blood vessels swell to allow for increased blood flow and the weight of the breasts can double. This makes the breasts dense and lumpy. As a result, it's difficult to examine the breasts, and mammography has an increased rate of false-negative results, meaning it doesn't detect cancer when cancer is present.

A careful examination of your breasts by your doctor is recommended at your first prenatal visit so that he or she can be alert to any abnormalities that might occur later.

If a lump is detected during pregnancy, your doctor may do an ultrasound of your breast to see if the mass is a cyst or solid lump. If mammography or other radiological procedures are necessary, they usually can be done safely by shielding your abdomen from radiation. Even if a mammogram comes back normal, but a worrisome mass can be felt, the mass should be biopsied. A biopsy is the surest way to determine if the lump is cancerous. A biopsy is usually done as a needle procedure (see Chapter 7 for a description of biopsies). If you're breast-feeding when the lump is detected, your doctor may advise that you stop before the biopsy is

performed to reduce the risk of complications. Be assured, there's no evidence that cancer can spread to your baby through breast milk.

Pregnancy itself doesn't appear to worsen your prognosis if you have breast cancer. Most studies show that the prognosis for women who are pregnant is similar to that for women at a similar age and with a similar stage of breast cancer who aren't pregnant. But diagnosis may be delayed because a pregnant woman's breasts are naturally swollen and tender during pregnancy, making a cancerous lump more difficult to detect. Delayed detection may mean that the cancer is diagnosed at a later stage, decreasing the chances of successful treatment and survival. Termination of the pregnancy hasn't been shown to improve prognosis and is generally unnecessary.

Treatment

Treatment for breast cancer in a pregnant woman is similar to that for a nonpregnant woman, and is based on such factors as the size of the lump, its grade and the extent of lymph node involvement. But modifications may be made to protect the fetus, depending on the trimester you're in. The first trimester is when fetal organ development takes place and is the period of greatest risk. Most medication is avoided during this time, if possible.

Surgery
If the cancer is stage I or II, surgery is usually the recommended therapy and is generally safe for both mother and fetus, especially after the first trimester. In the

first trimester, anesthesia can be harmful. Traditionally, the procedure of choice has been a mastectomy along with removal of the underarm (axillary) lymph nodes. This is because a mastectomy may decrease the need for radiation therapy, which can be dangerous to a fetus.

Some women diagnosed in the late stages of their pregnancies choose to have lumpectomies, followed by radiation after delivery of their babies. Even if you're far from delivery, lumpectomy may be an option, followed by chemotherapy after the first trimester and then radiation after the birth of the baby.

Surgery carries a slight risk of miscarriage or preterm labor, but it doesn't increase the risk of birth defects.

Radiation therapy

Radiation therapy generally isn't recommended in pregnant women because of possible risks to the fetus, such as miscarriage, birth defects and childhood cancer. It may also result in poor cosmetic results because of breast changes that occur during pregnancy.

Chemotherapy

In the first trimester, chemotherapy can cause miscarriage and fetal abnormalities, but this risk decreases substantially in the second and third trimesters, making its use an option in later stages of pregnancy. The chemotherapy drug methotrexate should be avoided, though, because it can have toxic effects on the placenta.

The long-term effects of chemotherapy on the child are unknown, but existing data suggest that it doesn't affect later growth and development. Because

chemotherapy drugs can come through in your breast milk, breast-feeding isn't recommended during chemotherapy.

Hormone therapy

Hormone therapy generally isn't recommended for a woman who's pregnant, primarily because hormones can influence the pregnancy and may cause side effects in the fetus. After delivery, though, hormone therapy may be used in a woman whose cancer is hormone receptor positive. See Chapter 9 for more information on hormone therapies.

Laura's Story

Laura was 34 years old, and she and her husband were expecting their second child when she found out that she had breast cancer. Her local doctor suggested termination of the pregnancy, but he also mentioned that he had read some articles in which pregnant women were able to continue their pregnancies while undergoing cancer treatment. Laura and her husband wanted to continue the pregnancy if at all possible, and they sought a second opinion with a cancer specialist.

After much discussion, explanation and careful consideration of the options, Laura, her husband and her doctors decided to continue the pregnancy and to proceed right away with a mastectomy. At the time of her surgery, Laura was five and a half months pregnant.

Laura's prognosis was very poor. The surgery revealed a very large — 15-centimeter (about 6-inch) — tumor. The laboratory report also indicated cancer cells in 21 of 22 underarm (axillary) lymph nodes.

Knowing that chemotherapy was important to her survival chances, and with the assurance of her medical team that chemotherapy drugs probably wouldn't harm the fetus, Laura agreed to have a couple of cycles of chemotherapy while she was still pregnant.

Approximately 10 weeks after her diagnosis, Laura gave birth to a healthy baby girl by way of Caesarean delivery. Later, Laura received additional chemotherapy and then radiation.

Laura says that the happiness of the pregnancy and the promise of another child made it easier for her to deal with her cancer. "I knew I had to be there to raise my children," Laura says.

After completion of her treatment, Laura's doctor continued to monitor Laura's health with trepidation, concerned that the cancer would recur. At each checkup, Laura reported feeling fine, and there were no indications of a cancer recurrence. At a recent checkup, Laura was accompanied by her 15-year-old daughter — the baby whose life Laura was determined to save.

Finally, Laura's doctor felt comfortable that Laura would be OK.

Pregnancy after breast cancer

One of the issues related to breast cancer and pregnancy is the question of whether it's safe to become pregnant after a diagnosis of breast cancer. In the past, there was concern about a later pregnancy because during pregnancy levels of female hormones increase, and these hormones are known to influence breast cancer development. The current feeling among doctors is that pregnancy following a diagnosis of breast cancer is generally safe. However, because many breast cancer recurrences tend to happen within the first few years after treatment, most doctors recommend waiting at least five years after treatment to become pregnant.

Sometimes, though, waiting so long may not be an option because doing so may place a woman outside the childbearing age. Ultimately, the decision is a personal one. The most important consideration usually revolves around your own risk of relapse.

Breast Cancer in Men

Breast cancer in men is quite rare. Approximately 1 percent of all breast cancers occur in men, and male breast cancer accounts for less than 1 percent of all male cancers.

In general, male breast cancer is similar to female breast cancer with a few differences. While hormone levels appear to influence the development of breast cancer in men, just as they do in women, in men, the influence appears to be related, in part, to an imbalance in the hormones estrogen and androgen. Approximately 85 percent of male breast cancers are estrogen receptor positive, and 70 percent are progesterone receptor positive. Men also tend to be older when they're diagnosed.

Risk factors

Factors that might increase a man's risk of breast cancer include:

- Testicular abnormalities, such as an undescended testicle, congenital

inguinal hernia, inflammation of the testicle, removal of the testicles
- Infertility
- Klinefelter's syndrome, a sex chromosome abnormality present at birth
- A family history of breast cancer
- Benign breast conditions, such as nipple discharge or breast cysts
- Radiation exposure
- Age
- Ashkenazi Jewish ancestry

A mutation of the BRCA2 gene increases a man's risk of breast cancer, but a BRCA1 mutation doesn't appear to have as much effect on male breast cancer risk.

In families with a significant history of breast cancer and in which at least one male has been diagnosed with breast cancer, the chances of a BRCA2 mutation being present are reported to be greater than 50 percent.

Diagnosis and staging

The predominant sign of male breast cancer is a painless breast mass. Other signs and symptoms include nipple retraction, pain or tenderness, an open sore on the nipple, nipple discharge and nipple bleeding. Sometimes, no signs or symptoms are present.

Because men don't have much breast tissue, a mass can usually be easily felt. In some cases, mammography may be helpful in distinguishing between a benign mass and a malignant one. A biopsy is used to diagnose a mass that appears suspicious. If cancer is present, it's staged in the same way as female breast cancer — according to the tumor's size and spread.

Treatment

The standard treatment for male breast cancer is surgical removal of the tumor, if possible. The procedure most often recommended is a modified radical mastectomy, which involves removal of the breast tissue and the underarm lymph nodes. The advent of sentinel lymph node evaluation may reduce the need for more extensive lymph node removal in some men (see Chapter 9 for more on sentinel lymph node biopsy). Radiation therapy also may be recommended to reduce the risk of local recurrence.

Because so many male breast cancers are hormone receptor positive, hormone therapy is often recommended. The success of tamoxifen in female breast cancer has also led to its use in men. Although no randomized clinical trials have been done to study the benefits of tamoxifen in men, existing data suggest that it may increase survival. Side effects of tamoxifen may include hot flashes and impotence. For men at high risk of recurrence, chemotherapy is also commonly recommended after surgery.

If the cancer has spread (metastasized) to a distant part of the body, hormone therapy, chemotherapy or both may be recommended. For hormone receptor positive breast cancers, hormone therapy is usually given first.

Before tamoxifen came into widespread use for treatment of male breast cancer, the recommended hormone therapy was androgen ablation, which is essentially the removal of testosterone from the body. This was routinely done by removal of the testicles. Today, men are more commonly given drugs, such as luteinizing hormone-releasing hormone (LH-RH) agonists, to suppress testosterone production. These are the same medications used to suppress ovarian estrogen production in premenopausal women. If one type of hormone therapy doesn't work, another may be used. If there's no response to any hormone therapies, chemotherapy may be considered.

Prognosis

Survival rates for men with breast cancer are similar to those of women with the same stage of breast cancer. Unfortunately, in men, breast cancer tends to be diagnosed at a later stage than in women, in part, perhaps because of a lack of awareness.

As with women, prognostic factors that influence survival in men include lymph node status, tumor size and grade. Whether the cancer has spread to the lymph nodes is usually the most important prognostic factor.

Chapter 12: Breast Cancer

Follow-up & Surveillance

Finally, treatment of your breast cancer is over. For the past number of months, the diagnosis and treatment of your cancer has been an active and tangible part of your everyday life. During your treatment, you may have undergone surgery, radiation therapy, drug therapy or a combination of these approaches. You've likely interacted with a team of health care professionals on a regular basis, at times even daily.

But when the flurry of treatment activity is over, you may wonder, "Now what?" Certainly, you're grateful to be done with treatment, but now you may begin to worry about a cancer recurrence, and find new concerns taking the place of old ones. Many questions may come to mind. Is there something that you can do to prevent the cancer from coming back, or to catch it early if it does? How often should you see your doctor? Will you need to take tests? Which tests are most effective, and how often should you have them?

Monitoring for recurrent cancer is an important component of follow-up care. However, it's only one part of a follow-up program. Other important goals include addressing complications of treatment, meeting physical rehabilitation needs, monitoring your overall health and providing you with psychological support. Addressing all of these needs will help you as you attempt to return to your normal routine.

An important point to keep in mind is that while guidelines are established for routine follow-up care after breast cancer treatment, each breast cancer survivor is unique. Just as with diagnosis and treatment, you and your doctor will ultimately decide together what's best for you once your treatment is complete.

Understanding Recurrent Cancer

One of the primary goals of follow-up care is to detect a possible return (recurrence) of your breast cancer. To understand which tests may be the most helpful in detecting a recurrence, it's important to know a bit about recurrent cancer.

When a cancerous tumor is first diagnosed, the cancer is known as a primary cancer. Recurrent cancer refers to cancer that later develops from cells that originally came from the primary tumor. The cells weren't visible at the time of diagnosis, and they weren't eliminated during treatment to destroy the primary cancer. Risk of a recurrence is dependent on the size of the original tumor and the number of lymph nodes that contained cancerous cells (lymph node involvement). Women with a very small tumor and no lymph node involvement have a lower chance of recurrence. Women with a large tumor

and many involved lymph nodes have a higher risk.

Types of recurrences

Breast cancer recurrences are divided into three categories — local, regional and metastatic — depending on where the cancer returns.

Local
A local recurrence refers to the growth of cancer cells at the site of the original tumor. In women who had a previous lumpectomy, a local recurrence may take place in remaining breast tissue. Among women who had a mastectomy to treat a primary tumor, the cancer may recur locally along the mastectomy scar or in chest wall tissue. With a local recurrence, the cancer cells are still contained within the area where the cancer first began and may be responsive to local therapy such as surgery or radiation.

Sometimes, a new cancer — a new primary tumor — will develop in the other breast. Almost always, this new cancer is not a recurrence but rather a second primary cancer. Second primary cancers are generally treated in the same manner as a first primary cancer.

Regional
When cancer cells travel from the original site of the tumor and they settle in nearby lymph nodes — in the armpit or collarbone area — this is known as a regional recurrence. With a regional recurrence, the chances of treatment curing the cancer are lower than with a local recurrence, but a cure may still be possible.

Recurrent Cancer or a New Cancer?

When cancer is detected in a breast that had previously been treated with a lumpectomy, two possible scenarios need to be considered.

One possibility is that the new tumor stems from cells that were leftover from the original tumor. When the cancer was originally treated, not all the cancer cells were removed or destroyed. This is known as recurrent breast cancer (in-breast recurrence). The other possibility is that the tumor is a new cancer that has developed in the breast. In this case, the cancer would be referred to as a second, or new, primary cancer.

In some instances, it can be difficult to determine if a new tumor in a previously treated breast is a recurrent tumor or a new primary tumor. Some factors, though, can provide clues. The tumor is more likely to be recurrent cancer if the following are true:

- The new tumor developed less than five years after the original diagnosis.
- The new tumor developed in the same area of the breast as the original tumor.
- When examined under a microscope, the new tumor has an appearance similar to that of the original tumor.

Metastatic

In the case of a metastatic recurrence, cancer cells from the original site have traveled to distant parts of the body. The bones, lungs and liver are organs commonly affected by metastatic breast cancer. With metastatic recurrence, a cure generally isn't possible, although effective treatment is available that can prolong survival.

Detecting recurrent cancer

The real question regarding screening for recurrent cancer is this: Will early detection — identification of recurrent cancer before it produces signs or symptoms — result in a woman living longer or better?

For localized and regional recurrences, the answer seems to be yes. Treatments such as mastectomy and radiation may be able to cure the cancer. For regional recurrences, the chance of a cure is lower.

For metastatic recurrence, to date, no evidence suggests that early detection of the disease and early initiation of treatment, results in longer life expectancy or better quality of life. This reality has come to have a significant effect on recommendations for follow-up care after treatment.

Follow-up Care

The purpose of follow-up care is to monitor your overall physical and emotional health, respond to complications from your treatment, and watch for indications that your cancer may have returned. Monitoring for recurrent cancer may sound like an involved process, but it includes fewer tests than you might expect.

BREAST CANCER

Signs and Symptoms to Watch For

One of the most important things to recognize is that you are your body's best guardian. You know your body best, and you know what feels normal and what doesn't. Most women discover a cancer recurrence themselves, before their doctors do. Therefore, it's important to be aware of signs and symptoms that may suggest a recurrence. If you experience any of the following, talk to your doctor. He or she can evaluate your signs and symptoms further, and together the two of you can decide on the appropriate plan.

Signs and symptoms of breast cancer recurrence may include:

- New, unexplained, persistent pain — such as in your bones, chest or abdomen
- Changes or new lumps in your breasts or surgical scars, or in surrounding tissue
- Unexplained changes in your weight, particularly weight loss
- Any shortness of breath, difficulty breathing or unexplained cough
- Any other persistent, abnormal sensation or occurrence that bothers you

Check your breasts monthly to look for changes. If you have questions, ask your doctor for instructions on how to examine your breasts after cancer treatment, especially if you've had breast surgery or breast reconstruction.

In the past, follow-up testing usually involved various blood tests, chest X-rays and bone scans. But the trend has been toward limiting testing to detailed medical histories, physical examinations and regular mammograms. As a result, a wide range of practices exists. Some women undergo all the tests available, and others receive only a few.

Because of these differences, some women wonder if they're not getting enough tests — if their doctors should be doing more. The truth is, when a recurrence occurs, most women discover it on their own. It's not test results that most often lead to a diagnosis of recurrent cancer but rather changes in how a woman feels or development of a new lump. Tests often used to help identify recurrent cancer — blood tumor marker studies, liver function tests and X-rays — haven't been found to be effective or useful in prolonging survival or improving quality of life.

In the following sections, we'll take a look at which follow-up tests are recommended by the American Society of Clinical Oncology — an organization that has developed guidelines for follow-up care after breast cancer treatment — as well as which tests this group doesn't recommend.

If you've already discovered a recurrence of your breast cancer, a different set of guidelines applies (see Chapter 13).

Recommended tests

The American Society of Clinical Oncology recommends the following steps for routine follow-up care in women who've been treated for early-stage breast cancer and who have no signs or symptoms of cancer.

Medical history

For the first three years after completion of your initial treatment, you'll likely see your doctor every three to six months. Chances are, your visit will begin with a detailed medical history. You'll most likely be asked about your general health since your last appointment, any changes in your body that you may have noticed and any concerns you may have. This is a good time to ask questions about issues such as diet, exercise and hot flashes, as well as questions regarding breast reconstruction or prostheses. You may want to write down your questions and bring them to your appointment.

After the first three years, your checkups may become less frequent. You may need to see your doctor only every six to 12 months for the next two years, and annually after that. If you were treated for noninvasive cancer, such as ductal carcinoma *in situ*, your follow-up exams may be less frequent, such as twice a year for the first five years and yearly after that.

Physical exam

After your doctor takes your medical history, a physical examination generally follows. Like medical histories, a physical exam is recommended every three to six months for the first three years after primary treatment, every six to 12 months for the next two years and annually after that. For women who've had a lumpectomy, breast examinations at six-month intervals may be recommended for up to 10 years.

During your physical exam, your doctor will check for any signs of cancer recurrence. This may include:

- A careful examination of the area where the cancer originally occurred, including the incision site, remaining breast tissue and the chest wall
- A careful examination of your other breast
- An examination of the area around your armpits, collarbone and neck to check for swollen lymph nodes

Your doctor may also listen to your lungs for any breathing abnormalities and check for liver enlargement and any sign of bone tenderness.

If you've been taking the medication tamoxifen and you haven't had a hysterectomy, your doctor will likely recommend a yearly Pap test and pelvic examination, because tamoxifen slightly increases the risk of uterine cancer.

Mammography

An annual mammogram is recommended for all women who have had breast cancer. In addition to a medical history and physical examination, this is the only other procedure that's routinely recommended after primary treatment. A mammogram can detect a local recurrence in the affected breast or a new tumor in the other breast. Studies have shown that there's no advantage to doing mammograms more than once a year, provided no peculiar areas showed up on past mammograms, which might prompt more frequent examinations.

If you've had a lumpectomy, your doctor may want you to have a mammogram of that breast six months after completion of your radiation treatment and yearly after that. If you've had a mastectomy, you still need to have a yearly mammogram on your other breast.

Tests that aren't recommended

For some women — perhaps even you — follow-up visits to the doctor involve a barrage of tests, including some or all of the following:

- A chest X-ray to check for lung tumors
- An ultrasound to check for liver tumors
- A bone scan to check for bone cancer
- A computerized tomography (CT) scan or magnetic resonance imaging (MRI) to look for cancer in the soft tissues and organs of the chest, abdomen and pelvis
- A blood test (blood tumor marker study) to check for certain substances in the blood that may be elevated in people with cancer
- A complete blood count (CBC) to check levels of white and red blood cells and blood platelets
- Liver and kidney function tests to check that these organs are functioning normally

These tests are done in an effort to detect a metastatic recurrence before it produces signs and symptoms. Unfortunately, though, there's no evidence, despite multiple studies, that the tests prolong survival or improve quality of life. At best, some of the tests appear only to increase the amount of time during which you know you have a recurrence, not the actual length of your life. In addition, these tests aren't always accurate — they may miss indications of a recurrence or, just the opposite, suggest the presence

of cancer when none exists. Finally, test results that are inconclusive can cause a lot of anxiety, perhaps needlessly.

A look at the research

A number of investigations have been done to try to assess the role of intensive testing in the routine follow-up care of women with no evidence of breast cancer after treatment. So far, the evidence indicates that such testing doesn't have a significant effect in helping to prolong survival or improve quality of life.

Key studies

The strongest evidence supporting the conclusion that most follow-up tests generally aren't beneficial comes from two large Italian studies that focused on intensive screening for breast cancer recurrences.

In the first study, 622 women received intensive follow-up testing including regular physical exams and yearly mammograms, plus chest X-rays and bone scans every six months. Another 621 women followed the same schedule for physical exams and yearly mammograms, but received no other tests. This was known as the clinical follow-up group. The investigators found that even though cancer that recurred in bone and the lungs was detected earlier in the intensive follow-up group than in the other group, there was no difference between the two groups in the detection of metastatic recurrences at other sites or in the detection of local and regional recurrences.

Even though in the intensive follow-up group, the cancer was detected earlier in bone and the lungs, there wasn't any improvement in survival five years later (see graph below). A 10-year update found no significant difference in death rates between the intensive follow-up group and the clinical follow-up group. The conclusion was that intensive follow-up with chest X-rays and bone scans doesn't offer any survival advantage to breast cancer patients.

The second study involved a similar number of participants, enrolling 655 of them in intensive follow-up consisting of regular physical exams, a yearly mammogram and bone scan, liver ultrasound, a chest X-ray and blood tests every six months. Another 665 women were enrolled in clinical follow-up consisting of only regular physical exams and yearly mammograms. After six years, there was no significant difference in death rates between the two groups. The trial also measured quality of life and found no difference there either.

Blood tumor markers

Tumors can make unique proteins or other substances that can be measured in the bloodstream. These are usually referred to as tumor markers. To date,

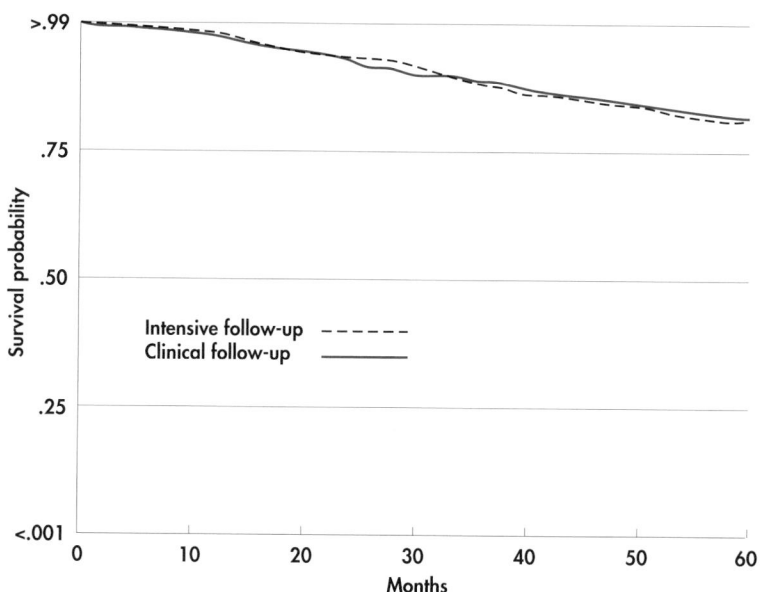

Intensive vs. clinical follow-up

In this follow-up study, even though cancer in bone and the lungs was detected earlier in the intensive follow-up group, there was no improvement in survival five years (60 months) later. A 10-year update found no significant difference in death rates between the intensive follow-up group and the clinical follow-up group.

Adapted from the *Journal of the American Medical Association*, May 5, 1999

there's no ideal tumor marker or combination of markers that's specific for breast cancer, but some markers may suggest the presence of breast cancer. Examples include CA 15-3, CA 27-29 and carcinoembryonic antigen (CEA). The question arises: Would these blood tests be helpful in detecting recurrent breast cancer? Currently, no available data suggest that these tests are accurate enough to detect cancer recurrence early enough to improve chances of survival.

In addition, these substances also exist in healthy people who don't have cancer, meaning a woman could receive a positive test result, indicating cancer recurrence when, in fact, there's no recurrence. This is what's known as a false-positive test result. Such tests may also miss certain recurrences.

Finally — even when they work accurately — it appears that blood markers indicate a cancer recurrence only a couple of months before the recurrence would be detected in other ways, such as by a medical history or physical examination.

As a result, the best use of blood tumor markers is to help diagnose a cancer recurrence when signs and symptoms suggest the cancer may be back.

Imaging tests

Some imaging tests may be better at detecting recurrent breast cancer than is mammography or ultrasound, but they haven't been fully evaluated in clinical trials to determine their potential benefits. These include such tests as computerized tomography (CT) scans, magnetic resonance imaging (MRI) and positron emission tomography (PET) scans.

For women who aren't experiencing any signs or symptoms of recurrent cancer, these tests generally aren't recommended because there's no conclusive evidence that they're beneficial.

However, if you do develop signs or symptoms suggestive of a cancer recurrence, your doctor may order an imaging test to help determine if cancer is present, and where.

Dealing With Uncertainty

One of the most difficult aspects of follow-up care after primary breast cancer treatment is dealing with the uncertainty of whether the cancer will come back. Some women feel that testing will help them deal with this uncertainty. When asked, most women say they want to be tested for a possible recurrence. And why not? Getting back normal test results can relieve a lot of anxiety and let you breathe a sigh of relief, at least until the next round of testing.

But testing has its pitfalls. Often tests will reveal a slight deviation or small abnormality that may need to be evaluated. And tests often lead to more tests, especially because very few are able to produce certain results by themselves.

For example, the results of your liver function test may come back a few points above the upper normal limit. Your doctor may tell you that this likely doesn't signify a cancer recurrence, but you probably should have it rechecked in a couple of months just to make sure it isn't going up.

Caring for Your Whole Self

In addition to the physical aspects of follow-up care, it's important to remember the emotional and spiritual components. Adjusting to life after breast cancer takes time and requires the strong support of family and friends. Many women find it helpful to join a support group where they can learn about the experiences of other breast cancer survivors and share their own experiences. Another important aspect of caring for yourself after breast cancer is learning to trust your body to tell you when something is wrong.

For some women, adjusting to life after cancer treatment also means concentrating on those aspects of their lives they can control. This includes eating well, exercising, getting enough rest, and learning to deal with stress and anxiety.

For more information on life after cancer, see Part 3, "Living With Cancer."

If the next test shows that the results are slightly higher, you and your doctor will likely want to investigate further and do a more definitive test, such as a CT scan. The CT scan might note a normal liver but suggest a worrisome shadow around the pancreas. An ultrasound might then be obtained, revealing a normal pancreas. You feel great relief at these final results, but waiting for them may have caused a great deal of additional and, in the end, unnecessary anxiety.

Musa Mayer, a breast cancer survivor and nationally known breast cancer advocate, illustrates this all-too-common scenario in her book *After Breast Cancer:*

Musa's Story

My own love-hate relationship with testing came to a head about two years ago, when my oncologist referred me to a cardiologist because of some minor chest pain I had while exercising. A stress test showed nothing, nor did a thallium stress test, where a radioactive isotope helped with imaging the blood vessels. ...

"It's probably indigestion," said the cardiologist, unconcerned. But if I wanted a further level of certainty, he told me, there was a new test available, called an ultra-fast CT scan of the heart. ... I went ahead with the scan, without a thought in the world about how it might relate to my breast cancer history.

My coronary arteries were, blessedly, completely clear of calcium deposits. But in the report, the radiologist made notations about nodules in my lungs. And there were unexplained "densities" in my liver. ... I remember sitting there with the report in my hand, my heart pounding. I could feel the blood draining from my face. Now what? I had no symptoms, and I felt fine. Or I had until I'd read the test results.

My oncologist thought the nodules would likely be from my smoking history, although I'd quit 25 years before. He recommended an MRI of my liver, to further check the "densities." ... Days later came the definitive

answer: I had hepatic cysts, a benign condition that probably would never have
caused me any problems. Mixed with a
huge sense of relief was a growing convic-
tion that this sequence of tests, and the
weeks of anxiety attending them, had probably been unnecessary. Yet once set in
motion, the progression of events had been
impossible to stop.

It's also important to remember that just
as tests can sometimes find more than you
want them to, they can also miss things,
such as a cancer recurrence. Negative
results aren't a guarantee that no cancer
is present.

An insecure future

Margaret Gilseth was first diagnosed
with breast cancer in 1957. In the decades
that have followed, she has had multiple
local and regional breast cancer recurrences and, as a result, has run the gamut
of testing.

After years of undergoing blood tests
and chest X-rays at almost every doctor's
visit, she began seeing a new oncologist
who relied mostly on medical histories
and physical examinations and requested
other tests only occasionally. At first, this
made Margaret uncomfortable, worried
that her doctor wasn't making an effort to
keep track of what was happening inside
her body.

After talking with her doctor about her
concerns and doing some research of her
own, Margaret, an accomplished author
of several books, wrote an article on follow-up testing, which was published in
a 1996 issue of the *Journal of Clinical*
Oncology. Following is an excerpt from
that article:

Margaret's Story

We live in a culture that worships technology, and the voice of the testing
is more credible than the voice of our doctor. Because testing is frequently performed,
we are conditioned to believe that a test will
detect an early recurrent cancer and bring
hope for our survival. I believe it is impera-
tive that patients be informed of recent
research that pertains to their situation. We
need to learn to discriminate as new
research results are available — to re-exam-
ine our myths. ...

For me reassurance came with new
understanding, and that came with learning
the truth from my doctor. Routine testing for
(recurrent) breast cancer is not very helpful,
because it seldom detects cancer before a
doctor can, and in those cases in which it
does, there is no substantial benefit from
early institution of chemotherapy. Nothing
can take the place of a good doctor-patient
relationship. As I learn to live with insecuri-
ty, the minimal assurance given by routine
testing becomes irrelevant.

Today, Margaret is 86 years old. She still
sees her doctor for regular checkups, and
she's no longer concerned that he's not
taking good care of her.

If the Cancer Comes Back

Cancer recurrence refers to the return of cancer. Most women who are treated for early-stage breast cancer remain disease-free, but some do experience a recurrence. When a cancer recurs, it means that some cancer cells remained in the body after cancer treatment and these cells have begun to grow.

Recurrence may occur weeks, months, years or even decades after an initial diagnosis. Sometimes, the cancer returns in the same location as the original tumor. Other times, it recurs in a different location. For example, a few cells from a breast tumor may have spread to bone by way of the bloodstream. These cells weren't eliminated during treatment, and eventually they grew to a size that could be detected.

For many women, dealing with a cancer recurrence can be more difficult than dealing with an initial diagnosis. Recurrence is often a breast cancer survivor's greatest fear. If your cancer does come back, you may feel as if you've lost the battle against the disease and that all your efforts were in vain. But this is not necessarily the case. The treatments you received may have actually delayed the cancer recurrence, giving you additional time you might not have had otherwise.

Although it's true that most breast cancer recurrences aren't curable, for some, there is potential for a cure, depending on where the cancer is located. Even if a cure isn't possible, treatments can help maintain your quality of life and control the cancer, sometimes for many years.

Types of Recurrence

Breast cancer recurrence is generally categorized by location. It can be local, regional, distant or a combination of these.

Local recurrence

A local recurrence means the cancer redevelops in the same spot or vicinity as the primary tumor. For example, if you had a lumpectomy in your right breast and the cancer recurs in that same breast, that's a local recurrence. This type of local recurrence is called an in-breast recurrence.

It's possible that a new primary tumor may develop in the breast of a woman who has had a lumpectomy. A new primary tumor isn't the same as a recurrent tumor, although the two can be difficult to distinguish. A general rule of thumb is that if cancer is found in the same breast 10 or more years after the first tumor, it's considered a new primary tumor. Recurrent cancer tends to develop sooner — less than 10 years from the initial diagnosis. In some cases, a new primary tumor may develop in the opposite breast. This isn't a recurrence either. Rather, it's treated as a new primary breast cancer.

If you've had a breast removed (mastectomy) and cancer appears in your chest wall near where the breast had been, that also is a local recurrence.

Regional recurrence

A regional recurrence means that cancer cells have broken away from the original tumor site and are appearing in nearby lymph nodes, such as those under your arm, near your breastbone or above your collarbone. Local and regional recurrences may occur simultaneously. The two are often lumped together and termed local-regional recurrences. In this situation, there isn't any proof that the cancer has spread to more distant parts of the body.

Distant recurrence

A distant recurrence is when the original cancer cells have managed to travel to other organs or tissues in your body besides your breast, chest area or nearby lymph nodes. This type of cancer is called distant recurrence because the cancer has been identified in places distant from the original tumor site. Other terms that are sometimes used are *metastatic* and *systemic recurrence*, because the cancer is now affecting more than one part of your body. Most often breast cancer cells spread to bone. Other sites of metastases include the lungs and liver. Less often, the cancer spreads to the brain or other areas of the central nervous system.

Although it seems logical that a local recurrence would come first, then a regional recurrence and then a distant one, it isn't always this orderly. Many times a distant recurrence will occur without a local or regional recurrence.

How Cancer Cells Spread

The manner in which cancer spreads to your lymph nodes and other parts of your body is a long and complicated process. Most cancer cells don't make the journey, but some of the ones that do are hardy enough to establish themselves in other tissues and survive there.

Normally, the cells that make up the organs and tissues of your body, including your breasts, are held in place by a substance called an extracellular matrix. For cancer cells to travel outside of your breast, they must first break through this extracellular matrix. They appear to do this by breaking down the matrix with enzymes or by altering the adhesiveness of their own cell surface.

Once they're free of this matrix, cancer cells can invade nearby tissues or travel through the lymphatic system or blood-stream to other more distant organs and tissues. Your lymphatic system is a network of channels throughout your body, similar to your circulatory system, but instead of carrying blood, it carries lymphatic fluid and immune cells.

With breast cancer, cancerous (malignant) cells that have broken free of the original tumor may be swept along with the lymphatic fluid that drains from your breast tissue and eventually may end up in your axillary lymph nodes — bean-shaped structures of lymph tissue located under your arm. Some of the cancer cells may be destroyed in the lymph nodes, which are full of scavenging white blood cells that ingest and destroy foreign

Is It Now Bone or Lung Cancer?

Breast cancer cells have a different makeup from bone, lung or liver cancer cells. They evolve differently, progress differently and respond differently to various therapies. When breast cancer cells spread to another part of your body — such as your bones, lungs or liver — they're still breast cancer cells, but they're growing in a different area. Breast cancer cells that are found in your bones don't become bone cancer. You still have breast cancer, only now it's called metastatic breast cancer in your bones.

One doctor uses the following analogy to explain this concept to his patients: If dandelions are growing in the yard and they go to seed, and wind spreads this seed to the rose garden, allowing the dandelions to grow in the rose garden, these flowers aren't called roses. They're dandelions that have spread to the rose garden. In the same manner, if breast cancer cells spread within the body and start growing in the bone, they wouldn't be called bone cancer, but breast cancer spread to bone.

This is an important distinction because breast, bone, lung and liver cancers behave differently and are treated differently. For example, lung cancer cells aren't affected by estrogen in the way that breast cancer cells are. Therefore, lung cancer wouldn't respond to estrogen-related drugs such as tamoxifen, but breast cancer cells in your lungs may.

substances. But some cancer cells may evade immune cells and survive and grow in the lymph nodes, or they may travel on within the lymph system.

To get into your bloodstream, cancer cells may burrow their way through a blood vessel wall (see the color illustration on page 259). Once the cells are in the bloodstream, they're swept along with the flow of blood and may be carried to parts of your body far from your breast. Like your lymphatic system, however, your bloodstream is also full of immune cells capable of destroying cancer cells that make their way in. Still, some cancer cells may survive the ride. These cells can become lodged in the smaller branches of your blood vessel network. From there, they burrow their way out of the blood vessel into nearby tissue — such as bone, lung or liver — where they may survive and grow in a different environment from which they originated.

Local Recurrence

Breast cancer can recur in your remaining breast tissue after a lumpectomy or in your chest wall tissue after a mastectomy. There are some differences between the two, so we'll discuss each separately. Some general factors, though, that might increase your risk of recurrence after initial treatment with either lumpectomy or mastectomy include:

- A young age (less than 40) at diagnosis
- A primary tumor that's 5 centimeters (about 2 inches) or more in diameter
- A high tumor grade, indicating markedly abnormal cancer cells

- Cancer in the lymph nodes
- Cancer cells at the margin of the removed tissue or close to it
- Tumors that involve breast skin, such as inflammatory breast cancer, or the chest wall

Some factors that may be in your favor if you have a local recurrence, regardless of your initial treatment, include:

- A long interval — a period of more than five years — from when your cancer was first diagnosed until it recurred. This is called the disease-free interval.
- An isolated local recurrence.

Characteristics such as these are called prognostic factors, which can help predict disease outcome. Keep in mind, though, that these are generalizations about a complex disease, and your individual outcome isn't based solely on such factors. Prognostic factors are mentioned throughout this chapter, but remember they serve only to give you a general picture. Nobody can absolutely know what will happen in your future.

Local recurrence after lumpectomy

Within 10 years after undergoing lumpectomy and radiation for stages I and II breast cancer, approximately 10 percent to 20 percent of women have a local recurrence in the same breast (in-breast recurrence). About 75 percent to 90 percent of these women appear to have an isolated local recurrence, meaning the recurrence isn't widespread throughout the breast and there isn't evidence the cancer has spread (metastasized) to distant locations.

Among women whose initial cancer was invasive and who experience an in-breast recurrence, in about 90 percent of cases the recurrent cancer is also invasive. About 10 percent of the time, it's noninvasive (carcinoma *in situ*). Among women who initially had ductal carcinoma *in situ* and who experience an in-breast recurrence, the recurrent cancer is invasive in about 75 percent of cases.

Signs and symptoms

About one-third of in-breast recurrences are detected by mammography before they can be felt. Another third are detected by self- or clinical examination and another third by a combination of the two.

The signs of an in-breast recurrence are generally the same as those of a new primary breast cancer, such as an unusual lump or a new change in your breast skin. But cancer can be a bit subtle the second time around, and sometimes it may be confused with a noncancerous (benign) abnormality. For one thing, surgery can produce changes in your breast, including mass-like areas of scar tissue, lumps of fatty tissue (fat necrosis) and scar tissue around the stitches used to close the incision (suture granulomas). Radiation can result in general swelling of your breast, thickening of your breast skin and increased density of breast tissue. Most often, breast changes that occur soon after treatment — for instance, within the first year — are most likely benign, and often a result of treatment. However, it's still important to point out the change to your doctor so that it can be monitored.

Occasionally, some women develop a breast infection (mastitis), which is characterized by inflammation, swelling and redness. Mastitis is easily treated with

antibiotics, but your doctor will want to make sure that it's not inflammatory breast cancer, a type of breast cancer that involves the skin and has features similar to mastitis.

So what should you watch out for? In general, report to your doctor any changes you notice in your breast, if only for your own peace of mind. Be particularly aware of these signs and symptoms:

- A new, firm lump or nodule in your breast or an irregular area of firmness
- A new thickening in a breast area
- A new pain in your breast
- Dimpling or indentation in your breast
- A skin rash, swelling or inflammation
- Progressive flattening of your nipple or other nipple changes

If you notice any of these signs and symptoms, tell your doctor right away so that they can be evaluated further.

Tests

If you and your doctor suspect an in-breast recurrence because of results of a mammogram or physical examination, your doctor may use another imaging test, such as ultrasound, to try to determine whether the suspicious finding is benign or malignant. You'll likely need a biopsy to confirm the presence or absence of cancer. Because the hormone receptor status of your cancer may change with a recurrence, if cancerous tissue is found during a biopsy, it may again be tested for the presence of estrogen and progesterone receptors. The specimen may also be tested for signs of overproduction of the HER-2/neu protein, especially if this testing was not performed during your first diagnosis. Both the hormone receptor status and HER-2/neu status are important in determining what types of therapy would be appropriate to treat the cancer.

Because some women who develop an in-breast recurrence also have distant metastases, other tests may be done to determine if the cancer has spread to other parts of the body. These tests may include a chest X-ray and other imaging tests, such as a computerized tomography (CT) scan or bone scan, as well as a complete blood count and liver function tests.

Treatment

Treatment for an in-breast recurrence after lumpectomy may include surgery, radiation therapy or drug therapy.

Surgery

Assuming there's no evidence of cancer spread to distant sites, an in-breast recurrence is usually treated by mastectomy. In some cases, a lumpectomy may be done, but using a lumpectomy to treat this type of recurrence is controversial. A lumpectomy carries a higher risk of yet another recurrence that may be more serious.

Because a local breast recurrence may be accompanied by hidden cancer in nearby lymph nodes, your doctor may remove some or all of the lymph nodes under your arm (axillary dissection) during surgery if they weren't removed during your initial treatment.

Radiation therapy

If you haven't had any previous radiation, your doctor may recommend it now. However, most women who undergo lumpectomy for their initial cancer also receive radiation, so radiation may not be an option for an in-breast recurrence.

Not much data exist on the use of repeat radiation in women who received radiation to treat their original tumors. Studies that have been done don't suggest that additional radiation is helpful in preventing future recurrences. Plus, receiving additional doses of radiation may increase your risk of radiation-related side effects.

Drug therapy

If an in-breast recurrence is so extensive that surgery isn't an option, your doctor may recommend chemotherapy, hormone therapy or both to treat the cancer. Most local recurrences, however, can be treated with surgery.

A decision to use chemotherapy, hormone therapy or both depends on a number of factors, including whether you received either to treat your initial cancer, and what type of treatment you had. Other important factors include your menopausal status, how long it has been since your initial diagnosis (your disease-free interval), details regarding your tumor, such as its hormone receptor status and HER-2/neu status, and whether you have other health problems.

Prognosis

Having an in-breast recurrence is a sign the disease is still active and is associated with a fairly high risk of subsequent recurrences in distant sites. Between 45 percent and 80 percent of women are alive five years after treatment, and between 40 percent and 65 percent survive 10 years later. Factors that may predict outcome include:

- **Longer time between treatment and recurrence.** The longer the time between your initial cancer and the recurrence, the better. In general, an interval greater than five years is considered favorable for long-term survival, but some studies have shown that intervals of even two years or more can signify a better outcome than if the recurrence occurred sooner. This is because the sooner a cancer returns, the more likely it is to be fast-growing (aggressive) with a higher risk of distant metastasis.
- **Noninvasive recurrence.** A noninvasive cancer recurrence signifies a better outcome than does an invasive one.
- **Isolated recurrence.** Recurrent cancer that's isolated to a small area of the breast is better than is a widespread in-breast recurrence or a regional recurrence involving the lymph nodes.

Local recurrence after mastectomy

Among women who have a mastectomy to treat breast cancer, about 5 percent to 10 percent experience a cancer recurrence in their chest wall tissue, either alone or in combination with other recurrences. Cancer recurrence on the chest wall is more likely in women whose original breast cancer had spread to lymph nodes. A local chest wall recurrence tends to occur within 10 years of initial treatment, but some local recurrences have been reported 15, 25 and even 50 years after a mastectomy.

In about two-thirds of the women who experience a chest wall recurrence after mastectomy, at the time the recurrence is

diagnosed there are no indications that the cancer has also spread to distant locations. In the other third, there's evidence the cancer has spread to other areas of the body.

Signs and symptoms

A local recurrence after a mastectomy usually appears as a painless nodule in or under your chest wall skin. It most often develops in or near the mastectomy scar. About half the local chest wall recurrences appear as a solitary nodule, while the rest show up as multiple nodules. Occasionally, a chest wall recurrence may appear as a red, often itchy skin rash.

Among women who've had tissue flap breast reconstruction, a recurrence may develop near the area where the stitches were placed or in the remaining chest wall skin, but a recurrence in the flap itself is rare. Recurrences in the chest wall muscle only also are rare. Benign lumps and fat necrosis, another benign condition, are fairly common with breast tissue reconstruction. If a lump occurs, a doctor may want to do a biopsy to make sure the diagnosis is correct.

Tests

Almost all chest wall recurrences after mastectomy are detected by physical examination. In a tissue-reconstructed breast, mammography or magnetic resonance imaging (MRI) may help distinguish between a cancerous mass and a noncancerous mass. A biopsy can confirm the presence of cancer. The biopsy specimen will likely be tested for estrogen and progesterone receptor status and possibly HER-2/neu status.

Because of the possibility of distant recurrence, your doctor may also request other tests, including a chest X-ray and other imaging tests, such as a CT scan and bone scan, as well as blood tests, including liver function tests.

Treatment

A chest wall recurrence after a mastectomy is typically treated with surgery, if possible, as well as radiation and medication — chemotherapy, hormone therapy or both.

Surgery

If the recurrent cancer is a solitary nodule that can be fairly easily removed, surgery may be done. If the disease is more extensive, surgery usually isn't recommended.

Radiation therapy

If you haven't received radiation before, your doctor will likely recommend it now. Surgery followed by radiation therapy may provide the most effective treatment for a chest wall recurrence after mastectomy. Usually, the whole chest wall area is treated. You and your doctor may also choose to include the area around your collarbone to reach nearby lymph nodes, which are at increased risk of recurrence. Sometimes — especially if some cancer still remains in the chest wall after surgery — an additional boost of radiation is given directly to the area of recurrence.

Chemotherapy and hormone therapy

Medication (systemic therapy) may be recommended after surgery and radiation to reduce the risk of another local recurrence or a metastatic recurrence. There aren't any good studies to direct doctors regarding the use of systemic therapy in preventing additional recurrences, but some studies suggest it can be helpful.

Photodynamic therapy

Photodynamic therapy is an experimental treatment that's being tested in some women with chest wall recurrence. This therapy involves injecting light-sensitive chemicals into the body. Cancer cells in the body absorb the chemicals. A doctor then uses a laser light to activate the chemicals, which destroy the cancer cells.

Prognosis

Compared with an in-breast recurrence after lumpectomy, a chest wall recurrence after mastectomy carries a considerably higher risk of eventual spread of the cancer to distant sites. Nonetheless, certain factors may indicate a better prognosis:

- **Longer time between treatment and recurrence.** This is very important. The longer the time between when you were initially diagnosed with cancer and your recurrence, the better the situation.
- **Isolated recurrence.** An isolated chest wall recurrence, particularly a single nodule, often has a better outcome than does a widespread local recurrence.
- **Complete excision.** Removal of the recurrent tumor, with no cancer cells located in the margins of the removed tissue, signifies a better outcome.
- **Estrogen receptor status.** A recurrent cancer that's estrogen receptor positive is more responsive to hormone therapy and, therefore, may result in improved survival.

Regional Recurrence

After a mastectomy or lumpectomy, it's possible for cancer to recur in the lymph nodes near the breast that was treated. This is known as a regional recurrence. A regional recurrence can occur by itself, but often it occurs simultaneously with a local recurrence and is referred to as a local-regional recurrence.

Types

Regional breast cancer recurrence is usually divided into one of three categories:

- **Axillary node recurrence.** Cancer is present in underarm lymph nodes.

- **Supraclavicular node recurrence.** Cancer is present in the lymph nodes above your collarbone. Occasionally, the cancer may also recur in lymph nodes just below your collarbone (infraclavicular lymph nodes).
- **Internal mammary node recurrence.** Cancer is present in a group of lymph nodes located along your breastbone in the center of your chest.

Signs and symptoms

The first sign of a regional recurrence is usually a swelling or lump in the affected lymph nodes, such as under your arm, in the groove above your collarbone or in

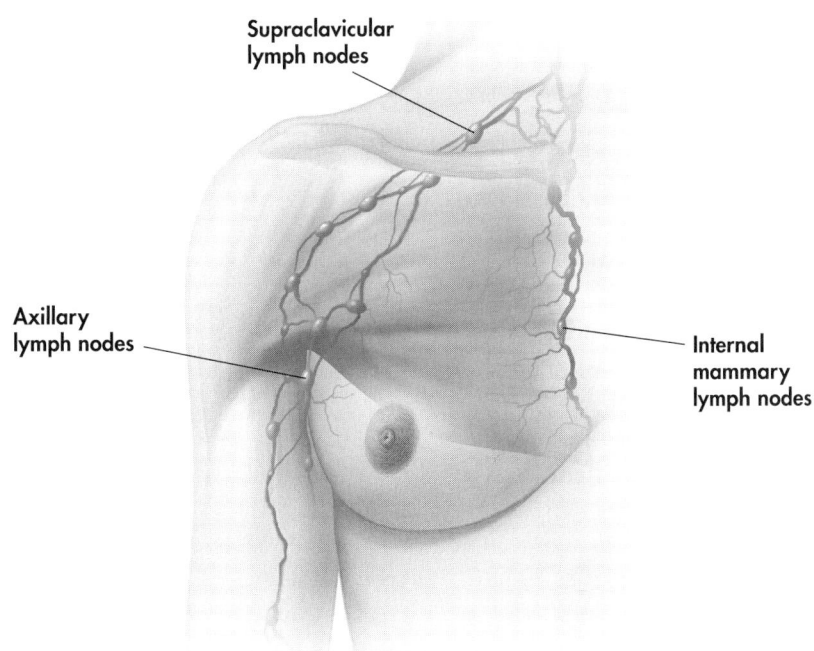

Supraclavicular
lymph nodes

Axillary
lymph nodes

Internal
mammary
lymph nodes

the area around your breastbone. Because your internal mammary nodes are located deep within your chest, a small recurrence in this area is more difficult to detect.

Regional recurrences aren't always accompanied by signs or symptoms. One study found that signs and symptoms occurred in only 30 percent of women with an isolated regional recurrence. Signs and symptoms that may indicate a regional recurrence include:

- Swelling of your arm
- Persistent arm and shoulder pain
- Increasing loss of sensation and motor skills in your arm and hand
- Persistent chest pain
- Difficulty swallowing

If you experience any of these, tell your doctor so that they can be evaluated.

Tests

A regional recurrence may be detected when your doctor asks you about your symptoms since your last appointment and gives you a physical examination.

Computerized tomography (CT) scans, magnetic resonance imaging (MRI), or positron emission tomography (PET) scans may be helpful in evaluating a suspected recurrence in the axillary nodes. These tests may also help detect an internal mammary node recurrence. Sometimes, your doctor may perform surgical exploration of a lymph node region to obtain a tissue sample for evaluation.

Because a regional breast cancer recurrence carries a high risk of distant recurrence, your doctor will likely have you undergo other tests to check for spread of cancer to other areas of your body.

Treatment

If it's possible, surgery may be the best option for removing the recurrence and controlling the cancer. In some cases, radiation therapy may be used after surgery to further destroy any cancer cells. If surgery isn't feasible, radiation therapy may be used as the primary form of treatment. Other nearby lymph node areas may also be radiated to try to prevent further recurrence. Because of significant risk of distant recurrence, chemotherapy or hormone therapy may be recommended after surgery, radiation or both to prevent recurrence of the cancer at other sites.

Prognosis

With a regional recurrence, the prognosis generally depends on where the recurrence is located, whether it's isolated, how long it was from the time you were first diagnosed with breast cancer until the recurrence, and certain characteristics of the cancer. Most women with regional breast cancer recurrences aren't cured. If the cancer has spread to regional lymph nodes, it likely has spread to other parts of the body, too. However, even when a cure isn't possible, with appropriate therapy it's still possible to live for years.

Distant Recurrence

When breast cancer cells reappear in parts of your body other than your breast or nearby lymph nodes, the cancer is considered a distant (metastatic) recurrence. Breast cancer most commonly spreads to the bones, lungs and liver. Other sites include the brain, scalp, lymph nodes, abdomen and ovaries.

Signs and symptoms

Metastatic disease usually becomes apparent through signs and symptoms.

Breast cancer metastasis to bone may be signaled by bone pain. Signs and symptoms of metastasis to the lungs may include:
- Persistent, dry cough
- Difficulty breathing
- Shortness of breath
- Chest pain

Liver metastasis may be signaled by:
- Loss of appetite
- Abdominal tenderness or discomfort
- Persistent nausea, vomiting or weight loss
- Jaundice

Brain metastasis may be signaled by:
- Severe headaches
- Visual disturbances
- New seizures or symptoms such as weakness, numbness or imbalance
- Persistent nausea not explained by another problem

Biopsy

A diagnosis of metastatic breast cancer needs to be made with as much certainty as possible. Often, this involves a biopsy of a tumor at a distant site. The tissue collected is tested for certain characteristics, such as estrogen and progesterone receptors and HER-2/neu receptors.

In some situations, though, a biopsy is either dangerous or unnecessary. For example, if you have a history of breast cancer and multiple new masses (tumors) occur in your bones or lungs and there's no other explanation for these masses, then a diagnosis of metastatic breast cancer can be made with reasonable certainty without the need for an invasive surgical biopsy. However, because breast cancer treatment is dependent upon the characteristics of the tumor cells, sometimes a biopsy is done in such situations so that your treatment can be tailored to the characteristics of your cancer.

Other tests

If your doctor suspects a metastatic recurrence, he or she may use a number of tests to confirm the presence or absence of cancer cells in different areas of your body.

Laboratory tests

Among women with metastatic breast cancer, laboratory tests may include:
- **Complete blood count.** A complete blood count is a common blood test that's often part of a general physical examination. It measures your red and white blood cells and your platelets to help determine your general health.
- **Blood tumor marker tests.** Some cancers produce certain substances (tumor markers) that can be detected in blood. These substances usually are present in low concentrations in healthy individuals. In case of certain cancers, their levels may increase. Some cancer markers associated with breast cancer include carcinoembryonic antigen (CEA), CA 15-3 and CA 27-29. A blood test may be done to test for these markers. Blood

tumor marker tests are generally inadequate for detecting cancer in women without signs or symptoms, but they may help confirm a cancer recurrence in women with symptoms.

- **Liver function tests.** When liver cells are damaged, enzymes normally found inside the cells leak into blood. Your blood may also contain higher than normal amounts of waste products, because the waste isn't being removed by your liver as it should be. In addition, your blood may contain abnormal amounts of certain liver proteins.

Imaging tests

Your doctor may use one or more of the following tests to check your lungs, liver, bones and abdomen for any unusual masses or structural abnormalities:

- **X-ray.** Chest X-rays may detect a tumor in your lungs. Bone X-rays may be able to detect bone metastases.
- **CT scan.** A CT scan can provide more detailed pictures than can ordinary X-rays. CT scans may be used to examine your head, chest, abdomen and bones for evidence of metastases.
- **MRI scan.** Similar to CT, MRI provides views of the inside of your body in cross-sectional slices. But it uses an extremely strong magnet instead of X-rays. An MRI may detect metastases to the brain or around the spinal cord.
- **Bone scan.** A bone scan is a type of nuclear medicine scan. It can provide a picture of your whole skeleton and may be used to check for metastases in your bones. During a bone scan, a small, safe amount of radioactive material is injected into your bloodstream. The material

binds to your bone cells. A gamma camera then records the pattern of radioactive absorption in your bones. In areas with bone metastases, generally more of the tracer is absorbed and the area "lights up" on the scan.

- **PET scan.** A PET scan also uses radioactive material injected into your body to produce an image of your body. Tissues using more energy — exhibiting increased metabolic activity — absorb greater amounts of the radioactive material. Tumors are often more metabolically active than are healthy tissues and generally appear more prominent on the scan.
- **Liver ultrasound.** An ultrasound exam can often help detect if the cancer has spread to your liver.

Prognosis and treatment

Because metastatic cancer is characterized by the spread of cancer cells throughout the body, systemic therapy — therapy that treats the whole body — is generally the recommended treatment. This may involve use of chemotherapy, hormone therapy or both. The main goal of treatment for an individual with a metastatic breast cancer recurrence is to prolong life and maintain as good a quality of life as possible.

In general, metastatic breast cancer isn't considered curable, but the prognosis for individual women can vary widely.

Treatment and prognosis of metastatic breast cancer is discussed in detail in the next chapter.

Chapter 14: Breast Cancer

Treating Advanced Breast Cancer

When breast cancer spreads to distant sites, such as the bones, lungs or liver, it's referred to as advanced breast cancer. Other terms commonly used are *metastatic cancer* or *stage IV cancer*. Although some women have advanced breast cancer when they're first diagnosed, more often it develops when the cancer recurs.

Usually, women with metastatic breast cancer have been through diagnosis and treatment before, when their original tumors were first found. The process of diagnosis and treatment this time has some similarities to that first experience, but it also has some key differences. This chapter focuses on evaluation and treatment of women with metastatic breast cancer.

Whether or not this is your first experience with breast cancer, you may be thinking that not much can be done for advanced breast cancer. In fact, treatment options are available for breast cancer in its later stages. Even though the goals of treatment aren't to cure the cancer, treatment may provide long-term control of the disease. As breast cancer treatments become more and more effective, women are surviving longer with breast cancer, even to the point where some have come to view it as a chronic disease rather than a terminal illness.

Determining Prognosis

Metastatic breast cancer isn't a simple, uniform disease. Instead of viewing it as a single entity, picture it as a spectrum. At one end of the disease spectrum is a rapidly progressive disease with extensive spread to organs such as the liver and brain. At this end, the disease may be resistant to hormone therapy and chemotherapy. Average survival is most often measured in terms of a few months.

At the other end of the spectrum are instances where the cancer follows a long, slow (indolent) course. Women in this situation generally have cancer spread to bone or soft tissue, and their internal organs aren't affected. At this end of the spectrum, the disease tends to be more sensitive to hormone therapy and chemotherapy. Women with this type of recurrence may live for years or even decades. Very rarely, a person will even do well for decades without any treatment aimed at halting the disease's progression.

In general, the average length of survival for women who have received a diagnosis of metastatic breast cancer is between two and three years. But survival may vary considerably, based on various tumor behaviors.

In predicting how a woman's cancer will behave and the disease's likely outcome, doctors rely on a number of factors (prognostic factors). These involve not only characteristics of the disease but also factors related to the person being treated and the type of treatment received.

Disease characteristics

Characteristics related to the cancer can help determine how it may behave:

Disease-free interval

The disease-free interval refers to the time from initial diagnosis to recurrence. This is often one of the best predictors of how the cancer will act after it has recurred.

Women who develop evidence of metastatic breast cancer early on, while they're still receiving initial treatment for breast cancer or soon after treatment ends, generally have a very poor prognosis. If, on the other hand, metastatic breast cancer becomes apparent 10 to 15 years after the initial diagnosis, the course of the disease is often slow and the prognosis better.

Hormone receptor status

Women with hormone receptor positive breast cancer — estrogen receptor positive, progesterone receptor positive or both — generally have a slower disease course than do women with hormone receptor negative cancers.

HER-2/neu status

In the past, it was generally noted that women with HER-2/neu positive cancers had a poorer prognosis than did women

Prognostic factors in metastatic breast cancer

Disease characteristics	Personal and treatment factors
Disease-free period between initial diagnosis and metastatic recurrence	Ability to get around (performance status) and presence of other medical conditions
Hormone receptor status	Prior treatment
HER-2/neu status	Response to prior treatment
Locations of disease	Age
Extent of disease	

whose tumors were HER-2/neu negative. The former is more aggressive and less sensitive to hormone treatments.

However, the drug trastuzumab (Herceptin) provides a new form of treatment for women with HER-2/neu positive cancers. This drug may cancel out HER-2/neu positive status as a negative prognostic factor.

Sites of disease
Women with metastatic disease that's limited to the skin, lymph nodes or bones have an improved prognosis, compared with women who have tumors in multiple sites or in the liver or brain. Women with cancer in the lungs or the tissue surrounding them have an intermediate prognosis.

Extent of disease
Women with only small amounts of metastatic disease tend to do better than do women with extensive disease.

Personal and treatment factors

A number of personal and treatment factors also can affect your prognosis, includ-

ing mobility and other medical conditions, prior treatment and age.

Mobility and other medical conditions
Mobility (performance status) refers to your ability to be up and about and to carry on normal activities. Your mobility helps determine how well you may tolerate certain treatments and how likely these treatments are to help. Performance status is usually measured using a tool such as the Eastern Cooperative Oncology Group (ECOG) Performance Status or the Karnofsky Scale.

In addition to mobility, the presence of other medical conditions, such as heart disease, stroke and diabetes, can affect your prognosis.

Prior treatment
How well a person with metastatic disease will do, may be affected by the extent of the treatment she received when her breast cancer was originally diagnosed.

Your doctor will review your breast cancer history, including whether your primary tumor was hormone receptor positive or negative as well as your HER-2/neu status. He or she will also look at the speed at which your cancer has progressed.

For example, did the cancer's spread become apparent 10 years after your initial diagnosis? Or did it occur two months after the completion of your initial treatment? These are two very different scenarios that have different effects on prognosis and treatment decisions.

Age

Whether age affects the course of breast cancer after it becomes metastatic is a matter of debate. Some data suggest that particularly young women or older women have poorer prognoses.

Treatment Options

Because the cancer has spread to other parts of the body, treatment for metastatic breast cancer generally involves whole body (systemic) therapy rather than local therapy, such as surgery or radiation. Within the arena of systemic therapy, several options are available, including:

- Hormone therapy
- Chemotherapy
- Biologically based therapy, such as trastuzumab (Herceptin)
- A combination of therapies

As you go along, you may find that there are easily 10 to 20 different options that may be used to treat metastatic breast cancer. You'll want to work with your doctor to decide which option is most appropriate for you. In addition, if one treatment doesn't work or stops working, you may be able to try other treatments.

Treatment goals

When devising a therapy plan, you and your doctor will want to address two questions:

1. Is being cured a realistic goal among women with metastatic breast cancer?
2. Are women with metastatic cancer occasionally cured?

The answer to the first question generally is no. Curing metastatic breast cancer isn't a realistic goal. In this sense, some people and their doctors have come to view metastatic breast cancer as a chronic disease and are treating it as such, similar to how incurable diabetes or heart disease might be treated. This means trying to control symptoms related to the cancer while minimizing toxic effects from the drugs. The goal of therapy then becomes to help you live as well as possible for as long as possible.

This doesn't mean, though, that women have never been cured of advanced breast cancer — meaning that the answer to the second question may be yes. Although being cured typically isn't a goal of metastatic breast cancer treatment, occasionally — maybe 2 percent to 3 percent of the time — women with metastatic breast cancer will experience a complete remission of their disease that lasts 10 to 15 years or longer.

Hormone therapy

It's well known that the female hormones estrogen and progesterone influence the growth and development of a majority of breast cancers. As a result, breast cancers that make receptors for estrogen and

Working Off Assumptions

Whether hormone therapy or chemotherapy actually prolongs survival in women with metastatic breast cancer has never been put to a proper scientific test. Doing so would mean that half the participants in the trial would receive drug therapy and the other half would receive no treatment. Because drug therapy appears to benefit the vast majority of women with breast cancer, it's generally considered unethical to conduct a trial that would deny treatment to half the participants.

Based on available information, it appears that women who receive hormone therapy or chemotherapy or a combination of the two do live longer than do women who don't receive such treatment. How much of a benefit is achieved? An average improvement in survival of a year or two appears to be a reasonable estimate. This average includes some women who clearly live many years longer than would have been expected if they had never received such treatment.

progesterone — referred to as hormone-receptor positive cancers — can be treated with hormone therapy.

Your menopausal status is generally the first thing a doctor evaluates in determining what hormone therapy options are available. Treatment options are different for premenopausal and postmenopausal women primarily because of the difference in the levels of estrogen in their bodies. Premenopausal women have high levels of estrogen. In postmenopausal women, the ovaries no longer produce estrogen or progesterone, but the body still continues to produce some estrogen, although in reduced amounts.

Premenopausal women

There are different ways to moderate the influence of estrogen and progesterone in premenopausal women whose ovaries are still fully functional. Treatment options include ovarian suppression, tamoxifen or both.

Ovarian suppression

One of the oldest methods of hormone therapy is ovarian suppression — keeping the ovaries from producing estrogen and progesterone. This can be done by surgically removing the ovaries (oophorectomy) or by radiating the ovaries or with use of medications.

- **Oophorectomy.** The first description of the use of oophorectomy to treat metastatic breast cancer dates back to 1896 by Sir George Beatson. He had previously noted hormone changes in animals when their ovaries were removed. So he performed an oophorectomy in a young woman with recurrent breast cancer who was willing to try the experiment. Within months, there was a dramatic shrinkage of the young woman's cancer.

  For many decades following, oophorectomy became the mainstay of treatment for premenopausal women with metastatic breast cancer, with approximately one-third of the women responding to the therapy.

When medical scientists found a way to identify the presence or absence of estrogen and progesterone receptors on breast cancer cells — indicating whether the cancer was sensitive to hormones — responses could be better predicted. Women with estrogen receptor positive cancers have approximately a 60 percent response rate to oophorectomy, whereas only about 10 percent or less of women with estrogen receptor negative cancers respond to this therapy. The highest response rates to ovarian suppression are generally seen in women who have cancers with both estrogen and progesterone receptors and long disease-free intervals.

Although oophorectomy is a century-old procedure, it's still a viable and effective treatment option.

- **Radiation therapy.** Radiating the ovaries also can cause ovarian suppression, but this method can take weeks to become effective. Today, it's rarely used.
- **Medications.** Another method of suppressing the ovaries is with a group of drugs called luteinizing hormone-releasing hormone (LH-RH) agonists. These include drugs such as goserelin (Zoladex), leuprolide (Lupron, Viadur) and triptorelin (Trelstar Depot).

The medications, given by injection once a month or every three months, effectively shut off ovarian function. They're used instead of surgery in a large number of women. This means ovarian suppression may be reversible by stopping the medications. However, depending on how close to menopause a woman is and how long she takes these drugs, her ovaries may shut down permanently.

Tamoxifen

The medication tamoxifen (Nolvadex) is another form of hormone treatment for women with metastatic breast cancer. It differs from drugs used in hormone suppression in that it doesn't prevent the ovaries from producing female hormones. Tamoxifen is a synthetic hormone belonging to a class of drugs known as selective estrogen receptor modulators (SERMs). It works by keeping estrogen from attaching

---

QUESTION & ANSWER

Q: **How do you know when you're past menopause?**

A: The definition of menopausal status varies. One definition that's commonly used is the absence of any menstrual period for at least 12 months. In some situations, such as if your period has ceased for other reasons, this may not apply. For example, in women whose ovaries are intact but who no longer have a uterus, this definition isn't useful. If your menopausal status is unclear, blood tests may be obtained to determine your hormone status. This will reveal whether you're premenopausal or postmenopausal.

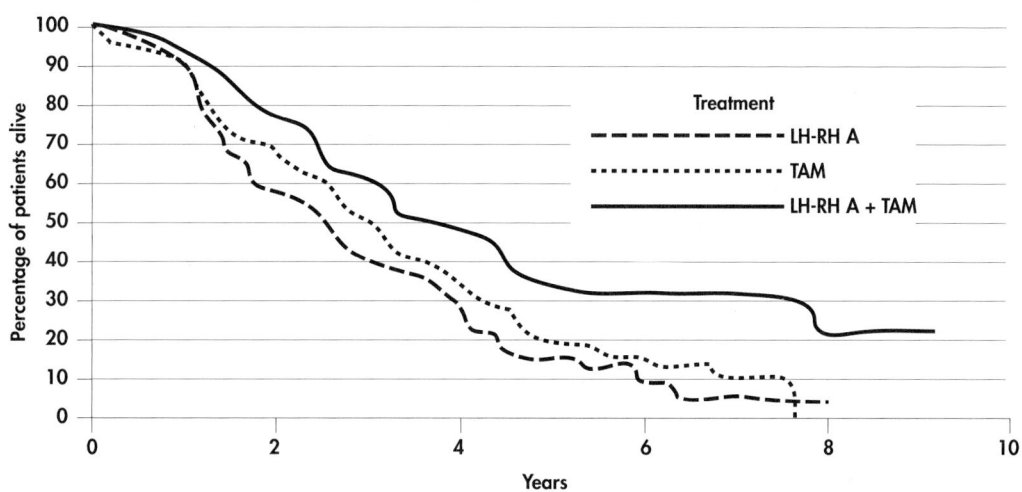

Combination treatment improves survival

LH-RH A = luteinizing hormone-releasing hormone agonist (buserelin). TAM = tamoxifen.
LH-RH A + TAM = buserelin plus tamoxifen.

Source: J. G. Klijn et al., "Combined Treatment with Buserelin and Tamoxifen in Premenopausal Metastatic Breast Cancer: A Randomized Study," *Journal of the National Cancer Institute*, 92:11 (June 7, 2000), pages 903-911

to estrogen receptors on breast cancer cells, thus blocking estrogen's influence on the tumor's growth (see page 182).

Tamoxifen is about as effective as oophorectomy among women with metastatic breast cancer, and because it's less invasive than is oophorectomy, it became the standard form of hormone therapy for premenopausal women with metastatic breast cancer. For more information on tamoxifen, see Chapter 9.

Tamoxifen and ovarian suppression
A recent clinical trial conducted in Europe tested the idea of combining tamoxifen and the LH-RH agonist buserelin to see if the combination would improve treatment results. In the trial, 161 pre-

menopausal estrogen receptor positive women with metastatic breast cancer were randomly selected to receive one of three treatments: tamoxifen only, buserelin only or both tamoxifen and buserelin.

After about seven years of follow-up, the results show an overall benefit in survival for the group that received the combination of agents, compared with the group that received only one medication (see the graph above). Improvement in average survival with the combination approach, as compared with the single-agent approach, was approximately one year. Thirty-four percent of the participants receiving the drug combination were still alive five years after they started their treatment, compared with approximately 15 percent of the participants who received only one of the drugs.

Based on this information, the current standard treatment approach for premenopausal women with hormone receptor positive metastatic breast cancer is a combination of ovarian suppression and tamoxifen.

Other options

If the combination of ovarian suppression and tamoxifen isn't effective and your doctor thinks that it's reasonable to consider another form of hormone therapy, several approaches are possible. The drug megestrol acetate (Megace), which is a progesterone medication, and the androgenic agent fluoxymesterone, which is similar to testosterone, have been used. More often, though, doctors are prescribing medications called aromatase inhibitors in combination with continued ovarian suppression. In women who are premenopausal, aromatase inhibitors are

Should You Consider Hormone Therapy?

The goal of treatment for metastatic breast cancer is to have you do as well as possible for as long as possible. Finding therapies with the best response rate and the fewest side effects is important.

Hormone therapy is generally less toxic than is chemotherapy. A common initial impression from some people is that chemotherapy is better and more powerful than is hormone therapy and therefore should be used first.

In some situations, though, hormone therapy may have a better chance of fighting the cancer than will chemotherapy. In addition, several studies have shown that people receiving hormone therapy as initial treatment for metastatic breast cancer do as well in terms of survival and life quality as do women who receive chemotherapy as their initial treatment.

Here's an example. A woman with estrogen receptor positive and progesterone receptor positive breast cancer develops a couple of small metastatic tumors in a lung 10 years after she was initially diagnosed with breast cancer. Chances are that this woman may have a higher response rate to hormone therapy (about 80 percent) than to chemotherapy (60 percent to 70 percent).

Factors that tend to predict that hormone therapy will be helpful include:
- A positive hormone receptor status
- No prior hormone therapy
- A long disease-free interval between diagnosis of the initial cancer and diagnosis of metastatic breast cancer
- Disease that doesn't involve the liver or brain

In general, hormone therapy is recommended if you have a reasonable chance of responding well to it, and the extent of the cancer is such that you can safely wait a month or two to see if the therapy is working.

effective only when other treatment is included that stops the ovaries from functioning. The drugs aren't effective if your ovaries are still making estrogen.

Postmenopausal women

In postmenopausal women, ovarian suppression isn't necessary because the ovaries have already stopped producing estrogen. However, a number of other treatment options are available to them.

Treatment for postmenopausal women with hormone-responsive breast cancer has changed dramatically over the past 40 years. Tamoxifen has been the first-line agent for approximately 30 years, but newer agents are just as promising, if not more so. Accumulating evidence suggests that compared with tamoxifen, aromatase inhibitors produce better response rates.

Following are hormone therapies that have been tested and shown to be effective in the treatment of hormone-responsive metastatic breast cancer.

High-dose estrogen vs. tamoxifen

Three or four decades ago, the primary form of hormone therapy for postmenopausal women with metastatic breast cancer was high doses of estrogen in the form of a hormone called diethylstilbestrol (DES). Although this sounds strange because estrogen can stimulate cancer growth, in a substantial percentage of women very high doses of estrogen causes tumors to shrink.

When tamoxifen became available, studies found both methods to be similarly effective. But tamoxifen became the standard treatment approach because it was less toxic than was DES. In some

Withdrawal Phenomenon

Interestingly, one way of shrinking breast cancer tumors is to take away a hormone medication that was previously effective. Although this may seem like a paradox, it does seem to work.

This type of response was initially observed when high doses of estrogen, in the form of diethylstilbestrol (DES) therapy, were used to treat metastatic breast cancer in postmenopausal women.

In women who received this therapy and experienced tumor shrinkage but later experienced regrowth, stopping the DES therapy caused the cancers to shrink again. This was called DES withdrawal.

What seems to be occurring is that after long exposure to hormone treatment, the cancer cells figure out how to grow during the treatment and are even stimulated by the medication. This same phenomenon has been seen with other types of hormone therapy, including tamoxifen, for women with breast cancer. It also has been seen in men with prostate cancer, another type of hormone-responsive cancer.

What all this means is that sometimes just stopping use of a previously effective hormone medication can in itself be an effective form of treatment.

BREAST CANCER

situations, however, high-dose estrogen treatment may still be used.

Aromatase inhibitors

Before the availability of tamoxifen, another type of hormone therapy for post-menopausal women was surgical removal of the adrenal glands — the organs located just above the kidneys. The adrenal glands produce a variety of hormones including androgens. An enzyme called aromatase found in fat cells and breast tissue turns androgen into estrogen. In post-menopausal women, this becomes one of the main sources of estrogen.

Eventually, this surgical procedure was replaced by the invention of a class of medications called aromatase inhibitors, which suppress aromatase enzymes, pre-venting the enzymes from converting androgen to estrogen. Currently, three aromatase inhibitors are in use: anastro-zole (Arimidex), letrozole (Femara) and exemestane (Aromasin).

In randomized trials comparing aromatase inhibitors and tamoxifen, aromatase inhibitors appear to suppress the cancer's growth rate for a longer period of time than does tamoxifen. One study showed a small survival advantage in favor of the aromatase inhibitor letrozole, compared with tamoxifen. Based on these studies, many doctors now recommend aromatase inhibitors as initial treatment for postmenopausal metastatic breast cancer that's hormone receptor positive.

However, other factors may influence which medication your doctor recom-

Chemotherapy for Metastatic Breast Cancer

Classes of chemotherapy drugs used to treat metastatic breast cancer include:

Anti-tumor antibiotics

Different from antibiotics used to treat bacterial infections, anti-tumor antibiotics inhibit the replication of cancer cells by interfering with DNA and by blocking RNA and key enzymes.

- Doxorubicin (Adriamycin)
- Epirubicin (Ellence)
- Mitomycin (Mutamycin)
- Mitoxantrone (Novantrone)

Taxanes

Taxanes, also known as mitotic inhibitors, disrupt division of individual cells by interfering with the specific cellular machinery that separates dividing cells into daughter cells.

- Paclitaxel (Taxol)
- Docetaxel (Taxotere)

mends first. These include the type of side effects produced by each drug, their cost — currently tamoxifen is much cheaper — and whether one of the medications was already used when the cancer was first diagnosed and treated.

Other options

A new hormone medication called fulvestrant (Faslodex) is an estrogen receptor antagonist that may be helpful for women whose cancer has become resistant to tamoxifen.

Whereas tamoxifen works by blocking estrogen, and aromatase inhibitors work by preventing the production of estrogen, fulvestrant works by destroying estrogen receptors in breast cancer cells. Clinical trials involving this medication show its

benefits to be similar to those of aromatase inhibitors.

Older hormone therapies also may be considered in postmenopausal women with metastatic breast cancer if other therapies don't work. These include megestrol acetate (Megace) and fluoxymesterone. Exactly how older therapies suppress tumor growth isn't known.

Chemotherapy

Chemotherapy is most often used to treat metastatic breast cancer when hormone therapy doesn't appear promising or when the cancer is life-threatening because it has spread so widely or because it's progressing rapidly. Multiple chemotherapy options are available.

Vinca alkaloids

Vinca alkaloids are another form of mitotic inhibitors. They work similarly to taxanes.
- Vinorelbine (Navelbine)
- Vinblastine (Velban)

Anti-metabolites

Anti-metabolites are medications that block enzymes vital to cancer cell growth by interfering with the synthesis of DNA.
- 5-fluorouracil, or 5-FU (Adrucil)
- Capecitabine (Xeloda)
- Gemcitabine (Gemzar)
- Methotrexate (Rheumatrex)

Alkylating agents

Alkylating agents interfere with the rapid growth of cancer cells by forming direct chemical bonds with DNA, inhibiting its function.
- Cyclophosphamide (Cytoxan, Neosar)
- Cisplatin (Platinol)
- Carboplatin (Paraplatin)

Single-agent vs. combination

Chemotherapy refers to a group of drugs that, when ingested or given intravenously, are toxic to cancer cells. Chemotherapy treatment may consist of taking just one drug (single-agent chemotherapy) or, quite often, a combination of drugs (combination chemotherapy). Combination chemotherapy uses multiple drugs, with each drug attacking the cancer in a different way. The medications each have different side effects, and the combinations are devised to try to increase efficacy and minimize side effects.

Doctors have long debated the merits of using individual chemotherapy agents among women with metastatic breast cancer versus combining two to four agents into a combination chemotherapy regimen. This debate still continues, particularly as new information becomes available from clinical trials.

In general, combination chemotherapy, when compared with single-agent chemotherapy, has a higher chance of causing the cancer to shrink and remain smaller for a longer period of time. But combination chemotherapy also tends to produce more side effects.

At the same time, a fair amount of evidence suggests that using single agents sequentially — that is, using one drug until it stops working and then using another one — leads to a similar length of survival and fewer side effects, when compared with combination chemotherapy.

It's generally agreed that women with rapidly progressing, life-threatening disease should be treated with combination chemotherapy, assuming that they're otherwise healthy enough to withstand the side effects of the drugs. Among women with breast cancer that's not as aggressive,

Combination Chemotherapy

Chemotherapy drugs are often given in combination in order to fight cancer cells in different ways. Some combinations used for metastatic breast cancer include:
- **AC:** Doxorubicin (*A* for Adriamycin, a brand name) and cyclophosphamide
- **CAF:*** Cyclophosphamide, doxorubicin (Adriamycin) and 5-fluorouracil
- **FAC:*** 5-fluorouracil, doxorubicin (Adriamycin) and cyclophosphamide
- **CMF:** Cyclophosphamide, methotrexate and 5-fluorouracil
- **CEF:** Cyclophosphamide, epirubicin (similar to doxorubicin) and 5-fluorouracil
- **AT:** Doxorubicin (Adriamycin) and docetaxel (Taxotere)
- **AC + paclitaxel:** Doxorubicin (Adriamycin), cyclophosphamide, then paclitaxel (Taxol)
- **TC:** Paclitaxel (Taxol) and cyclophosphamide
- **TAC:** Docetaxel (Taxotere), doxorubicin (Adriamycin) and cyclophosphamide
- **TX:** Docetaxel (Taxotere) and capecitabine (Xeloda)
  *CAF and FAC differ by dose and frequency.

many doctors prefer single-agent chemotherapy.

A recent study addressed the question of single-agent chemotherapy versus combination chemotherapy. Women participating in the trial received either doxorubicin (Adriamycin) alone or paclitaxel (Taxol) alone or a combination of the two. The trial found that no one treatment approach was superior to the others.

Drug options

An array of chemotherapy drugs may be used to treat metastatic breast cancer. They're grouped into categories based on how they work against cancer cells. Some factors that you and your doctor may consider in deciding which drug to use include:

- Whether you've already received chemotherapy to treat your cancer, and which drugs you received.
- How you responded to the drugs.
- The side effects of each drug. Each person is affected differently, and some side effects may be more problematic for you than for others.

One of the newer chemotherapy medications for metastatic breast cancer is called capecitabine. This medication is similar to 5-fluorouracil, one of the older chemotherapy drugs. Unlike many chemotherapy medications, which are given intravenously, capecitabine is given in the form of a pill.

Multiple combination chemotherapy regimens also might be considered by your doctor. You may start off with a well-established combination regimen, which usually has a good balance between potency and side effects. If this doesn't work, your doctor may suggest other combinations.

To learn more about chemotherapy medications and their side effects, see Chapter 9.

Herceptin

About 25 percent of women with breast cancer have cancer cells that overproduce a protein called HER-2/neu. This protein is normally produced by a gene that regulates cell growth.

In certain breast cancers, the gene produces too much HER-2/neu protein. As a result, cells that are sensitive to the protein are overstimulated, aiding in the development and growth of a tumor. Women whose breast cancers are characterized by an overproduction of the HER-2/neu protein are referred to as HER-2/neu positive. For more information on HER-2/neu, see Chapter 3.

Medical scientists have developed a drug called trastuzumab (Herceptin) — a type of drug known as a monoclonal antibody — to fight HER-2/neu positive cancers. Herceptin is the only form of antibody therapy for breast cancer that has been approved by the Food and Drug Administration. The drug works by attaching to the HER-2/neu receptors on cancer cells, thereby blocking the action of the receptor. This inhibits the growth of HER-2/neu positive cancer cells and, in many cases, is able to shrink the tumor.

Studies also show additional benefits when Herceptin is combined with chemotherapy. One recent study found that in comparison to women taking chemotherapy alone, those taking Herceptin and chemotherapy:

- Had slower tumor growth
- Had greater tumor shrinkage
- Maintained their tumor shrinkage for a longer period of time
- Lived longer

Based on this evidence, Herceptin has become an important part of therapy for women with advanced HER-2/neu positive cancers.

If your tumor is HER-2/neu positive and you're about to start chemotherapy, your doctor may consider Herceptin. For women who also have estrogen receptor positive cancer, it's not clear that Herceptin needs to be started while they're still receiving hormone therapy, because hormone therapy may work for a considerable period of time. At this time, there's no proof that combining hormone therapy and Herceptin is better than using these medications sequentially.

Monitoring Treatment

Once you begin treatment, your doctor will frequently monitor the status of your cancer. This can be done in basically three ways: continued updating of your medical history, regular physical exams and periodic tests.

The most important of these is probably the medical history, which includes how you've felt since your last appointment and any new signs or symptoms you've noticed. Many times this provides the best information for your doctor to determine the effectiveness of treatment. A physical examination is probably the next most important determinant of how you're doing. Various tests can also shed light on how your cancer is responding to treatment. These may include blood tests, such as liver function or tumor marker tests, and imaging procedures, such as X-rays or ultrasound.

Discontinuing Herceptin

In general, medications aimed at halting cancer progression are stopped once convincing evidence indicates that the disease is progressing while you're taking them. But whether to discontinue Herceptin in women who are HER-2/neu positive is a subject of considerable debate. In women whose tumors continue to grow while receiving Herceptin alone, the medication may be continued with the addition of chemotherapy. That's because evidence indicates that chemotherapy combined with Herceptin works better than does chemotherapy alone.

For women who experience progression of their cancer while receiving a combination of Herceptin and chemotherapy, the issue is less clear. Some doctors continue Herceptin while switching to an alternative chemotherapy agent. Other doctors stop the combined treatment and proceed to use an alternative chemotherapy regimen alone. Results of ongoing clinical trials may provide better direction in future years as to the best approach.

After completing his or her assessment, your doctor should be able to place your tumor status into one of three categories:

1. The tumor has clearly shrunk since you started treatment.
2. The tumor has clearly grown since you started treatment.
3. The cancer is stable, a condition often referred to as stable disease.

This last category can be subdivided even further:

- The disease looks like it hasn't changed at all.
- There's some suggestion that the cancer may be shrinking, but the evidence isn't conclusive. Generally, an oncologist likes to see a 50 percent reduction in tumor size before indicating a definite response to treatment.
- There's some indication that the cancer is a bit worse, but the status hasn't changed enough to clearly declare it so.

In addition to monitoring your tumor status, your doctor will also look at how you're tolerating the treatment and its side effects. Based on all this information, you and your doctor can decide whether to continue your treatment. If you decide to stop it, the two of you then need to decide whether to try another form of treatment.

Localized Treatments

Depending on where a cancer has spread and what symptoms it may be causing, a number of treatments may be directed toward specific sites of your body, as opposed to the systemic treatment approaches already described.

Deciding on Drug Therapies

As you try to make some decisions about using various drug therapies for treating metastatic breast cancer, it may be helpful to try to address the following questions:

1. What's the goal of the therapy?
2. What's the likely response rate with the therapy? That is, what is the chance that the cancer will shrink? In addition, what is the chance that there will be no evidence of cancer growth for at least six months?
3. In those patients whose cancers shrink or don't grow, what's the average time that this response lasts? This may be called the response duration.
4. Is there evidence that the proposed treatment will prolong survival? If it's expected to prolong survival, what would be the average length of prolonged survival?
5. Will this therapy, on average, improve your quality of life? This is a difficult question to address scientifically, yet some estimates can be made. The effect on quality of life generally depends on how well the therapy works against the cancer, its side effects (toxicities), and the psychological and social considerations of the person receiving therapy.
6. What are the potential side effects of the therapy?

Bone metastases

A group of medications (bisphosphonates) used to treat osteoporosis is also used to treat women with metastatic breast cancer to their bones. Osteoporosis is a disease that causes bones to become weak and prone to fracture.

In one study, participants with breast cancer that had spread to bone were randomly assigned to receive a bisphosphonate or an inactive pill (placebo) in addition to their standard cancer treatment. Women receiving the bisphosphonate were less likely to develop subsequent bone fractures or to need radiation therapy to relieve bone pain. Based on this evidence, bisphosphonates are now commonly used in women with metastatic breast cancer in their bones.

It's not certain, though, how long the therapy should be continued. Bisphosphonates can cause kidney damage and can lower blood calcium levels. If you're receiving a bisphosphonate, your doctor will likely monitor your kidney function and follow your calcium levels during the course of the therapy.

Pleural effusions

At times, cancer can develop in the pleural lining of the lungs, leading to the development of fluid buildup around the lungs (pleural effusion). This may require removal of the fluid by draining it with a needle or by a more extensive process where the fluid is removed either through a chest tube or a surgical procedure. Your doctor may then insert a chemical irritant into the pleural space to create scar tissue and close up the space (pleurodesis). This is done to decrease the chance that the fluid buildup will recur.

Central nervous system metastases

If metastatic cancer develops in the brain or around the spinal cord, steroid medications are generally used to try to decrease the swelling and the resulting pain. Radiation may also be used to treat the

---

QUESTION & ANSWER

Q: **Are bone marrow transplants ever used to treat advanced breast cancer?**

A: In the 1980s and 1990s, there was a lot of enthusiasm about the use of high-dose chemotherapy combined with bone marrow transplantation as treatment for women with breast cancer. The treatment was based on the idea that if some chemotherapy is good, then more would be better. Randomized clinical trials were set up, and in one trial women with metastatic breast cancer were randomly assigned to receive either standard chemotherapy or standard chemotherapy followed by high-dose chemotherapy with bone marrow transplantation. The results of this trial didn't suggest any survival benefit in using high-dose chemotherapy with bone marrow transplantation, and as a result, enthusiasm for the treatment has waned considerably.

tumor. Sometimes a neurosurgeon may be called upon to try to remove some of the cancer.

When Treatment Stops Working

Unfortunately, there are no guarantees that any particular treatment will work. When there's evidence that the disease is progressing despite treatment, it's a reasonable choice to go back to the beginning and reanalyze what your next maneuver might be — similar to what you and your doctor did when you first learned you had metastatic breast cancer and were deciding on treatment.

With metastatic breast cancer, the value of each subsequent treatment tends to decrease. For example, in a woman who starts off with chemotherapy, the initial response rate might be around 50 percent to 70 percent, and the benefits may last for an average of 10 to 12 months. If the disease progresses, a second chemotherapy regimen might have only a 30 percent to 35 percent response rate, with an average response duration of just four to six months.

There may come a time when the potential benefits of treatment are no longer meaningful to you. At this point, it's certainly appropriate for you to say no to further treatment. For some women and their doctors, this may seem like giving up. But this assumption is generally incorrect. If the treatment is more likely to cause troublesome side effects — and not prolong survival or improve quality of life — declining treatment is a reasonable choice. This shouldn't be construed as giving up.

At this point, the goals of your treatment change. The focus of treatment is no longer on controlling the cancer but, instead, on controlling your symptoms and making you as comfortable as possible. For additional information on making the transition to supportive care, see Chapter 36.

Clinical Trials

This chapter discusses the benefits and the risks of treatments for metastatic breast cancer. All this information has become available because of women who have participated in clinical trials. For some of the treatments you may be considering, there may be a clinical trial in which you can participate.

These trials, as a rule, are safe and they provide access to the newest ideas and approaches. They're the best way to continue to identify new treatment options for women with metastatic breast cancer.

You can find out about specific clinical trials by asking your doctor or a member of your health care team or by visiting the National Cancer Institute's Web site at *www.cancer.gov/clinicaltrials*. For general information on clinical trials, see Chapter 2.

BREAST CANCER

Three Different Outcomes

This book includes many personal stories of women who have survived cancer, who are undergoing treatment or who have taken steps in hopes of preventing cancer. The women discuss why they made the decisions they did and, in many cases, how well they've done.

Unfortunately, though, not all women do well with their cancers. It's important that we tell you not just the good-news stories, but also the ones that didn't have such happy endings.

The pages that follow contain the stories of three women with advanced breast cancer. The first story is of a young woman who died prematurely from a very aggressive cancer. It needs to be noted that this story does not depict a typical case. Rather, it represents one end of the spectrum of metastatic breast cancer. In addition, it illustrates the fortitude of this young woman as she dealt with her disease. If you don't think that you're ready to read this story now, skip over it and consider coming back to it later.

The second story is a hypothetical one that combines parts of several actual cases. The story describes a more typical outcome for a woman diagnosed with recurrent breast cancer. It tells of a woman who does eventually die of her disease, but only after living with it for a relatively lengthy period. We'll call the patient Jane.

The third story is of a woman who continues to amaze her doctors. She lives with recurrent breast cancer — just as she has for well over 40 years!

Carol's Story

In April 2002, at the age of 31, Carol was diagnosed with cancer in her left breast. The diagnosis came just a few weeks after she noticed a lump in the breast. Carol underwent a lumpectomy, and her surgeon removed the lymph nodes under her left arm. The tumor was 2.5 centimeters (about an inch) in diameter — not particularly large — and all the lymph nodes tested negative for cancer. The tumor was also estrogen receptor positive and HER-2/neu receptor negative. Based on the characteristics of her tumor and the laboratory results, it was estimated that with just surgery alone, Carol had a 75 percent chance of living disease-free for at least 10 years.

At the time of Carol's diagnosis, for a tumor like hers, it was standard practice to recommend chemotherapy after surgery. Carol agreed to the treatment and, during the summer of 2002, she received chemotherapy with the medications doxorubicin (Adriamycin) and cyclophosphamide. With chemotherapy, Carol's chances of living disease-free for another 10 years increased to an estimated 80 percent.

After completing treatment with Adriamycin and cyclophosphamide, Carol discussed with her doctor the potential benefit of receiving additional chemotherapy with a medication called paclitaxel (Taxol). Based on the information available at the time, it was estimated that Taxol might boost her 10-year survival chances by a couple more percentage points. Because Carol was young and had a young child, she wanted to be aggressive in treating her cancer. So Carol decided to undergo an additional two months of treatment with Taxol.

In December 2002, upon completion of chemotherapy, Carol met with her doctor to discuss radiation therapy to her left breast. During her visit, her doctor noticed a change in her left breast, which led to further tests. To everyone's dismay, a computerized tomography (CT) scan revealed a large recurrent tumor in her left breast and cancer in some remaining lymph nodes under her left arm and her breastbone (sternum).

Her doctor recommended that Carol begin taking a hormone medication to turn off production of estrogen by her ovaries, as well as the medication tamoxifen. She also received radiation therapy to her left chest wall to try to control the disease, knowing that there was a good chance the radiation wouldn't be very successful.

During a visit to her doctor in March of 2003, Carol had more fullness in her left upper breast region. A CT scan showed enlarging tumor masses in the breast and lymph node areas, in addition to spots in her liver, consistent with the spread of breast cancer to the liver.

Before her death, Carol began writing poetry as a way to cope with her illness. Following is one of her poems:

I had a dream

I dreamed the other night
I married the man I love so
For better, for worse, in sickness, in health
We live, we love, and we grow

I dreamed the other night
A beautiful boy was born
Thanks, praise, adoring him so
We live, we love, and we grow

I dreamed the other night
A cancer crept within
Faith, prayer, strength, hope
We live, we love, and we grow

I dreamed the other night
I was a survivor that had made it through
For better, for worse, in sickness, in health
We lived, we loved, and we grew

Carol Alcalá-Samaniego

At this juncture, Carol had to make some tough decisions regarding future treatment. Knowing that there wasn't any chance of curing the cancer, and that the chance of chemotherapy shrinking the cancer was quite small, Carol, with input from her medical team and her husband, decided to try another chemotherapy medication.

Within a month, however, it was clear that not only was the cancer in her liver growing, but also it had spread to her spine, where it was causing considerable pain. To help control the pain, Carol received a course of radiation therapy to her spine. Over the next few weeks, she received more radiation therapy to painful sites in her spine, and she had a mastectomy because the tumor in her breast continued to grow and was causing considerable pain. After the mastectomy, Carol decided to try yet another chemotherapy drug, but it was stopped within two weeks because the cancer continued to grow and the drug was causing side effects that only added to her discomfort.

BREAST CANCER

Carol continued to receive supportive care from her health care team to ensure that she was as comfortable as she could be. On July 27, 2003 — a little more than a year from when she was diagnosed with cancer — Carol died at home with her extended family present. Despite the relentlessly aggressive course of her disease, Carol lived her life as fully as was feasible. Although they did plan for her likely death, up to the very end, Carol and her husband never gave up hope.

Jane's Story

Jane was diagnosed with breast cancer in 1993 at the age of 58. On a mammogram, doctors noticed abnormal calcifications in one of her breasts. A biopsy revealed invasive ductal cancer. Imaging tests didn't find any evidence of cancer anywhere else in her body, and Jane was otherwise healthy. After discussing potential treatment options with her doctor, Jane decided to have a lumpectomy, to be followed by radiation therapy.

During her surgery, Jane also underwent a procedure called a sentinel node biopsy to check for cancer spread to nearby underarm (axillary) lymph nodes. The test revealed cancer cells in the sentinel lymph node. In light of this finding, other lymph nodes under Jane's arm were removed.

The pathology report following her surgery indicated that Jane had a tumor in her breast that was 2.5 centimeters (about an inch) in diameter and that two of 18 lymph nodes from under her arm contained cancer cells. Jane's tumor was also found to be estrogen and progesterone receptor positive and HER-2/neu negative.

After her surgery, Jane met with her oncologist who estimated that with surgery and radiation alone, she had an estimated 50 percent chance of living disease-free for the next 10 years. With the addition of chemotherapy and the hormone drug tamoxifen to her treatment regimen, her estimated 10-year survival rate increased to 63 percent. Jane chose to have chemotherapy and was given four cycles of the medications Adriamycin and cyclophosphamide. After chemotherapy, she began taking tamoxifen and also received radiation therapy to her breast. She completed her five years of tamoxifen in January 1999.

Jane continued to do well until January of 2001, when she developed back pain. A bone scan revealed metastatic breast cancer in her bones. Jane received radiation therapy to a painful area in her lower back where the cancer had spread. She was also started on the hormone medication anastrozole.

The radiation therapy helped relieve Jane's pain, and for 14 months anastrozole controlled the spread of the cancer. Eventually, Jane developed some shortness of breath caused by fluid around one of her lungs. The fluid was drained and found to contain cancer cells. A surgical procedure was performed to help keep the fluid from re-accumulating. The anastrozole was stopped, and Jane was given another hormone medication. Six months later she developed some pain in her right upper abdomen, and subsequent tests indicated that the cancer had spread to her liver.

At this point, Jane and her doctor decided to stop hormone therapy and switch to chemotherapy. The chemotherapy initially shrank the tumors in her liver, but eight months later the cancer began to grow again. She switched to a different chemotherapy medication, which had the same results. The tumors initially regressed, but started to grow again eight months later. A couple more chemotherapy medications were tried over the next three months, but her cancer didn't respond well to them.

Jane discussed the pros and cons of additional treatment with her doctor, and it was clear to both of them, and to her family, that the risk of serious side effects from the medications was greater than any potential benefit they might bring. Jane decided to stop all efforts to control the cancer, and her medical team concentrated on making sure that Jane was as comfortable as possible. Jane received hospice care, and five months later, in September 2004, she died in her home with her family present.

Although Jane did eventually die of her breast cancer, it's important not to forget that she lived for more than a decade after her initial diagnosis. And, for many of those years, she led a full life, keeping the disease from interfering with her life as much as was possible.

Margaret's Story

To say that Margaret Gilseth has lived with breast cancer most of her life is true. Margaret first noticed a lump in her breast when she was 39 years old. That was in 1957. Today, Margaret is 86, and she's still living with breast cancer — as she has for 47 years.

In 1957, when her cancer was first diagnosed, Margaret had a mastectomy to remove her left breast. Two years later, a small growth appeared on her incision scar.

It would be the first of many such tumors. Initially, the tumors were limited to her left chest wall, but eventually they began to spread across her chest wall and developed in her right breast as well.

Margaret handled each of the recurrences as she did her initial diagnosis. "I took them one at a time, and was glad to get rid of them. And then I went on living each time. I think you make use of each day. "

"Getting rid" of her tumors has required many major and minor surgeries and radiation therapy. She has had more than 25 separate surgical procedures, which have removed more than 65 tumor nodules.

To keep new tumors from developing, or at least slow their growth, Margaret has taken multiple anti-cancer hormone therapies. She has done this on and off for well over 20 years. When the effects of one medication begin to wear off — signaled by the appearance of new growths — her hormone therapy is changed.

In addition to her strong faith, one of Margaret's biggest allies in her lifelong battle with cancer has been a pen and paper, which eventually gave way to a computer.

An English teacher for 25 years, Margaret enjoyed writing and always kept a journal. Her journal helped her face, and then let go of, her worries and fears. It was her therapy. "I tell people if they have something bothering them — anxieties that persist — there's nothing better than writing."

After her retirement, with more time on her hands, Margaret's writing took on a broader scope. She wrote a novel about the lives of several generations of a Norwegian immigrant family, based, in part, on her own family's experiences. Additional books and collections of poetry followed.

Eventually, she wrote a book about her personal battle with breast cancer, called *Silver Linings*.

When not writing, Margaret finds other ways to keep busy. She has volunteered at the local nursing home, read to children in the Head Start program and taught Norwegian in community education classes. She and her husband, Walter, have traveled when they could, often as part of a volunteer organization. For Margaret, volunteer work has been another part of her therapy, her way of coping and carrying on. "I think taking an interest in other people makes a lot of difference. If you just go around thinking about yourself, it can cause you problems."

Over the years, whenever Margaret was facing another surgery or a change in treatment — times when she wondered if "this was the one," the one recurrence that she wouldn't be able to overcome — her son Steve would offer her comfort by telling her in his lighthearted manner that she was going to live to a ripe, old age. Steve was right.

So, why has Margaret done so well despite her breast cancer that keeps recurring? Her oncologist for the past decade — Margaret having outlived the 30-year career of her previous oncologist — readily admits that he doesn't know. Under the microscope, Margaret's cancer looks like a routine type of breast cancer. Why it has acted so differently from 99+ percent of other such cancers is a real mystery. Hopefully, it's a mystery that can one day be solved to help doctors better understand cancer and better help patients. Margaret is a great reminder to doctors to never say never, and never say always.

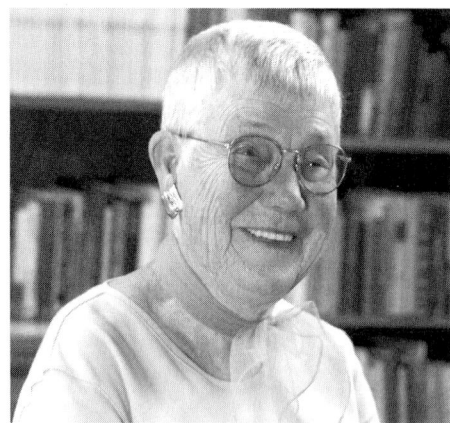

Margaret Gilseth at home in her den, where she keeps busy writing and communicating with family and friends.

Visual Guide

Cancer biology

The normal functioning of a cell is controlled at many levels, including its surface (cell membrane), interior (cytoplasm) and growth control center (nucleus). Changes that may lead to cancer development and growth can occur at any of these levels.

Cell membrane

At the cell surface, chemical messengers that signal a cell to divide (growth factors) and nutrients bind to receptors on the cell surface. Cancer cells overexpress receptors that capture growth factors and nutrients.

Cytoplasm

Signals from growth factors are sent to the cell nucleus by way of a cascading series of so-called secondary messengers. Cancer cells can cause numerous growth-promoting changes in these signaling pathways.

Nucleus

Within the tightly coiled DNA of each cell are the genetic instructions to make all of the proteins a cell needs to carry out its work. Which genes are turned on depends on the signals received from the cytoplasm, conveyed by transcription factors. Transcription factors bind to the DNA of targeted genes.

Cell division is controlled within the nucleus, too. Before a cell can divide, it must pass through a tightly governed cycle with several checkpoints. This is to ensure that an injured cell doesn't divide until damaged DNA has been repaired. Cancer cells lack these checkpoint mechanisms, allowing altered cells to grow and proliferate.

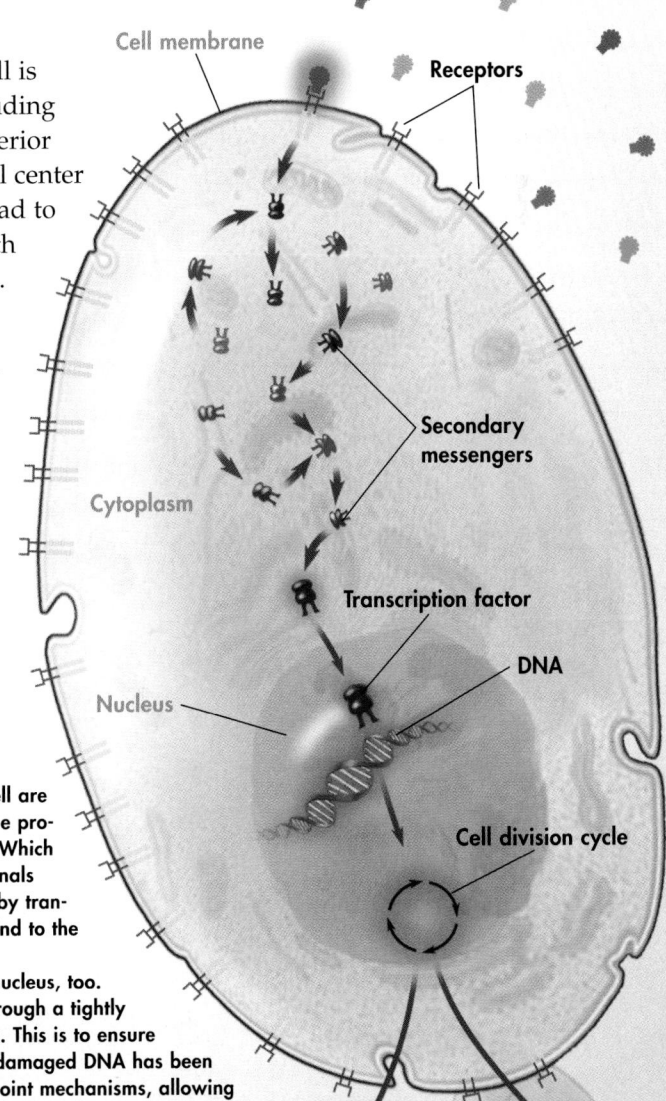

Growth factors

Cell membrane

Receptors

Secondary messengers

Cytoplasm

Transcription factor

DNA

Nucleus

Cell division cycle

Cancer development

Cancer is characterized by the overgrowth of abnormal cells, a multistep process called carcinogenesis. Over time, the abnormal cells accumulate into a mass, called a growth or tumor, that can invade nearby normal tissue and spread.

Atypical hyperplasia
As the excess cells stack upon one another, some start taking on an abnormal appearance.

Hyperplasia
The intricate system of cell development and growth is disrupted, causing an overproduction of normal-appearing cells.

Normal cell
Normal cells grow and divide in an orderly fashion.

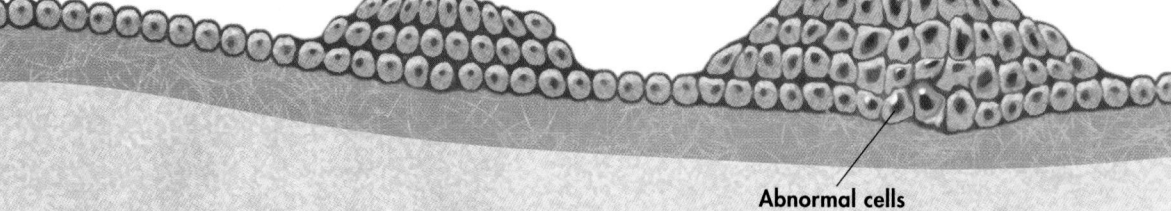

Abnormal cells

Noninvasive cancer
The abnormal cells continue to change in appearance and multiply, evolving into cancer. The cancer remains confined within normal borders.

Invasive cancer
As the cancer cells invade deeper into surrounding tissue, eventually they can spread to nearby lymph channels and tiny blood vessels (capillaries), which can carry cancer cells to other parts of the body.

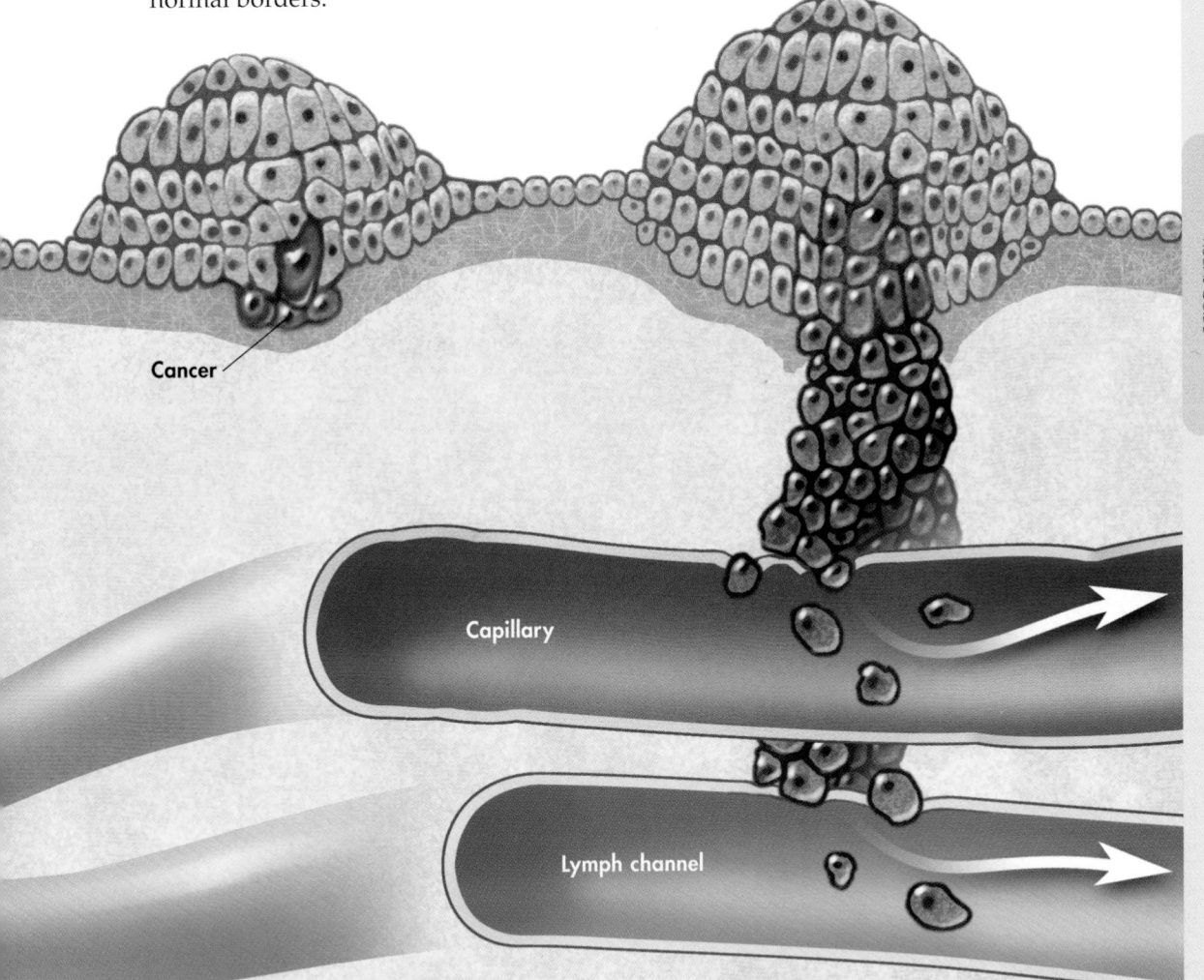

Cancer

Capillary

Lymph channel

Cancer spread

Cancer cells from a breast tumor can spread throughout the body by way of tiny blood vessels (capillaries), which empty into veins, and by lymph channels, which drain into lymph nodes. Fluid and cancer cells from the lymphatic system eventually empty into large veins, which in turn empty into the heart. From the heart, the cancer cells can spread to the rest of the body by way of the arteries.

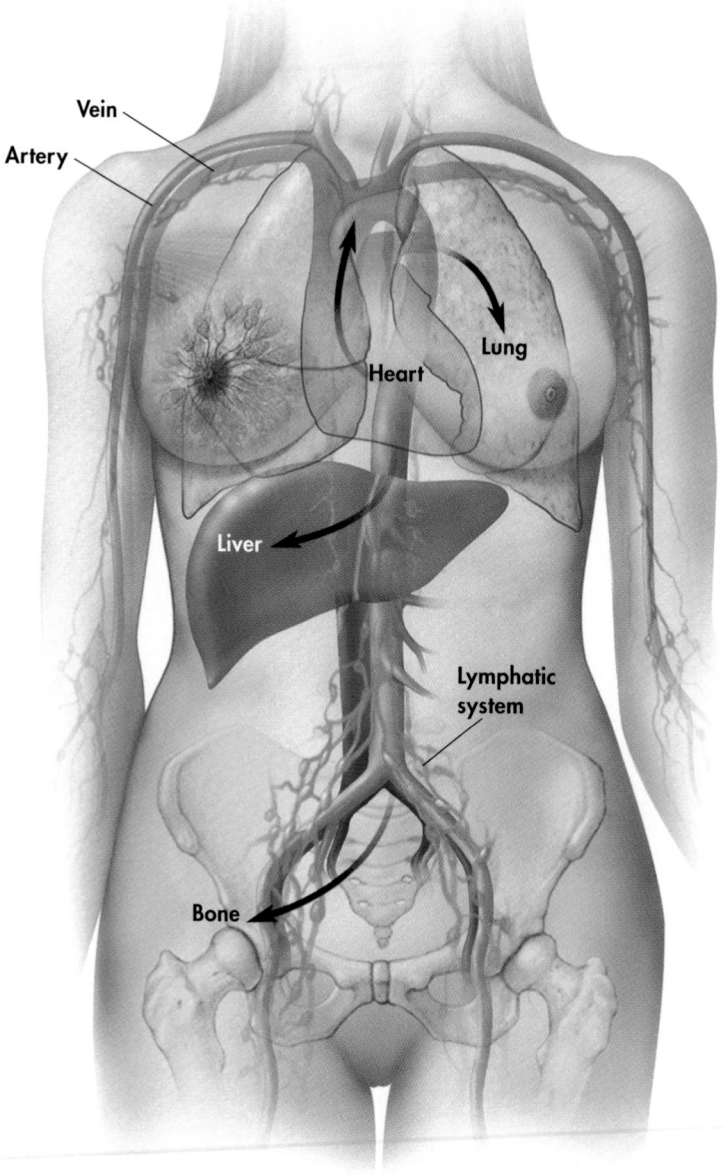

Vein

Artery

Lung

Heart

Liver

Lymphatic system

Bone

Sentinel node biopsy

In this procedure, a dye is injected into the area of the tumor. The dye is absorbed into nearby lymph channels. The first lymph nodes to collect the dye, called the sentinel nodes, likely are the first to receive drainage from the breast tumor. The sentinel nodes are removed and examined for cancer cells. Alternatively, a radioactive material may be used instead of a dye.

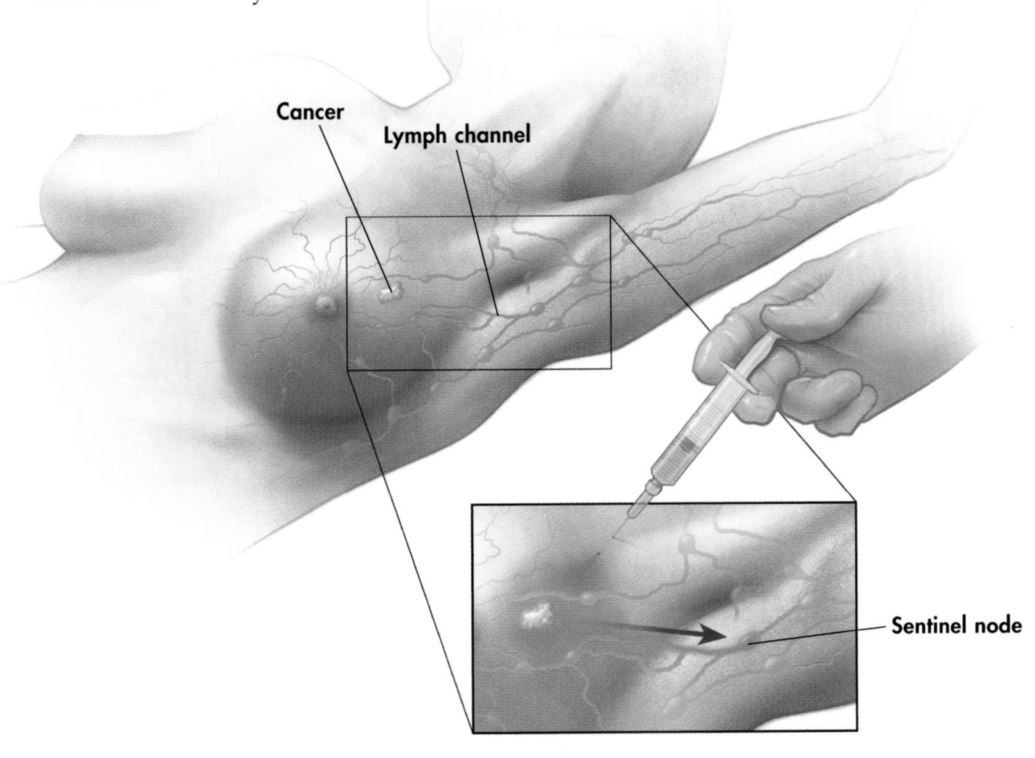

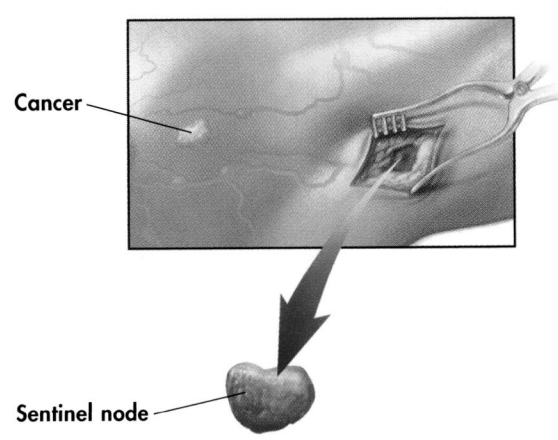

Cancer

Lymph channel

Sentinel node

Cancer

Sentinel node

Breast cancer stages

Stage I

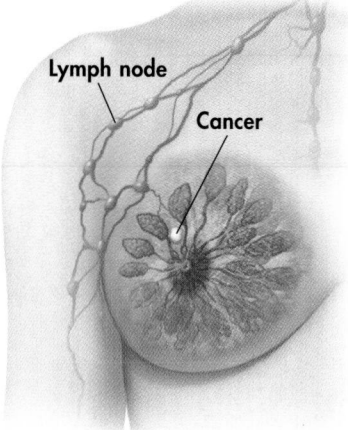

Cancer is 2 centimeters (cm) in size or less. No spread to the lymph nodes.

Stage II

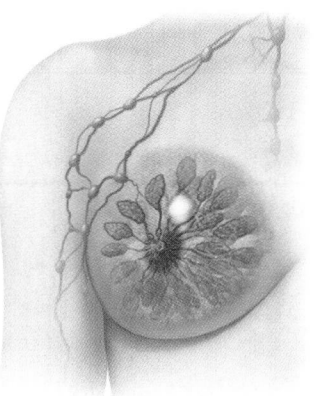 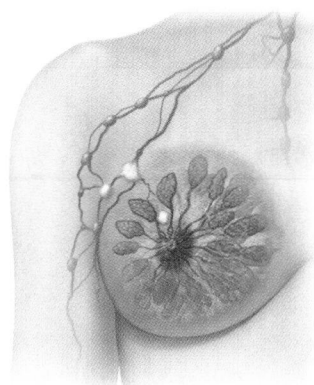

Cancer is 2.1 cm to 5 cm in size, or has spread to lymph nodes under the arm or both.

Stage III

A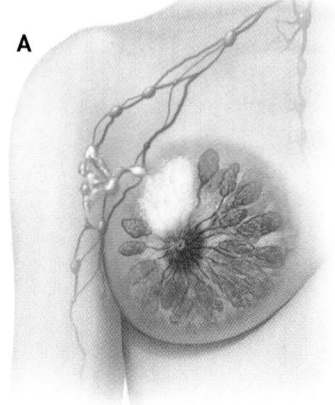

B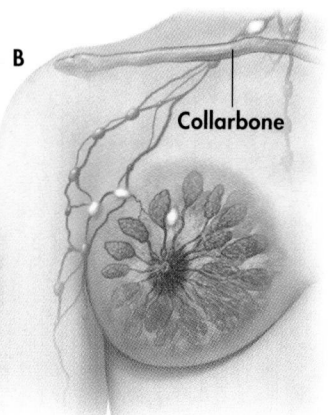

C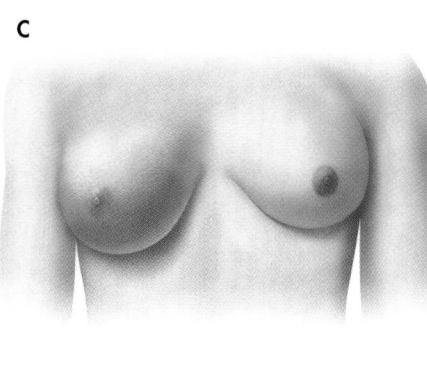

Stage III cancers include a number of criteria that make it a broad category. Here are three examples: tumor greater than 5 cm in size (A); spread to lymph nodes above the collarbone (B); spread to breast skin causing swelling and redness, known as inflammatory breast cancer (C).

Stage IV
Cancer has spread to distant
sites, such as the lungs, liver
or bone.

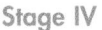

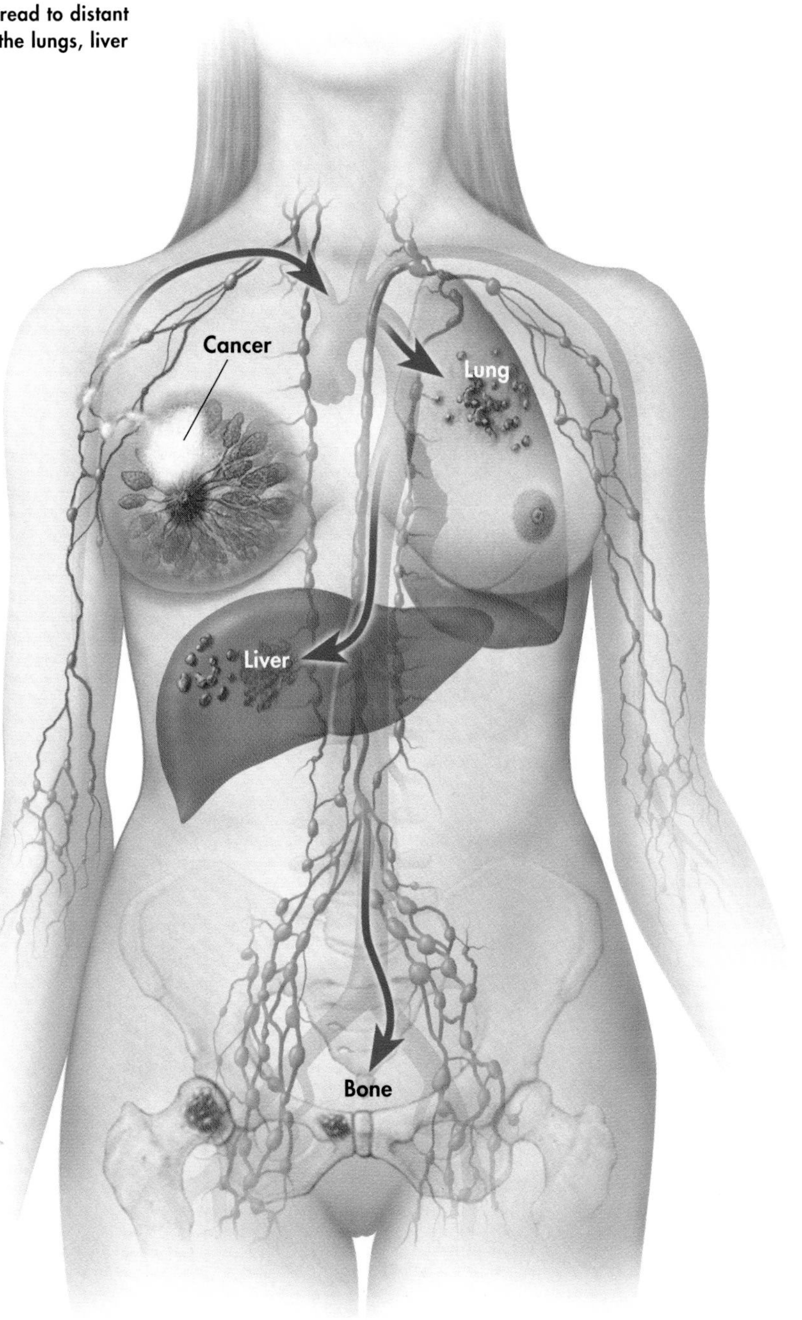

Cancer

Lung

Liver

Bone

Gynecologic anatomy

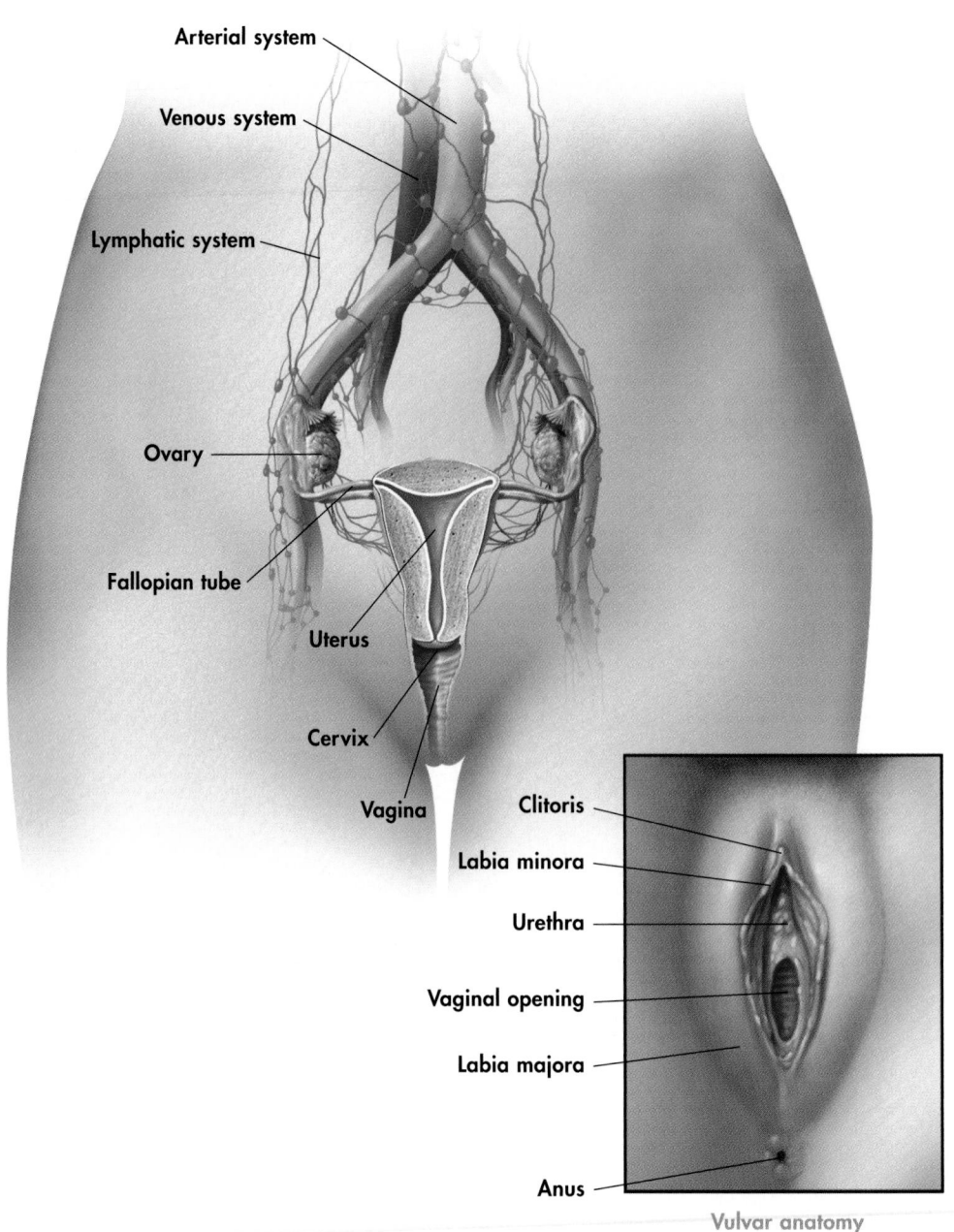

Arterial system

Venous system

Lymphatic system

Ovary

Fallopian tube

Uterus

Cervix

Vagina

Clitoris

Labia minora

Urethra

Vaginal opening

Labia majora

Anus

Vulvar anatomy

Ovarian cancer stages

Stage I

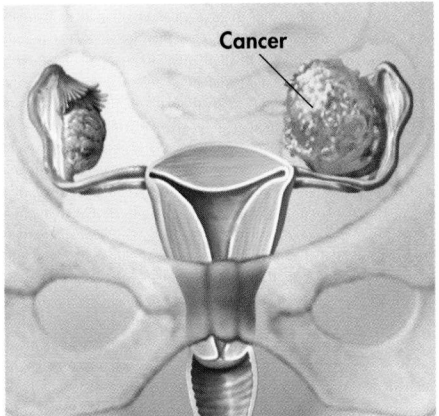

Cancer

Cancer is confined to one or both ovaries.

Stage II

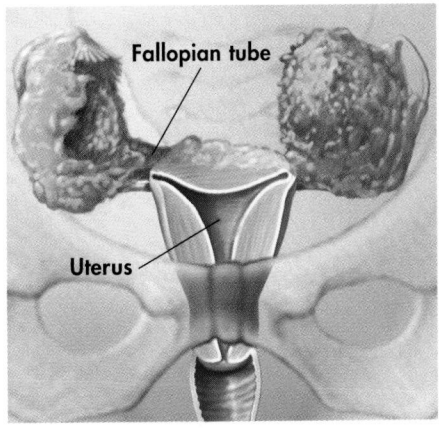

Fallopian tube

Uterus

Cancer has spread from one or both ovaries to another site(s) in the pelvis.

Stage III

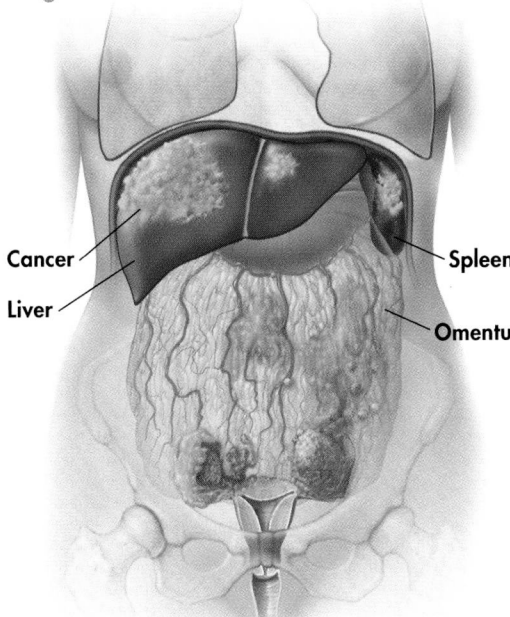

Cancer

Liver

Spleen

Omentum

Cancer has spread beyond the pelvis to the upper abdomen, including the omentum and the surfaces of the liver or spleen.

Stage IV

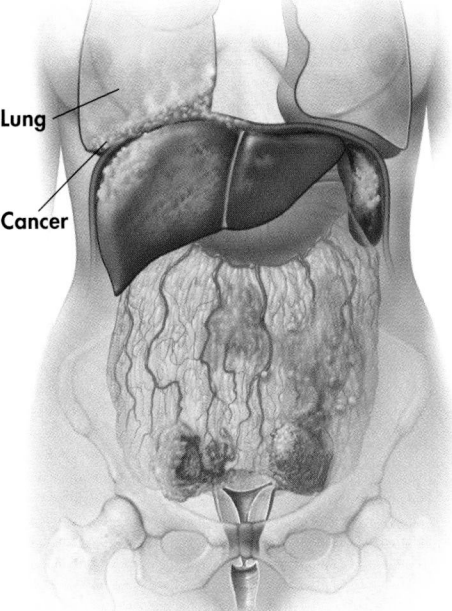

Lung

Cancer

Cancer has spread outside the abdominal cavity to organs such as the lungs, or has invaded the interior of the liver or spleen.

Endometrial cancer stages

Stage I

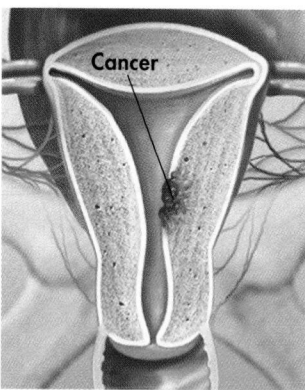

Cancer is limited to the inner lining (endometrium) of the uterus.

Stage II

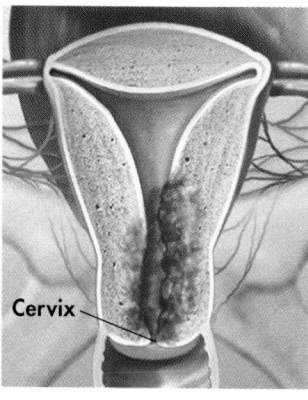

Cancer involves both the uterus and cervix.

Stage III

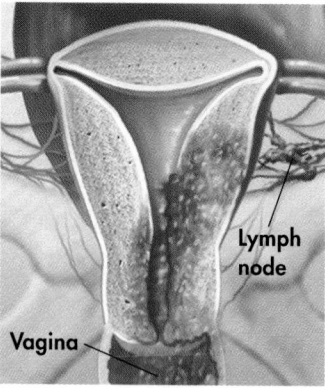

Cancer has spread to the surface of the uterus or to the vagina or nearby lymph nodes.

Stage IV

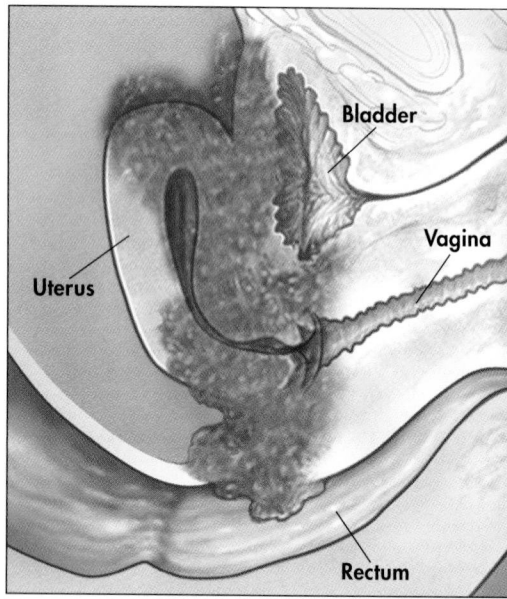
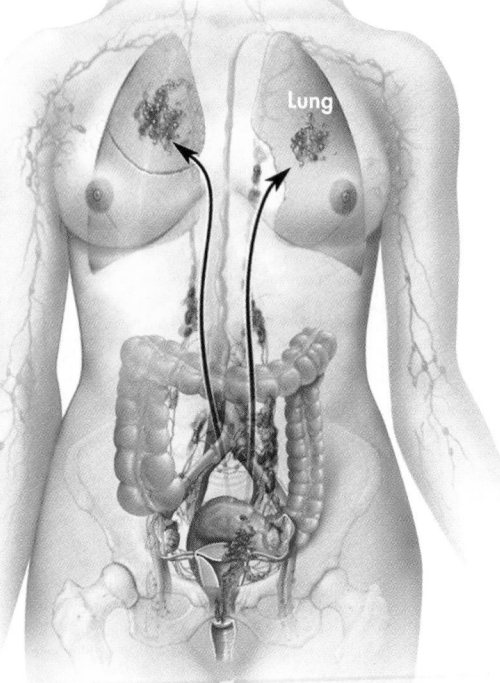

Cancer has spread to the rectum or bladder (side view above) or to sites outside of the pelvis, such as the lungs (right).

Cervical cancer stages

Stage I

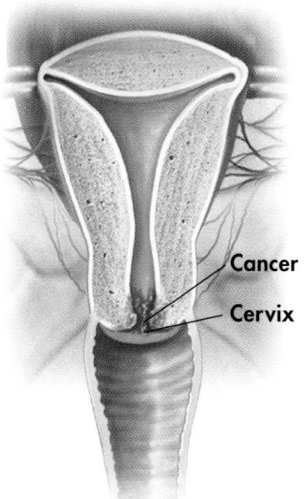

Cancer is limited to the cervix.

Stage II

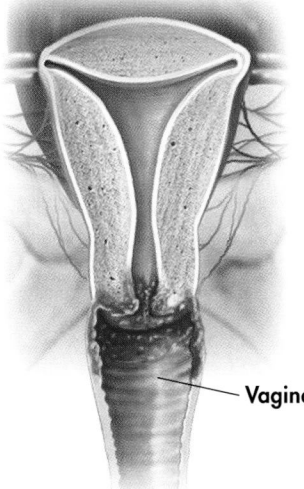

Cancer has spread to the upper vagina or sideways to nearby tissue.

Stage III

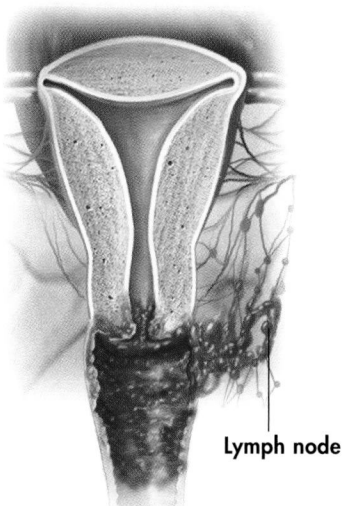

Cancer has spread to the lower vagina or to the pelvic wall or lymph nodes or to both.

Stage IV

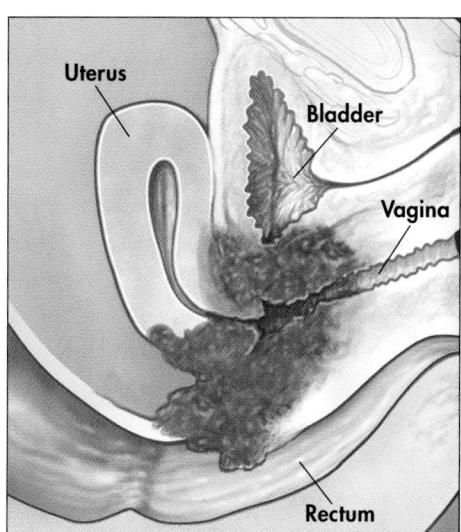

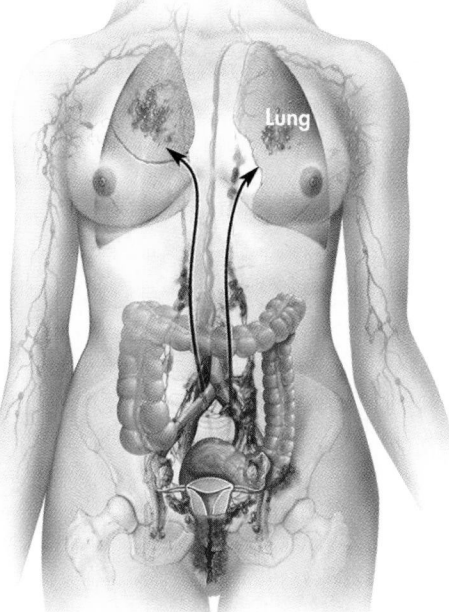

Cancer has spread to the bladder or rectum (side view above) or to distant sites, such as the lungs (right).

Vaginal cancer stages

Stage I

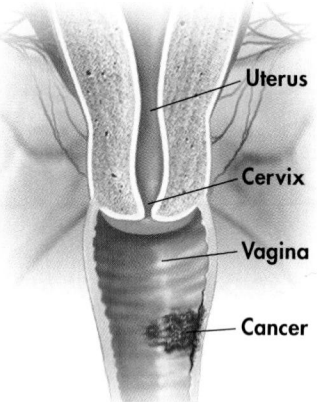

Uterus

Cervix

Vagina

Cancer

Cancer is limited to the
vaginal wall.

Stage II

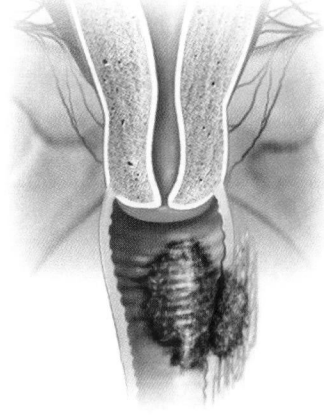

Cancer has spread to tissue
next to the vagina.

Stage III

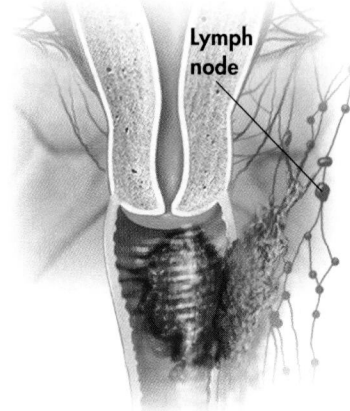

Lymph
node

Cancer has spread to nearby lymph
nodes, or to the pelvic wall or both.

Stage IV

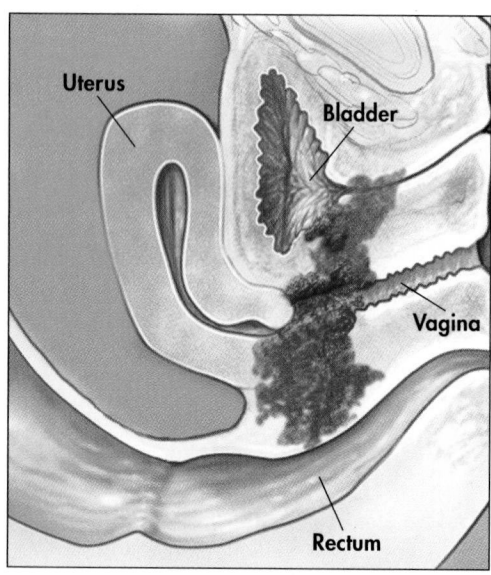

Uterus

Bladder

Vagina

Rectum

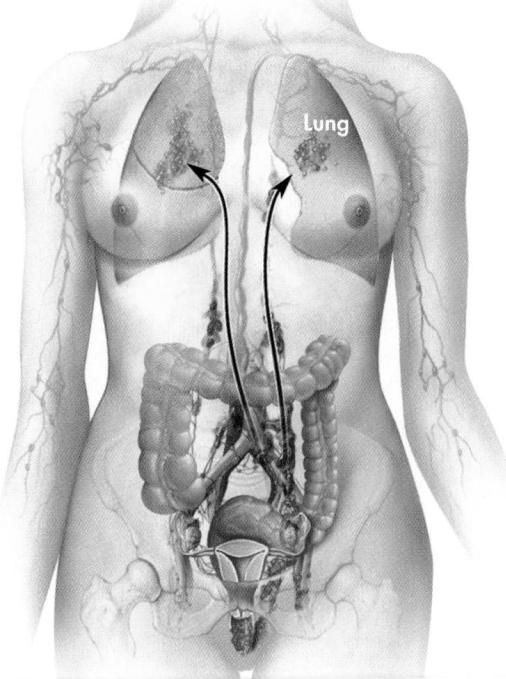

Lung

Cancer has spread to nearby organs (side view
above), to lymph nodes on both sides of the pelvis,
or to distant organs such as the lungs (right).

Vulvar cancer stages

Stage I

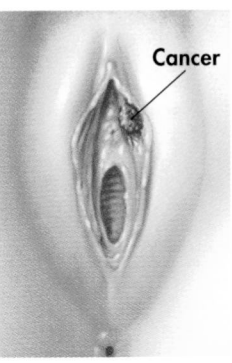

Cancer is less than 2 cm and is limited to the surface of the vulva.

Stage II

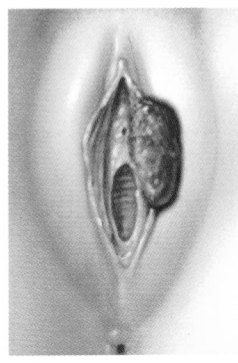

Cancer is larger than 2 cm and is limited to the vulva.

Stage III

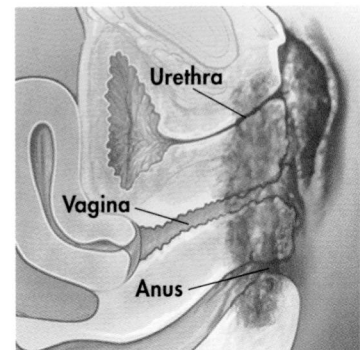

Cancer has spread beyond the vulva to nearby groin lymph nodes or to nearby structures such as the urethra, vagina and anus.

Stage IV

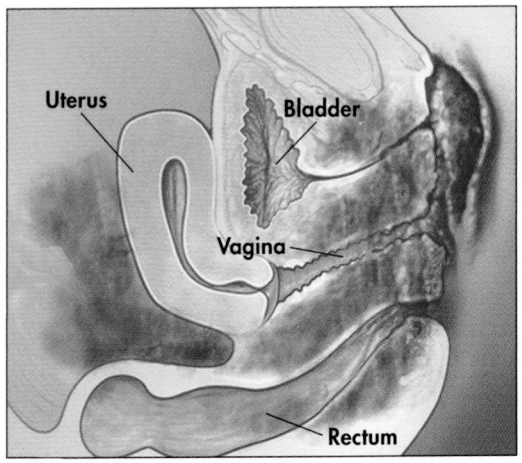

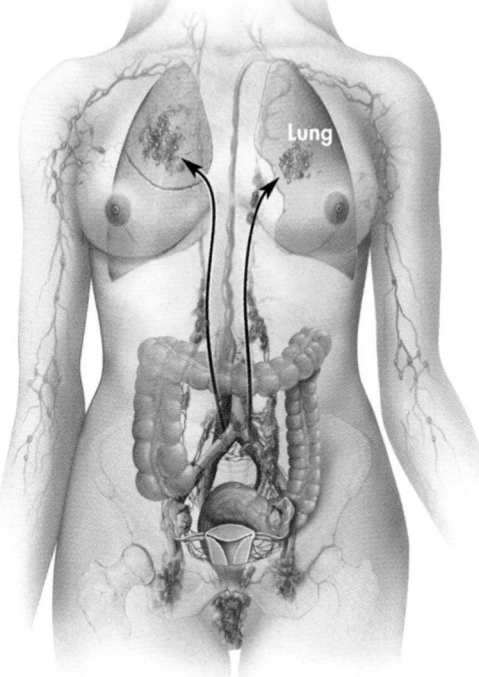

Cancer has spread to organs such as the bladder or rectum (side view above), or to lymph nodes on both sides of the groin, or to distant organs such as the lungs (right).

Surgery

A common surgery for treatment of ovarian cancer, as well as some other gynecologic cancers, is a total abdominal hysterectomy with bilateral salpingo-oophorectomy. This surgery involves removal of the uterus, including the cervix, as well as both ovaries and both fallopian tubes. The vagina remains intact.

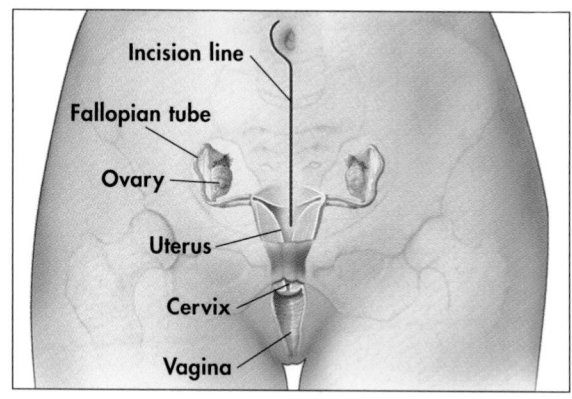

1. Female reproductive organs before surgery

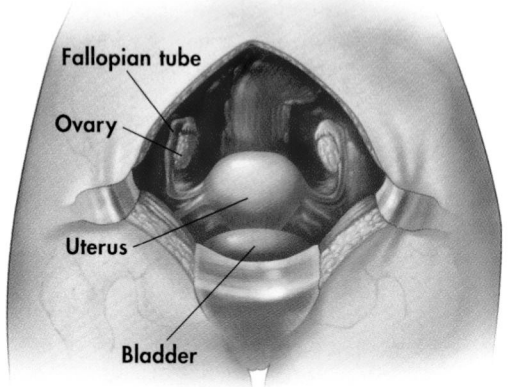

2. View of the lower abdomen during surgery

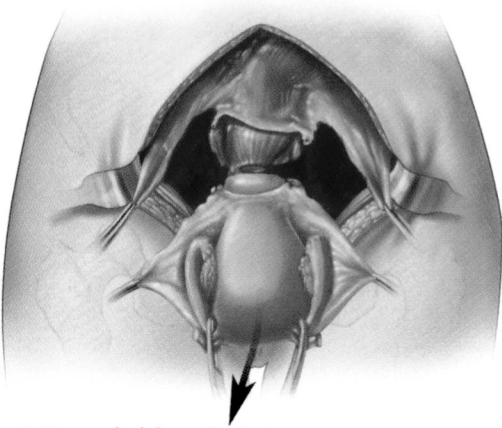

3. Removal of the reproductive organs

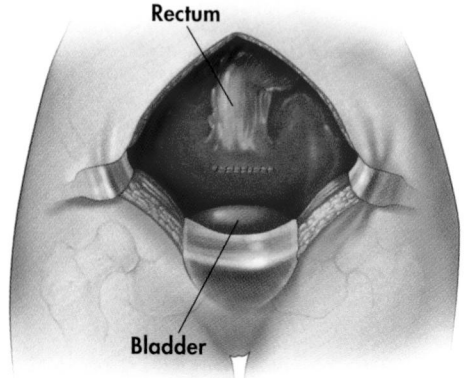

4. Surgeon's view after removal of the organs

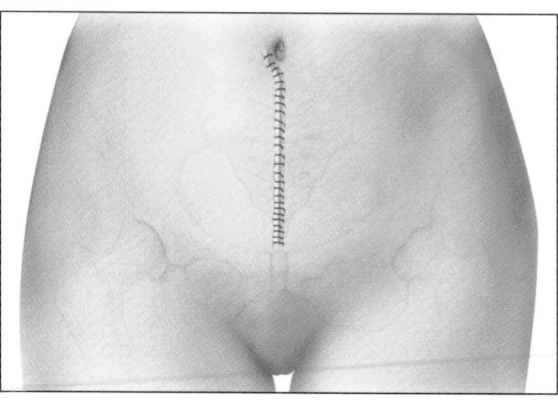

5. Incision site after surgery

Radiation therapy

Radiation therapy uses a high-energy radiation source to kill cancer cells or interfere with their ability to grow and divide. Radiation may be delivered two different ways.

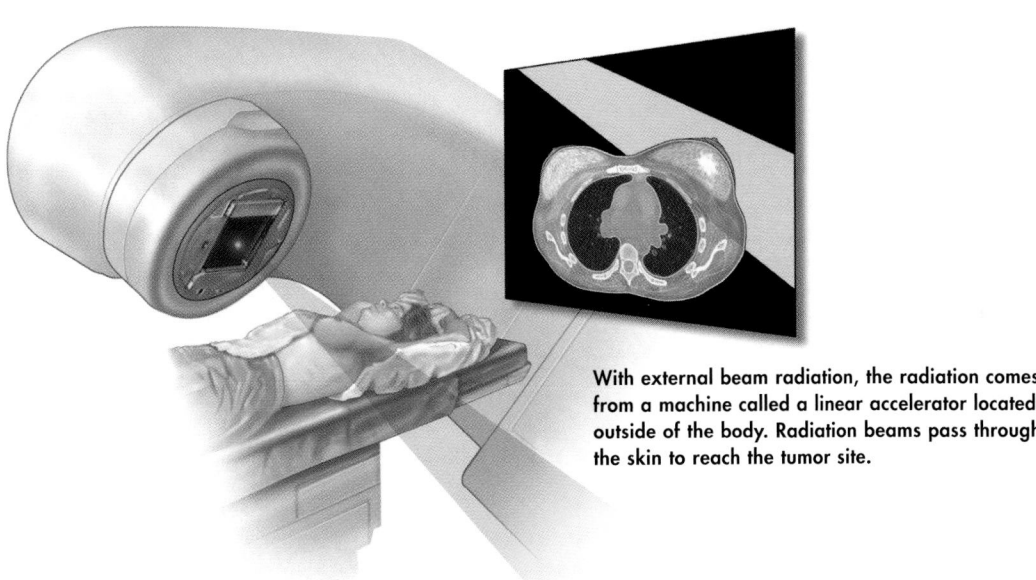

With external beam radiation, the radiation comes from a machine called a linear accelerator located outside of the body. Radiation beams pass through the skin to reach the tumor site.

With internal radiation (brachytherapy), an applicator containing a radioactive substance is placed within the body, at or near the site where the tumor is located or was removed.

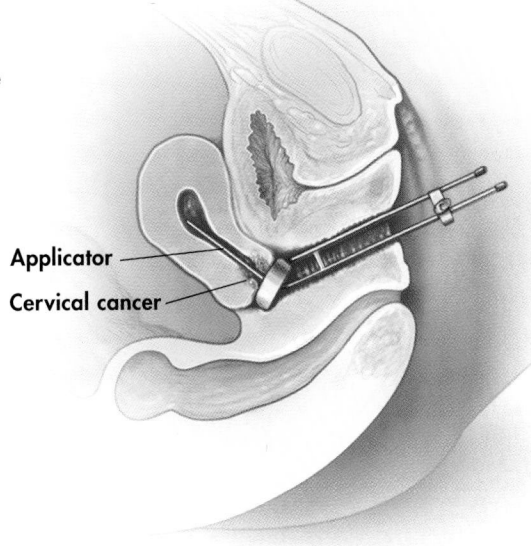

Applicator

Cervical cancer

Drug therapy

Medications (therapeutic agents) that kill or slow down cancer cells work at many sites within the cell. They can interfere with processes at the cell membrane. They can block the signaling cascades occurring within the cytoplasm that stimulate cell growth and division. And they can interfere with the normal functioning of DNA so that new proteins can't be made and new cells can't be formed.

Cell membrane

Medications that act at the cell membrane block the binding of growth factors to their receptors, or they bind to the receptors but inhibit their activation. This prevents the transmission of growth signals to the interior of the cancer cell. The drug Herceptin is an example. It's a monoclonal antibody that binds to HER-2/neu, a growth factor receptor on the cell membrane, shutting down the receptor. Newer medications being tested inhibit the erbB1 receptor, which is important in several cancers.

Cytoplasm

Several new drug therapies target the secondary messengers that transmit growth signals to the nucleus. Examples include farnesyl transferase inhibitors that block the ras pathway, an important signaling system in multiple types of cancer.

Nucleus

Many therapeutic agents work directly at the nucleus, the control center of the cell. Most chemotherapy medications, for example, interfere with the function of DNA. Cisplatin and carboplatin bind directly to DNA, preventing it from unfolding to manufacture proteins or to be duplicated for new cancer cells. Other chemotherapy drugs cause breaks in the DNA structure and inhibit the enzymes needed to repair the damage. The drug tamoxifen interferes with the ability of the receptor for the hormone estrogen to act as a transcription factor and turn on relevant downstream genes. Other agents work within the nucleus to induce cancer cells to undergo cell death.

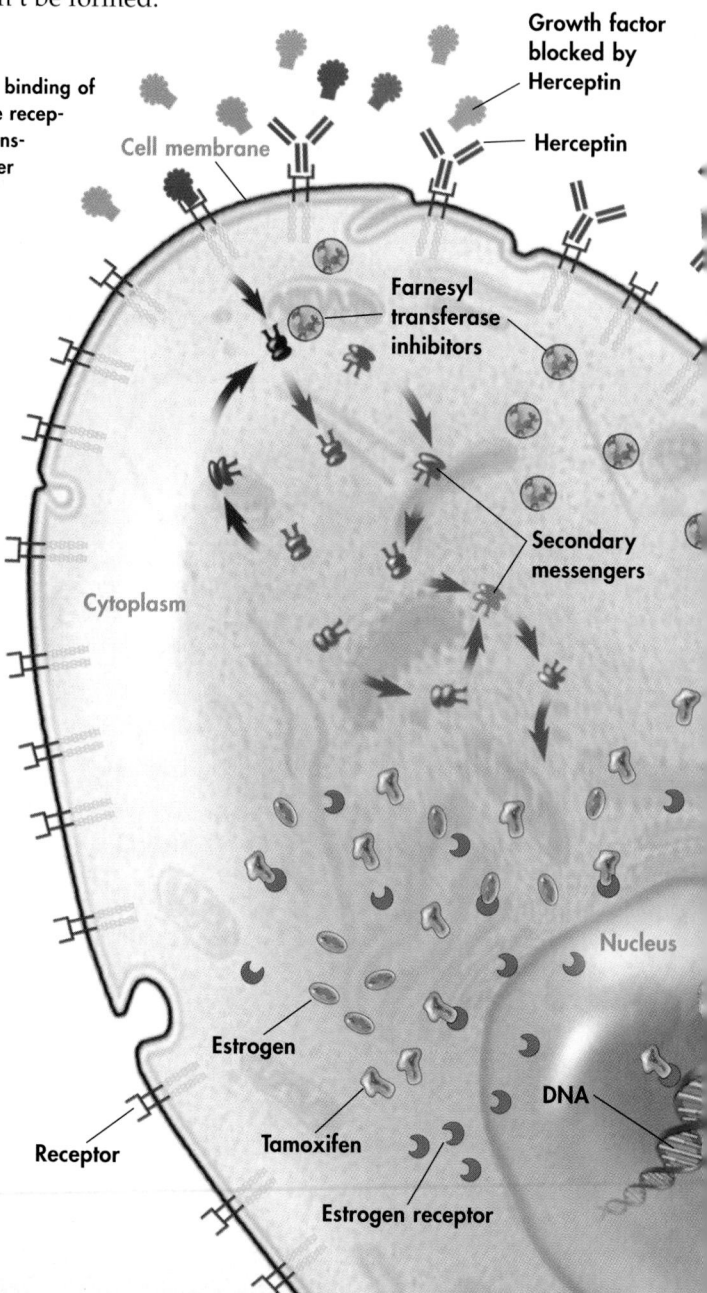

Growth factor blocked by Herceptin

Herceptin

Cell membrane

Farnesyl transferase inhibitors

Secondary messengers

Cytoplasm

Nucleus

Estrogen

DNA

Receptor

Tamoxifen

Estrogen receptor

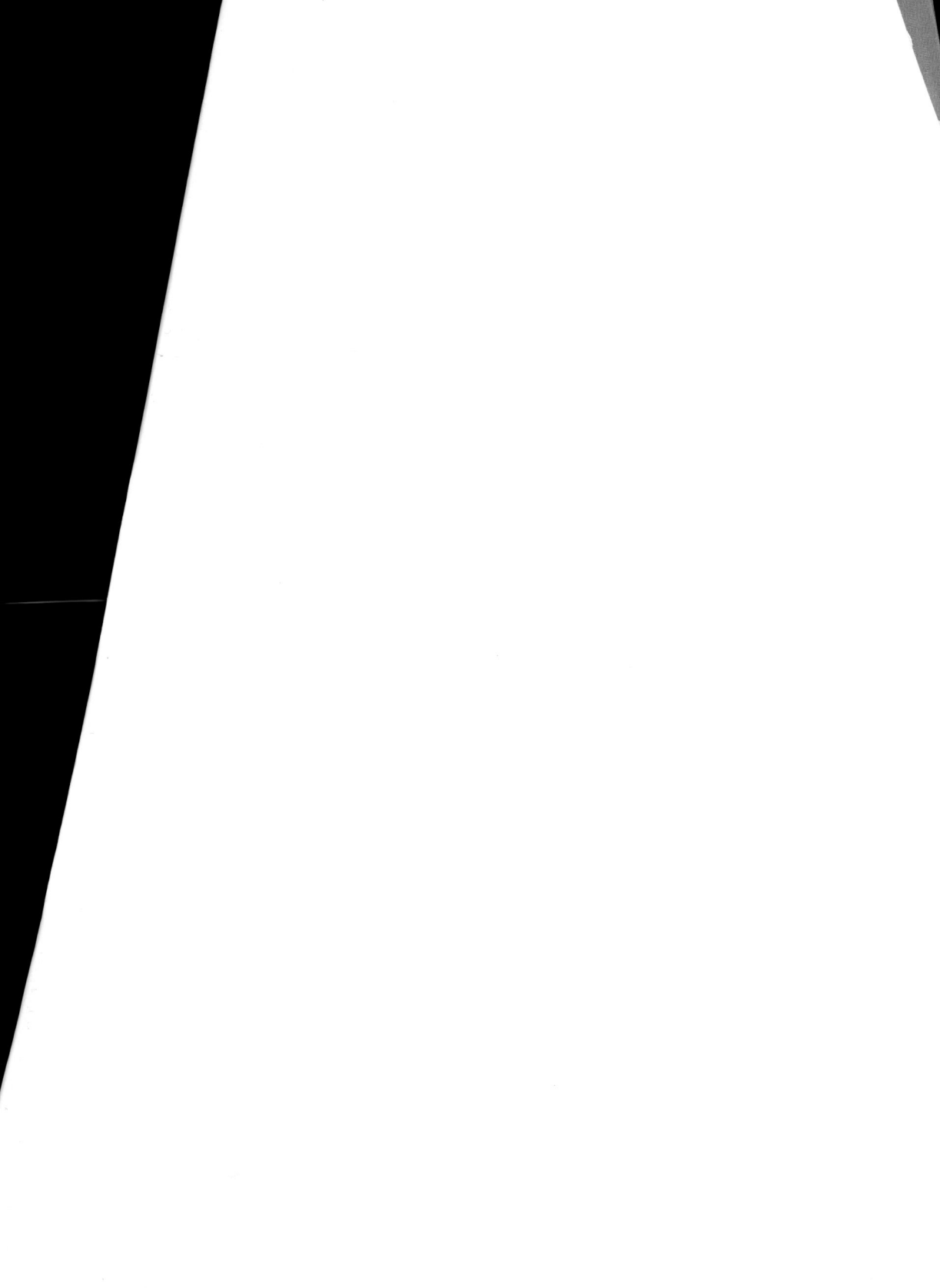

Gyneco
Car

Chapter 15: Gynecologic Cancers

Ovarian Cancer Overview

The ovaries are a source of life. They produce the eggs (ova) that enable a woman to have children. For some women, the ovaries are also a threat to life. In the ovaries, cancer can develop and grow quietly and unnoticed for years.

Ovarian cancer isn't the most common cancer to affect women, but what makes this cancer so frightening is its track record. It causes more deaths than any other gynecologic cancer, mainly for two reasons. In its early stages, ovarian cancer produces few, if any, signs and symptoms. And when they do occur, they can easily be confused with those of other conditions. In addition, no effective test to screen for ovarian cancer is available. Screening tests are a type of test used to catch diseases in their early stages.

In more than 70 percent of women with ovarian cancer, the disease has already spread (metastasized) beyond the ovaries at the time it's diagnosed — it has advanced to the point where treatment is less likely to cure the cancer. By comparison, when ovarian cancer

FASTFACT

The most common cancers among American women

Type	Estimated number of new cases each year
1. Breast cancer	215,990
2. Lung cancer	80,660
3. Colorectal cancer	73,320
4. Uterine cancer	40,320
5. Ovarian cancer	25,580
6. Non-Hodgkin's lymphoma	25,520
7. Melanoma	25,200
8. Thyroid cancer	17,640
9. Pancreatic cancer	16,120
10. Bladder cancer	15,600

Source: American Cancer Society, "Cancer Facts and Figures 2004"

is caught in its early stages, the five-year survival rate is greater than 75 percent.

However, there is some good news to report. The incidence of ovarian cancer has been slowly decreasing since 1991. Incidence refers to the number of new cases diagnosed each year. According to the American Cancer Society, from 1989 to 1999, ovarian cancer incidence declined at a rate of 0.7 percent a year. In addition, women with ovarian cancer now have more treatment choices and longer durations of survival than ever before.

Ten years ago, long-term survivors of ovarian cancer were rare. Today — even when the disease recurs — more women are living longer. Among women with all stages of ovarian cancer diagnosed between 1992 and 1997, more than half lived at least five years. That's a significant improvement from the early 1970s, when the five-year survival rate was just 36 percent.

Learning that you have ovarian cancer can be devastating, but don't lose hope.

Ovarian cancer is a serious disease, but it can be treated. Although many women experience persistent or recurrent disease, they're often able to live with the cancer for years. Some long-term survivors view ovarian cancer as more of a chronic condition — in spite of their cancer, they're still living reasonably well.

Your Ovaries

The ovaries are situated in the lower portion of your pelvis on each side of your uterus (see the color illustration on page 264). During your menstrual cycle, your ovaries can change in size, varying from the size of an almond to the size of a walnut. After menopause, they shrink to less than half their premenopausal size.

The ovaries produce eggs (ova). When a baby girl is born, her ovaries contain all the eggs that she'll need throughout her life. Each month, beginning when a girl reaches puberty and continuing until

An ovary

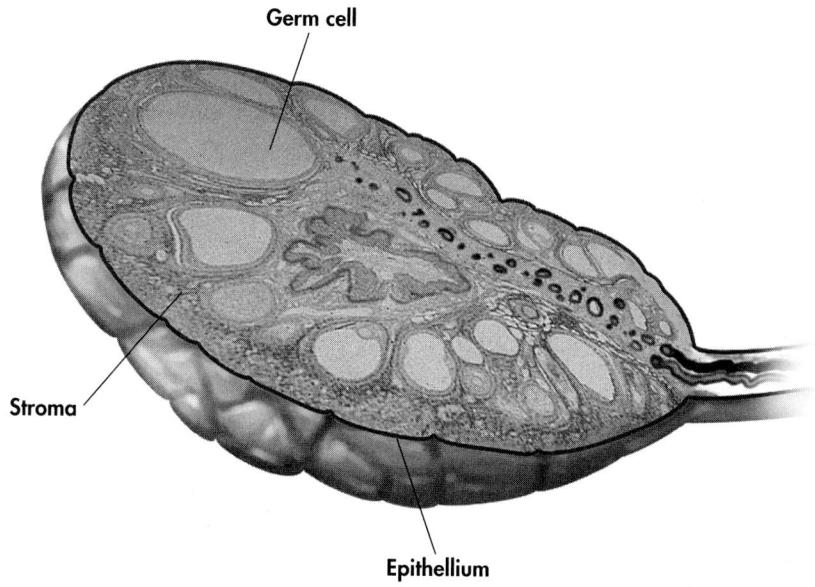

Germ cell

Stroma

Epithellium

The ovaries are situated on each side of your uterus. Each month between puberty and menopause the ovaries grow cyst-like structures called follicles that release an egg (ovum) into a fallopian tube. The ovaries are composed of three types of cells: epithelial, stromal and germ.

menopause, the ovaries grow cyst-like structures called follicles. During ovulation, one follicle releases an egg into a fallopian tube, which connects the ovary to the uterus.

The ovaries are also the primary source of the female sex hormones estrogen and progesterone. These hormones influence the development and maintenance of feminine physical characteristics, such as breast development, body shape and body hair. Estrogen and progesterone also help regulate menstrual cycles and pregnancy. At menopause the ovaries stop producing eggs and these hormones.

The ovaries contain three categories of cells: epithelial, stromal and germ. The epithelium is the thin layer of cells that covers the outside of the ovaries. The stroma is the connective tissue that holds the ovaries together. Stromal cells produce most of your estrogen and progesterone. Germ cells, which are located within follicles, develop into eggs.

Ovarian Cancer

Like other cancers, ovarian cancer results from the loss of control of normal cell growth and regulation. Over time, abnormal cells in the ovary accumulate into a mass of tissue called a growth, or tumor. An ovarian tumor may be noncancerous (benign) or cancerous (malignant). Although benign tumors are made up of

Types of ovarian cancer

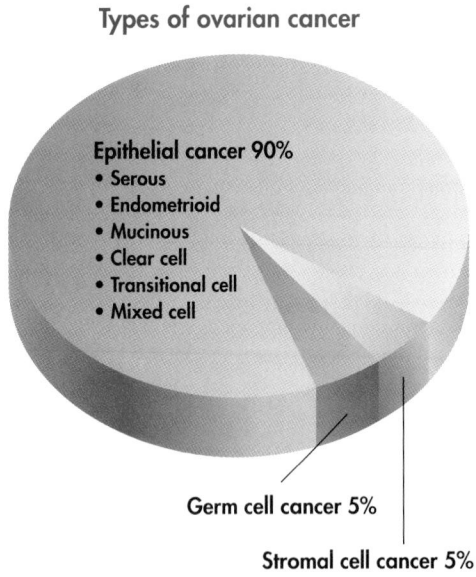

Epithelial cancer 90%
- Serous
- Endometrioid
- Mucinous
- Clear cell
- Transitional cell
- Mixed cell

Germ cell cancer 5%

Stromal cell cancer 5%

cells that are growing in excess numbers, they don't spread (metastasize) to other body tissues. Malignant cells may spread directly to nearby tissues in the abdominal cavity, or they may detach from the original tumor site and spread throughout your body by way of your blood vessels or lymphatic system.

Any type of cell in the ovary can become cancerous. The three main categories of ovarian cancer are named according to where they originated in the ovary. Most ovarian tumors arise from cells in the layer of tissue that covers the surface of the ovaries (epithelium). These are known as epithelial tumors. When the term *ovarian cancer* is used, it usually refers to this epithelial type. The other types of ovarian tumors are germ cell tumors, which arise in the egg-producing cells, and stromal tumors, which occur in the connective tissue (stroma).

Epithelial tumors

Epithelial tumors may be noncancerous, cancerous or borderline (sometimes called low malignant potential tumors).

Most epithelial ovarian tumors are noncancerous. There are several types of benign epithelial tumors, including serous adenomas, mucinous adenomas and transitional cell tumors. These tumors don't spread and usually don't lead to serious illness. They can be treated with surgery to remove the affected ovary or the part of the ovary where the tumor is located. Benign ovarian tumors are different from simple ovarian cysts, which are fluid-filled sacs that usually go away without treatment.

Epithelial cancer is by far the most common type of ovarian cancer, accounting for 85 percent to 90 percent of all ovarian cancers. Epithelial cancer can be further divided into subtypes, which are classified according to how the cancerous cells appear under a microscope. These subtypes, discussed in the next chapter, include serous, mucinous, endometrioid, clear cell and transitional cell cancers.

Some types of epithelial tumors are neither benign nor malignant. They fall into a gray zone in between. The cells of these so-called borderline tumors, when viewed under a microscope, don't appear normal, but they aren't as abnormal as cancer cells typically are. In addition, they don't invade the supporting tissue (ovarian stroma) or other structures. Generally, borderline tumors don't become truly cancerous, but in some instances they can behave more aggressively. Therefore, these types of tumors need to be moni-

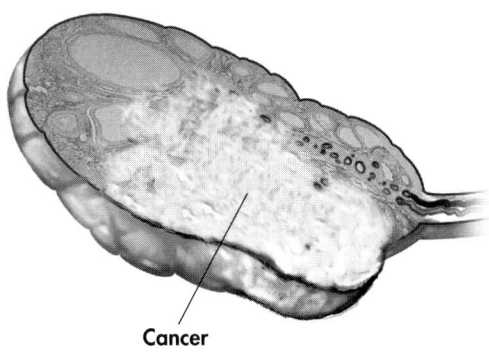

Cancer

Epithelial ovarian cancer, the most common form of ovarian cancer, results when cells on the surface of the ovary undergo malignant change and begin to grow in an uncontrolled manner.

tored closely. For more information on borderline tumors, see Chapter 19.

Spread of epithelial cancer

Epithelial ovarian cancer can spread by a unique process called seeding. As the tumor grows on the surface of the ovary and becomes larger, it can shed cells like seeds directly into the abdominal cavity. The shed cells can become implanted on the surrounding tissues and organs, such as the membrane that lines the abdominal cavity (peritoneum), diaphragm, fallopian tubes, uterus, bladder, spleen and liver. The seeded cells form new tumors in these sites.

One of the most common sites for the spread of ovarian cancer is the fatty apron that covers the stomach and intestines (omentum). This seeding within the peritoneal cavity is the most common mode of spread for ovarian cancer.

Ovarian cancer can also spread by entering the bloodstream or lymphatic channels. Lymph nodes most likely to contain ovarian cancer cells are those in the pelvis and surrounding the major blood vessel leading from the heart to the lower torso (aorta). Once cancer cells are in the bloodstream or lymphatic system, they can travel and form new tumors in other parts of the body, such as the pleural cavity around the lungs.

As ovarian cancer spreads, it may cause fluid to collect in the abdominal cavity. The tumor nodules themselves may cause formation of excessive fluid. Or a collection of tumors may interfere with normal fluid drainage from the abdominal cavity. This abnormal fluid collection is known as ascites. In some women, several quarts of excess fluid may accumulate.

Primary Peritoneal Carcinoma

Closely related to epithelial ovarian cancer is a cancer called primary peritoneal carcinoma. It forms from cells that make up the lining of the abdominal cavity (peritoneum) and pelvis. These cells are very similar to those on the surface of the ovaries (epithelial cells). Under a microscope, peritoneal cancer looks just like epithelial ovarian cancer. It also acts in a manner similar to ovarian cancer. Women who have had their ovaries and fallopian tubes removed still have a slight risk of developing primary peritoneal carcinoma.

Germ cell tumors

Germ cell tumors form out of an ovary's egg-producing cells. These types of tumors are uncommon and often benign. About 5 percent of ovarian cancers are the germ cell type.

Unlike epithelial ovarian cancer, which is most common in older women, germ cell tumors affect mainly girls, teenagers and young women. Another important difference is that a high percentage of cancerous germ cell tumors can be cured.

Treatment for these tumors typically involves surgery and chemotherapy. For more information on germ cell tumors, see Chapter 19.

Sex cord-stromal tumors

Sex cord-stromal tumors, also called stromal tumors, account for about 5 percent of ovarian cancers. They form in connective tissue cells of the ovaries. Many women who develop sex cord-stromal tumors are younger than age 40,

Ovarian Cysts

Most women have ovarian cysts at some point. Ovarian cysts are fluid-filled sacs in an ovary or on its surface. In women who are still menstruating, cysts typically occur as a normal and expected part of ovulation. Each release of an egg (ovulation) leaves behind a cyst about an inch in diameter. Normally, these cysts disappear without any treatment. In rare cases, though, they persist and grow larger. Some ovarian cancers can have cyst-like components, but most ovarian cysts aren't cancerous and produce few or no symptoms.

Unlike malignant tumors, ovarian cysts don't invade neighboring tissue. However, if an ovarian cyst is large, it can cause pelvic discomfort. In some cases, it may interfere with the production of normal ovarian hormones, which could result in irregular vaginal bleeding or an increase in body hair. If a large cyst presses on your bladder, it may reduce

your bladder's capacity, causing you to urinate more frequently.

Some specific types of ovarian cysts include:

- **Follicular cysts.** Your ovaries normally grow cyst-like structures called follicles each month as part of the menstrual cycle. Follicles hold eggs and release them during ovulation. Sometimes, a monthly follicle doesn't release its egg. It just keeps growing and becomes a cyst. Follicular cysts rarely cause pain and usually disappear on their own within two or three menstrual cycles.
- **Corpus luteum cysts.** Another type of cyst develops from the empty follicle that's left after the egg is released (corpus luteum). Sometimes after the egg is released, the corpus luteum expands into a cyst. Although it usually disappears within a few weeks, such a cyst can grow large enough to twist the ovary, causing pelvic or abdominal pain. If the cyst fills with blood, it may rupture, causing sudden, sharp pain.

but these tumors can occur in women of all ages. Indications of a possible sex cord-stromal tumor typically depend on a woman's age and menstrual status.

Some sex cord-stromal tumors make sex hormones. As a result, such a tumor could cause a young girl to begin having her menstrual period or developing breasts earlier than normal.

In a mature woman, a sex cord-stromal tumor can cause irregularities in the menstrual cycle. Less frequently, the tumors may produce male hormones, which can disrupt normal periods and promote the growth of facial and body hair.

In women past menopause, a hormone-producing tumor can cause a return of vaginal bleeding.

Sex cord-stromal tumors generally aren't fast growing, and they don't spread rapidly. Because most are discovered before they've spread outside the ovary, treatment for this form of ovarian cancer is often successful. For more information on sex cord-stromal tumors, see Chapter 19.

- **Dermoid cysts.** These cysts are noncancerous germ cell tumors known as teratomas. They may contain tissue such as hair, skin or teeth because they form from cells that produce human eggs. They can become large and cause painful twisting of the ovary and fallopian tube.
- **Endometriomas.** Endometriosis is a condition in which cells that normally make up the uterine lining grow outside the uterus. In women with endometriosis, some endometrial tissue may attach to the ovary and form a cyst called an endometrioma.
- **Cystadenomas.** These cysts develop from ovarian tissue and may be filled with a watery liquid or mucous material. They can become very large and cause twisting of the ovary and fallopian tube.

For younger, menstruating women, ovarian cysts are common, usually harmless and will resolve spontaneously. When a cyst develops after menopause, there's a higher chance that it may be associated with cancer. For a woman age 50 or older, the likelihood that an ovarian cyst is associated with cancer is 25 percent. For a woman in her 80s, the chance increases to about 60 percent.

In addition, the larger the cyst, the greater the likelihood that it will be cancerous. The vast majority of cysts smaller than 5 centimeters (about 2 inches) aren't cancerous. When a cyst is larger than 10 centimeters, the chances of it being cancerous are 40 percent to 65 percent.

Cysts that don't cause any signs or symptoms may be found when a doctor performs a pelvic examination. Changes in your monthly menstrual cycle — signs or symptoms accompanying menstruation that aren't typical for you or that persist — also may signal development of a cyst.

Treatment options may range from taking a wait-and-see approach to undergoing surgery to remove the cyst.

GYNECOLOGIC CANCERS

How Common Is Ovarian Cancer?

The incidence of ovarian cancer — the number of new cases diagnosed each year — is relatively low. Ovarian cancer accounts for about 4 percent of all cancers that occur in women in the United States. Among gynecologic cancers — cancers of the female reproductive tract — ovarian cancer is the second most commonly diagnosed cancer, after uterine cancer. It's diagnosed in about 25,000 women in the United States each year, and more than 16,000 women in the United States die of the disease annually.

To put these figures into perspective, you have about a one in 70 chance of getting ovarian cancer during your lifetime, provided you live to age 80. Compare that with the incidence of breast cancer. One in 10 women who live to age 80 will develop breast cancer at some point in their lives.

Across the world, about 190,000 new cases of ovarian cancer are diagnosed each year, and 114,000 deaths occur. Ovarian cancer rates are the highest in Scandinavia, Europe, the United States and Canada. The lowest rates for this type of cancer are found in Africa and Asia. Rates are increasing in the countries of Japan, Italy and Spain.

The disease is more common in Jewish women of Ashkenazi (Eastern and Central European) descent. In the United States, the incidence of ovarian cancer is slightly higher among white women than it is among black, Asian-American and Hispanic women.

What Causes Ovarian Cancer?

The causes of ovarian cancer remain unknown. Over the years, several theories have been proposed. One is that cycle after cycle of uninterrupted ovulation may lead to an increased risk of ovarian cancer. Ovulation is the monthly process in which the ovary releases an egg (ovum) into the fallopian tube for travel to the uterus and possible fertilization by a sperm.

When an ovary releases an egg, the egg breaks through the epithelial layer covering the ovary. This creates a small rupture that needs to be repaired. This repeated rupturing is followed by inflammation and the creation of new epithelial cells. The formation and division of new cells may set up a situation in which genetic errors can occur. In addition, as the wound is being repaired, some epithelial cells can become trapped below the surface of the ovary, forming an inclusion cyst. Some scientists think this type of cyst contributes to the development of ovarian cancer.

This theory may explain why events that prevent ovulation, such as pregnancy, breast-feeding and use of birth control pills, are associated with a reduced risk of ovarian cancer. However, some researchers believe that it's the increased hormone levels before and during ovulation, and not the rupturing of the ovarian surface, that lead to higher risk of ovarian cancer among women whose menstrual cycles aren't interrupted by pregnancy or other events. According to this theory, high levels of certain reproductive hormones may stimulate the growth of abnormal epithelial cells.

Researchers are still trying to understand all the changes that occur on a molecular and genetic level that lead to ovarian cancer. Most cancers involve many alterations (mutations) to genes that control the human cell. Genetic alterations may either be inherited or develop spontaneously. Inherited mutations are those you were born with — a defective gene that one of your parents passed on to you. Inherited mutations are present in all the body's cells but they may create a cancer risk only in specific cells.

Spontaneous (sporadic) mutations occur during a person's life and aren't passed on to the next generation. Spontaneous mutations are common, and they're harmful only if they're passed on to newly generated cells. Most ovarian cancers likely involve several gene mutations. It's thought that an initial gene mutation is followed by subsequent mutations that gradually progress to cancer.

Risk Factors

Although the causes of ovarian cancer are still being uncovered, researchers have identified a number of factors that increase a woman's odds of developing ovarian cancer.

Just because you have one or more risk factors for ovarian cancer doesn't guarantee that you'll get it. In fact, most women have one or more risk factors for ovarian cancer, but only a small number of them actually get the disease. Most of the common risk factors increase your risk only slightly, so they don't completely explain the occurrence of the disease.

The risk factors discussed here apply to epithelial ovarian cancer, not to the two other less common types of ovarian cancer. Much less is known about risk factors for germ cell or stromal tumors.

Genetic factors

In some families, people may inherit genes that make them more susceptible to certain cancers, such as ovarian cancer.

BRCA genes increase risk

	BRCA1 mutation carriers	BRCA2 mutation carriers	General population
Risk of developing breast cancer by age 70	65%	45%	8%-11%
Risk of developing ovarian cancer by age 70	39%	11%	1.5%

Women who inherit BRCA1 or BRCA2 gene mutations are at significantly higher risk of developing breast and ovarian cancers than are women in the general population. Underlying BRCA1 or BRCA2 mutations are present in about 10 percent of women with ovarian cancer.

Most ovarian cancers are sporadic, with no family pattern. About 10 percent result from an inherited predisposition.

Inherited cancers

The most significant risk factor for ovarian cancer is having an inherited mutation in one of two genes called breast cancer gene 1 (BRCA1) and breast cancer gene 2 (BRCA2). These genes were originally identified in families with multiple cases of breast cancer, which is how they got their names, but they're also responsible for about 10 percent of ovarian cancers. You can inherit a BRCA gene mutation from either your mother or your father.

Women with a BRCA1 or BRCA2 mutation have an estimated 39 percent to 11 percent chance, respectively, of developing ovarian cancer during their lifetimes, compared with a 1.5 percent chance for the general population of women. Estimates vary considerably due to differences in the gene involved, the location of the mutation and the groups of women who participated in the research studies.

Women of Ashkenazi Jewish ancestry have a higher incidence of BRCA mutations than does the general population of women. For women not of Ashkenazi descent, the prevalence of a BRCA mutation is one in 800. For women of Ashkenazi decent, it increases to one in 40.

Certain factors suggest the possibility of an inherited genetic mutation:
- Two or more women in the family with ovarian cancer or breast cancer before age 50
- Breast and ovarian cancer in the same individual
- Male breast cancer

- Ashkenazi Jewish women with early-onset (before age 50) breast cancer

For more information on the BRCA genes and genetic testing, see Chapter 4.

Another known genetic link involves an inherited syndrome called hereditary nonpolyposis colorectal cancer (HNPCC). Individuals in HNPCC families are at increased risk of cancers of the uterine lining (endometrium), colon, ovary, stomach and small intestine. Risk of ovarian cancer associated with HNPCC is lower than that associated with BRCA mutations.

Noninherited cancers

Sometimes, ovarian cancer occurs in more than one family member but isn't the result of an inherited gene alteration. Having some family history of ovarian cancer increases your risk of the disease, but not to the same degree as does having an inherited genetic defect. If you have one first-degree relative — a mother, daughter or sister — with ovarian cancer, your risk of developing the disease is five percent over your lifetime, which means there's still a 95 percent chance that you won't develop the disease.

Having other relatives, such as a grandmother, aunt or cousin, with ovarian cancer also increases your risk above that of the general population, but not as high as does having a first-degree relative with the disease. A family history of other cancers, such as breast cancer, also increases the risk of ovarian cancer.

Age

Ovarian cancer is more common in older women. Epithelial ovarian cancer, the most common ovarian cancer, is uncommon in women under 40. The average age at diagnosis is 61. Incidence increases from about 16 per 100,000 women in the 40 to 44 age group and peaks at 57 per 100,000 women in the 70 to 74 age group.

Hormonal and reproductive factors

The number of times you ovulate during your lifetime appears to affect ovarian cancer risk. Studies show that reduced ovulations during a woman's lifetime is associated with a lower risk of ovarian cancer. For example, women who've taken oral contraceptives have a reduced risk of ovarian cancer, as do women who've given birth. The more children a woman has had, the less likely she is to develop ovarian cancer. Oral contraceptives and pregnancy prevent ovulation.

Reproductive factors associated with increased risk of ovarian cancer include:

Childbearing status
Women who've never had children or who had their first child after age 30 are more likely to get ovarian cancer. During pregnancy, a woman doesn't ovulate.

Infertility
If you've had trouble conceiving, you may be at increased risk. Studies indicate that infertility increases the risk of ovarian cancer, even without use of fertility drugs. The risk appears to be highest for women with unexplained infertility and women with infertility who never conceive. The link between infertility and increased ovarian cancer risk is poorly understood, and research in this area is ongoing.

Use of fertility drugs
Some studies suggest that use of clomiphene (Clomid, Serophene) for longer than a year — especially without becoming pregnant — may contribute to an increased risk of ovarian cancer. However, a study published in 2002 that pooled and analyzed the results of eight studies conducted over several years indicated that fertility drugs don't increase the risk of invasive ovarian tumors. The study did find, though, that the incidence of borderline tumors was higher among women who took fertility drugs and who didn't become pregnant.

Early onset of menstruation and late menopause
Although experts have long thought that a relationship exists between a long menstrual life — that is, one with more ovulatory cycles — and increased risk of ovarian cancer, some studies have cast doubt on this theory. More research is needed.

Estrogen therapy after menopause
Findings regarding use of the hormones estrogen and progestin after menopause (hormone replacement therapy) and ovarian cancer risk have been inconsistent. Some studies indicate a slightly increased risk of ovarian cancer in women taking estrogen after menopause; others don't.

Researchers from the National Cancer Institute followed 44,241 postmenopausal women for approximately 20 years. In a report published in 2001, they indicated that the women who took estrogen alone, without progestin, for 10 years or more had a significantly higher risk of developing ovarian cancer than did women who

GYNECOLOGIC CANCERS

Don't Blame Yourself

If you've recently learned that you have ovarian cancer, you can drive yourself to distraction thinking about what you could have done differently in your life that might have prevented the cancer. You might blame yourself for your cancer because you chose not to or were unable to have children, took fertility drugs or relied on estrogen to help you through symptoms of menopause.

Keep in mind that most women who have the same risk factors — who made choices similar to the ones you made — don't have ovarian cancer. Your illness isn't your fault. Ovarian cancer results from an interplay of many factors, not one thing you did or didn't do.

In addition, don't blame yourself if you've been diagnosed with ovarian cancer that has already spread. This is a particularly insidious disease, with signs and symptoms that are similar to more common, less serious problems.

It's important not to spend too much time and emotional energy on what-ifs. Look ahead. From now on, the most important thing that you can do is to take the best possible care of yourself and act as a partner with your doctor in your treatment.

---

never used estrogen. However, the researchers found no increased risk for women who took estrogen combined with progestin, the most common form of hormone replacement therapy. Other studies have not found a link between taking estrogen alone after menopause and development of ovarian cancer.

The Women's Health Initiative, a study of thousands of postmenopausal women, found that combined estrogen and progestin therapy doesn't reduce the risk of ovarian cancer and may even increase it. Although the results weren't statistically significant, researchers saw a trend toward increased ovarian cancer risk among women taking the combination.

Ovarian cysts

Women who develop ovarian cysts between the ages of 50 and 70 are at higher risk of ovarian cancer. Cysts that form after menopause have a greater chance of being cancerous. Doctors aren't certain why ovarian cysts form after menopause.

Certain conditions of the reproductive tract

Some studies have suggested that a history of endometriosis, pelvic inflammatory disease or polycystic ovarian syndrome may increase a woman's risk of ovarian cancer. More research is needed to determine if there's a connection and, if so, to what extent.

Other factors

Studies haven't identified any major environmental or dietary factors linked to an increased risk of ovarian cancer. Besides family history, age and reproductive issues, other factors that may increase a woman's risk of ovarian cancer include:

Personal history of breast or colon cancer

If you've had breast or colon cancer, you also have an increased risk of developing ovarian cancer.

Use of talcum powder

Some studies have shown a slight increase in the risk of ovarian cancer among women who used talcum powder on the genital area or on sanitary napkins. In the past, talc (magnesium silicate), which is the basis of talcum powder, contained asbestos, a known cancer-causing substance. When applied directly to the genital area or sanitary napkins, talc particles can enter the vagina and travel up the genital tract to the ovaries. For more than 20 years, body and face powder products have been legally required to be free of asbestos. But proving the safety of newer products will require follow-up studies of women who've used them for many years. Currently, no evidence links cornstarch powders with any female cancer.

Obesity and weight gain

Several studies have examined the relationship between a woman's weight and her risk of ovarian cancer, with varying results. In the Nurses' Health Study, researchers examined weight changes among almost 110,000 participants. Study results, published in 2002, found no association between body weight and ovarian cancer risk. Researchers did, however, observe a connection between obesity at age 18 and premenopausal ovarian cancer, highlighting the importance of a healthy weight in adolescence to help prevent disease in later years. Another large study published in the same year suggested a possible association between excess weight and ovarian cancer deaths.

More studies are needed to clarify the relationship between obesity and ovarian cancer. In the meantime, achieving and maintaining a healthy weight is good for your overall health.

Smoking

Some studies have found that smoking increases the risk of mucinous ovarian tumors, a type of epithelial cancer. The risk is higher for current smokers and goes up with the number of cigarettes smoked.

Reducing Your Risk

There isn't anything you can do to completely eliminate your risk of ovarian cancer. But, just as certain factors may increase your risk of this cancer, others may reduce it. Some of these strategies reduce your risk only slightly, and others reduce it more significantly. If you're concerned that you may be at high risk of ovarian cancer, talk to your doctor about your situation.

Following are factors shown to lower risk of epithelial ovarian cancer.

Birth control pills

Multiple studies have shown a protective benefit from use of birth control pills. Use of oral contraceptives for three or more years reduces a woman's risk of ovarian cancer by 30 percent to 50 percent, compared with women who have never used them. Risk decreases even further with longer use, and the protective effect continues for at least 10 to 15 years after you stop taking the pill.

Birth control pills work by suppressing hormones needed for ovulation. Because these hormones may promote the development of cancerous cells, suppressing them with birth control pills may help prevent ovarian cancer.

If you have a strong family history of breast cancer or carry a known BRCA mutation, talk with your doctor about whether it would be beneficial for you to take oral contraceptives. Along with the benefits, there are some risks. Some studies have suggested that birth control pills may slightly increase breast cancer risk in women at high risk of the disease.

Pregnancy and breast-feeding

Having at least one child lowers your risk of developing ovarian cancer, especially if you deliver your first child before age 30. Your risk decreases further with each subsequent delivery. Breast-feeding a child for a year or longer also may reduce the risk of ovarian cancer.

But experts don't recommend that women base their childbearing decisions on possible prevention of ovarian cancer. Pregnancy and breast-feeding reduce risk,

---

RESEARCH UPDATE

Chemoprevention

Another preventive measure that's receiving increasing attention is chemoprevention — the use of specific drugs to reduce the risk of cancer in people at high risk. Two chemopreventive agents under study are the medication fenretinide and oral contraceptives.

Fenretinide
Retinoids are vitamin A-derived substances that inhibit cell growth and have other properties that suggest they may help prevent the growth of cancer. Unfortunately, to have a therapeutic effect, the medications need to be taken in high doses, which can be toxic to the body. Fenretinide was developed as a less toxic synthetic derivative of vitamin A. It's being evaluated in clinical trials

as a potential chemopreventive agent for breast, lung and ovarian cancers.

Oral contraceptives
It's been estimated that more than half the ovarian cancer cases in the United States could be prevented by use of oral contraceptives for four to five years or more. Although it's well-known that birth control pills decrease the risk of ovarian cancer, experts don't fully understand how they do so. The pills reduce the number of ovulatory cycles a woman has, but the mechanism by which they reduce ovarian cancer risk is likely more complex.

One study is investigating the effectiveness of oral contraceptives, fenretinide or both as chemoprevention agents for ovarian cancer.

but they don't guarantee protection against ovarian cancer. Oral contraceptives may afford equal or greater benefits.

Tubal ligation or hysterectomy

Tubal ligation, commonly referred to as having your tubes tied, is a surgical procedure designed to prevent pregnancy by sealing the fallopian tubes, thereby keeping sperm from reaching the egg. Studies suggest that tubal ligation may reduce ovarian cancer risk. The Nurses' Health Study, which followed thousands of women for 20 years, found a substantial reduction in ovarian cancer risk in women who had had tubal ligations. Tubal ligation has also been shown to reduce ovarian cancer risk among women with mutations in the BRCA1 gene. How the procedure reduces risk is uncertain.

The Nurses' Health Study also indicated that surgical removal of the uterus (hysterectomy) may reduce ovarian cancer risk, but not by as much as tubal ligation.

Removal of your ovaries

Women who are at very high risk of developing ovarian cancer may elect to have their ovaries removed as a means of preventing the disease. This surgery, known as preventive (prophylactic) oophorectomy, is recommended primarily for women who've tested positive for a BRCA gene mutation or women who have a strong family history of breast and ovarian cancer, even if no genetic mutation has been identified. Studies indicate that prophylactic oophorectomy lowers ovarian cancer risk by up to 95 percent for women

who have the surgery. It also reduces the risk of breast cancer by 50 percent, if the ovaries are removed before menopause.

Prophylactic oophorectomy doesn't completely eliminate cancer risk because despite having both ovaries removed, some women still develop cancer in the cells lining the abdominal and pelvic cavity, a condition called primary peritoneal carcinoma (see page 279).

Generally, the surgery involves removal of both ovaries as well as the fallopian tubes (salpingo-oophorectomy). The fallopian tubes are removed because women at high risk of getting ovarian cancer also have an increased risk of developing cancer of the fallopian tubes.

The optimal age at which to have prophylactic oophorectomy depends on whether you're a BRCA carrier, the age at which other family members received a diagnosis of ovarian cancer and whether you have other health risks, such as the bone-thinning disease osteoporosis. Removal of the ovaries in premenopausal women results in premature menopause, which increases the risk of osteoporosis.

Prophylactic oophorectomy isn't an option for a younger woman who wants to maintain her fertility. Many experts recommend that high-risk women have the procedure after age 35 or when childbearing is complete.

The main drawback of prophylactic oophorectomy is that it causes early menopause. Menopausal signs and symptoms include hot flashes, vaginal dryness, sleep disturbances and sexual problems.

The decision to have this surgery is a major one. Before you make a final decision, discuss the pros and cons of the

GYNECOLOGIC CANCERS

Prophylactic oophorectomy

Advantages	Disadvantages
Reduces ovarian cancer risk by up to 95 percent	Causes premature menopause and accompanying signs and symptoms
Reduces breast cancer risk by 50 percent if done before menopause	Increases risk of osteoporosis
	Causes loss of fertility in premenopausal women

surgery in detail with your doctor. It's key that you have an accurate understanding of your risk of ovarian cancer. Genetic testing may be an option to help define your risk (see Chapter 4).

Oophorectomy is discussed in further detail in Chapter 17.

Future Directions

Research is progressing along several fronts as doctors and scientists seek better detection, treatment and prevention methods for ovarian cancer. One of the most positive developments in the last decade has been the explosion of information about the molecular and cellular processes involved in a cell's transformation from normal to malignant. This information has led to new technologies that open the possibility for new targets for detection and treatment.

Detection methods under investigation include blood markers. These are substances in blood that may indicate the presence of an early ovarian cancer. One new approach to testing blood, called proteomics, has shown promise in this regard. In this method, patterns of proteins in the blood may provide clues about whether a woman has early-stage ovarian cancer. Other specific markers also are being studied.

Several new treatment options are being explored, including new chemotherapy drugs, vaccines, gene therapy and immunotherapy, which boosts the body's own immune system to help combat cancer. The discovery of genes that are mutated in ovarian cancer also may lead to the development of drugs that specifically target the function of these genes.

Research has also suggested that tests to identify changes in specific individual genes or panels of genes may help predict a woman's response to chemotherapy and her prognosis. More research is needed in this area.

In addition to working on better methods of detection and more effective treatments, researchers and doctors continue to study how to reduce the risk of ovarian cancer and how to improve the quality of life for women with ovarian cancer.

Chapter 16: Gynecologic Cancers

Diagnosing Ovarian Cancer

Ovarian cancer is sometimes referred to as a silent killer or the cancer that whispers, because all too often it isn't accompanied by easily recognizable signs and symptoms. Yet, according to recent studies, many women with ovarian cancer, even in its early stages, do have symptoms. The problem is, the symptoms aren't specific to ovarian cancer — they tend to mimic those of other conditions, such as gastrointestinal disorders.

Often, symptoms such as abdominal discomfort or indigestion stem from a digestive problem or stress. But these commonplace complaints can also signal the presence of ovarian cancer. Being aware of signs and symptoms associated with ovarian cancer may lead to earlier detection. Unfortunately, too many women are diagnosed too late. Only about 25 percent of ovarian cancers are found at an early stage. The earlier cancer is detected, generally the better the prognosis.

Adding to the difficulty of early detection is the lack of a reliable, standardized method of screening for ovarian cancer. Pelvic examinations, blood tests and vaginal ultrasounds are used to help detect ovarian cancer, but none of these methods can reliably detect the disease at an early stage in the general population. One of the most urgent priorities for cancer researchers is to develop a better screening test for ovarian cancer. New approaches that are in the early stages of testing show promise.

Until a new screening method is available, your best bet is to become aware of the signs and symptoms of ovarian cancer and to see your doctor if you're concerned you may have the disease. Regular pelvic exams also are important for detecting cancers of the reproductive tract. For women at high risk of developing ovarian cancer, additional screening procedures are recommended.

Signs and Symptoms

Most of the signs and symptoms of ovarian cancer relate to abdominal bloating or discomfort and other gastrointestinal disturbances. Common signs and symptoms that women with ovarian cancer may experience include:

- Abdominal or pelvic pressure, discomfort or pain
- Persistent indigestion, gas or nausea
- Feeling full even after a light meal
- Unexplained changes in bowel habits, including diarrhea or constipation
- Abdominal swelling or bloating, which can cause your clothing to feel tighter
- Changes in bladder habits, including a frequent or urgent need to urinate
- Loss of appetite

- Unexplained weight loss or gain, especially in the abdominal area
- Pain during intercourse

Less common symptoms include:

- A persistent lack of energy
- Low back pain

Because these signs and symptoms are associated with many diseases and disorders, they're said to be nonspecific. A woman or her doctor may assume that a more common condition is to blame. In fact, it's not unusual for women with ovarian cancer to be diagnosed with another condition before finally learning they have cancer. The key seems to be persistent or worsening signs and symptoms. With a digestive disorder, they tend to come and go, or they occur in certain situations or after eating certain foods. With ovarian cancer, there's typically little fluctuation — signs and symptoms are constant and may gradually worsen.

To gain a better understanding of the signs and symptoms associated with ovarian cancer, the authors of a 2001 study asked women about their experience with eight signs and symptoms — bloating, fullness and pressure in the abdomen or pelvis, abdominal or low back pain, lack of energy, nausea, diarrhea, loss of appetite, constipation, and frequent, urgent or burning urination. Among the participants, 168 women had recently been diagnosed with ovarian cancer and 251 were healthy. Although the eight signs and symptoms were fairly common among all the women questioned, each sign or symptom — except for nausea — was considerably more prevalent among the women with ovarian cancer. The most prominent indication of

Signs and symptoms study

Symptom	Women with ovarian cancer	Women without cancer
Any of the following signs or symptoms	93%	42%
Bloating, fullness and pressure in the abdomen or pelvis	71%	9%
Abdominal pain or low back pain	52%	15%
Lack of energy	43%	16%
Frequent, urgent or burning urination	33%	12%
Constipation	21%	7%
Loss of appetite	20%	3%
Diarrhea	16%	6%
Nausea	13%	9%

Source: *Obstetrics & Gynecology*, 98:2 (August 2001), pages 212-217

ovarian cancer was abdominal bloating, fullness and pressure. In women with cancer, these sensations were more likely to be constant rather than intermittent.

If you're experiencing any of these signs or symptoms, especially if they're persistent, talk to your doctor. If you've already seen a doctor and received a diagnosis other than ovarian cancer, but you're not getting relief from the treatment, schedule a follow-up visit with your doctor or get a second opinion. In particular, don't ignore persistent abdominal bloating or discomfort. Unusual bloating may indicate that ovarian cancer has spread to your upper abdomen, causing a buildup of fluid, a condition known as ascites.

A pelvic examination, a CA 125 blood test, and an ultrasound exam or computerized tomography (CT) scan may help to rule out ovarian cancer as the cause of your symptoms. These tests are discussed later in this chapter.

Screening for Ovarian Cancer

Screening for a disease or disorder involves looking for it before any signs or symptoms appear. Routine screening methods have been developed for several cancers, including mammograms for breast cancer, colonoscopy for colon cancer and the Pap test for cervical cancer. Screening helps save lives by detecting diseases in their early stages, when they're most curable. For example, since women have been getting Pap tests, deaths from cervical cancer have dropped dramatically.

So why don't doctors routinely screen for ovarian cancer? In a nutshell: Researchers haven't yet found a screening tool that's sensitive enough to detect ovarian cancer in its early stages and specific enough to distinguish ovarian cancer

GYNECOLOGIC CANCERS

from other, noncancerous conditions. Developing a good screening test for ovarian cancer is hampered by two key factors.

1. Ovarian cancer isn't very common. Compared with several other cancers, its incidence is relatively low. The more common a disease is, the more beneficial screening becomes. If a disease is uncommon, unless the test is 100 percent accurate — which no test to date is — it will identify more false-positives than true-positives. False-positives are test results that indicate cancer may be present when it really isn't. False-positives can cause needless worry and expense and the possibility of unnecessary surgery.

2. No precancerous (pre-malignant) stage of ovarian cancer has been identified. With colon cancer, for example, polyps are known to be precursors of cancer. If polyps are discovered during your colonoscopy exam, they can be removed and you'll be monitored more closely. Another example is precancerous changes in the cells of the cervix that can be detected by a Pap test. The changes are an indicator of possible cancer. For ovarian cancer, there's no recognizable indicator that the cancer may be developing.

Ongoing efforts

Of those screening methods that have been tested or are in use on a limited basis, a major flaw is that they produce too many false-positives. In addition, the tests miss many early cancers. Such results are called false-negatives.

CA 125

One screening tool that has been studied is a blood test that measures the level of a circulating protein called CA 125. This protein is produced by a variety of cells, including most ovarian cancer cells, especially in their later stages. Most healthy women have CA 125 levels below 35 units per milliliter of blood. In women with ovarian cancer, the level is often, but not always, elevated.

However, measuring a woman's CA 125 level isn't a reliable screening tool for ovarian cancer, for a couple of reasons:

• Only about 50 percent of women with stage I ovarian cancer have elevated CA 125 levels. That means the test misses about half the early-stage cancers.

• Several other benign and malignant conditions also can cause elevated CA 125 levels. Among them are nonovarian cancers and noncancerous (benign) conditions such as endometriosis, ovarian cysts, menstruation, pregnancy and pelvic inflammatory disease. Thus, CA 125 screening can produce false-positives, indicating cancer when it isn't present. This often leads to unnecessary worry and diagnostic surgery.

For a woman at high risk of ovarian cancer or for someone who's experiencing signs or symptoms of the disease, a doctor may recommend a CA 125 test. But the test isn't sensitive or specific enough to be used routinely for the general public.

Pelvic ultrasound

Another example is ultrasound (sonography or ultrasonography), which uses high-frequency sound waves to produce images of the inside of the body. Although

Q: **What about the Pap test? Can't it detect ovarian cancer?**

A: The Pap test is a screening test to identify cancer of the cervix (cervical cancer). During the test, a sample of cells from the cervix is removed by gently scraping the cervix with a small spatula, brush or cotton swab. The sample is then sent to a laboratory, where it's examined under a microscope to look for cell abnormalities. Because the cells that give rise to ovarian cancer typically aren't found in the cervix, the Pap test isn't an acceptable tool for diagnosing ovarian cancer.

pelvic ultrasound can help find an ovarian mass, it doesn't accurately determine whether the mass is benign or malignant. This is a real problem because benign ovarian cysts are common. This limits the test's effectiveness as a screening tool.

Recommendations

Because of the limitations of screening tests for ovarian cancer, the National Institutes of Health doesn't recommend screening for ovarian cancer among women without known risk factors for the disease.

Experts do recommend, though, that all women have a regular pelvic exam. Occasionally, an ovarian mass can be felt on such an examination, although if it's detected this way, the cancer may already be advanced. Even though pelvic exams aren't generally useful for early detection of ovarian cancer, they're important to have because cancer in the uterus, cervix or vagina may be discovered at earlier stages. It's recommended that women begin having regular pelvic exams at approximately age 18. Women who've had their uterus removed but still have

their ovaries should continue to have pelvic exams.

Screening women at high risk

Routine screening for ovarian cancer is done only for women who are at high risk of the disease. This is the recommendation of an expert panel of the National Institutes of Health that reviewed all the studies on ovarian cancer screening.

Women at high risk include those who carry breast cancer gene (BRCA) mutations or have a significant family history of ovarian or breast cancer, such as two or more family members with ovarian cancer. Even for this group, there's no good evidence that screening saves lives, but it's the best option available for finding ovarian cancer early, when the chance of a cure is greatest.

For women at high risk of ovarian cancer, several procedures are used to help detect the disease. Doctors recommend that a woman at high risk have a pelvic exam, a CA 125 blood test and ultrasound twice a year beginning at age 30 and continuing for the rest of her life, or until she has her ovaries removed. Depending on

Pelvic exam

You lie on an examining table with your knees bent and your heels in metal supports (stirrups). After examining your external genitals, your doctor performs the following:

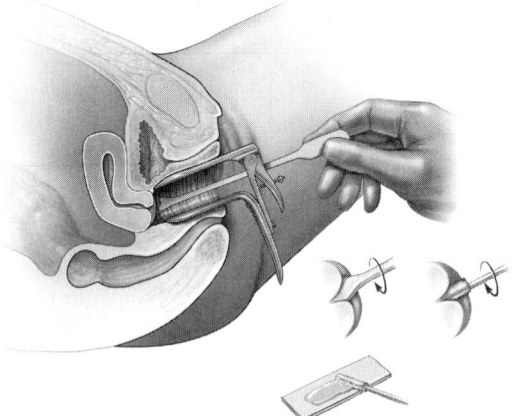

Pap test

To see the inner walls of your vagina and cervix, your doctor inserts into the vagina an instrument called a speculum. When in the open position, the speculum holds the vaginal walls apart so that the cervix can be seen. Your doctor then shines a light inside to look at the walls of the vagina for lesions, inflammation, abnormal discharge and anything else that's unusual. During a Pap test — which is generally included in a pelvic exam — a sample of cells is taken from your cervix.

Vaginal exam

To check the condition of your uterus and ovaries, your doctor inserts two lubricated, gloved fingers into the vagina and presses down on your abdomen with the other hand. This allows your doctor to locate your uterus, ovaries and other organs, judge their size and confirm that they're in the proper position. While exploring the contours of these organs and the pelvis, your doctor feels for any lumps or changes that may signal a problem.

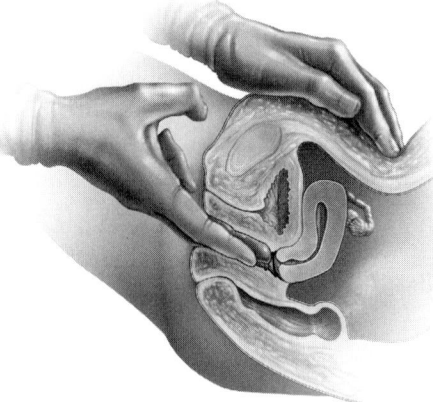

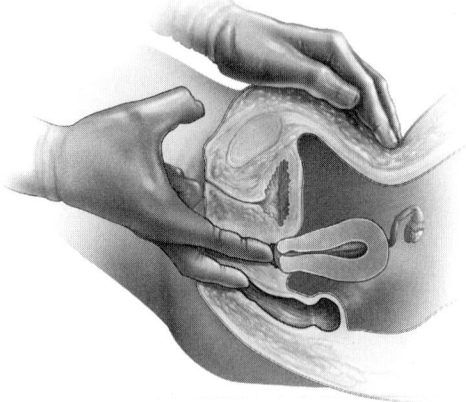

Rectovaginal exam

A rectovaginal exam checks the same organs as the vaginal exam, but from a different angle. For this exam, your doctor inserts one finger into your rectum while another remains in your vagina.

the results of the tests and a woman's individual circumstances, other tests also may be recommended.

Pelvic examination

During a pelvic examination, a doctor examines your vagina, uterus, rectum and pelvis, including the ovaries, for masses or growths (see the opposite page). A pelvic exam can be done by your gynecologist or primary care doctor.

CA 125 blood test

Though not recommended as a general screening tool, in a woman at high risk of ovarian cancer, a doctor may use the CA 125 blood test (see page 294).

Ultrasound

Ultrasound can detect ovarian growths, such as a tumor or cyst. In transabdominal ultrasound, a transducer is slowly moved over the abdomen to look for a suspicious mass. In transvaginal ultrasound, a transducer about the size of a tampon is inserted in the vagina. To examine the ovaries, most doctors prefer to use transvaginal ultrasound because the probe can be placed closer to the ovaries, and it produces a better image than does transabdominal ultrasound.

In women at high risk, ultrasound is a safe, noninvasive way to evaluate the size, shape and configuration of the ovaries. But if a mass is found, ultrasound can't reliably differentiate a cancerous growth from one that's not cancerous.

Color-Doppler imaging

A procedure called color-Doppler imaging (transvaginal color-flow Doppler) may be

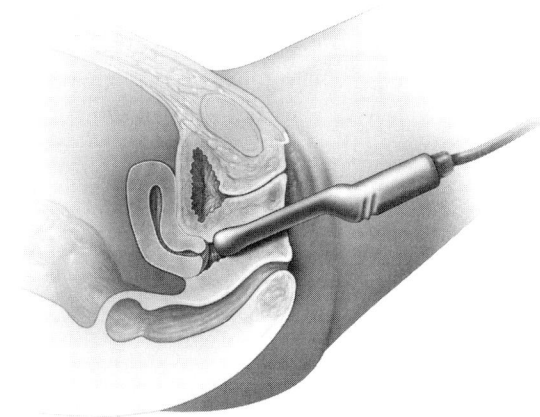

In transvaginal ultrasound, the ultrasound probe, which is about the size of a tampon, is inserted into the vagina. This method often allows for better views of the ovaries.

used in conjunction with ultrasound imaging to help determine whether an ovarian mass is cancerous. Benign ovarian cysts are nourished by normal blood vessels. Malignant tumors need new blood vessels to keep growing. These newly formed vessels don't behave like normal blood vessels — they're smaller and weaker and blood flow is often abnormal. Color-flow Doppler can detect changes that suggest new blood vessels and a cancerous tumor. However, this test is expensive and isn't completely accurate.

Other measures

Women at high risk of ovarian cancer are often advised to consider the following steps, in addition to regular screening:

- Seek genetic counseling to determine if you may have a hereditary form of the disease, which could be detected with BRCA testing.
- Consider participating in research studies (clinical trials) of new screening

approaches. One such study is the National Cancer Institute's National Ovarian Cancer Early Detection Program.

- Give consideration to surgery to remove the ovaries, a procedure called preventive (prophylactic) oophorectomy.

Combination screening

Sometimes, combining two screening approaches can improve results. Researchers are studying the combination of the CA 125 blood marker test and an ultrasound exam as a screening strategy for women at high risk of ovarian cancer. The hope is that the combination may result in fewer false-positives than are found with either of the methods alone.

One ongoing clinical trial designed for women at high risk of ovarian cancer compares a combination screening strategy of CA 125 testing and ultrasound with preventive oophorectomy. In this study, participants choose which approach they want to follow. The study will assess the effectiveness of the screening combination

Can Screening Save Lives?

Although it may seem obvious that screening for a cancer would automatically save lives, research finds that for some conditions screening has little effect on disease outcomes. In the case of ovarian cancer, two large, long-term studies are currently under way to try to determine if screening can alter this disease's deadly grasp.

The National Cancer Institute is sponsoring the Prostate, Lung, Colorectal and Ovarian Cancer Screening Trial. Starting in 1992, more than 154,000 men and women joined the study through 10 centers across the United States. At the start of the trial, participants were between the ages of 55 and 74, didn't have any of the cancers for which the trial is screening and weren't receiving treatment for any other cancer. Participants were divided randomly into two groups: those who would receive routine health care from a primary care doctor and those to be screened. In the screening group, upon entry into the trial women had both a CA 125 blood test and transvaginal ultrasound to screen for ovarian cancer. The ultrasound is repeated annually for three years, and the blood test is repeated annually for five years. Participants will undergo exams for six years and then be followed for 10 years after that.

In 2001, in Great Britain, the United Kingdom Collaborative Trial of Ovarian Cancer Screening began recruiting 200,000 postmenopausal women between the ages of 50 and 74 who are at average risk of ovarian cancer. Some women are receiving CA 125 and transvaginal ultrasound screening, others are receiving ultrasound screening alone, and the remainder aren't being screened at all. The study is expected to take 10 years to complete.

in reducing deaths from ovarian cancer, compared with the effectiveness of risk-reducing surgery. In the screening group, the CA 125 test is repeated every three months and transvaginal ultrasound is given once a year. If screening tests are abnormal, ultrasound is repeated. The trial plans to include 3,400 women.

Making a Diagnosis

If you have signs or symptoms suggestive of ovarian cancer or if your doctor discovers an ovarian mass during a routine pelvic exam, the next step is to determine if cancer is present. Keep in mind that of the thousands of women hospitalized yearly in the United States for ovarian growths, the majority don't have cancer.

If it turns out that the tumor is cancerous, it's important to know the type of cancer and whether it has spread beyond the ovaries.

Diagnosing ovarian cancer generally involves several steps. If your pelvic examination or other tests suggest possible ovarian cancer, you'll need to talk to a doctor or surgeon who specializes in treating women with this type of cancer. A gynecologic oncologist is a gynecologist who's specially trained in treating cancers of the female reproductive system.

Medical history and examination

Your doctor will likely ask you about any signs and symptoms that you're experiencing. Other questions may relate to your general health and your risk of ovarian cancer, including whether other people in your family have had ovarian cancer or breast cancer. A physical exam is usually next. In addition to the screening and diagnostic measures already discussed — pelvic exam, ultrasound and CA 125 blood test — your doctor may perform one of the following:

Computerized tomography
A computerized tomography (CT) scan uses X-ray images and computer technology to produce multiple, detailed, cross-sectional views of the part of your body being scanned. A CT scanner takes many pictures from different angles as it rotates around you. Sometimes a dye (contrast agent) is injected into your veins so that your organs show up more clearly on the X-rays. You may be asked to drink a liquid that temporarily stays in your stomach and intestines, enabling your doctor to differentiate these organs from abnormal tissue. CT scans can provide information about the size, shape and position of a tumor and identify enlarged lymph nodes, which might indicate if the cancer has spread. They can also identify the presence of a buildup of fluid in the abdominal cavity (ascites).

Magnetic resonance imaging
Magnetic resonance imaging (MRI) uses magnetic fields and radio waves to generate multiple cross-sectional images of the inside of the body, such as the pelvis and abdominal organs. For this test, you're placed on a motorized table that's moved into the tunnel (cylinder) of the scanner. The scanner houses a powerful magnet that surrounds the cylinder. When atoms in your body are exposed to a very strong

GYNECOLOGIC CANCERS

magnetic field, they line up with one another. The radio waves briefly knock the atoms out of alignment. As they realign, the atoms emit tiny signals that are picked up and passed on to a computer. The computer converts these signals into an image. An MRI scan can help identify a potentially cancerous tumor and its spread.

X-rays

Your doctor may also order a chest X-ray to determine if the cancer has spread to the lungs or to the pleural space surrounding the lungs where fluid can accumulate, a condition called pleural effusion. If fluid is present, a needle may be inserted into the space to remove it (tho-

racentesis). The fluid is then checked in the laboratory for cancer cells.

Positron emission tomography

A positron emission tomography (PET) scan is different from a CT or MRI scan in that it records tissue activity rather than tissue structure. Cancer cells often exhibit more metabolic activity than do normal cells. During a PET scan, your doctor injects into your body a small amount of a radioactive tracer — typically a form of blood sugar (glucose). All the tissues in your body absorb some of this tracer, but tissues that are using more energy — exhibiting increased metabolic activity — absorb greater amounts. Tumors are usually more metabolically active and tend to

The Search for a Better Marker

In an effort to improve the cure rate for ovarian cancer, researchers are looking for new ways to detect the disease earlier, before it has spread beyond the ovaries. This research includes finding substances in blood that signal the presence of ovarian cancer. These substances are called blood markers, or biomarkers. Discovering such a marker for ovarian cancer could make it possible to use a simple blood test as a screening tool for the disease.

Several studies are being conducted in hopes of finding more specific and sensitive markers. Some promising possibilities include:

- **Lysophosphatidic acid.** This substance, found in blood, may prove to be a more sensitive marker for ovarian cancer than is CA 125. In one study, lysophosphatidic acid (LPA) levels were elevated in all women with advanced ovarian cancer, in all women with recurrent ovarian cancer and in nine of 10 women with stage I ovarian cancer.
- **Protein patterns.** Among the most exciting recent discoveries is that a simple blood test may be able to detect protein patterns (proteomics) in blood that identify ovarian cancer, even in its early stages. These proteins may be produced by the tumor itself or may reflect the body's response to an early tumor. In an initial study, researchers were able to distinguish blood protein

absorb more of the sugar tracer, which allows the tumors to light up on the scan.

Use of PET scans in the diagnosis of ovarian cancer is still experimental.

Surgery

If your signs and symptoms, physical exam and test results indicate that you might have ovarian cancer, you'll need surgery to confirm the diagnosis and treat the cancer. The only way to know for certain if a woman has ovarian cancer is to remove samples of tissue from suspicious areas and have them examined under a microscope. This is known as a biopsy.

For many cancers, a biopsy is done before surgery. But for an ovarian tumor,

surgery is necessary to obtain tissue samples because the ovaries lie deep in the pelvis, and it's difficult to obtain tissue from them using a needle biopsy.

In addition, surgery serves not only to establish a diagnosis of ovarian cancer but to determine the extent of the cancer and to treat it by removing as much of it as possible. This is all done in the same surgical procedure, called a laparotomy.

What's involved?

For a laparotomy, you're placed under general anesthesia. Once the anesthesia takes effect, the surgeon makes a vertical incision from the bellybutton to the pubic area. If cancer is present, the incision will likely need to be extended above the

patterns in women with ovarian cancer from those in women with noncancerous disorders. The test used an artificial intelligence computer program to sort through thousands of proteins found in blood to detect key patterns. The research still needs to be confirmed by other studies. The Food and Drug Administration and the National Cancer Institute, sponsors of the study, believe that proteomics might be applicable to other diseases as well.

- **Osteopontin.** Early research results indicate that blood levels of the protein osteopontin appear to be significantly higher in women with ovarian cancer than they are in healthy women. However, osteopontin isn't specific to ovarian cancer. Elevated levels have been documented in several cancers. In

women with ovarian cancer, osteopontin levels appear to rise before CA 125 levels, suggesting that this could be a promising blood marker for early detection.

- **Macrophage colony-stimulating factor.** This is another substance found in blood. Macrophage colony-stimulating factor may prove to be a valuable indicator of ovarian cancer when used in combination with CA 125.

Although these and other potential screening biomarkers appear promising, the studies so far have been small, and the results need to be validated by other, larger studies. Nevertheless, the research offers hope that in the future we will be able to identify ovarian cancer earlier in more women.

GYNECOLOGIC CANCERS

bellybutton to allow access to upper abdominal structures.

Generally, the surgeon first examines the abdominal cavity for signs of cancer, looking for excess fluid or growths on other organs. He or she collects samples of abdominal fluid, which are analyzed for the presence of cancer cells. If no free-floating fluid is present, samples are gathered by instilling a small volume of fluid to wash over the area and then removing the fluid. The samples are sent to a pathologist, a specialist in diagnosing disease in tissue samples, for examination.

Often, the next step is removal of an ovary for examination by a pathologist. If cancer is present in the removed material, the surgeon continues with the staging process to determine if and how far the cancer has spread. He or she takes small amounts of tissue from various sites within the abdomen. Lymph nodes in the pelvis or near the aorta may be removed. If the samples confirm cancer is present, several other procedures may be done.

Removal of the ovaries, fallopian tubes, uterus, omentum and any visible cancerous tissue is the primary treatment for ovarian cancer. This surgery is discussed in more detail in Chapter 17.

Staging

Based on the results of your surgery and laboratory tests, your doctor or team of doctors gathers all the information needed to classify the stage of your cancer.

Ovarian cancer spread

Ovarian cancer typically spreads when the tumor sheds cancerous (malignant) cells into the abdominal cavity (seeding). These cells can then implant in the lining of the abdominal cavity (peritoneum) or on the surface of other organs. Ovarian cancer may also spread to lymph nodes in the groin and pelvic area, or near the aorta, or travel to other parts of the body by way of the bloodstream.

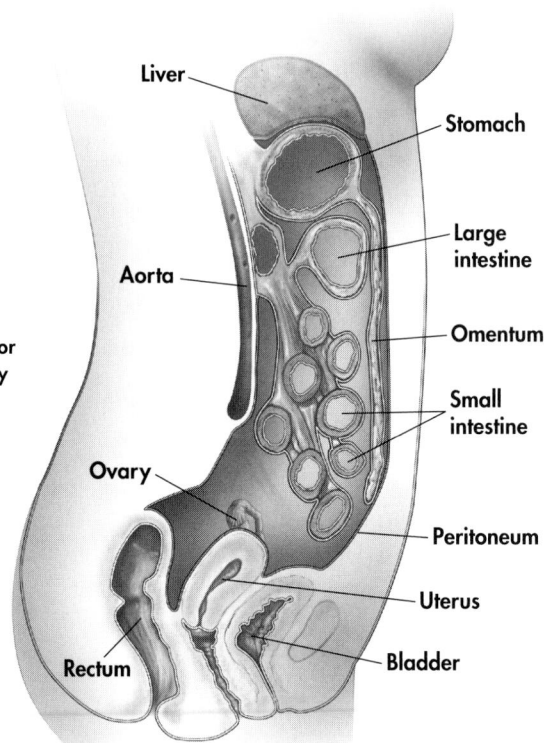

Staging is a key factor in determining prognosis and treatment.

The system that's most commonly used to stage ovarian cancer comes from the International Federation of Gynecology and Obstetrics. It's called the FIGO system.

With the FIGO system, which is similar to other staging systems, a lower number indicates that the cancer is still in an early stage, and a higher number reflects a more advanced stage with extensive cancer spread.

Stage I

Stage I cancer is confined within the ovary or ovaries.

Stage IA

The cancer is contained within one ovary.

Stage IB

The cancer is in both ovaries but confined within them.

Stage IC

The cancer is in one or both ovaries and one or more of the following conditions apply:

- Cancer has been found on the surface of at least one ovary.
- A fluid-filled (cystic) tumor has burst.
- Cancer cells have been found in fluid from the abdominal cavity.

Stage II

In stage II ovarian cancer, the cancer has spread from one or both ovaries to another organ in the pelvis. This may include the uterus, fallopian tubes, bladder or rectum.

Stage IIA

The cancer has spread to or invaded the uterus, fallopian tubes or both. Cancer cells aren't seen in abdominal fluid.

Stage IIB

The cancer has spread to at least one other pelvic organ, such as the bladder or rectum, with no cancer cells found in the abdominal fluid.

Stage IIC

The cancer has spread to at least one other pelvic organ, and one or more of the conditions listed in stage IC are present.

Stage III

The cancer is in one or both ovaries and has spread beyond the pelvis to the upper abdomen or to the lymph nodes.

Stage IIIA

The surgeon saw no visible cancer outside the pelvis during surgery, but the pathologist finds small, microscopic deposits of cancer in the lining of the upper abdomen (peritoneum). The cancer hasn't spread to the lymph nodes.

Stage IIIB

The surgeon can see cancer deposits outside the pelvis, but they're smaller than 2 centimeters (cm), which is about ¾ inch. There's no spread to the lymph nodes.

Stage IIIC

The cancer has spread to the lymph nodes, or the surgeon can see deposits of cancer in the abdomen larger than 2 cm. A tumor may be on the surface of — but not inside — the liver or spleen.

diagnosis of ovarian cancer, the better her prognosis. According to a 2003 report by the American Cancer Society, women younger than age 65 are about twice as likely as are women older than age 65 to survive five years after a diagnosis of ovarian cancer.

- **Extent of residual disease.** During surgery, the surgeon makes every attempt to remove as much of the cancer as possible. The less cancer that's left, the greater the likelihood of a complete response to chemotherapy and the better the prognosis. For these reasons, it's important that the procedure be performed by a gynecologic oncologist, a specialist trained in these operations.

Survival statistics

When ovarian cancer is detected and treated before it spreads beyond the ovaries, the five-year survival rate is good, ranging from 75 percent to 90 percent, depending on the tumor grade. However, because ovarian cancer is only detected early about 24 percent of the time, just a small group of women receive such a good prognosis. The overall five-year survival rate for all stages of ovarian cancer is 53 percent.

Survival statistics can be frightening. Remember, though, that statistics don't tell the whole story. They only provide a general picture and a standard way for doctors to discuss prognosis. Every woman's situation is unique.

If you have questions about your own prognosis, discuss them with your doctor or other members of your health care team. They can help you determine

5-year survival rates for ovarian cancer

Stage	Percentage diagnosed	5-year survival rate
Stage I	24%	75%-90%
Stage II	6%	65%
Stage III	55%	15%-30%
Stage IV	15%	Less than 15%
Overall	100%	53%

Source: American Cancer Society

how these statistics relate, or don't relate, to you.

Even if the numbers don't appear to be in your favor, remember that steps can be taken to try to control the cancer. At any stage, treatment options are available. You likely will want to take an active role with your doctors in making choices about your treatment.

Pat's Story

Pat Goldman considers herself a child of the women's movement. Fittingly, her own life provides a striking illustration of the feminist maxim "The personal is political." Pat transformed her personal experience with ovarian cancer into a national effort to increase awareness of and attention to this previously silent disease.

A former airline executive, Pat was the founding president of the Ovarian Cancer National Alliance (OCNA). The organization was launched in 1997 to bring ovarian cancer issues to national political and health care agendas. Today, Pat is president emeritus of OCNA.

Pat's journey from survivor to activist began in 1992, when she was 50 years old. In November of that year, she saw a gynecologist because she had had some breakthrough spotting between her regular periods. The doctor did an endometrial biopsy, which found nothing, and an ultrasound, which revealed gallstones. The doctor told her that everything seemed to be fine and recommended regular checkups.

Early the following year, Pat got a call from a resident at the hospital where she had had the ultrasound. The resident had seen Pat's ultrasound and suspected that she might have adenomyosis, a noncancerous (benign) thickening of the outside of the uterus. Pat was offered a free magnetic resonance imaging scan as part of a study the resident was conducting on diagnosing adenomyosis.

Pat had the test, and the resident confirmed that she had the condition. "I was not the aggressive or informed consumer prior to my ovarian cancer diagnosis that I am today," she reflects. "When the resident said that was what I had, I accepted it, never asked for a written report or copy of the pictures. With today's knowledge, I certainly wouldn't have accepted a phone diagnosis. I would have insisted on seeing her, the records and my gynecologist for a follow-up."

Pat was told she may need a hysterectomy, but it wasn't urgent. Over the next few months, she experienced more discomfort. "I'd roll over in bed and feel a twinge," she recalls. "In the car, driving over bumps made my stomach hurt." She went up two

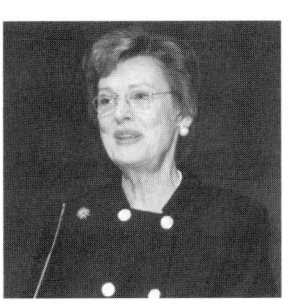

Pat Goldman speaking at a meeting of the Ovarian Cancer National Alliance, the ovarian cancer awareness organization she helped establish.

dress sizes and could no longer fit into her pants because she was so bloated.

By early July, Pat was so uncomfortable that she could barely eat. She went back to her regular doctor and had another ultrasound. This time it showed a mass. She was referred to a gynecologic oncologist. Pat had surgery and was diagnosed with stage IIA ovarian cancer.

"I was devastated … because the only thing I knew was that Gilda Radner had it, and she died," Pat says. "First you expect you're going to die, then you have to figure out how to live."

That wasn't easy at first. After she finished her treatment in 1994, she kept expecting to have a recurrence, even though her surgeon told her that her relatively early stage at diagnosis improved her odds. Pat even postponed needed hernia surgery, figuring she was going to have another operation for cancer anyway, so she could take care of everything at once.

Meanwhile, she began educating herself about ovarian cancer. She read a lot and looked for a support group. To her disappointment, she couldn't find one. She told a friend involved with a breast cancer organization, who said, "You can't do this alone. You're going to have to find others."

Gradually, Pat connected with other ovarian cancer survivors. In 1997, Pat and a few other women in the Washington, D.C., area put a notice in the *Washington Post* announcing a meeting on ovarian cancer advocacy. To their surprise, 30 people showed up. They formed a group called the

GYNECOLOGIC CANCERS

Ovarian Cancer Coalition of Greater Washington.

From there, Pat, representing the Washington group, and leaders from six other organizations established the Ovarian Cancer National Alliance. From the beginning, OCNA's foremost goal has been to raise awareness of ovarian cancer among the public, physicians and policymakers. As Pat's experience demonstrates, ovarian cancer often goes undetected or misdiagnosed at an early stage. Alliance members have worked to promote earlier detection. The group's slogan has been, "Until there's a test, awareness is best."

Pat and other alliance members are eagerly awaiting the development of an ovarian cancer screening test that's based on the study of patterns of proteins in human blood or other tissues (proteomics). Such a test will soon enter clinical trials (see "Genomics and proteomics," page 31).

"The situation is a lot better than it was 10 years ago," Pat says, noting that better therapies and increased understanding of ovarian cancer signs and symptoms have resulted in improved survival. "But we still have a long way to go in increasing awareness among general physicians."

For Pat, having ovarian cancer has brought the gift of meeting many wonderful women. She encourages other women with ovarian cancer to make contact with others in the same situation. And these days, thanks to OCNA and other organizations, ovarian cancer support and advocacy groups exist throughout the country.

However, the gift of new friendships has also brought sadness. "The hardest part of the whole experience has been losing so many friends," Pat says. "As I say when I'm doing public speaking, it's a lousy way to make good friends."

She stays optimistic, though. Not only has she remained cancer-free, but she notes that more and more women are living far beyond the five-year survival mark. "Even with advanced cancer, you can get good therapies and have many more years of life," she says. "It's really important to have a sense of hope."

Chapter 17: Gynecologic Cancers

Treating Ovarian Cancer

With ovarian cancer, surgery plays a central role both in diagnosis of the disease and its treatment. For most women, treatment of ovarian cancer involves surgery followed by chemotherapy. For some women, radiation therapy may be an option. More often, though, radiation is used in the management of recurrent disease, as discussed in Chapter 18.

This chapter details treatment for newly diagnosed ovarian cancer. It focuses on the most common form, epithelial cancer. Treatment of germ cell and sex cord-stromal cancers are discussed in Chapter 19.

Early vs. Advanced Disease

As with most cancers, the prognosis and treatment of ovarian cancer depend on how far the cancer has spread, what's known as its stage. The information gained during surgical staging is crucial in helping to determine your prognosis and whether you'll need additional (adjuvant) therapy after the operation.

For early-stage ovarian cancer, depending on the tumor grade — that is, how aggressive the cancer appears under a microscope — surgery alone may be adequate. This is only the case when a thorough surgical staging procedure and the results of multiple biopsies indicate no cancer spread. If a surgeon simply looks in the abdomen and feels the organs without taking multiple biopsies, the staging is considered insufficient because about 40 percent of the time the surgeon will miss cancer that has spread.

For advanced ovarian cancer, the standard treatment is surgery to remove as much of the cancer as possible and follow-up chemotherapy. Because only about 25 percent of ovarian cancers are diag-

nosed at an early stage, most women with the disease receive chemotherapy. In cases of advanced ovarian cancer, studies have consistently shown that women who have as much of the cancer removed as possible — leaving only minute amounts of the cancer remaining — have a better probable outcome (prognosis) than do women in which larger amounts of cancer remain.

This chapter describes the general guidelines for treatment of ovarian cancer based on cancer stage. Keep in mind, though, that not all cancers of the same stage have the same prognosis. Other factors related to the tumor also influence whether the outlook is favorable and what treatments should be considered. For example, tumors that are low-grade (well differentiated), that is, the cells are more normal looking, have a better prognosis than do high-grade (poorly differen-

Selecting Your Surgeon

One of the most important decisions that needs to be made before surgery to diagnose and treat ovarian cancer is who will be performing the operation.

Surgery for ovarian cancer is extensive and complex, requiring a high level of specialized skill. Accurately determining how far the cancer has spread (staging) and removing as much of the cancer as possible are crucial to the effectiveness of follow-up treatment and long-term survival.

The specialist with the necessary skills and experience to perform this task is a gynecologic oncologist, a surgeon who

specializes in the care and treatment of women with cancers of the reproductive tract.

The best surgery is key to the best outcome. A 1999 study found that women whose surgery was performed by a gynecologic oncologist had a significant survival advantage. Women with ovarian cancer who were treated by gynecologic oncologists had 25 percent fewer deaths than did women with ovarian cancer who were treated by other surgeons.

If you've been told that you may have ovarian cancer or another type of gynecologic cancer, ask for a referral to a gynecologic oncologist.

Understanding Your Treatment Options

It's important to understand your treatment options before you have your initial surgery. Take time to consider treatment recommendations without feeling rushed, and make sure you get the opinion of a gynecologic oncologist.

If you don't understand something, ask. You're likely to have many questions and concerns about your treatment options. Most women want to know how they'll function after treatment and whether they'll have to change their normal activities.

Some questions you might have about treatment include:

- What is the standard treatment for my situation?
- Are there other options?
- What are the side effects of the treatment?
- Are there new treatments or clinical trials that I should consider?
- How will we know if the treatment is working?
- What are my chances of being cured?
- How will this treatment affect my daily life?
- What are the chances that the tumor will come back?

Taking an active role may give you a greater sense of control and peace of mind. This can help with your recovery and quality of life.

tiated) tumors. Other factors associated with a less favorable prognosis in early-stage disease include a tumor growing on the outside of the ovary, cancerous cells found in fluid within the abdominal cavity and rupture of the tumor contents into the abdominal cavity.

In determining your treatment regimen, your doctor or team of doctors considers a number of factors, including cancer stage, tumor grade, your general health, and your personal views and wishes.

Stage I

In stage I disease, the cancer is confined to one or both ovaries (see the color illustration on page 265). The standard surgical approach for stage I ovarian cancer is to remove both ovaries, both fallopian tubes, the uterus, pelvic and para-aortic lymph nodes, and the fatty layer of tissue in front of the abdomen (omentum). Cancer cells can collect in the omentum. In addition, the surgeon performs multiple biopsies throughout the abdominal cavity to check for cancer spread.

Younger women with stage IA tumors that are low-grade may want to preserve their ability to have children. In such situations, the surgeon may be able to remove just the cancerous ovary and its fallopian tube and leave the other ovary or just the uterus in place. However, this type of situation is rare (see "Fertility and ovarian cancer treatment" on page 316).

Whether chemotherapy is recommended after surgery is based on a number of

GYNECOLOGIC CANCERS

Surgery-Speak

The medical terms for the surgical procedures used to treat gynecologic cancers stem from the Greek and Latin names of the organs that are removed. The medical name for an operation that removes something usually ends with *ectomy*, which is from the Greek word for "excision." Medical terminology used in relation to ovarian cancer surgery includes:

- **Bilateral oophorectomy.** Removal of both ovaries
- **Bilateral salpingo-oophorectomy.** Removal of both ovaries and fallopian tubes
- **Cytoreduction.** Removal of as much cancer as possible (debulking)
- **Laparotomy.** The abdominal surgery used most often to diagnose and treat ovarian cancer
- **Lymphadenectomy.** Removal of the lymph nodes (lymph node dissection)
- **Omentectomy.** Removal of the fatty layer of tissue in the front of the abdomen (omentum)
- **Salpingectomy.** Removal of one (unilateral) or both (bilateral) fallopian tubes
- **Total abdominal hysterectomy.** Removal of the uterus and the cervix
- **Unilateral oophorectomy.** Removal of one ovary

factors, especially the grade of the cancer. The higher the grade, the greater the likelihood chemotherapy will be used.

Stage II

In stage II disease, the cancer has spread from the ovaries to one or more adjacent pelvic structures, including the fallopian tubes, uterus and pelvic wall.

Treatment for stage II ovarian cancer includes surgery to remove both ovaries, both fallopian tubes, the uterus, pelvic and para-aortic lymph nodes, and the omentum. If the surgeon sees deposits of cancer, he or she will attempt to remove as much of the cancer as possible during an often lengthy process called debulking (cytoreduction).

Chemotherapy is recommended after surgery for stage II cancer.

Stage III

In stage III disease, the cancer has spread to the upper abdomen or nearby lymph nodes. Treatment for stage III cancer includes surgery to remove both ovaries, both fallopian tubes, the uterus, pelvic and para-aortic lymph nodes, and the omentum. The surgeon also removes as much of the remaining cancer as possible. Chemotherapy is recommended after surgery. Occasionally, doctors advocate a second surgery after chemotherapy (second-look surgery), to evaluate the effect of the treatment, but this is a matter of debate (see page 322).

Stage IV

In stage IV disease, the cancer has spread to structures outside the abdomen —

most commonly, the pleural space around a lung — or into the interior of the liver or spleen. Treatment for stage IV disease usually involves surgery to remove as much of the cancer as possible followed by chemotherapy.

Surgery

The most common surgery for simultaneously diagnosing and treating ovarian cancer is laparotomy. During this procedure, a surgeon is able to:

- Confirm that cancer is present
- Determine how far the cancer has spread (stage the cancer)
- Remove the primary tumor as well as cancer that may have spread to adjacent tissues (debulk the cancer)

In certain cases, a less invasive surgical procedure called laparoscopy may be used. Laparoscopy requires only a couple of small incisions, through which a lighted instrument and other small cutting tools are inserted to perform the surgery. Laparoscopy may be used if a surgeon wants to remove a tissue mass to determine whether it's cancerous before proceeding with more invasive surgery. The potential role of laparoscopy in staging ovarian cancer hasn't been adequately evaluated. Additional research about its effectiveness and safety for the management of ovarian cancer is needed before it can be used more commonly.

What's involved?

The extent of your surgery will depend on whether the cancer has spread and how

far. More often than not, a surgeon doesn't know precisely what needs to be done until he or she is in surgery and can see and evaluate the situation.

It's important to have all the possible surgical scenarios explained to you before your surgery. Have a member of your surgical team describe the planned operation and explain the goals, risks and possible outcomes. He or she should also tell you how successful the surgery is expected to be and the side effects that some women experience after the operation. You may have a number of questions. Don't hesitate to ask them.

Before surgery

Preparation for a laparotomy is similar to that for many surgeries performed under general anesthesia. Your surgeon will review your medical history and look for medical conditions that may affect the surgical outcome. You'll likely be given a laxative to clean out your bowels. Tests such as a complete blood count or chest X-ray may be done to assess the general state of your health. If you have a medical condition such as diabetes or high blood pressure, your doctor will want to make sure that your condition is stable enough for you to undergo surgery.

Your anesthesiologist will likely visit with you to explain how the anesthesia will be administered and determine whether you have any conditions that will affect your reaction to the medications that will be used. Just before your surgery, you'll receive — either through a mask, intravenously or both — medications that render you unconscious, serve as painkillers and relax your muscles.

GYNECOLOGIC CANCERS

During surgery

Once you're unconscious, the surgeon will make a vertical incision that begins above your bellybutton and runs down the center of your abdomen to just above the pubic bone. This large incision allows the surgeon to view abdominal and pelvic structures, including the ovaries and the tissue and organs surrounding them and the upper abdomen. Depending on what your doctor finds, he or she may extend this incision to just below the rib cage.

Often, the first step is to remove samples of tissue and abdominal fluid, which are analyzed for the presence of cancer cells. Samples are taken from multiple sites inside the abdomen. If the samples confirm the diagnosis of ovarian cancer, several other procedures will be done, including removing the ovaries and other organs and removing as much of the cancer as possible (see the color illustration on page 270).

Based on the results of laboratory tests and the extent of the cancer spread, surgery will likely involve:

- Removing the uterus, including the cervix, as well as both ovaries and both fallopian tubes, a procedure called total abdominal hysterectomy with bilateral salpingo-oophorectomy.
- Removing the fatty tissue in front of the abdomen (omentum), a common site for ovarian cancer to spread.
- Removing adjacent lymph nodes for analysis.
- Removing visible cancer from adjacent tissues and organs (debulking).
- Relieving bowel obstructions, if any exist. Because ovarian cancer can spread widely throughout the abdominal cavity, essentially coating the surfaces of all structures, it commonly extends to the intestines, where it can interfere with bowel function.
- Removing the appendix and, occasionally, the spleen.

Removing deposits of ovarian cancer is a laborious process that may take many hours. The surgeon's goal is to remove as much visible cancer as possible, striving to leave no growth that measures more than 1 centimeter in diameter.

Women who have minimal tumor deposits remaining after surgery — that is, whose cancer is considered to be optimally debulked — generally experience longer survival than do women who have larger amounts of cancer remaining after surgery. This is why it's crucial to have a surgeon with experience in treating this type of cancer perform your operation.

After surgery

Once the surgery is complete, you'll be taken to a recovery area where staff will monitor your blood pressure, heart rate and breathing as you emerge from the anesthesia. You're likely to remain in the hospital for four or five days.

Ovarian cancer surgery involves not only anesthesia and the administration of strong pain medication but also extensive handling of your intestines. As a result, it slows down bowel function for a time. After surgery, a tube is threaded through one of your nostrils and your esophagus into your stomach to suction stomach contents for a few days until your bowels start to move again. You'll know your bowels are functioning when you're able to pass gas.

Survival based on cancer remaining after surgery

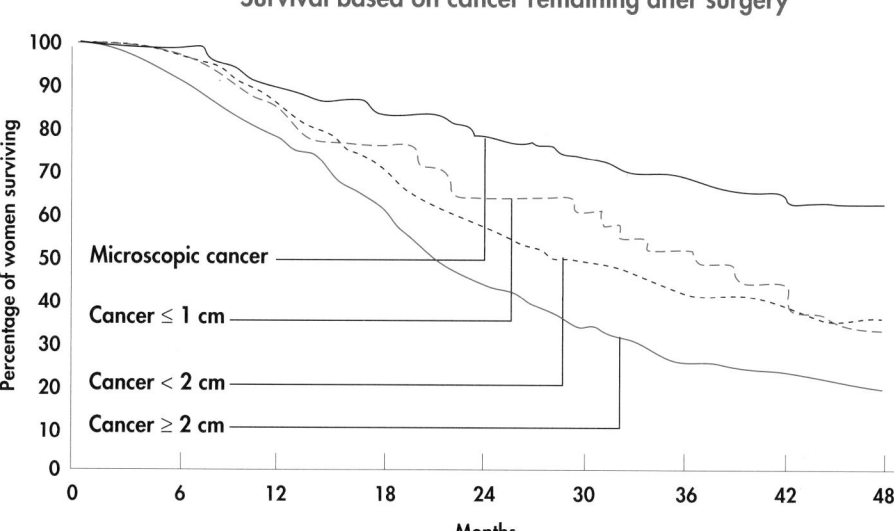

The quality and extent of surgery to treat ovarian cancer are key to the best outcome. This graph shows survival curves for women with ovarian cancer, based on the amount of cancer that remains after surgery (residual disease). There's a significant survival advantage for women who have no or only minimal (microscopic) cancer remaining after surgery. All of these women were treated with chemotherapy after surgery.

Source: Gynecologic Cancer Foundation, 2000

After surgery, some women experience urinary difficulties, such as frequent urination, limited bladder capacity and pain during urination. You may have a urinary catheter inserted temporarily to drain your bladder. You may also have ongoing trouble with constipation, requiring stool softeners and dietary changes. Some women who've had portions of their bowel removed experience just the opposite — diarrhea and occasional loss of control of their bowel movements.

You can expect to experience abdominal discomfort and vaginal discharge for a few weeks. You may also feel tired or weak for a while. If you were having menstrual periods before your surgery, removal of your ovaries and uterus will result in menopause, and you may experience signs and symptoms such as hot flashes, sleep disruption, sweating and vaginal dryness. Complications of surgery can include infection, bleeding, and injury to the bowel, rectum, bladder or ureter, and formation of blood clots in a leg.

Your doctor can prescribe medication to reduce pain after surgery and will work with you to manage other side effects you may experience, such as nausea and menopausal symptoms.

How long it takes to fully recover from surgery varies for each woman, but most women can resume their usual activities in four to six weeks. It's generally recommended that you not have sexual intercourse for six weeks after surgery.

Fertility and Ovarian Cancer Treatment

Most women with ovarian cancer are past menopause, so they're beyond the age of having children. However, the disease can also affect younger women.

Unfortunately, almost all the treatments for ovarian cancer take away a woman's ability to bear children. Surgery to remove the ovaries and uterus is standard practice in the treatment of ovarian cancer. This results in menopause and loss of the ability to get pregnant.

Depending on their tumor stage and grade, some younger women who want to preserve the option to have children may be able to have a more conservative surgery. If the cancer is confined to one ovary (stage IA) and it's low-grade, it may be possible to leave the other ovary and uterus in place.

In some cases, only the uterus can be preserved. Although normal fertilization is no longer possible, preserving the uterus gives a woman the option of using assistive reproductive technology to achieve pregnancy.

If you would like to have children, discuss this issue with your doctor before your surgery. Unfortunately, for the large majority of women with ovarian cancer, to cure or control the cancer it's necessary to remove both ovaries and the uterus.

Chemotherapy

For most stages of ovarian cancer, even if all the visible cancer is removed, it's likely that microscopic cancer cells remain after surgery. That's why for most women with ovarian cancer, doctors recommend chemotherapy after surgery. This is referred to as adjuvant chemotherapy.

The purpose of adjuvant chemotherapy is to kill any remaining cancer cells. Most often, chemotherapy involves not just one drug but a combination of two or more drugs. The medications attack cancer cells that have spread throughout your abdominal cavity or entered your bloodstream or lymphatic system and traveled to other parts of your body.

Sometimes, the cancer is so extensive that debulking surgery can't effectively remove the majority of the cancer. In those cases, chemotherapy may be recommended before debulking surgery, in an attempt to reduce the size of the tumor. The hope is that the drugs can shrink the cancer enough to improve chances of removing all or most of the cancer during a later surgery. This is known as neoadjuvant chemotherapy. It's sometimes used for women who can't tolerate extensive surgery or who are thought to have stage IV ovarian cancer, based on diagnostic tests and imaging.

Early-stage disease

An ongoing question has been whether all women with ovarian cancer might benefit from chemotherapy or if some women with early-stage disease can be cured with surgery alone. Not all stage I tumors are alike — some have features that are associated with a higher risk of recurrence. Tumors that are higher grade, of the clear cell type, or are on the external surface of the ovary all carry a higher risk. Several clinical trials have investigated which women with early-stage ovarian cancer might benefit from chemotherapy.

In early trials, women with stage I, low-grade cancer did very well with surgery alone. More than 90 percent survived for five years or more, indicating this group is unlikely to achieve much benefit from chemotherapy.

But what about women with early-stage disease who are at higher risk of recurrence? European investigators recently published the results of two randomized clinical trials. Both studies included women with high-risk, early-stage ovarian cancer and compared the effects of two postsurgical treatment options: chemotherapy and observation only. After five years, 74 percent of the women who had observation only were still alive, compared with 82 percent of the women who received chemotherapy after surgery.

A U.S. study of women with early-stage ovarian cancer at high risk of recurrence compared three cycles of the chemotherapy drugs cyclophosphamide and cisplatin with a certain type of internal radiation. Comparing the two treatment approaches, the likelihood of recurrence was slightly less in the chemotherapy group, but the difference was not statistically significant. There were some problems, though, with the delivery of radiation, including inadequate distribution and catheter problems.

Considering all of the data, most experts recommend chemotherapy for the majority of women with early-stage ovarian cancer with high-risk features.

Types of chemotherapy

More than 40 different chemotherapy drugs are used to treat cancer. These drugs work in different ways. For example, medications called alkylating agents form chemical bonds with DNA, the principal carrier of a cell's genetic information. When bound to DNA, these drugs prevent cells from dividing properly. Blocking cell division is most harmful to rapidly dividing cells, such as cancer cells. Another class of chemotherapy drugs, called antimetabolites, cause rapidly dividing cancer cells to create new DNA that's flawed and lethal to the cell.

Combining chemotherapy medications that work in different ways can have a greater effect against a tumor. In addition, this approach may decrease the chance that cancer cells will develop resistance to any one drug over time. Another advantage of combination chemotherapy is that the dosages used when combining two or more drugs may produce fewer or less severe side effects than would higher dosages of a single drug.

The types of chemotherapy medications most often used to treat ovarian cancer include the following:

- **Platinum complexes.** Platinum-based compounds, including cisplatin (Platinol) and carboplatin (Paraplatin), bind directly to DNA and RNA, interfering with normal function.
- **Mitotic inhibitors.** Mitotic inhibitors such as taxanes and vinca alkaloids disrupt cell division by interfering with the

cellular machinery that separates a dividing cell into two daughter cells. Examples are paclitaxel (Taxol) and docetaxel (Taxotere). Vinorelbine (Navelbine) is a vinca alkaloid.

- **Alkylating agents.** These medications interfere with the reproduction of cancer cells by forming direct chemical bonds with DNA, inhibiting its function. Examples include melphalan (Alkeran) and cyclophosphamide (Cytoxan, Neosar).

- **Antimetabolites.** Antimetabolites interfere with the synthesis of new DNA. Gemcitabine (Gemzar) is an antimetabolite used to treat ovarian cancer.
- **Anti-tumor antibiotics.** Different from antibiotics used to treat bacterial infections, these chemotherapy medications interfere with DNA and block RNA and key enzymes. One such drug is liposomal doxorubicin (Adriamycin).
- **DNA topoisomerase inhibitors.** These medications inhibit the enzyme topo-

Chemotherapy Breakthroughs

In looking for new chemotherapy medications, scientists screen natural and manufactured (synthetic) materials to see if they display anti-tumor properties. Substances that show potential in destroying cancer cells growing in laboratory cultures and then animal models are tested in clinical trials.

The most important chemotherapy drugs used today to treat ovarian cancer resulted from two key research breakthroughs — the discovery of the anticancer properties of the metal platinum and the discovery of a valuable compound in the bark of the Pacific yew tree.

Platinum

Platinum's anti-cancer properties were discovered by accident in 1965. Researchers were studying the effects of electricity on bacterial cell growth. In the

process, they found that the electrodes they were using — which were made of platinum — inhibited cell division in bacteria. This lead to further testing in which platinum was found to be highly lethal to cancer cells. Platinum is a highly reactive compound that binds directly to DNA and RNA. In so doing, it impairs the function of these molecules, essential for the function and division of rapidly growing cells.

In the late 1970s and early 1980s, the platinum drugs cisplatin and its synthetic look-alike, carboplatin, revolutionized the treatment of epithelial ovarian cancer. At the time, the alkylating agents melphalan (Alkeran) and cyclophosphamide (Cytoxan, Neosar) were the most effective drugs available. Cisplatin (Platinol), the first platinum drug to receive Food and Drug Administration approval, significantly improved response rates in ovarian cancer, and it practically doubled the average survival time.

A downside of cisplatin, though, is that it can cause a number of serious side

isomerase, which permits the uncoiling of DNA — a necessary step for DNA to be duplicated or read, to be made into RNA and proteins. Examples include etoposide (Etopophos, VePesid, VP-16) and topotecan (Hycamtin).

Developing a drug regimen

The initial chemotherapy regimen for ovarian cancer includes the combination of carboplatin and paclitaxel. Years of clinical trials have proved this combination to be the most effective, though studies continue to look for ways to improve on it. The two drugs act on cancer cells in different ways, and their potential side effects are different.

With the carboplatin-paclitaxel combination, around 80 percent of women whose cancer is newly diagnosed achieve at least a 50 percent reduction in tumor volume. Studies have also shown that the combination results in longer survival, effects, including hearing loss and kidney and peripheral nerve damage. Carboplatin (Paraplatin), a synthetic derivative of platinum, was developed in the 1980s. Carboplatin is considerably less toxic than cisplatin.

In addition to improving response rates and survival time for women with epithelial ovarian cancer, cisplatin also has revolutionized the treatment of germ cell tumors of the ovary and, in men, testicular cancer. Before cisplatin became available, only about 5 percent of individuals with ovarian germ cell tumors or testicular cancer survived long term. With cisplatin, 80 percent to 90 percent now experience long-term, disease-free survival.

Paclitaxel

The next major advance in ovarian cancer chemotherapy was the introduction of the drug paclitaxel (Taxol). In screening natural products, scientists found potent anti-cancer activity in the bark of the relatively rare and slow-growing Pacific yew tree. This was in 1971. But the production of what was to be paclitaxel was fraught with difficulties.

First, researchers had to determine which molecule within the crude extract from the tree bark was responsible for the anti-cancer activity. Then they had to overcome the problem of obtaining sufficient amounts of the drug. Initially, a single 300-milligram dose required the sacrifice of a 100-year-old tree. It took years before scientists could reliably manufacture paclitaxel in the laboratory. The synthetic drug was finally introduced in the mid-1990s, and supplies are now plentiful.

Paclitaxel, a type of medication known as a mitotic inhibitor, stops cell division in a unique way. It interferes with the process that separates duplicated DNA from one cell into two daughter cells. The medication belongs to the group of drugs known as taxanes.

compared with previously used chemotherapy drugs and combinations. The
outcome depends in large part on the
amount of cancer remaining after surgery.
The less cancer remaining after debulking
surgery, the fewer tumor cells there are
for chemotherapy to eradicate.

What's involved?

Chemotherapy for ovarian cancer is typically started one to four weeks after surgery. Most commonly, chemotherapy is
given in cycles — a schedule of regular
doses of the drugs, followed by a rest
period. Because chemotherapy targets
rapidly growing cells, it can also affect
normal cells that divide rapidly. Hair follicles, white blood cells and mucous membranes are especially vulnerable to the
drugs. Thus, your body needs time
between treatments to rest and produce
new, healthy cells.

For ovarian cancer, chemotherapy usually is administered one day every three
or four weeks, allowing for a recovery
period after each treatment. The standard
approach is six to eight cycles.

Chemotherapy is most often administered in an outpatient setting. Some
women, depending on the drugs given
and their overall health, need to be hospitalized for a time to receive treatment.

Before treatment

Before you begin chemotherapy, your
doctor should explain the treatment to
you, including the drugs you'll be receiving and the side effects they may cause.

You'll want to let your doctor know all
the medications you take, including over-
the-counter products such as vitamins,
herbal supplements, laxatives, allergy
medications and pain relievers. Your doctor will tell you if you should stop taking
any of these substances before your
chemotherapy. After your treatments
begin, check with your doctor before taking any new medications, vitamins or
herbal supplements.

A substance used in the preparation of
paclitaxel can cause severe allergic reactions in some people, even though they've
never been exposed to it before. To reduce
the chance of an allergic reaction, before
chemotherapy with paclitaxel you'll be
given a steroid medication.

During treatment

Most often chemotherapy is administered
through a vein (intravenously). The medications may be injected through a needle
that's inserted into a vein in your forearm
or hand or through a thin plastic tube
(catheter). Some people who need many
intravenous (IV) treatments have a semipermanent catheter inserted so that an IV
doesn't have to be started every time. The
catheter may be attached to a device
called a port, which is a small plastic or
metal disc placed under the skin. The
port can be used for as long as it's needed. These catheters are usually placed
in a large vein in your chest (central
venous catheter).

For intravenous chemotherapy, it takes
from 30 minutes to several hours for the
medications to drip into your vein,
depending on the drugs you receive. You
can spend that time reading, sleeping, listening to music or watching television.
Afterward, depending on how you feel,

Chemotherapy advances improve survival in women with advanced disease

Drug	Time period	Average survival
Melphalan	1970s	17 months
Platinum	1980s	31 months
Platinum plus paclitaxel	1990s	38 months

The discovery of platinum-based drugs and the drug paclitaxel, derived from the bark of the Pacific yew tree, has significantly increased survival times for women with advanced epithelial ovarian cancer.

you'll most likely be able to go about your regular routine. It's usually a good idea to have someone drive you to and from treatments, at least until you see how they affect you.

Side effects

Chemotherapy medications travel through your entire body. They target not only cancer cells but also any rapidly dividing cells. Fortunately, most normal cells aren't dividing rapidly and are largely unaffected by chemotherapy. But some healthy cells do grow and reproduce quickly, and chemotherapy can affect these cells, too. They include hair follicle cells, the cells that produce blood cells in your bone marrow and the cells lining your mouth and digestive tract.

The medications paclitaxel and carboplatin can also cause damage to nerve endings in your fingers and toes. This can result in bothersome numbness or tingling.

Before you begin treatment, your health care team will tell you what you might expect and suggest ways to manage potential side effects. Let your nurse or doctor know about any side effects you experience.

Hair loss

Hair loss is a universal side effect of paclitaxel and carboplatin and, for many women, one of the more difficult aspects of ovarian cancer treatment.

The hair loss starts 10 to 14 days after the first dose. Over just a few days, most of your hair will fall out. Some women decide to have their hair cut short before chemotherapy to lessen the effect when they lose their hair. Other women have their hairdressers shave their head when the hair starts to fall out.

Chemotherapy doesn't damage your hair permanently. If anything, it's often thicker when it grows back and may have a bit of a curl if you didn't have it before. Or your hair may be slightly different in color. Within a few weeks of your last treatment, your hair should gradually begin to grow back.

Nausea and vomiting

Nausea and vomiting aren't very common with paclitaxel and carboplatin. If they do occur, excellent anti-nausea (anti-emetic) medications are available to prevent or lessen nausea and vomiting. Changing your eating habits — avoiding big meals and certain foods — also may help reduce nausea and vomiting.

GYNECOLOGIC CANCERS

Lower blood cell counts

Both paclitaxel and carboplatin can cause a temporary lowering of blood cell counts. The drugs' effect on blood cell production can result in:

- Anemia and fatigue, caused by low red blood cell counts.
- Increased risk of infection due to a shortage of white blood cells. Be sure to promptly report any fever over 101 F or a shaking chill.
- Uncommonly, increased bruising or bleeding due to a shortage of platelets, a blood component essential to clotting.

For information on strategies for managing chemotherapy side effects, see Chapter 34.

Intraperitoneal Chemotherapy

Ovarian cancer, even when it spreads, tends to remain in the abdominal cavity. So one way of administering chemotherapy medications is to inject them directly into the abdominal (peritoneal) cavity. The drugs are administered by way of a catheter that's implanted in the abdomen. The procedure requires surgery to place a device called a port under the skin. A port is a small plastic or metal disc that a catheter can be attached to.

Intraperitoneal chemotherapy offers the advantage of delivering concentrated doses of medications directly to the cancer cells located within the abdominal cavity. But much of the chemotherapy

Second-Look Surgery

In the 1970s when the drug melphalan (Alkeran) was commonly employed to treat ovarian cancer, it was critical to discontinue the medication as soon as the cancer had fully responded to the drug. This is because long-term use of the medication could result in leukemia. The problem was knowing when a response had occurred.

The need to find out if the chemotherapy had worked led to the use of a procedure called second-look laparotomy, also known as reassessment, or second-look, surgery. Although widely used years ago, today its use is controversial.

still gets into the bloodstream from the abdomen, so the drugs also reach cancer cells that aren't in the abdomen.

Women who are the most likely to benefit from intraperitoneal chemotherapy are those with small amounts of disease left after surgery because the drugs can penetrate only a very small distance into the tumor. Intraperitoneal delivery generally isn't used in women whose cancer has spread outside the peritoneal cavity, unless it's combined with chemotherapy that's administered through the veins (intravenously).

Some studies have suggested that intraperitoneal chemotherapy may halt progression of the disease or slightly increase survival, compared with chemotherapy that's administered intravenously. So why isn't intraperitoneal delivery used more routinely for ovarian cancer?

Some doctors still recommend and practice the surgery. Others don't support its use.

Because there's no evidence that second-look surgery affects survival, the procedure is no longer considered a part of standard care for women with ovarian cancer. The National Cancer Institute recommends its use only on a limited basis, mainly among individuals participating in clinical trials. If your doctor recommends second-look surgery, make sure you consider the pros and cons of the procedure. And don't be afraid to get a second opinion from another surgeon if doing so would make you feel more comfortable.

What's involved?

The purpose of second-look surgery is to determine if any cancer remains after your initial surgery and chemotherapy treatment. The surgery is generally performed in women who have no signs or symptoms or other evidence of persistent disease. Second-look surgery is usually scheduled as soon as your blood counts have recovered satisfactorily after completing your final cycle of chemotherapy.

Just as with your initial surgery, for second-look surgery you're placed under general anesthesia. Your surgeon again makes a vertical incision in your abdomen, cutting along the previous scar,

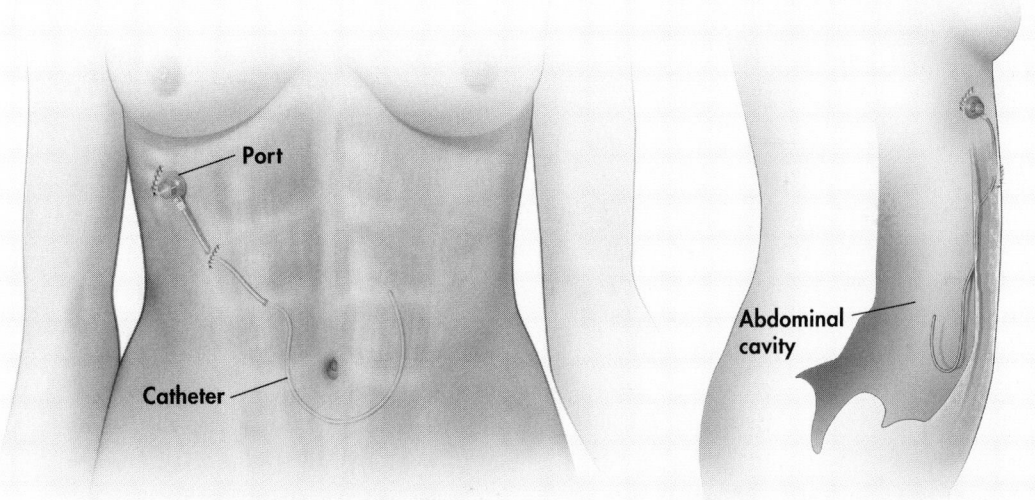

There are practical factors to consider, such as difficulties inserting and managing the catheter and the possibility of greater toxic effects from the drugs with this more direct delivery route. Studies on the use of intraperitoneal delivery

have raised as many questions as they've answered. They haven't made clear the optimal drugs, dosages and delivery times. More studies are needed to define the procedure's role.

and carefully explores the entire area, looking for any signs of remaining cancer. Tissue samples from any suspicious-looking areas are biopsied. Samples are also taken from sites that appear normal.

All in all, 50 or more biopsies may be taken during a second look to assess as many areas as possible. The surgeon again collects fluid samples from the abdominal cavity to be examined under the microscope for the presence of cancer cells.

If the surgeon finds visible cancer in the abdominal or pelvic cavity, he or she may try to remove as much of the cancer as possible. You're more likely to have visible cancer at the time of second-look surgery in the following situations:

- You had significant amounts of visible cancer remaining — greater than 2 centimeters — after your initial surgery.

- You had a high-grade (grade 3 or 4) tumor.
- Your CA 125 level remained elevated throughout most of your chemotherapy treatments.

If no disease is found, chemotherapy is generally stopped and surveillance begins. If cancer cells still are present, your doctor is likely to recommend that you continue treatment, but with a different chemotherapy regimen. Sometimes, radiation therapy is recommended in this situation.

Advantages

Second-look surgery is the most accurate way to determine if there's persistent cancer after initial treatment. Imaging techniques such as computerized tomography,

Clinical Trials

Clinical trials provide a means to test new treatment approaches. Thanks to clinical trials, new and effective treatments continually make it from the laboratory to the doctor's office.

Clinical trials have resulted in several improvements in the treatment of ovarian cancer:

- Women with ovarian cancer used to be given cyclophosphamide (Cytoxan, Neosar) and cisplatin (Platinol) for a whole year after surgery. Clinical trials showed that six cycles were just as effective as 12.
- Clinical trials found that carboplatin (Paraplatin), a less toxic platinum

medication, could be substituted for cisplatin.
- Early trials found paclitaxel (Taxol) to be very effective for ovarian cancer.

Many other new drugs and treatment approaches are being studied, including a worldwide study by the Gynecologic Oncology Group that's investigating whether treatment outcomes would be improved by the addition of a third drug, such as gemcitabine (Gemzar), doxorubicin (Adriamycin) or topotecan (Hycamtin), to the standard paclitaxel-carboplatin regimen.

To find out more about clinical trials that might benefit you, ask your doctor or contact the National Cancer Institute (see page 601).

ultrasound, magnetic resonance imaging and positron emission tomography aren't sensitive enough to detect small tumors. The CA 125 blood test, if elevated, usually indicates persistent disease, but a woman may have normal levels of CA 125 and still have remaining cancer.

However, second-look surgery isn't foolproof. It's possible that microscopic disease that can't be seen is present in areas that your surgeon didn't biopsy.

Second-look surgery provides your doctor with valuable information to help determine your overall chances for long-term survival (prognosis).

Disadvantages

Laparotomy is a major surgery, and it carries risks of infection and other complications that come with invasive surgery. In addition, although second-look surgery may offer valuable information, no study has shown that it improves overall survival rates. Women who have second-look surgery don't live longer than those who don't.

Even though a doctor may not find cancer during second-look surgery, there's no guarantee that cancer isn't present.

About 40 percent of women who undergo second-look surgery are found to be free of any evidence of cancer at the time of the surgery. This is called a negative second look. However, among this group, 30 percent to 50 percent will eventually experience a recurrence. That means that at the time of second-look surgery there was cancer present but, because of its microscopic size or its location, it wasn't discovered.

Surveillance and Follow-up

Once you've completed your treatment, you'll receive follow-up care to monitor your status. Although it's hoped that you're disease-free after initial treatment, there's no way to know for certain that the cancer has been completely destroyed. Even with a negative second-look surgery, lack of visible cancer isn't a guarantee that none is present.

So how will you know your disease status? Regular follow-up examinations can help provide that information. There are no set guidelines as to how often you should have a checkup, but most doctors schedule visits every three to four months the first couple of years after treatment. If you remain cancer-free for two years, your doctor may extend the length of time between checkups to every six months. After five years, annual exams are recommended. With ovarian cancer, recurrences after five years are uncommon.

During these appointments, your doctor looks for changes that may indicate a cancer recurrence. You'll have a physical examination, including a pelvic exam. During this exam, your doctor feels for abnormalities in your pelvis that might indicate a cancerous growth. In addition, you'll likely have a blood test to monitor the level of the protein CA 125 in your blood. If your doctor has any concerns, he or she may request an ultrasound exam or computerized tomography scan.

Be sure to tell your doctor about any signs or symptoms you're concerned about, especially if they're similar to problems you had when you received your first diagnosis.

CA 125 blood test

The CA 125 blood test measures the level of a specific protein produced by most ovarian tumors, especially in their later stages. The test is used primarily to monitor the status of women with ovarian cancer. Most healthy women have a CA 125 level below 35 units per milliliter of blood. In 85 percent of women with advanced ovarian cancer, the level is high.

The reason doctors monitor CA 125 levels is that an increase may signal cancer regrowth before the recurrence can be picked up by another test or procedure. A rising CA 125 level accurately predicts cancer recurrence in more than 95 percent of women.

But monitoring CA 125 for recurrence of ovarian cancer has drawbacks. First, it's far from certain that beginning another chemotherapy regimen on the basis of a rising CA 125 level alone is advantageous. To date, there's no evidence that initiating chemotherapy early rather than waiting for signs and symptoms to develop improves survival. In fact, beginning chemotherapy or other treatments before they're necessary can compromise your quality of your life at a time when you're feeling well.

We've stated often in this book that treating a cancer early is the best chance for a cure. However, that pertains to a new cancer diagnosis, not to a recurrence. Unfortunately, if ovarian cancer cells survive the original chemotherapy, it means that they're at least partially resistant to it.

So a second or third attempt at chemotherapy, even with different drugs, probably won't destroy all of these cells. Rather, the medications then become a means of controlling the disease and its symptoms, rather than a cure. For more information on recurrent cancer, see Chapter 18.

Another limitation of monitoring CA 125 after treatment is that it can be very stressful. Many women feel anxious each time they have the test, knowing that an increase in CA 125 may mean their cancer is back. Instead of making the best of the time they have, some women live by the numbers — breathing a sigh of relief every time a lab test shows no rise in CA 125, only to anxiously await the next test result.

Chapter 18: Gynecologic Cancers

Ovarian Cancer Recurrence

For too many women with ovarian cancer — especially those with later-stage disease or an aggressive type — the cancer persists or recurs after initial surgery and chemotherapy. Unfortunately, even with the most thorough surgery to remove the cancer (debulking, or cytoreduction) and the best chemotherapy, sometimes cancer cells manage to survive and eventually regrow. For some women, the cancer returns within months after initial treatment. For others, it may be two to three years. For women with stage III disease (see page 303) who develop recurrent cancer, the average time from initial diagnosis to recurrence is about 20 months.

If you've had your ovaries and other reproductive organs removed, you may wonder how ovarian cancer can come back. Most of the time, the disease recurs where it first occurred — within your abdominal (peritoneal) cavity. Because ovarian cancer tends to spread by shedding cells, which then seed (implant) throughout the peritoneal cavity, the surfaces of all the abdominal organs are vulnerable sites for disease recurrence. Less often, ovarian cancer cells travel through the blood or lymphatic system, and the disease recurs in more distant locations, such as the lungs or within the liver.

Recurrence can be devastating because once the cancer returns, it's generally not curable. Developing new therapies for recurrent ovarian cancer is a high priority, but for now, the focus of treatment after a recurrence isn't on curing the disease but on extending life, relieving symptoms and maintaining quality of life.

Even after a recurrence of ovarian cancer, increasing numbers of women are living longer with the disease than ever before. The increased life expectancy for women with advanced ovarian cancer — average survival now a period of three years instead of the previous one year — is a major step forward, attributable largely to more effective chemotherapies.

Some women with recurrent ovarian cancer view it as a chronic condition with signs and symptoms that can be managed. You'll have choices to make about your treatment, and you'll play a major role in deciding how to best manage your cancer while maintaining your comfort, well-being and dignity.

Signs and Symptoms

For many women, the first indication of a recurrence may be a rising CA 125 level (see page 326). Other signs and symptoms that may signal the cancer's return are often similar to the original signs and symptoms of ovarian cancer. They include:

- Abdominal or pelvic pressure, discomfort or pain
- Persistent indigestion, gas or nausea
- Feeling full after a light meal

Maintaining Quality of Life

With recurrent ovarian cancer, the quality of your life should be of primary importance. Think about how you want to live your life, and express your preferences to your doctor.

Only you can decide what your goals are, how you want to spend your time and what you're willing to tolerate in terms of treatments and side effects. For instance, if your doctor recommends additional chemotherapy, discuss your

options: Which drug or drugs will you receive? How will the medications be delivered — intravenously, by pill or directly into the abdominal cavity? What will the treatment schedule be, and how will it fit in with your life?

Also discuss side effects of the medications or other treatments that your doctor suggests. Are you willing to tolerate the side effects? If you become too tired or sick to do some of the things you would like to do, is the treatment worth it to you? Is there another treatment that you might find more tolerable? It's important to recognize that starting a

- Unexplained changes in bowel habits, including diarrhea or constipation
- Abdominal swelling or bloating, especially if it comes on suddenly
- Changes in bladder habits, including a frequent or urgent need to urinate

These signs and symptoms are fairly common and can come and go in women without cancer. However, if you have a history of ovarian cancer and your symptoms persist, let your doctor know.

Deciding on Treatment

When ovarian cancer recurs, the focus of treatment shifts from curing the disease to controlling it. You and your doctor will discuss options for extending your life while trying to preserve the highest quality of life possible.

Many treatment options are available to optimize survival time and quality of life.

The treatment your doctor recommends depends on several factors. One of the most important is the amount of time between completion of your initial chemotherapy and the cancer recurrence. This is a good measure of how well chemotherapy worked for you. How well you may respond to a new round of treatment depends on how well it worked before.

In general, if you had no sign of disease for 12 months or longer between when you stopped the initial chemotherapy treatments and the recurrence, your disease is considered chemotherapy-sensitive (also called platinum-sensitive). This means the cancer cells were responsive to the drugs' effects. The longer you remained free of recurrence, the greater your chances of responding to chemotherapy again.

On the other hand, if your cancer recurred early — less than six months

certain treatment doesn't mean that you must complete it. If the treatment schedule or its side effects are interfering with your life more than you consider acceptable, you always have the option of stopping or changing the treatment.

Throughout the process, you have options. If you try one treatment and your cancer either doesn't respond or stops responding after a time, your doctor might suggest that you try other treatments. New therapies are being developed and tested. At some point, you may choose not to try more chemotherapy because the side effects

outweigh possible benefits. For more information on supportive cancer treatment, see Chapter 36.

With recurrent cancer, there's often a fine balance between treatment to extend your life and the ability to live your life to the fullest. Expressing your wishes and preferences to your doctor allows him or her to help you develop a treatment strategy that fits your wants and needs. It's your life, and these are your decisions to make. Talk with your doctor and other members of your health care team about your goals and how best to achieve them.

GYNECOLOGIC CANCERS

after you finished initial chemotherapy — your disease may be chemotherapy-resistant (platinum-resistant). That is, the medication had little effect on the cancer. If your disease progressed during your initial chemotherapy or recurred soon after therapy ended, it may be resistant to other chemotherapy drugs as well. In this situation, it's unlikely that re-treatment with the same medications will work. If your cancer recurred between six and 12 months after completing chemotherapy, it's generally considered to be more chemotherapy-sensitive than it is chemotherapy-resistant.

Other factors that you and your doctor may consider when making a decision about how to treat your recurrence include:

- The severity (toxicity) of side effects you experienced with your initial chemotherapy and the expected side effects of new agents
- How and when the treatment is administered
- Other health problems you may have
- The extent of your signs and symptoms
- How fast the cancer is growing and how much is present
- Your priorities and goals
- How different treatments might affect your lifestyle and quality of life
- The availability of promising clinical trials

Because recurrent ovarian cancer usually isn't curable, most doctors recommend that chemotherapy and other treatments be reserved for cancer that's causing symptoms, rather than initiating treatment based solely on a rising CA 125 level. If your only sign of recurrence is an elevated CA 125 level but you feel uncomfortable not doing anything, you may be able to participate in a clinical trial.

Treatment Options

Treatment for recurrent ovarian cancer is generally individualized to each woman's situation. Treatment options may include another operation to remove the cancer, chemotherapy, hormone therapy and radiation. Some women decide to participate in clinical trials of new or investigational treatments. Other women, meanwhile, choose not to pursue any further treatment and opt for supportive care only. This is an individual decision that can be made only by weighing the potential benefits, risks and side effects of various treatments.

As you consider your options, be sure to ask your doctor about the chances of your cancer responding to a particular treatment. Realistically, only a small percentage of women with recurrent ovarian cancer will achieve long-term remission. More commonly, women go through a series of treatments, remissions and recurrences. Some women will have "stable disease" on a particular treatment for a period of time. This means that although the cancer doesn't shrink, for a while it doesn't appear to grow, either.

Repeat surgery

A certain group of women may benefit from a second debulking surgery before beginning second-line chemotherapy. Similar to the first surgery, the goal is to remove as much of the cancer as possible. This type of treatment is aggressive and is generally considered only in women who meet specific criteria.

Repeat surgery usually is recommended only for women who've been disease-free for at least a year after finishing their initial treatments. Some surgeons feel a disease-free period of two years is more appropriate. Repeat surgery isn't appropriate for women with extensive cancer deposits. It also generally isn't recommended if a lot of fluid has collected in the abdomen or if the bowel has become obstructed. These conditions are often associated with widespread cancer throughout the abdomen. A second surgery won't affect survival or quality of life unless all cancer larger than 1 centimeter in diameter is removed.

Candidates for surgery should have minimal amounts of visible cancer, as assessed by imaging tests such as computerized tomography (CT). The surgeon has a better chance of completely removing the cancer if he or she is dealing with smaller, isolated cancer deposits rather than larger, more widespread deposits. Unfortunately, only a small percentage of women meet these criteria.

Repeat debulking surgery is a complex and difficult procedure that carries a higher risk of complications than does the first surgery. Possible complications include infection, bleeding and damage to the bowel that may result in a prolonged hospital stay. You can expect to experience discomfort for a few weeks and be tired for a few months after the operation.

In order for the surgery to be effective, it should be followed by additional thera-py. Usually it's chemotherapy, but occasionally it may be radiation therapy.

Chemotherapy

Several options for second-line chemotherapy are available, and the regimen is tailored to each woman. The option you and your doctor choose depends on several factors, including how much you benefited from your initial chemotherapy. Other factors are your preferences and concerns regarding the drugs' side effects, delivery schedule and ease of administration. For example, is a weekly schedule or a monthly schedule more convenient for you? Have you had any problems with intravenous access or particular side effects?

One chemotherapy option is to go back to the same drugs you received initially, such as a combination of a platinum (usually carboplatin) and paclitaxel. Another is to use these agents one at a time, thereby reducing side effects. A third possibility is to introduce a new drug.

If your disease is chemotherapy-sensitive — meaning that the cancer cells were responsive to the treatment — then retreatment with the same agents is commonly the first choice.

Among women who are chemotherapy-sensitive, 40 percent to 50 percent will respond to second-line treatment with these medications. This means that they'll have significant cancer shrinkage, defined as at least a 50 percent decrease in the amount of disease, judged by a physical exam, computerized tomography scan or CA 125 blood test. The longer the interval between your first-line chemotherapy and the cancer recurrence, the greater your response to second-line chemotherapy is likely to be. For women who've been off chemotherapy for more than two years, response rates to second-line chemotherapy are as high as 70 percent to 80 percent.

If your disease is resistant to chemotherapy, several other medications may be considered. There's no single drug that's considered better or more effective than any other because many factors have to be taken into consideration. In general, response rates run about 20 percent, and responses last on average six to eight months. In other words, for about one-fifth of the women treated, the cancer decreases in size by at least 50 percent for an average of about six months.

Here's a list of some of the chemotherapy drugs used to treat recurrent ovarian cancer, along with their most common side effects:

- **Carboplatin.** Carboplatin (Paraplatin) is a synthetic derivative of the platinum drug cisplatin. Side effects include lowered blood counts, which can result in increased risk of infection. Another side effect is some tingling and numbness in the fingers and toes (peripheral neuropathy). Carboplatin is typically given intravenously every three weeks.

- **Paclitaxel or docetaxel.** Paclitaxel (Taxol), a natural product originally derived from the Pacific yew tree, now is synthesized instead of extracted from its natural source. Side effects include hair loss, allergic reactions, peripheral neuropathy, lowering of white blood cell counts and muscle aches that come and go. Docetaxel (Taxotere) is another taxane drug that works in the same way

as paclitaxel. Paclitaxel and docetaxel are given intravenously. Paclitaxel may be given once a week or every three weeks, depending on the dose. Docetaxel is given every three weeks.

- **Doxorubicin liposome injection.** Contained within a fatty protective coating, liposomal doxorubicin (Doxil) remains stable in the bloodstream longer than do most chemotherapy drugs, giving the agent more time to gain access to cancer cells and destroy them. Side effects include skin peeling and redness on the palms of the hands and the soles of the feet. Liposomal doxorubicin is administered intravenously once a month.

- **Topotecan.** Topotecan (Hycamtin) belongs to a group of medications known as topoisomerase inhibitors. Side effects include a lowering of blood counts. This medication is given intravenously once a day for five days every three weeks.

- **Gemcitabine.** Gemcitabine (Gemzar) prevents rapidly dividing cells from making functional DNA and ribonucleic acid (RNA). This drug is generally well tolerated. Side effects include lowered blood cell counts. Gemcitabine is given intravenously once a week for three weeks, with one week of rest.

- **Etoposide.** Etoposide (Etopophos, VePesid, VP-16) inhibits DNA synthesis. Side effects include a reduction in white blood cells and hair loss. It can be taken intravenously or by mouth as a capsule once a day for three weeks, followed by one week of rest.

- **Ifosfamide.** Ifosfamide (Ifex) is in the class of drugs called alkylating agents, which bind directly with DNA to inhibit its function. The medication can cause hair loss and bladder irritation. It's given intravenously for three days every four weeks.

- **Altretamine.** Altretamine (Hexalen) is thought to act similar to an alkylating agent. The drug can cause nausea and loss of appetite. Altretamine is taken by mouth once a day for 14 days every four weeks.
- **Vinorelbine.** Vinorelbine (Navelbine) is a vinca alkaloid and is part of the class of medications known as mitotic inhibitors. These medications cause a delay in cell division. The medication can cause tingling of the hands and feet and constipation, as well as hair loss and low blood counts.

Regardless of which medication is used, initially you'll probably receive two or three cycles of treatment. Your doctor will closely monitor your response to the drug. If the medication is helping you by reducing your symptoms or lowering your CA 125 level and you tolerate the drug reasonably well, your doctor may suggest that you continue it. If the medication isn't helping or if it's causing significant side effects, your doctor will likely suggest that you stop taking it. You can then try an alternative medication, or you may choose to stop chemotherapy.

The more cycles of chemotherapy you have, the more side effects related to treatment accumulate (cumulative toxicity). In addition, if you've had several different kinds of chemotherapy previously, you have less chance of responding to yet another drug.

Hormone therapy

Hormone therapies may be used to treat breast, ovarian and uterine cancers. These medications have been used to treat breast cancer for many years. One of the drugs that's most commonly used is the synthetic anti-estrogen agent tamoxifen (Nolvadex), which belongs to a class of drugs known as selective estrogen receptor modulators (SERMs).

In breast tissue, tamoxifen works against the effects of the female hormone estrogen. More recently, tamoxifen has been found to have some anti-tumor effect on ovarian cancer and has been used to treat women with a cancer recurrence. Tamoxifen is typically recommended for women whose only evidence of recurrence is a rising CA 125 level.

Although some women with recurrent ovarian cancer respond to tamoxifen, there's no reliable way to predict who will benefit. In breast cancer, tamoxifen is used in women whose tumors are estrogen receptor positive, meaning the tumors feed on estrogen. In ovarian cancer, the presence or absence of estrogen receptors hasn't proved useful in determining which tumors will respond to tamoxifen.

For approximately 10 percent to 15 percent of women with recurrent ovarian cancer who take tamoxifen, the disease responds to the drug — that is, their tumors shrink. In another 10 percent to 15 percent of women who use it, the cancer remains stable for a period of time, neither growing nor shrinking. Side effects of tamoxifen are milder than those of chemotherapy medications. The side effects are similar to symptoms of menopause and include hot flashes. Less common side effects include an increased risk of uterine cancer — which isn't a risk for women who've had a hysterectomy — and a slightly increased risk of blood clots. Unlike chemotherapy medications, tamoxifen doesn't cause hair loss or affect production of white blood cells.

Several other types of hormone therapies are available. However, response rates to these drugs are usually low, less than 10 percent.

Radiation therapy

Radiation therapy uses high-energy X-rays to kill cancer cells. Because ovarian cancer tends to remain localized in the abdominal and pelvic cavities, radiation therapy to the abdomen and pelvis is one option for treating the disease. However, its use in the treatment of ovarian cancer is somewhat controversial, and over the last 10 years radiation has been used less often in women with ovarian cancer. It's not clear that radiation adds major value beyond what chemotherapy provides, and delivering radiation to the abdomen can cause serious side effects.

Radiation therapy may be a consideration for women who have a fairly localized recurrence and for women who don't tolerate chemotherapy, which is rare.

Delivery

Radiation to treat ovarian cancer can be delivered internally or externally to the abdomen, the pelvis or both.

With internal radiation, radioactive phosphorus is inserted as a liquid directly into the abdominal cavity (peritoneal cavity), where it comes in contact with the tumor and your organs. With this type of radiation, called intraperitoneal radiation, a radioactive material called P 32 is used.

The radiation is given by way of a catheter, similar to the way intraperitoneal chemotherapy is administered. Because P 32 emits a radioactive particle that travels only a couple of millimeters, this treatment is only for women thought to have very small amounts of cancer left behind after surgery.

It takes about 70 days from when P 32 is administered until the radioactive isotope is completely "out of your system." P 32 can be toxic. Side effects can include abdominal pain and bowel damage.

External radiation is the most common form of radiation therapy. With external radiation, a machine outside the body produces a beam that delivers radiation to the abdomen. External radiation for the treatment of ovarian cancer is also referred to as whole abdominal radiation therapy (WART).

During the procedure, radiation is delivered to the entire abdominal cavity and pelvis using external radioactive beams that pass into the body. It's similar to having a diagnostic X-ray, except the X-rays are more powerful. Treatment typically is administered five days a week for several weeks. Each treatment lasts only 30 to 60 seconds. It takes more time to position you than it does to administer the radiation. This ensures that the X-rays are aimed at the precise location that needs treatment. Because your liver and kidneys have a relatively low tolerance for radiation, they may be shielded during treatment.

Like chemotherapy, WART kills healthy cells in addition to cancer cells, so you may experience some side effects. Initially, you may experience nausea and vomiting. To help prevent this, your doctor may give you anti-nausea medications before your treatment. About 10 percent to 15 percent of women are unable to complete WART because of severe nausea and vomiting.

Around the third week, you might begin to experience diarrhea, which again may be controlled with medication. Other common side effects include fatigue and dry skin. Fatigue may increase over the course of your treatment. Your doctor will also monitor your blood counts during treatment because radiation can cause them to decrease. Because about 40 percent of your functional bone marrow (in your spine and pelvic bones) is in the treatment field, a long-term side effect of WART can be loss of bone marrow reserve. Although this shouldn't affect your normal daily routine, it may make it more difficult for your blood counts to recover from additional chemotherapy.

Radiation may also worsen chronic bowel problems, including scarring and obstruction, which may result from the cancer itself or prior abdominal surgeries.

Experimental treatments

Ovarian cancer is one of the most drug-sensitive cancers — 80 percent of women with newly diagnosed disease will respond to chemotherapy. Unfortunately, just because a tumor responds to chemotherapy and it shrinks significantly doesn't necessarily mean the cancer is cured or that it will never return. Although ovarian cancer is quite chemosensitive, the medication typically doesn't cure the cancer.

Chemotherapy resistance

One area of study involves specific tests that are done before chemotherapy treatment begins to determine which chemotherapy medications may not be beneficial. Over time, cancer cells can develop resistance to chemotherapy drugs — that is, the cells become immune to the drugs' effects.

A major focus of ovarian cancer research is to take advantage of the disease's natural chemosensitivity whenever possible and to better understand what enables tumors to become resistant to chemotherapy. By learning what makes tumors chemo-resistant, researchers can try to modify or block that resistance.

In a laboratory, there are ways to culture and grow a person's tumor cells that were obtained during surgery and then to test them by exposing them to different chemotherapy agents. The goal is to avoid giving a person chemotherapy that will cause side effects when there's little chance that the drug will effectively fight the tumor. This may sound simple and straightforward, but it's not. Not all factors — such as immune system activity or how each individual processes (metabolizes) different chemotherapy drugs — can be included in this analysis. Clinical trials that will address the issue of chemotherapy-resistance testing are now in planning stages.

At the same time, newer chemotherapeutic agents are being developed, including those that can be used to treat recurrent ovarian cancer. These experimental therapies are in various stages of testing.

Immunotherapy

For years, researchers have been working on ways to get the body's immune system to attack cancer cells, an approach called immunotherapy. Other names for this approach include biological therapy, biotherapy and biologic response modifier therapy.

Your body's immune system protects you by watching out for and destroying foreign substances. For instance, if your immune system detects the presence of a virus, it produces binding proteins (anti-bodies) and specialized immune killer cells that destroy the virus. Unfortunately, the system doesn't work as well when the invader is a cancer that has arisen from your own cells. Your immune system often doesn't perceive the cancer as foreign, and the cancer grows unchecked.

Immunotherapy research involves several areas of investigation.

Monoclonal antibodies

Antibodies are proteins produced by your immune system to help attack and get rid of foreign invaders. Antibodies can also be designed and produced in the laboratory to seek out and bind to a specific target. Monoclonal antibodies — so called because they're produced (cloned) from a

---

Targeting the Folate Receptor

For immunotherapy to work, there needs to be some kind of marker or target on cancer cells that isn't present on healthy cells so that the immune system can recognize and target the cancer cells. There also needs to be a way to jump-start a person's immune system to get it to attack the target. Here's a look at one approach being studied for treatment of recurrent ovarian cancer:

Folate, a B vitamin, is essential for biochemical reactions in all human cells, especially those that are producing new DNA, ribonucleic acid (RNA) and proteins. Cancer cells need more folate (called folic acid in its synthetic form) than do normal cells, and they have a unique way of capturing as much folate as possible, enabling them to beat out normal cells in competition for the vitamin. Ovarian cancer cells have a surface receptor that captures folate molecules from the environment. Called the folate receptor, it's rarely present on normal cells. Because of its abundance on cancer cells and scarcity on normal cells, this receptor is an appealing target for immunotherapy agents.

Several clinical trials testing strategies that target the folate receptor are being developed. It's still too early to tell if this approach will be successful. However, even if this particular approach has limitations, it illustrates the promise of the next generation of immune therapy agents.

The Measles Virus and Ovarian Cancer

Researchers are testing the use of a vaccine strain of the measles virus as a potential treatment for ovarian cancer. Normally, measles causes rash, fever, cough and other signs and symptoms. In the 1950s, researchers created vaccines from weakened strains of the measles virus. The vaccine protects (vaccinates) people against a severe strain of measles, reducing the incidence of measles worldwide. More recently, researchers discovered that these vaccine strains also have an effect on some cancers.

How does this work? Certain cancer cells, including ovarian cancer cells, make a receptor protein called CD46 on their cell surface. The CD46 receptor is produced by all human cells, but ovarian cancer cells overexpress it — that is, they produce more than do normal cells. The protein has several functions, but one of them is to act as a receptor for the measles virus. Once the measles virus binds to a cancer cell and enters it, the virus uses the cell's own mechanisms to make viral proteins. One of these proteins causes the cell to fuse with its neighbors. In the treatment of cancer, when 50 to 100 cancer cells fuse together, the cell cluster can't divide and thus dies.

A 2002 study looked at the effects of delivering a vaccine strain of the measles virus directly into the abdominal cavity of mice that had been infected with human ovarian cancer cells. The mice treated with the measles virus survived significantly longer than did the untreated animals. The next step is to test the vaccine strain in humans.

single cell — attach themselves to recognizable proteins or pieces of proteins produced by cancer, known as antigens. The antibodies either directly attack the cancer cells bearing the antigen or stimulate your immune system to recognize the antigen as abnormal, so your immune system killer cells will attack the cancer cells.

Antibodies can serve multiple purposes. They can attack the tumor directly, as described above, or they can be used as delivery agents. For this purpose, they can be bound (conjugated) to a radioactive agent or toxin. The antibodies deliver the toxic substance to the cancer cells, where, the hope is, the radioactive agent or toxin will destroy them.

One example of a monoclonal antibody developed for the treatment of ovarian cancer is oregovomab (OvaRex). It targets the antigen CA 125, which is produced by the majority of ovarian tumors. The hope is that by binding with CA 125, oregovomab will stimulate the body's immune system to attack cells that produce CA 125. Although some studies suggest beneficial immune responses after the administration of oregovomab, other studies show no improvement. The drug is still being tested in clinical trials.

GYNECOLOGIC CANCERS

Interferons

Your body produces specific immune system stimulants called cytokines. Specific cytokines known as interferons are produced in response to viral infection to help attack the virus. Interferons may have anti-tumor activity as well. In clinical trials, some interferons have been shown to have an effect against ovarian cancer. These drugs are most likely to be used in combination with other approaches to enhance the effect of those therapies.

Gene therapy

Tumors grow because normal regulatory genes become damaged, allowing healthy cells to turn cancerous. Gene therapy aims to repair or replace defective genes and increase the production of healthy ones.

At its basic level, gene therapy involves delivering healthy copies of missing or defective genes to abnormal cells. A potential use of gene therapy for cancer is to introduce a specific gene into cancer cells so that either the cells produce a toxic protein that causes them to self-destruct, or they become vulnerable to drugs that kill cancer cells.

One of the greatest challenges in gene therapy is finding ways to deliver genes to the appropriate target cells efficiently, effectively and safely. A number of methods are being studied, including the use of viruses as transporters (vectors). Viruses have the natural ability to insert their own genes into human cells.

For gene therapy, researchers first remove disease-causing genes from a virus and then insert therapeutic genes. The viruses are then delivered to a specific area, such as a tumor, where, it is

hoped, they will take up residence in tumor cells and coerce them to produce the desired proteins. The hope is that the viruses will produce proteins that destroy cancer cells. Various viruses are being studied, including the herpes virus and viruses that cause the common cold. Another area of research involves a strain of the measles virus (see page 337).

Progressive Cancer

Most women with advanced ovarian cancer remain mentally alert and free of severe pain. But as ovarian cancer progresses, tending to spread throughout the abdominal cavity, it can cause signs and symptoms that may include abdominal swelling (distention) and pressure and a reduced ability to eat, which may progress to nausea and vomiting. Two of the most troublesome problems associated with progressive ovarian cancer are bowel obstruction and an accumulation of fluid in the abdomen (ascites).

Bowel obstruction

Ovarian cancer typically recurs within the abdominal cavity, where it commonly causes intestinal problems. Cancer cells growing on the outside of the intestines can press on the intestine, blocking passage of fluids and waste. Cancer cells can also coat the nerve supply to the intestines, slowing the movement (motility) of digested food through the bowel. When food can't pass through your intestines properly, eating can be very difficult, even painful. As the area just before a blockage

---

MYTH vs. FACT

Myth: **Drug companies and the Food and Drug Administration are blocking or withholding new cancer treatments.**

Fact: Going through cancer treatment is never easy. Even when things are going well, it's natural to become frustrated and wish for a magic cure.

Scientific studies to determine a cancer treatment's safety and effectiveness take time. That may create the appearance, or lead to reports, that new treatments are being blocked. But the thorough testing required has kept many unsafe and ineffective drugs from being used in the United States.

Concerned health professionals and consumers have long advocated that doctors should be able to use new treatments in needy and willing patients, even if those treatments haven't completed the lengthy FDA approval process. The FDA has taken steps to respond to these concerns. In 1991, for example, the agency initiated an accelerated approval process for certain new drugs. The FDA has also shortened the time devoted to preapproval drug testing, without compromising requirements for safety and effectiveness. The risks and benefits of a more rapid approval process continue to be a topic of much debate.

---

stretches to accommodate the food, your abdomen may swell, and you may experience colic-like pain. Eating more only makes the pain and distention worse.

Interference with bowel function is a serious complication of ovarian cancer. In fact, cancerous (malignant) bowel obstruction is the most common cause of death from ovarian cancer. The majority of bowel obstructions in women with ovarian cancer are cancerous. Others are the result of scar tissue from previous surgery, radiation to the pelvis or abdomen, or chemotherapy that's administered directly to the lining of the abdominal cavity (intraperitoneal chemotherapy).

Bowel obstruction is a life-threatening physical problem, and it can be extremely difficult on an emotional and social level as well. Women who can't eat or drink in a normal way often feel frustrated and set apart from personal and social interactions. For these reasons, your doctor will try to help ease the problems associated with it.

Surgery

For some women, surgery to try to relieve the obstruction is an option. However, surgery generally is considered only for women whose obstruction isn't cancerous or for women whose bowels are obstructed in only one or two places and whose cancers are still responsive to chemotherapy. Imaging tests, such as X-rays or computerized tomography scans, help to determine whether obstructions are treatable by surgery.

Unfortunately, for most women with recurrent ovarian cancer and bowel obstruction, bowel function is impaired at many sites along the small and large intestines and, therefore, the condition can't easily be treated with surgery. The decision of whether to operate on a cancerous bowel obstruction can be very complicated and has to be made on an individual basis.

This type of operation typically is very difficult and associated with a high risk of complications, the most common being injury to the bowel. In many cases, women who undergo such surgery in this situation are found to have widespread ovarian cancer, and the only effective way to relieve the obstruction is to create a stoma before the blockage. A stoma is created by pulling a loop of colon or small intestine though an incision in the abdomen. Intestinal contents empty into a bag, which covers the stoma. Among women who are candidates for the procedure, a stoma often helps relieve obstructive symptoms, allowing the women to eat again.

Other approaches

Signs and symptoms of bowel obstruction, including vomiting, diarrhea, constipation and pain, often can be improved with medications, such as pain relievers and anti-nausea medications. Some women need to be hospitalized for gastric suction, in which a tube is inserted into the nose and threaded through the esophagus into the stomach. Suction through the tube relieves intestinal pressure by emptying stomach and intestinal contents. Another option is to place a draining tube (percutaneous endoscopic gastrostomy tube) directly into the intestinal tract by way of a small abdominal incision. This also allows the suction removal of bowel contents that can't pass through properly. Many women find this less objectionable than a tube through the nose.

Fluid in the abdomen

Another possible complication of recurrent ovarian cancer is the accumulation of fluid in the abdomen (ascites). When fluid buildup is caused by cancer, it's called malignant ascites.

Normally, your lymph system drains fluids from your abdomen, but cancer can cause excess fluid to build up within the abdominal cavity. Fluid can also collect around the lungs (pleural effusions), but excess fluid in the abdomen is more common.

A large volume of fluid can be quite uncomfortable, causing signs and symptoms that may include:

- Abdominal swelling or bloating
- An inability to eat or a feeling of fullness after eating very little food
- Nausea and vomiting

Your doctor may withdraw the excess fluid using a large needle attached to a tube that's inserted into your abdomen, a procedure called paracentesis. The procedure usually isn't painful, and it can provide a great deal of relief. Unfortunately, the fluid tends to re-accumulate rapidly, often in just a few days. Draining this fluid repeatedly depletes the body of needed proteins, and every procedure carries a risk of infection. For this reason, doctors are often reluctant to remove this fluid unless it's absolutely necessary to do so because of symptoms.

Low doses of medications that reduce the amount of water in the body (diuretics) may be tried. However, this approach can lead to dehydration, and it may not be helpful.

Carolyn's Story

Carolyn Webb says she could be the poster girl for ovarian cancer. Before she was diagnosed with the disease in June 1999, she sought help from a number of doctors. "I had been desperately trying for at least 18 months to figure out what was wrong with me," she says. "I knew something was amiss."

Carolyn's early symptoms were mostly gastrointestinal — indigestion, bloating, constipation and diarrhea. "I'd eat something, and I'd feel very full and uncomfortable," she recalls. She also had low back pain, and she urinated more frequently. Normally a high-energy person, she often found herself tired. But, she thought,

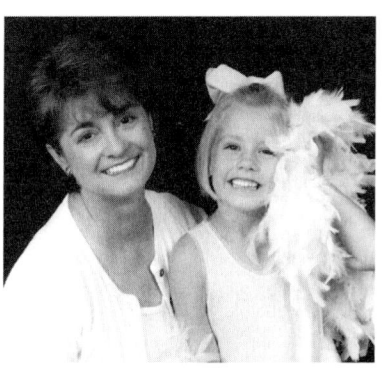

Carolyn and her granddaughter after Carolyn's cancer diagnosis in 1999.

getting older and having a stressful job might account for her fatigue.

Because of the nature of her symptoms, Carolyn went to a gastroenterologist. He mentioned the possibility of ovarian cancer and ordered a computerized tomography (CT) scan. Although one ovary wasn't visible on the scan, the imaging test was read as normal. Carolyn's husband, a pediatric surgeon, wondered about the other ovary. He suggested that Carolyn have a minimally invasive surgical procedure called laparoscopy to check her ovaries, but other doctors didn't see the need for it.

After that, Carolyn says, "No one mentioned ovarian cancer again, not even my gynecologist." She had several other tests and was given medication for irritable bowel syndrome. Her gynecologist suggested that she was going through a tough menopause and prescribed an anti-anxiety medication. She also saw a family practitioner who wanted to do a colonoscopy.

No one was coming up with an answer, and Carolyn's symptoms were getting worse. In May 1999, she traveled to England. She was miserable on the trip, with "hideous" gas and bloating. "I called my gynecologist and said, 'I look like I'm five months pregnant.'"

She had another CT scan, and the gynecologist ordered a CA 125 blood test. Carolyn was also scheduled to have a pelvic ultrasound, but when she arrived for her appointment, she was told she didn't need the test. In a few minutes, Carolyn's husband showed up. "I just took one look at his face, and I knew it was bad. He said you've got ovarian cancer, and it's very bad, very advanced."

At this point Carolyn was referred to a gynecologic oncologist. He was cruelly honest, Carolyn says. He told her the cancer, likely stage IIIC, was extensive, with spread to the colon and with a huge mass attached to her liver. He outlined some grim statistics, but he told her, "You can be one of those numbers that doesn't fit."

Carolyn was warned that the surgery would be tough — and it was. During the eight-hour operation, part of her stomach and liver were removed, along with her ovaries, uterus and fallopian tubes. She had an unusual reaction to the anti-nausea drugs she received after the surgery and was in the hospital for 15 days.

Soon after that, she began chemotherapy. She had an uncommon allergic reaction to paclitaxel (Taxol), and then started on seven cycles of cyclophosphamide (Cytoxan) and cisplatin (Platinol). The treatment was exhausting. "It was a fatigue that no one understands," Carolyn says, "Not a 'good' tired from housework or yardwork, but bone weary tired. I felt like I couldn't put one foot in front of the other."

After finishing chemotherapy, Carolyn had a second-look surgery. With no visible remaining cancer, she enrolled in a trial in which researchers were studying a drug designed to deliver radiation straight to a tumor. This treatment had a severe effect on Carolyn's bone marrow, knocking out her blood counts. Following it, she needed 20 blood transfusions. But so far, she's had no cancer recurrence in her abdomen.

Unfortunately, though, the cancer did come back in her lymph nodes. She's been on chemotherapy for the last year and a half, and in September 2002 she had a third surgery to remove more cancer near her aorta.

The rigors of treatment have taken a toll on Carolyn, physically and emotionally. "Having cancer is like having a hand grenade or a bomb thrown into your life," Carolyn says. "Not just you, but your whole family. They're worried about you, and you're worried about them."

At first, Carolyn says, she was frantic. Anxiety kept her up at night. But one thing that turned her around, she says, was realizing that things like heart attacks or accidents can happen to anyone at any time. "None of us know what our time is."

Her spirituality also provided solace. "I've come a long way in my religion," she reflects. "That's brought me comfort. Some people get very angry with God. It's made me question my beliefs. Do I think that God did this to me? No, I just think these things happen."

She's been buoyed by an outpouring of love, cards, prayers, food and flowers. "I've had great support, and I don't think you can do this alone."

Carolyn has connected with other women living with ovarian cancer. She started a support group and is president of her local chapter of the National Ovarian Cancer Coalition. Like other women with ovarian cancer, Carolyn wants to help increase awareness of the disease.

Despite everything she's been through, Carolyn keeps a positive outlook. "I view it as a chronic disease," she says. "I want to be one of those 20-year survivors."

Although she has some ongoing side effects from treatment, they don't keep her from doing the things she loves, such as reading, going to movies, participating in three book clubs and, above all, spending time with her family and friends.

"I have six grandchildren, five children and my parents who are still alive," she says. "My husband has fought like a tiger for me. I've got lots of reasons for being here. ... As I have said to my husband, 'I will not go quietly into that good night.'"

Chapter 19: Gynecologic Cancers

Special Cases

Most people know something about breast and ovarian cancers. But if your doctor tells you that you have a granulosa cell tumor or gestational trophoblastic disease, your first question may well be, "What is that?" That's where this chapter can be useful. It covers some of the more unusual gynecologic cancers.

For example, although invasive epithelial cancer is the most common type of ovarian cancer, other types of tumors can develop in the ovary. These include borderline tumors, germ cell tumors and sex cord-stromal tumors. In another less common scenario, some women develop ovarian cancer and endometrial cancer at the same time. Finally, this chapter discusses gestational trophoblastic disease, rare tumors that can develop in the uterus after conception.

This chapter provides an overview of some uncommon gynecologic cancers. Fortunately, while these cancers may be less common, many are highly responsive to treatment.

Borderline Tumors

Borderline ovarian tumors, also known as tumors of low malignant potential, develop in cells of the epithelium, the thin layer of tissue that covers the surface of the ovaries. These are the same cells that give rise to the more typical ovarian cancer. While borderline tumors have some cancerous (malignant) features, such as an abnormal cellular appearance and excess cell proliferation, they generally behave in a more benign manner than does standard epithelial ovarian cancer. When viewed under a microscope, borderline tumor cells appear abnormal, but unlike cancer cells, they don't invade an ovary's supporting tissue (stroma).

Borderline tumors also differ from cancerous epithelial tumors in other respects. For one thing, they tend to grow much more slowly. Although a borderline tumor can return after the initial tumor has been removed, recurrences may not occur until 10 or 15 years later. Even advanced borderline tumors grow very slowly, with long periods between recurrences.

About 25 percent to 30 percent of borderline tumors spread beyond the ovary to the lining of the abdominal cavity (peritoneum). The new tumor sites are referred to as peritoneal implants. However, unlike typical ovarian cancer implants, borderline peritoneal implants are usually noninvasive — meaning the cells are tacked onto the abdominal lining but don't invade underlying tissue. In fewer than 5 percent of borderline tumors, the implants invade below the peritoneal surface layer. A borderline tumor with invasive implants behaves more aggressively than does a borderline tumor with noninvasive implants.

Like epithelial ovarian cancer, borderline tumors are divided into subtypes based on the microscopic appearance of their cells. Among the subtypes, serous is the most common, followed by mucinous.

Endometrioid, clear cell and transitional cell (Brenner) borderline tumors are very uncommon.

Who gets borderline tumors?

Borderline ovarian tumors make up 10 percent to 15 percent of all epithelial ovarian tumors. About 3,000 women in the United States are diagnosed with borderline tumors each year. They can occur in women of all ages but are more likely to affect younger women than are epithelial ovarian cancers. Women who receive this diagnosis tend to be in their mid-40s.

Some of the risk factors for epithelial ovarian cancer are also associated with borderline tumors. For example, not bearing children increases risk slightly. And some of the protective factors are the same, such as having children and breast-feeding. But the use of birth control pills, another factor that's linked to reduced risk of epithelial ovarian cancer, doesn't appear to protect against borderline tumors.

The causes of borderline tumors are unknown. Because the number of cases is relatively small, few studies have been conducted to determine what might cause these tumors.

Diagnosis and treatment

Signs and symptoms of borderline tumors are similar to those of standard ovarian cancer, but women with borderline tumors are more likely not to have any signs and symptoms at the time of their diagnoses. In one study, nearly a quarter of the women who received a diagnosis of

Borderline Ovarian Tumors and Fertility

Because many women who get borderline tumors are still in their reproductive years, surgical treatment may aim to preserve a woman's ability to have children by sparing one ovary and the uterus.

A few studies have examined whether women who had such an operation were still able to become pregnant. In one study, half the women who had had fertility-sparing surgery for borderline tumors and later tried to conceive were successful. Although the research involved small numbers of women, the findings suggest that young women who have this type of surgery have a good chance of maintaining their fertility.

For women who have fertility-sparing surgery, follow-up is important to monitor for possible recurrence of the tumor.

a borderline tumor didn't have any signs and symptoms.

When signs and symptoms are present, those that are the most common are abdominal or pelvic pain, bloating or increased abdominal size, and a mass in the pelvis or abdomen. If you have signs or symptoms suggestive of an ovarian tumor, your doctor will likely do a pelvic examination and may order blood tests and an ultrasound of the pelvis. These diagnostic procedures are described in Chapter 16.

Surgery is the only way to tell for sure if you have a benign, malignant or border-line tumor. During surgery, your doctor is able to not only establish a diagnosis but also, if needed, remove the tumor and determine its stage. Tumor stage is determined by whether the tumor has spread and to what extent. Borderline tumors are classified (staged) in the same manner as are invasive ovarian epithelial cancers. This classification system is described on page 302.

Surgery to remove the tumor is the mainstay of treatment. For women who don't wish to have children, removal of both ovaries, the uterus and the fallopian tubes is the standard treatment. The surgeon will try to remove (debulk) as much of the cancer as possible. For women who hope to preserve their fertility, the uterus and uninvolved ovary might be left in place.

If you've received a new diagnosis of a borderline tumor, it's likely that surgery will be the recommended treatment. After surgery, every few months you'll likely have a checkup with a physical exam and CA 125 blood test (see page 326). These regular checkups will continue for approximately five years. For the small group of women with an advanced-stage tumor with invasive implants, treatment with chemotherapy — generally three to six courses of paclitaxel (Taxol) and carbo-platin (Paraplatin) — may be recommended. But the value of this treatment hasn't been clearly established, so it's important to talk to your doctor about its potential risks and benefits. Some women decide to have follow-up monitoring rather than chemotherapy. For more information on chemotherapy, see Chapter 17.

A favorable outlook

Borderline ovarian tumors generally have an excellent prognosis. In large studies, 70 percent to 80 percent of women with borderline tumors have stage I disease, with no spread to any other area.

Among women with stage I borderline tumors, the 10-year survival is greater than 95 percent. For women with non-invasive peritoneal implants, approximately 15 percent to 20 percent will have a relapse. For women with invasive implants, the risk of recurrence is about 35 percent.

When necessary, recurrent borderline tumors may be treated with surgery, hormone therapy or chemotherapy. In some cases, given the slow growth of this type of tumor, close follow-up alone is the best option, until signs and symptoms warrant intervention.

Germ Cell Tumors

Germ cell tumors begin in the reproductive cells of the body. In women the germ cells are the egg-producing cells in the ovaries, and in men the germ cells are the sperm-producing cells in the testicles.

Several different types of ovarian germ cell tumors can occur. They may be malignant or benign. Most are benign. As a group, germ cell tumors account

for about 25 percent of all ovarian tumors but only about 5 percent of malignant ovarian tumors.

Dermoid cysts (also called mature cystic teratomas) account for almost all benign germ cell tumors. Dermoid cysts occur most frequently in young women but may occur in females of any age. Because these tumors originate in the egg-producing cells, they can differentiate into numerous types of tissues and often contain various tissue elements such as hair, bone and teeth.

About 1 percent of dermoid cysts have malignant elements — usually a cancer called squamous cell carcinoma — essentially forming a cancerous tumor within a benign tumor. Cancerous tumors arising from elements of a dermoid cyst are rarely found in women under age 40.

Besides benign and malignant dermoid cysts, the third major category of ovarian germ cell tumors is known as primitive malignant germ cell tumors. The cells of these tumors resemble the primitive cells of an embryo and its surrounding structures. This type of tumor has several subtypes:

- **Dysgerminoma.** This is the ovarian counterpart of seminoma, a type of testicular cancer in men, although it's less common in women. About half of all primitive germ cell tumors are dysgerminomas.
- **Yolk sac tumors.** Also referred to as endodermal sinus tumors, these tumors account for 20 percent of primitive germ cell tumors.
- **Immature teratomas.** These also account for 20 percent of primitive germ cell tumors. Like dermoid cysts, imma-

ture teratomas may contain hair, bone and teeth, as well as cysts.

- **Others.** Less common primitive germ cell tumors include embryonal carcinomas, choriocarcinomas and mixed primitive germ cell tumors, which include a combination of subtypes, such as yolk sac and dysgerminoma.

Malignant germ cell tumors are most common in girls and young women. The tumors are most often diagnosed in females ages 16 to 20. Most often the tumor affects just one ovary.

Diagnosis

The most common signs and symptoms of germ cell tumors are abdominal or pelvic pain and a mass that can be felt in that area. You may experience no signs and symptoms in the early stages of the tumor's development, but a mass may be discovered during a regular gynecologic exam. Less common signs and symptoms include swelling of the abdomen and sharp, intense pain in the abdomen.

To detect and diagnose an ovarian germ cell tumor, your doctor will do a pelvic exam and may order imaging tests such as a computerized tomography (CT) scan of the pelvic area. Blood tests that measure the level of specific markers, including alpha-fetoprotein and human chorionic gonadotropin, may help with the diagnosis. Many germ cell tumors produce these substances, and increased concentrations of the substances can be detected in blood.

As with other forms of ovarian cancer, surgery serves to confirm the presence of a cancerous germ cell tumor and to assess the extent of the cancer. The usual surgical procedure for diagnosis and treatment of germ cell tumors is a staging laparotomy, which is discussed in Chapters 16 and 17. Information gathered during surgical staging determines the appropriate treatment. Cancerous ovarian germ cell tumors are staged using the same numeric system as is used for epithelial ovarian cancer (see page 302). About 60 percent to 70 percent of cancerous germ cell tumors are diagnosed at stage I, and another 25 percent to 30 percent at stage III. Stages II and IV are uncommon.

Treatment

Treatment depends on the type, stage and size of the tumor. Cancerous germ cell tumors are treated with surgery, often followed by chemotherapy or radiation.

Because many women with germ cell tumors are young, often a high priority for them is to preserve their ability to have children. For women who wish to preserve their fertility, malignant germ cell tumors that appear to be limited to an ovary can be safely treated by removing only the affected ovary and its fallopian tube, leaving in place the other ovary and the uterus. If the cancer has spread beyond an ovary, the uterus and opposite ovary also may need to be removed. In either instance, lymph nodes are removed to check for cancer spread, and tissue samples (biopsies) are taken from various sites within the pelvis and abdomen and sent to a laboratory for microscopic examination.

Unlike the much more common epithelial ovarian cancers, many ovarian germ cell tumors are curable with chemotherapy. The development of effective chemotherapy for testicular cancer, which was then applied to the less common ovarian germ cell cancers, is considered one of the triumphs of cancer treatment. The standard regimen for germ cell tumors is a combination of bleomycin (Blenoxane), etoposide (VePesid, Etopophos) and cisplatin (Platinol), sometimes referred to as BEP.

Virtually all women with early-stage germ cell tumors are expected to survive long term after treatment with surgery and, possibly, chemotherapy. Among women with advanced-stage disease, about 80 percent are cured with surgery and chemotherapy.

Like women with borderline ovarian tumors, women with germ cell tumors who are treated by removing only the affected ovary generally have an excellent chance of conceiving after treatment. Studies of women who've had fertility-sparing surgery found that the majority resumed their normal menstrual periods within six months of chemotherapy and were able to conceive. In addition, studies haven't found any increased risk of birth defects in the children born to women who had chemotherapy for this type of cancer.

For women with recurrent germ cell tumors, treatment options may include chemotherapy, additional surgery, radiation therapy or some combination of these treatments. Some women with recurrent cancer may be candidates for a clinical trial of high-dose chemotherapy medications with stem cell or bone marrow transplantation.

Sex Cord-Stromal Tumors

Cancerous (malignant) sex cord-stromal tumors (stromal tumors) represent about 7 percent of all ovarian cancers. These tumors form from cells in the connective tissue (stroma) of the ovaries. The different types of sex cord-stromal tumors are named for different types of cells found in this part of the ovary. The most common type is called a granulosa cell tumor, which accounts for 70 percent of malignant sex cord-stromal tumors.

Some sex cord-stromal tumors make sex hormones such as estrogen. As a result, these tumors may cause a girl to enter puberty early or a woman past menopause to have vaginal bleeding. Sex cord-stromal tumors generally aren't fast growing and don't spread rapidly. Because most are discovered before they've spread outside the ovary, treatment for this form of ovarian cancer is usually successful.

Granulosa cell tumors

Granulosa cell tumors arise from granulosa cells, which normally produce estrogen. Therefore, most granulosa cell tumors also secrete estrogen. The two forms of this tumor are adult and juvenile. The adult type is far more common. Most adult granulosa tumors are discovered at an early stage and have a favorable prognosis. Only 5 percent of these tumors are the juvenile type. Juvenile granulosa cell tumors usually occur in young girls or in women under age 30.

MYTH vs. FACT

Myth: **Exposing a tumor to air during surgery causes cancer to spread.**

Fact: Because you may feel worse during your recovery than you did before surgery, you might believe the surgery caused your cancer to spread. However, air hitting the tumor doesn't cause cancer to spread.

Although it's possible that during surgery your doctor may find the cancer to be more widespread than previously thought, an operation can't cause cancer to spread nor can it cause cancer to start. Surgically removing a cancer is often the first and most important treatment.

The adult type of granulosa cell tumor can occur at any age but is most often diagnosed in women between the ages of 50 and 54. The most common signs and symptoms are postmenopausal vaginal bleeding, abdominal pain and swelling. Premenopausal women may experience menstrual irregularities or abnormal bleeding.

If you have signs and symptoms such as these, your doctor will likely do a pelvic examination. Most women with this type of tumor have an abdominal or pelvic mass that can be felt during a pelvic exam. A pelvic ultrasound also may be done to gather more information about the mass. Surgery is necessary to confirm the diagnosis and to establish the stage of disease. The surgery and staging of granulosa cell tumors are generally the same as for epithelial tumors. Surgical and staging procedures are described in Chapters 16 and 17.

Granulosa cell tumors tend to grow slowly, and they don't usually spread outside the ovary. Because of this, 80 percent to 90 percent of these tumors are stage I at the time of diagnosis.

The primary treatment for granulosa cell tumors is surgery. For postmenopausal women, surgery typically includes removal of both ovaries, both fallopian tubes and the uterus. For younger women with early-stage disease who still want to have children, the uterus and unaffected ovary may be preserved. If the cancer has spread to other areas in the abdominal cavity, your surgeon will attempt to remove as much of the cancer as possible.

Women with stage I cancer — cancer that's confined to the ovary — generally need no treatment beyond surgery. Most women with higher stage disease are advised to have additional (adjuvant) therapy after surgery. This usually takes the form of platinum-based chemotherapy, although radiation may be an option in certain circumstances. Hormone-based therapies also may be considered. Because granulosa cell tumors grow slowly, a recurrence can occur years after the original diagnosis.

Because most women with granulosa cell tumors are diagnosed at stage I, their prognoses are excellent. The 10-year survival for stage I disease is approximately

GYNECOLOGIC CANCERS

90 percent. For women with more advanced tumors, survival figures range from 25 percent to 50 percent.

Others

Other types of stromal tumors are named for the cells in which they originate. Some sex cord-stromal tumors contain a mixture of cell types. In addition to granulosa cell tumors, other sex cord-stromal tumors include:

- **Thecomas.** Arising from theca cells, which normally surround the ovarian follicles, these tumors generally occur in women in their 60s and 70s. The tumors may cause postmenopausal bleeding, but they're usually benign.
- **Fibromas.** These tumors originate in the cells that form collagen in the supportive tissue of the ovary. Almost all fibromas are benign. They're most common during middle age.
- **Sertoli cell and Leydig cell tumors.** These extremely uncommon tumors arise from primitive cells that are similar to cells in the male testes and may produce male sex hormones (androgens). Tumors that make these hormones can cause conditions such as male-pattern hair growth in women.

Simultaneous Tumors

Some women develop ovarian cancer and endometrial cancer at the same time. Most often, the two tumors are thought to have developed independently, and they're referred to as independent primary tumors. Less commonly, cancer in the ovary may have spread (metastasized) from the endometrium, or vice versa.

Generally, doctors are able to distinguish between independent and metastatic tumors by examining the tumor cells under a microscope and taking into account factors such as tumor size and whether one or both ovaries are involved. Sometimes, though, it can be difficult to determine whether a tumor is an independent primary cancer or a metastatic cancer. Researchers are working on several new methods for distinguishing between the two by studying genetic changes in the tumors. This may help with planning appropriate treatment.

The development of simultaneous tumors in the endometrium and ovary is more common than would be expected given the frequency of these two types of cancer. One reason ovarian and endometrial tumors might develop at the same time is that the two cancer types share several of the same risk factors. For example, women who haven't given birth are at higher risk of both types of cancer. In addition, use of birth control pills can reduce the risk of both ovarian and endometrial cancer.

The discovery of a second simultaneous tumor typically comes to light when surgery is performed to treat a known cancer of either the ovary or the endometrium. When tissues from the other organ are examined in the laboratory, that organ also is found to be harboring a cancer.

Among women with simultaneous tumors of the ovary and endometrium, the prognosis is excellent when the tumors are confined to the ovary and uterus. In one study, even among women whose cancer had spread within the pelvis, only 15 percent had a cancer recurrence within five years of being treated.

Treatment for simultaneous tumors is generally surgery followed by chemotherapy, radiation therapy or both. The treatment plan will be tailored to whichever cancer appears most aggressive. Treatment for ovarian cancer is described in Chapter 17, and treatment for endometrial cancer is discussed in Chapter 23.

Gestational Trophoblastic Disease

Gestational trophoblastic disease (GTD) is a general term for a group of rare, interrelated tumors that start in the placenta. Unlike cervical or endometrial cancer, GTD doesn't develop from cells of the uterus. Rather, it results from abnormalities within the trophoblast, a special layer of cells surrounding the embryo. The trophoblast begins to develop immediately after conception and eventually forms the placenta, which protects and nourishes the growing fetus. The word *trophoblast* comes from the Greek words *tropho*, meaning "nutrition," and *blast*, which means "bud."

GTD includes several types of tumors. They account for less than 1 percent of all gynecologic cancers. Fortunately, all forms of GTD can be treated effectively. In the last 30 years, GTD has gone from being one of the most fatal cancers in women to one of the most curable, thanks to the development of effective chemotherapy. In most cases, treatment produces a com-

plete cure, even when the cancer has spread to other organs.

The most common type of GTD is called a hydatidiform mole. Another term for the condition is a *molar pregnancy*. This is a pregnancy in which there's an abnormal placenta without a normal fetus. A molar pregnancy can lead to the development of two other types of GTD — an invasive mole and a choriocarcinoma. Choriocarcinomas can also develop after a normal pregnancy and delivery, an abortion, a miscarriage, or a tubal (ectopic) pregnancy.

Hydatidiform mole

With a hydatidiform mole, instead of a normal embryo, an abnormal mass (mole) forms inside the uterus after fertilization. The mole has fluid-filled clusters of cyst-like swellings that look like bunches of grapes. Hydatidiform moles don't spread and aren't cancerous, but they can develop into cancer.

Hydatidiform moles are rare, occurring in only about one of every 1,500 pregnancies in the United States. The two types of molar pregnancies are complete and partial. A complete hydatidiform mole contains no fetal tissue, and a partial mole contains some tissue from an abnormal fetus. Some cases of molar pregnancy stem from abnormalities in fertilization, such as a sperm fertilizing an egg that contains no chromosomes or two sperm cells penetrating the egg, resulting in three sets of chromosomes rather than the normal two sets.

Molar pregnancies are almost always diagnosed in the first 12 weeks after

Molar Pregnancy: Who's at Risk?

Women older than age 40 and younger than age 20 are at higher risk of molar pregnancy. The eggs of older women may be more susceptible to abnormal fertilization, which is one cause of molar pregnancies. Why younger women are at increased risk is unknown.

Risk is also higher in women with a history of miscarriage and infertility. Having one molar pregnancy slightly increases your risk of having another one, and this risk continues to rise with each molar pregnancy.

conception. Vaginal bleeding is the most common sign. In addition, a molar pregnancy often results in higher than expected levels of a pregnancy hormone called human chorionic gonadotropin (HCG). This hormone is produced by trophoblastic cells of normal placentas and by a molar pregnancy. Because molar pregnancies and other forms of GTD usually release more HCG than does a normal placenta, higher than expected levels of HCG in the blood can indicate a problem. Other signs may include excessive vomiting caused by hormonal imbalance and abdominal swelling caused by a uterus that's enlarged beyond the expected size for the stage of the woman's pregnancy.

Often, a woman learns that she has a molar pregnancy when she has an ultrasound in early pregnancy, typically because of abnormal bleeding. In a molar pregnancy, the ultrasound reveals that there's no fetus. Sometimes, a diagnosis is made following a miscarriage by analyzing the tissue remaining from conception.

Treatment of hydatidiform mole consists of removal of the tumor, usually by suction curettage or dilation and curettage (D and C). A special instrument is used to stretch the opening of the uterus (cervix), allowing a vacuum-like device to be inserted to remove most of the material. A doctor then scrapes the lining of the uterus with a long, spoon-like instrument to remove any remaining molar tissue. For women who don't want to have any more children, removal of the uterus (hysterectomy) is an option.

After the mole is removed, you'll be monitored carefully. Your HCG levels will be checked frequently until they've returned to normal. Continued high levels of beta HCG after a molar tumor has been removed suggest a persistent problem. Despite apparent removal of a mole, invasion of the uterine wall occurs in 15 percent of cases, and 4 percent result in distant spread to other locations.

Women with molar pregnancy who are considered at high risk of persistent GTD are those who had a complete molar pregnancy, very high HCG levels and a markedly enlarged uterus.

Invasive mole and choriocarcinoma

In about 15 percent of women with complete molar pregnancies, and a smaller percentage of women with partial molar pregnancies, an invasive mole develops after treatment for the initial molar pregnancy. An invasive mole is a hydatidiform mole that penetrates the muscular wall of the uterus (myometrium). This can lead to heavy bleeding. Most invasive moles are only locally invasive — meaning they haven't spread beyond the uterus. About 15 percent of invasive moles spread (metastasize) to other sites, usually the lungs.

About 4 percent of women with a complete hydatidiform mole develop another type of gestational trophoblastic tumor, called choriocarcinoma, after removal of the initial tumor.

Choriocarcinoma is a malignant tumor that forms in the chorion, a layer of the trophoblastic membrane that surrounds the fetus. Only about half of all choriocarcinomas stem from a molar pregnancy, though. About 25 percent begin in tissue that remains in the uterus after a miscarriage, abortion or ectopic pregnancy. Another 25 percent occur after a normal pregnancy and delivery.

Choriocarcinoma tends to spread to other areas of the body, most commonly the lungs, vagina, pelvis, liver and brain.

Signs and symptoms of invasive mole and choriocarcinoma may include vaginal bleeding, elevated HCG levels in the blood, abdominal swelling or pain, and infection of the uterus. A tumor that has spread to other sites may cause signs and symptoms such as coughing, coughing up blood, chest pain and a mass in the vagina.

The treatment and prognosis for these tumors depend on several factors, including the type of tumor and whether it has spread to other locations. The tumors are staged from I to IV, and treatment varies by stage.

For invasive moles and choriocarcinomas that haven't spread to other parts of the body, treatment usually involves mild, single-agent chemotherapy. If a woman no longer wishes to have children, a hysterectomy may be performed.

For more advanced tumors that have spread (metastatic tumors), treatment usually includes combination chemotherapy. The choice of drugs depends on a woman's prognosis, which in turn depends on the extent and location of disease spread, how high the HCG level is and the amount of time that has passed since the pregnancy.

A highly curable disease

Gestational trophoblastic disease can be emotionally draining because you may also be dealing with the loss of a pregnancy. Many women with GTD experience anxiety, fatigue, anger and concerns about their fertility. But there are many reasons for optimism and hope.

Virtually 100 percent of women with molar pregnancy, nonmetastatic GTD and low-risk metastatic GTD are cured with appropriate treatment. Even among women with disease that has spread, 80 percent to 90 percent experience long-term survival after treatment.

Women who've had a molar pregnancy generally can have normal pregnancies later, though their risk of developing another molar pregnancy is slightly increased. For this reason, if you've had

GYNECOLOGIC CANCERS

a molar pregnancy and you become pregnant again, your doctor likely will do an ultrasound examination in the first trimester to make sure that the fetus is developing normally.

Women treated for GTD generally aren't at higher risk of having babies who are stillborn, premature or affected by birth defects.

Chapter 20: Gynecologic Cancers

Fallopian Tube Cancer

The fallopian tubes serve as the passageway between the ovaries and the uterus. They play a key role in reproduction as the site where fertilization takes place. Very rarely, cancer develops in these thin, muscular tubes. Fallopian tube cancer is the least common gynecologic cancer. It accounts for less than 1 percent of all cancers of the female reproductive tract. About 300 women in the United States are diagnosed with fallopian tube cancer each year.

Although cancer that starts in a fallopian tube is rare, the fallopian tubes are a relatively common site for the spread of other gynecologic cancers, particularly ovarian cancer. In up to half of women with ovarian cancer, the tumor spreads to a fallopian tube. Most tumors found on a fallopian tube have spread there from another site.

In many respects, fallopian tube cancer is similar to ovarian cancer. The two cancers look alike under a microscope, they're composed of similar types of cells, and they spread in the same way. Treatment of fallopian tube cancer has been modeled on the approach used for ovarian cancer. But the signs and symptoms of the two diseases are different, as are the criteria for diagnosis.

What Is Fallopian Tube Cancer?

It is in a fallopian tube that fertilization generally takes place when a sperm penetrates an egg that has been released from one of the ovaries. The fertilized egg then travels down the tube and implants itself into the uterus.

The fallopian tubes are made up of three layers of tissue. An inner lining of mucosal tissue is surrounded by a layer of muscle. The layer of muscle is surrounded by a coating tissue called the serosa. The mucosal lining of the inner surface of the fallopian tubes is referred to as the epithelium. It's similar to the epithelial tissue covering the surface of the ovaries.

The majority of fallopian tube cancers arise in the epithelium. But even though the epithelial surface area of the fallopian tubes is much greater than that of the ovaries, epithelial ovarian cancer is much more common than fallopian tube cancer.

Like ovarian cancer, fallopian tube cancer is classified according to the microscopic appearance of its cells. The main cell types are serous, mucinous, endometrioid and clear cell. Other, more rare subtypes are squamous, glassy cell and mixed cell. More than 90 percent of fallopian tube cancers are of the serous type. The medical term for this form of the cancer is *papillary serous adenocarcinoma*.

When viewed under a microscope, epithelial fallopian tube cancer of one cell type looks identical to that same type of epithelial ovarian cancer. The two cancers also spread in a similar way — cancer cells may be shed into the abdominal cavity and implant themselves on the lining of the cavity (peritoneum) and the surface of nearby organs. These cancers can also spread to distant sites through the lymphatic system or bloodstream.

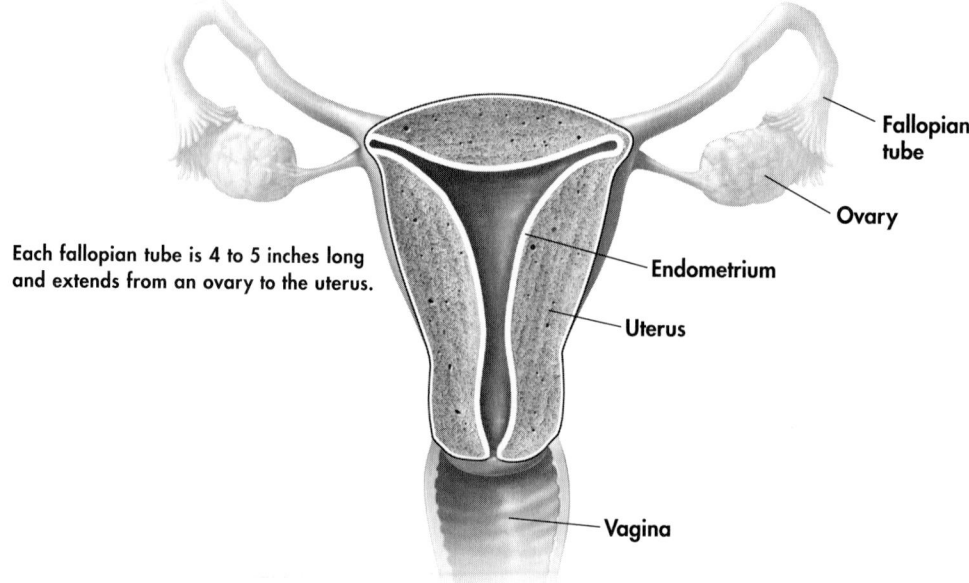

Each fallopian tube is 4 to 5 inches long and extends from an ovary to the uterus.

Fallopian tube

Ovary

Endometrium

Uterus

Vagina

Because fallopian tube cancer is so rare, little is known about its causes and risk factors. In about 10 percent of the women with this cancer, an inherited mutation in breast cancer gene 1 (BRCA1) or breast cancer gene 2 (BRCA2) is identified. These genes, which are involved in the repair of damaged DNA, are responsible for 5 percent to 10 percent of breast and ovarian cancers. For more information about BRCA gene mutations, see Chapter 4.

Some researchers have suggested that some ovarian cancers may actually arise in the fallopian tubes. According to this theory, cancerous (malignant) cells arise in the epithelial lining of a fallopian tube and then extend from the tube to involve the surface of the ovary.

This theory is unproved, but studies do show that tubal ligation — having your "tubes tied" — lowers the risk of ovarian cancer. Other evidence comes from studies of women who tested positive for a breast cancer gene (BRCA) mutation — meaning they were at increased risk of breast and ovarian cancer. In a few women who chose to have their ovaries and fallopian tubes removed to reduce their cancer risk, previously undetected fallopian tube cancer was discovered.

Diagnosing Fallopian Tube Cancer

Fallopian tube cancer can occur in any adult woman, but it's most common in women in their 50s and 60s. Although ovarian cancer may not cause noticeable signs and symptoms early on, a woman with a fallopian tube tumor may have early warnings. The most common sign is unexplained watery vaginal discharge. Other signs and symptoms are pelvic pain and abnormal vaginal bleeding. Many women with fallopian tube cancer have a pelvic mass that can be felt during a pelvic examination.

Surgery is generally necessary to diagnose fallopian tube cancer, which is also true of ovarian cancer. This is because the signs and symptoms of tubal cancer can resemble those of other conditions, such as inflammation of the fallopian tubes, an ovarian tumor and pelvic inflammatory disease. The only way to know for sure if the signs and symptoms are from cancer is to examine the tubes. In addition, no test can reliably detect the presence of fallopian tube cancer, although several different methods of detection and diagnosis are being investigated (see page 358).

The surgery used to diagnose and treat fallopian tube cancer is similar to that used to diagnose and treat ovarian cancer. The procedure is called a laparotomy. In some situations, a less invasive procedure called laparoscopy may be performed. These surgeries are discussed in detail in Chapters 16 and 17.

As is the case with ovarian cancer surgery, the initial surgery for fallopian tube cancer serves several purposes. The surgeon first verifies that cancer is present and, if it is, then determines whether it's confined to a fallopian tube or has spread (metastasized) to other areas. In addition, the surgeon tries to determine if the tumor started in the fallopian tube or in another organ. Because ovarian and fallopian tube cancers look alike, the

GYNECOLOGIC CANCERS

surgeon and pathologist rely on several criteria to help distinguish between the two cancers.

In the case of fallopian tube cancer, the main tumor should be in the tube. The ovaries and lining of the uterus (endometrium) are either normal or contain less tumor than the fallopian tubes. The pathologist may examine the tumor cells to see if they show a pattern that's typical of epithelial fallopian tube cancer. He or she also looks for an area of the epithelium that shows a transition from normal to malignant cells, which can indicate that the cancer originated in the tube.

Staging

The findings from surgery and the examination of the cancer cells removed during surgery are used to stage fallopian tube cancer. Staging refers to the process of determining whether the cancer has spread and, if so, how far. Staging is key

to determining treatment and the probable outcome of treatment (prognosis).

The system used to stage fallopian tube cancer is similar to the one most frequently used for ovarian cancer, the FIGO system of the International Federation of Gynecology and Obstetrics. On the four-stage FIGO scale, a lower number indicates that the cancer is still in its early stages, and a higher number reflects more extensive spread. Each of these stages also has several substages, such as stage IA, IB and IC. In one study that compiled reports on 558 patients with fallopian tube cancer, at diagnosis 33 percent had stage I cancer, 33 percent had stage II cancer, and 34 percent had stage III or IV cancer.

New methods of detection

No screening test can detect fallopian tube cancer at an early stage. Researchers are studying possible methods to do so. They include the following:

Fallopian tube cancer stages and 5-year survival rates

Stage	Description	5-year survival rate
Stage I	The cancer is limited to one or both fallopian tubes.	70%
Stage II	The cancer involves one or both fallopian tubes and has spread into the pelvic area.	40%-60%
Stage III	The tumor affects one or both fallopian tubes with spread into lymph nodes or outside the pelvic area to other parts of the abdominal cavity. The tumor may initially appear to be limited to the pelvic area, but samples of tissue taken from the upper abdomen show microscopic cancer deposits.	20%-30%
Stage IV	The cancer involves one or both fallopian tubes with spread to distant organs, such as to the lungs or liver.	Less than 15%

Ultrasound

Ultrasound (sonography or ultrasonography) uses high-frequency sound waves to produce images of the inside of the body. In transvaginal sonography, a transducer about the size of a tampon is inserted in the vagina. This ultrasound can show growths or tumors on the fallopian tubes.

During the last decade, researchers have reported success in diagnosing fallopian tube cancer using ultrasound imaging. Typically, a mass in a fallopian tube shows up in a distinct pattern similar in appearance to a cogwheel. A procedure called transvaginal color-flow Doppler may be used along with ultrasound to help determine whether the mass is more likely to be cancerous (malignant) or non-cancerous (benign) based on the way the blood vessels look. Ultrasound is used mainly in combination with other diagnostic techniques. Ultrasound is described in more detail in Chapter 16.

CA 125 blood test

CA 125 is a circulating protein that's produced by a variety of cells in the body as well as by certain cancer cells, including ovarian and fallopian tube cancers. A blood test can measure a person's level of CA 125. Most healthy women have CA 125 levels below 35 units per milliliter (u/mL) of blood. In women with fallopian tube cancer, CA 125 levels are usually above 65 u/mL. The problem is, several other benign and malignant conditions also can cause elevated CA 125 levels. For example, levels may be elevated in women with endometriosis or pelvic inflammatory disease or in early stages of pregnancy.

Researchers are studying the possibility of using CA 125 tests in conjunction with ultrasound to diagnose fallopian tube cancer. For now, this blood test is most commonly used to monitor a woman's response to treatment for fallopian tube cancer.

Magnetic resonance imaging

Magnetic resonance imaging (MRI) uses magnetic fields and radio waves to generate multiple cross-sectional images of the inside of the body, such as the pelvic and abdominal organs. An MRI scan can help identify a tumor and its spread.

Some studies have found that MRI is better than are ultrasound and computerized tomography (CT) in differentiating the fallopian tube from other pelvic organs. But ultrasound is still considered a superior test for evaluating a pelvic mass because it provides detailed close-up views and it's the most cost-effective method.

Positron emission tomography

A type of imaging test called positron emission tomography (PET) may be used to look for areas where the cancer may have spread. In this test, radioactive glucose (sugar) is injected into a vein. Because malignant tumors use sugar much faster than normal tissues do, the cancerous tissue takes up more of the radioactive material than the normal tissue does. A scanner can then detect the radioactive deposits. PET scanning is expensive and is still considered investigational. Whether it would add useful information must be decided on an individual basis.

Estimating Survival

The stage of the cancer is the most important factor in estimating the probable outcome of treatment, what's commonly referred to as prognosis. Another factor that affects survival is how much disease remains after surgery. The goal of surgery is to remove as much of the cancer as possible because this improves the chances of survival.

Doctors can use your disease stage to predict your estimated length of survival, and they can give you survival rates for women who have been diagnosed with cancer similar to yours.

But survival statistics don't tell the whole story. They only serve to provide a general picture and a standard way for doctors to discuss prognosis. Every woman's situation is unique. This is especially true for an uncommon disease like fallopian tube cancer, where the studies tend to be small and without well-defined patient groups.

Even if the statistic you receive is alarming, don't give up on your efforts to cure or control the cancer.

Treating Fallopian Tube Cancer

Treatment for fallopian tube cancer is similar to that for ovarian cancer. The first step is thorough surgical staging and removal of the tumor. For most women, chemotherapy is recommended after surgery. Radiation may be used only in very specific situations.

Surgery

For most women with fallopian tube cancer, surgery involves removing the fallopian tubes, ovaries and uterus. The medical term for this surgery is *total abdominal hysterectomy with bilateral salpingo-oophorectomy*. For some younger, premenopausal women with an early-stage, low-grade (slow-growing) tumor, another option may be less extensive surgery in which an ovary, a fallopian tube and the uterus are left in place. But this is a very uncommon situation.

Surgery usually also includes removal of the fatty apron in the front of the abdomen (omentum), where cancer cells can collect, and removal of lymph nodes in the pelvic and abdominal areas. If the surgeon finds that the cancer has spread within the abdominal cavity, he or she will try to remove as much visible tumor as possible, a process called debulking (cytoreduction). The goal is not to leave any tumor deposits larger than 1 centimeter in diameter. Women with smaller amounts of cancer remaining after surgery have higher survival rates than do women with larger amounts of remaining cancer.

A second surgery, called second-look laparotomy or second-look surgery, may be considered for some women with fallopian tube cancer after completion of chemotherapy. Second-look surgery allows the surgeon to see if any cancer remains after the chemotherapy. If the surgeon finds cancer, he or she may perform further surgery to remove all visible cancer, and additional chemotherapy may be given. Because second-look surgery

The Right Doctor

Because fallopian tube cancer is so rare, it may be difficult to find a specialist with experience in treating it. Surgery for fallopian tube cancer is complex, and staging the cancer accurately and removing as much of it as possible are crucial to the effectiveness of subsequent chemotherapy and long-term survival. It's important to get a referral to a gynecologic oncologist, a surgeon who specializes in the care and treatment of women with cancers of the reproductive tract.

has not been shown to improve overall survival in women with ovarian or tubal cancer, use of this procedure is controversial. Second-look surgery is discussed in further detail in Chapter 17.

Chemotherapy

Fallopian tube cancer responds relatively well to treatment with chemotherapy. Chemotherapy is a whole-body (systemic) treatment approach that uses drugs to try to kill any remaining cancer cells. Even if all visible cancer is removed during surgery, it's likely that microscopic cancer cells remain.

Chemotherapy for the treatment of fallopian tube cancer is similar to chemotherapy for ovarian cancer. Usually a combination of the drugs carboplatin (Paraplatin) and paclitaxel (Taxol) is used. The drugs target cancer cells that may have spread throughout your abdominal cavity or entered your bloodstream or lymphatic system and traveled to other parts of your body.

Other medications your doctor may recommend include cisplatin (Platinol), topotecan (Hycamtin) and doxorubicin (Adriamycin). These medications and

information about the way chemotherapy is administered and its possible side effects are discussed in Chapter 17.

Radiation therapy

Radiation therapy uses high-energy X-rays to kill cancer cells. Because fallopian tube cancer, like ovarian cancer, tends to remain localized in the abdomen and pelvis, radiation therapy to these areas is one option for treating the disease. However, use of radiation therapy for fallopian tube cancer is a matter of debate, just as it is for ovarian cancer. Generally, tubal cancers are treated with chemotherapy after surgery.

When radiation is used to treat fallopian tube cancer, it's generally delivered to the pelvis, the lymph nodes along the main blood vessel in the upper abdomen (aorta), or the whole abdomen. The radiation is tailored specifically to the person receiving it, depending on where cancer was found during surgery.

External beam radiation is more commonly used than is internal radiation. External radioactive beams are aimed at a specific target. The X-rays pass through your skin to reach the site

GYNECOLOGIC CANCERS

receiving radiation. The procedure is similar to having an X-ray except these treatment X-rays have much higher energy. Typically, treatment is administered five days a week for five to six weeks.

For more information on radiation therapy, see Chapter 17.

Surveillance and Follow-up

After you've been treated for fallopian tube cancer, you'll receive follow-up examinations to monitor your disease status. Although treatment aims to remove or kill all cancer cells, some microscopic cells may remain, causing a cancer recurrence.

You'll likely have follow-up exams every three to four months for the first couple of years after treatment. If you remain free of cancer for two years, the length of time between checkups may be extended. Most recurrences of fallopian tube cancer happen within three years of treatment.

During your follow-up appointments, you'll likely receive a physical examination, including a pelvic exam. During the pelvic exam, your doctor generally feels for any abnormalities in the pelvis that might indicate a cancerous growth. In addition, you may have a test to monitor the level of CA 125 in your blood.

If these tests raise any concerns, your doctor may also request an ultrasound or computerized tomography scan. Be sure to tell your doctor right away about any signs and symptoms you find worrisome,

especially if they're the same as those you had when you first received your diagnosis.

Chapter 21: Gynecologic Cancers

Endometrial Cancer Overview

Of all the cancers that affect the female reproductive tract, uterine cancer is the most common. About 40,000 American women receive a diagnosis of uterine cancer each year. Fortunately, approximately 80 percent to 85 percent of these women are cured of their disease.

Most cases of uterine cancer are discovered before the cancer has spread outside the uterus, when chances of a complete cure are the greatest. Vaginal bleeding after menopause — the most common sign of early-stage uterine cancer — usually prompts women to see a doctor.

Anatomy of the Uterus

The uterus is the hollow organ where a baby grows and develops during pregnancy. When you're not pregnant, it's about the size and shape of an upside-down, medium-sized pear.

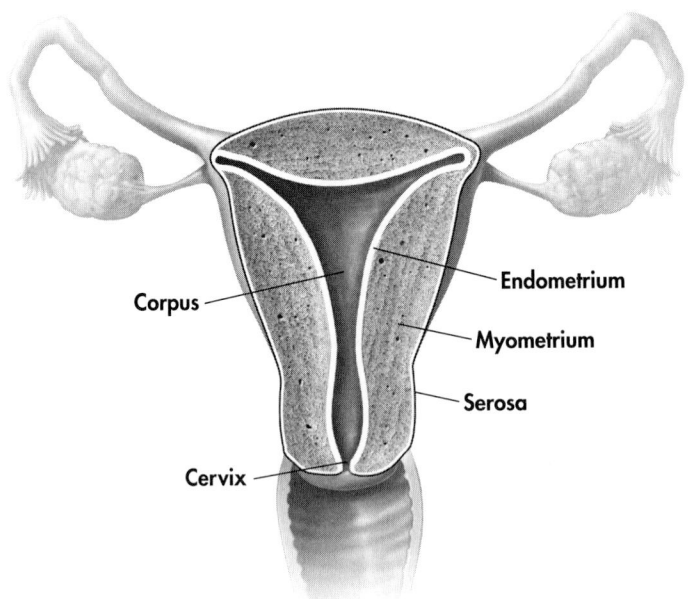

The uterine corpus has an inner lining known as the endometrium. The myometrium is a thick layer of smooth muscle tissue. Covering the myometrium is the serosa.

The uterus has two main parts. The lower, neck-like portion that extends into the vagina is called the uterine cervix. The upper, larger portion of the uterus is called the uterine corpus. It's also known as the body of the uterus.

The uterine corpus has an inner lining known as the endometrium. A portion of this thick, blood-rich lining is shed each month during your menstrual period. If fertilization has occurred, this is where the fertilized egg attaches and develops.

Two other layers of tissue make up the walls of the uterine corpus. The myometrium, a thick layer of smooth muscle tissue, contracts during menstruation as well as during childbirth. On top of the myometrium is the serosa, a thin, fibrous layer connecting the uterus to supporting ligaments.

Cancer can start in either the uterine corpus or the uterine cervix. In this book, we use the term *uterine cancer* to refer to cancers of the uterine corpus. Cancers affecting the cervix (cervical cancers) are discussed in Chapters 26 through 30. This chapter focuses on the most common form of cancer to affect the uterine corpus, endometrial cancer, which accounts for about 95 percent of all uterine cancers.

Types of Endometrial Cancer

The medical term for endometrial cancer is *endometrial carcinoma*. Within this broad category are subtypes classified by how the cells appear under a microscope.

Endometrioid adenocarcinoma

Endometrioid adenocarcinoma is the most common form of endometrial cancer, making up 80 percent to 85 percent of all cases. This type of cancer is often preceded by a condition called atypical hyperplasia, in which there's an increase in the number of tissue cells (hyperplasia) in the endometrium and the cells begin to take on abnormal features (atypia).

Papillary serous carcinoma

Papillary serous carcinoma is a more aggressive cancer. Fortunately, it's also rare, making up less than 5 percent of endometrial cancers. Unlike most other types of endometrial cancer, papillary serous carcinoma usually arises from an endometrium that's inactive (atrophic) rather than one in which endometrial cells are increasing in number.

Clear cell carcinoma

Clear cell carcinoma also is a relatively rare form of endometrial cancer, affecting about 4 percent of women with the disease. However, it's considered to be one of the more aggressive types.

Mixed cell type

When an endometrial cancer has two or more different cell types, each making up 10 percent or more of the tumor, it's called a mixed cell type. About 10 percent of women with endometrial cancer have a mixed cell type tumor.

Others

Very rare forms of endometrial cancer include mucinous carcinoma, squamous carcinoma and undifferentiated carcinoma. Each occurs in about 1 percent of women with endometrial cancer.

How Common Is Endometrial Cancer?

Endometrial cancer is the most common cancer of the female reproductive tract, and the fourth most common cancer among American women, after breast cancer, lung cancer and colorectal cancer.

The number of new cases of endometrial cancer declined steadily between the mid-1970s and mid-1980s. However, cases

GYNECOLOGIC CANCERS

QUESTION & ANSWER

Q: **Is uterine cancer the same thing as endometrial cancer?**

A: Because *endometrial cancer* is the most common type of *uterine cancer*, people often use the terms interchangeably. However, this isn't quite accurate.

Most cancers of the uterine corpus start in the endometrium and are appropriately referred to as endometrial cancers. These cancers are discussed in this chapter. About 5 percent of uterine cancers, though, get their start in nearby muscle or connective tissue, instead of the endometrium. These cancers, known as uterine sarcomas, are discussed in Chapter 25.

increased between the mid-1980s and 2000. Deaths from the disease also rose significantly — more than doubling. This dramatic rise in endometrial cancer deaths is an area of active research. Some researchers suspect it might have to do with increased use of the hormone estrogen — taken by itself without the hormone progesterone — to relieve signs, symptoms and conditions associated with menopause.

Endometrial cancer most often occurs after menopause, in women between the ages of 50 and 70, but it can occur earlier in life. About 25 percent of cases of endometrial cancer occur in women younger than 50. Endometrial cancer among women under age 40 is quite rare, accounting for only 2 percent to 5 percent of all cases.

Endometrial cancer is about twice as common among white women as it is among black women and other ethnic and racial groups in the United States. However, deaths from endometrial cancer are higher among minorities. The reasons for these trends aren't well understood.

What Causes Endometrial Cancer?

Healthy cells grow and divide in an orderly way to keep your body working normally. But sometimes this tightly regulated process goes awry. Cells keep dividing even when new cells aren't needed. At a very basic level, this is cancer.

In endometrial cancer, cancerous (malignant) cells develop in the inner,

Uterine cancer incidence and deaths

Year	Cases	Deaths
1987	35,000	2,900
2004*	40,320	7,090

*Estimated cases

Source: American Cancer Society, "Cancer Facts and Figures 2004"

These figures refer to cancers of the uterine corpus. About 95 percent of cancers of the uterine corpus begin in the endometrial lining. These are called endometrial cancers. The remaining 5 percent begin in uterine muscle or connective tissue and are called uterine sarcomas. In recent decades, uterine cancer deaths have risen significantly.

glandular lining of the uterus. Why these cancer cells develop isn't entirely known. Scientists believe that increased exposure to the female hormone estrogen plays a key role in the development of many endometrial cancers. Excess estrogen given to laboratory animals produces increased cell growth in the endometrium (endometrial hyperplasia), as well as endometrial cancer.

Does this mean that estrogen causes endometrial cancer? Yes and no. Although estrogen appears to be an important factor in the development of endometrial cancer, exactly what occurs to cause the cancer isn't known. One possible explanation is called the unopposed estrogen hypothesis. According to this theory, when the cells of your endometrium are exposed to estrogen that's not offset (opposed) by the hormone progesterone, these cells start dividing and accumulating more quickly. This background sets the stage for an increased number of DNA replication errors — genetic mistakes, if you will.

FAST FACT

Most common cancers among American women

	Type	Estimated number of new cases in 2004
1.	Breast cancer	215,990
2.	Lung cancer	80,660
3.	Colorectal cancer	73,320
4.	Uterine (endometrial) cancer	40,320
5.	Ovarian cancer	25,580
6.	Non-Hodgkin's lymphoma	25,520
7.	Melanoma	25,200
8.	Thyroid cancer	17,640
9.	Pancreatic cancer	16,120
10.	Bladder cancer	15,600

Source: American Cancer Society, "Cancer Facts and Figures 2004"

These mistakes can ultimately result in completely transformed, malignant cells.

This idea is consistent with what doctors and scientists know about endometrial cancer. But again, the details aren't as clear. Scientists aren't sure whether estrogen is a direct cancer-causing agent (carcinogen) or whether it plays more of a supporting role.

Scientists have identified several factors that are associated with increased estrogen levels, as well as other factors that seem to increase the risk of endometrial cancer. New risk factors continue to emerge as well.

Risk Factors

A risk factor is anything that increases your chances of getting a certain disease, such as endometrial cancer. Scientists determine risk factors by reviewing the medical histories and lifestyles of different groups of people. They then calculate which characteristics seem to be linked to increased incidence of a particular disease. They compare the incidence of a given disease among people who possess a certain characteristic with the incidence of that disease among people who don't have that characteristic. This comparison yields a statistic called relative risk.

For example, data show that women who smoke have a relative risk of developing lung cancer of about 25, compared with women who don't smoke. That means they're 25 times as likely to develop lung cancer as are women who don't smoke.

Here's another example: Studies show that women who've taken the hormone estrogen alone after menopause, without the hormone progesterone — even for a short time — have an increased risk of developing endometrial cancer, compared with women who've never used estrogen. How much the risk is increased depends on how long a woman took estrogen without progesterone. That means that for endometrial cancer, the relative risk associated with unopposed estrogen use can range from two to 10. For more information on relative risk and risk measurement, see Chapter 4.

When it comes to cancer, there are many different kinds of risk factors. Some, such as age, race and family history, can't be changed. Others, such as obesity and smoking, can be.

Demographic risk factors

Demographic risk factors include factors such as your age, race and ethnicity.

Age
As you get older, your risk of endometrial cancer increases. About 95 percent of cases of endometrial cancer occur in women age 40 or older, with most occurring in women between ages 50 and 70. The average age at diagnosis is 60.

Race and ethnicity
Compared with black women and women of other ethnic and racial minorities in the United States, white women have about twice the risk of endometrial cancer. However, black women who get endometrial cancer are more likely to have advanced-stage disease at the time of diagnosis. Perhaps because of this, black women are almost twice as likely to die of the disease, once diagnosed, as are white women.

Reproductive risk factors

Your ovaries produce the two main female hormones, estrogen and pro-

> ### FASTFACT
>
> **Endometrial cancer risk by age**
>
> | Age | Risk |
> | --- | --- |
> | 39 or younger | 1 in 1,881 (0.05 %) |
> | 40 to 59 | 1 in 137 (0.73 %) |
> | 60 to 79 | 1 in 63 (1.59 %) |
> | Lifetime | 1 in 37 (2.7 %) |
>
> Source: National Cancer Institute, 2002

gesterone. In your menstruating years, the balance between these two hormones changes during each month. These shifts help the lining of your uterus to thicken in case it needs to nourish a fertilized egg or to shed tissue through menstruation if an egg isn't present.

When the balance of the female hormones estrogen and progesterone shifts more toward estrogen, your risk of developing endometrial cancer increases. That's because estrogen stimulates growth of the cells lining your uterus, while progesterone shuts off this growth. In fact, high lifetime exposure to estrogen appears to be the main risk factor for developing endometrial cancer.

Any factor that increases your exposure to estrogen over time, especially if it's not offset (opposed) by progesterone, leads to an increased risk of endometrial cancer.

Early onset of menstruation and late menopause
If you got your first period before age 12 and continue to have periods after age 50, you're at greater risk of endometrial cancer than are women who menstruate for fewer years. Studies suggest women who go through menopause in their mid- to

RESEARCH UPDATE

The genetics of endometrial cancer

Scientists are conducting research into the root causes of endometrial cancer. One major effort involves studying changes in certain genes that may cause cells in the endometrium to become cancerous.

Scientists have known for several years that abnormalities (defects) can change genes that control cell growth. Recently, studies have shed light on how such changes can cause normal endometrial cells to become cancerous.

Mismatch repair genes
Some of what doctors and scientists currently know about the causes of endometrial cancer comes from families who have an inherited tendency to develop colon cancer, endometrial cancer and ovarian cancer. This genetic defect is called hereditary nonpolyposis colorectal cancer (HNPCC) syndrome.

Scientists have pinpointed what appears to be the primary cause of HNPCC-related cancers. These cancers are caused by defects in the genes, called mismatch repair genes, that help repair damaged DNA. When these genes are defective, it sets the stage for an accumulation of mutations and, hence, cancer.

Tumor suppressor genes
Another category of genes that contributes to the development of endometrial cancer is tumor suppressor genes, which help maintain normal growth and development of cells. In so doing, they suppress the growth of tumors.

Studies show that a tumor suppressor gene called PTEN is often partially or completely inactivated in endometrial cancers. The most commonly mutated gene in human cancers — a tumor suppressor gene called p53 — may also play a role in endometrial cancer.

late 50s have an increased risk of endometrial cancer, compared with women who experience menopause earlier.

Early menstruation is less of a risk factor if you also experience early menopause. Likewise, late menopause isn't a risk factor for endometrial cancer if you got your first period later in your teens.

Never having been pregnant
During pregnancy, the balance of female hormones shifts more toward progesterone, which helps protect you from endometrial cancer. If you've never been pregnant, you don't get the benefit of this protection. As a result, your risk of developing endometrial cancer is higher than that of women who have had children. Most studies suggest that women who've never been pregnant have about two to three times the risk of endometrial cancer as that of women who have given birth.

Infertility
For some women, not becoming pregnant is a personal choice. For others, it's the

result of infertility. Infertility is usually defined as the inability to achieve pregnancy after one year of frequent sexual intercourse without using contraception.

Some doctors and scientists think that infertility increases the risk of developing endometrial cancer — above and beyond the excess risk associated with never having been pregnant.

Irregular ovulation or menstruation

Ovulation — the monthly release of an egg from an ovary in menstruating women — is partly regulated by the hormones estrogen and progesterone. Failure to ovulate and infrequent ovulation, important factors in female infertility, are associated with a slight increase in risk of endometrial cancer. This could be because these conditions can increase your lifetime exposure to estrogen.

Irregular ovulation sometimes leads to ceased or irregular menstrual periods. This also may increase your risk of endometrial cancer. Without the regular monthly sloughing of the uterine lining, tissue may build up, a condition called endometrial hyperplasia. This can set the stage for the development of cancer.

Endometrial hyperplasia

Often, endometrial cancer evolves from a condition called endometrial hyperplasia, in which cells lining the uterus overgrow and cause it to thicken. There are four main types of endometrial hyperplasia: simple, complex, simple atypical and complex atypical.

Simple hyperplasia, the most common type, refers to an excess of normal-appearing cells. It's very unlikely to

develop into endometrial cancer. It can go away on its own or with hormonal treatment. Complex hyperplasia refers to an increased thickness of the endometrium, similar to simple hyperplasia, but the cells — though they appear normal — are more crowded and have a more complex structure.

The term *atypical* signifies that the excess cells appear abnormal. Simple atypical hyperplasia and complex atypical hyperplasia refer to endometrial cells that are enlarged and whose center (nucleus) is irregular in size, shape or composition. These conditions are more serious.

Studies have shown progression to endometrial cancer in 1 percent of women with simple hyperplasia, 3 percent of women with complex hyperplasia, 8 percent of women with simple atypical hyperplasia and 29 percent of women with complex atypical hyperplasia. Risk of endometrial cancer among women with complex atypical hyperplasia is 25 to 30 times that of women who don't have the condition (see the chart on page 371).

Heavy menstrual periods, bleeding between periods and bleeding after menopause are common signs of endometrial hyperplasia. Treatment includes hormone therapy and follow-up exams, or removal of the uterus (hysterectomy). For more information, see Chapter 23.

Polycystic ovarian syndrome

Polycystic ovarian syndrome (PCOS) is a condition in which hormonal imbalances prevent regular ovulation and menstruation. The ovaries develop cysts and fail to release eggs.

Endometrial cancer risk factors

Characteristic	Relative risk
Abnormal increase in the number of endometrial cells and cells that take on abnormal features (complex atypical hyperplasia)	25.0 to 30.0

Obesity
    More than 30 pounds over ideal weight
    More than 50 pounds over ideal weight
	
	3.0
	10.0

Estrogen use without progestin	2.0 to 10.0
Late menopause	4.0
Tamoxifen use	2.0 to 3.0
Never being pregnant (nulliparity)	2.0 to 3.0
Diabetes	2.0 to 3.0
High blood pressure (hypertension)	1.5

Source: Gynecologic Cancer Foundation, 2000

Women with PCOS have elevated estrogen levels and lower levels of progesterone. This imbalance can increase the risk of endometrial cancer. Studies show that young women with PCOS have a higher risk of endometrial cancer.

Treating PCOS can help restore a monthly ovulation and menstrual cycle, decreasing the risk of endometrial cancer.

Estrogen-producing ovarian tumors

Some uncommon ovarian tumors produce estrogen, increasing your estrogen levels and therefore your risk of endometrial cancer. Specifically, studies show that some women with ovarian tumors called granulosa cell tumors or granulosa-theca cell tumors have a higher risk of endometrial cancer.

Estrogen therapy after menopause

In the past, doctors commonly prescribed the hormone estrogen to treat symptoms of menopause, without also prescribing a synthetic form of the hormone progesterone (progestin). Studies show that taking estrogen alone after menopause, without also taking progestin, increases risk of endometrial cancer. Women who've used estrogen alone — even for a short time — have at least two to three times the risk of endometrial cancer as do women who've never used it. The longer you use it, the greater the risk. An analysis of 30 different studies found that women who took estrogen alone for 10 years or more had almost 10 times the risk of endometrial cancer as did women who never took it.

As a result of these and other findings, hormone replacement therapy (HRT), or menopausal hormone therapy, as it's also called, now generally consists of estrogen combined with progestin. (If a woman has had a hysterectomy and no longer has a uterus, it's safe to take estrogen alone.)

GYNECOLOGIC CANCERS

This combination therapy poses no increased risk of endometrial cancer. Recent studies, though, have shown that some combination hormone therapies may increase the risk of developing other health problems, including blood clots and breast cancer. Use of hormones after menopause should be determined on an individual basis.

Lifestyle-related risk factors

Lifestyle-related risk factors are, at least partly, related to your environment and choices you make in your daily life.

Obesity

Obesity, roughly defined as being 30 pounds or more overweight, is a major risk factor for endometrial cancer. Scientists estimate that it could account for about 25 percent of all cases of the disease. The heavier a woman is, the higher her risk. Studies suggest that obesity increases the risk of endometrial cancer by three to 10 times, depending on the degree of obesity.

What's the link between obesity and endometrial cancer? Your ovaries produce most of the estrogen in your body. However, fat tissue also can change some hormones — those produced by the ovaries and adrenal glands — into estrogen. Thus, having excess fat tissue can increase your estrogen levels, increasing your risk of endometrial cancer. If you're obese and have been through menopause, you're at even higher risk of endometrial cancer. Your fat cells are making estrogen, but your ovaries are no longer making progesterone to oppose the estrogen.

High-fat diet

A high-fat diet can add to your risk of endometrial cancer by promoting obesity. Some scientists believe that fatty foods themselves may directly affect how your body uses estrogen, further increasing your risk of endometrial cancer.

Health-related risk factors

Health-related risk factors are associated with your personal health and your family health history.

Hereditary nonpolyposis colorectal cancer

Endometrial cancer tends to occur in some families that also have an inherited tendency to develop a certain type of colon cancer. This uncommon, inherited condition is called hereditary nonpolyposis colorectal cancer (HNPCC) syndrome, and it accounts for about 5 percent of all cases of colorectal cancer. It's caused by defects in certain genes responsible for repairing errors in DNA.

Aside from colorectal cancer, endometrial cancer is the most common form of cancer in families with HNPCC. As many as half of women with an HNPCC-related genetic defect will develop endometrial cancer. A 70-year-old woman with an HNPCC-associated mutation has a 60 percent chance of developing endometrial cancer during her remaining lifetime. However, endometrial cancer linked to HNPCC typically occurs earlier in life than do noninherited cancers.

If several of your family members have had colorectal cancer or endometrial cancer, consider having genetic counseling and testing. This can help determine if you and your family members have a high risk of developing these cancers.

Breast cancer or ovarian cancer

If you've had breast cancer or ovarian cancer in the past, you may be at increased risk of endometrial cancer. Some of the same risk factors for breast cancer and ovarian cancer also increase your risk of endometrial cancer.

Tamoxifen use

Tamoxifen is an anti-estrogen drug used to treat breast cancer. It's also used to help prevent breast cancer in women who have a high risk of developing it. Although it acts as an anti-estrogen on breast cancer cells, it acts like estrogen on some tissues, including the uterus. It can cause your uterine lining to grow, increasing your risk of endometrial cancer.

Among women who take tamoxifen to treat or prevent breast cancer, each year about one in 500 (0.2 percent) will develop endometrial cancer.

Women taking tamoxifen who haven't had a hysterectomy are advised to have a yearly pelvic exam and report any unusual vaginal bleeding to their doctors.

Diabetes

Endometrial cancer is more common among women who have diabetes. Because type 2 diabetes (formerly called adult-onset or noninsulin-dependent diabetes) is common among women who are overweight, many doctors think that obesity, not diabetes, actually increases a woman's risk of endometrial cancer.

However, some studies have compared women who are both overweight and diabetic with those who are overweight but not diabetic. They've found that the risk of endometrial cancer is higher among women who have both conditions. This evidence is further bolstered by women with type 1 diabetes (formerly called juvenile or insulin-dependent diabetes), the type in which the pancreas doesn't produce insulin. These women have higher rates of endometrial cancer even though their diabetes isn't caused by obesity.

High blood pressure

Some studies have found an association between high blood pressure (hypertension) and an increased risk of endometrial cancer. Other studies have failed to confirm this link. As with type 2 diabetes, it's hard to determine whether high blood pressure itself increases the risk of endometrial cancer or whether underlying obesity is to blame. This is because many individuals with high blood pressure also are obese.

Putting risk in perspective

Having one or even several risk factors for a particular condition doesn't mean that you'll develop it. Most women who have known risk factors for endometrial cancer never get the disease. At the same time, many women who develop endometrial cancer have no major risk factors for it. In most cases, doctors can't explain why one woman develops endometrial cancer and another doesn't.

If you're at higher risk of endometrial cancer, it's particularly important to have a yearly physical and to be aware of signs and symptoms of the disease.

Reducing Your Risk

Unfortunately, most cases of endometrial cancer happen for reasons that are unknown or beyond a woman's control. But you can do certain things that may lower your risk of developing the disease.

Taking progesterone with estrogen

Taking progesterone or a synthetic form of the hormone (progestin) with the hormone estrogen protects the lining of the uterus. Hormone replacement therapy (HRT) that includes both estrogen and progestin lowers your risk of endometrial cancer, compared with use of estrogen alone. It appears that you need to take progestin for at least 10 days each month to get this protection. Newer combination drugs contain a daily dose of both estrogen and progestin.

In addition to prevention of hyperplasia, progestins may be beneficial if hyperplasia develops. Studies show that a progestin can reverse increased endometrial growth (endometrial hyperplasia) caused by taking estrogen alone.

But not all of the effects of HRT are positive. All combination HRT regimens can cause irregular vaginal bleeding, particularly during the first year of use. HRT may also increase your risk of blood clots, gallbladder disease and heart disease. And taking HRT as a combination therapy — estrogen with medroxyprogesterone (Prempro) — for several years or more appears to slightly increase your risk of breast cancer. The long-term benefits of HRT, therefore, are under intense scrutiny.

If you're considering HRT, talk with your doctor about the risks and benefits.

Taking birth control pills

Studies show that using combination birth control pills (estrogen plus a progestin) can reduce your risk of endometrial cancer. Taking the pill for longer time periods provides greater risk reduction. A review of 11 different studies found that women who took birth control pills (oral contraceptives) for 12 years had a 72 percent reduced risk of endometrial cancer, and women who took them for four years reduced their risk by 56 percent. Some studies suggest that you need to take oral contraceptives for at least a year to get a protective benefit.

In addition, research suggests that the protective effect of birth control pills continues for at least 15 years after you stop taking them.

The risk of endometrial cancer isn't the only factor you should consider when choosing a method of birth control. Talk with your doctor about the pros and cons of different types of contraceptives.

Prompt evaluation for abnormal vaginal bleeding

Most endometrial cancers develop over many years. Often, cancer follows a less serious endometrial condition, such as endometrial hyperplasia.

Abnormal vaginal bleeding is the most common sign of precancerous hyperplasia and endometrial cancer. If you begin having especially heavy menstrual periods, have bleeding between periods or have bleeding after menopause, talk with your doctor.

Chapter 22: Gynecologic Cancers

Diagnosing Endometrial Cancer

Endometrial cancer typically causes unusual vaginal bleeding, either between menstrual periods or after menopause — a potential sign of illness that's easy to notice and that prompts most women to see a doctor. Because of this, endometrial cancer is often detected early, when it's most likely to be cured.

When detected and diagnosed early, this slower growing form of cancer is generally confined to the uterus. About 75 percent of women who have the most common type of endometrial cancer receive a diagnosis when the disease is still in its earliest stages.

Signs and Symptoms

If you've experienced menopause, be especially alert to the signs and symptoms of endometrial cancer. Endometrial cancer — cancer of the lining of the uterus (endometrium) — is primarily a disease of postmenopausal women. The average age at diagnosis is 65. However, the disease can occur earlier in life. About 25 percent of endometrial cancer cases occur in women younger than 50.

Signs and symptoms of endometrial cancer may include:

- Vaginal bleeding or spotting after menopause or during the time around menopause (perimenopause)
- Heavy menstrual periods or bleeding between periods
- A watery pink or white discharge from the vagina
- Pain in the lower abdomen or pelvic area
- Pain during sexual intercourse

For most women with endometrial cancer, the first clue that something is wrong is abnormal vaginal bleeding. This sign of illness occurs in more than 90 percent of women who have the disease. If you've gone through menopause, you may have a watery discharge that precedes bleeding by several weeks or months. In about 10 percent of cases, vaginal discharge associated with endometrial cancer is white instead of pink or blood-tinged.

The older you are when post-menopausal bleeding occurs, the more likely it is that the cause is endometrial cancer. Postmenopausal bleeding in a 50-year-old woman is associated with a 9 percent chance of endometrial cancer. In a 70-year-old woman, the likelihood increases to 28 percent. In an 80-year-old woman, the odds jump to 60 percent.

If you have abnormal vaginal bleeding or any other sign or symptom of endometrial cancer, see your doctor soon for an evaluation. It may be that your signs and symptoms are associated with a non-cancerous condition, such as a vaginal infection, uterine fibroid or uterine polyp. But it's still important to bring them to the attention of your doctor.

If it turns out that you do have endometrial cancer, chances are good that your disease will be found at an early stage.

Screening for Endometrial Cancer

When doctors and scientists talk about screening people for cancer, they're referring to something very specific. Screening for cancer means testing people for early stages of a disease, even though the people being tested have no signs or symptoms. Some cancer screening tests are relatively simple, such as a Pap test to check for cervical cancer. Others are more involved, such as a colonoscopy exam to detect the early stages of colon cancer.

Unfortunately, in the case of endometrial cancer, there's no effective screening test yet available.

With endometrial cancer, scientists have studied whether techniques used to diagnose the cancer, such as endometrial biopsy and transvaginal ultrasound, might be worthwhile as screening tests. But results suggest that they're not. In one study of 800 women with no signs or symptoms of endometrial cancer, endometrial biopsy detected only one

Early detection improves the chances that your cancer will be successfully treated. Some endometrial cancers can reach an advanced stage before they display signs and symptoms, but this is uncommon.

Diagnosing Endometrial Cancer

If your primary care doctor suspects that you have endometrial cancer, you may be referred to a gynecologist, a doctor who specializes in conditions affecting the female reproductive system. A gynecologist or your primary care doctor will likely perform a general physical examination, including a pelvic exam, and talk with you about your signs and symptoms, risk factors and family medical history. He or she may request tests and procedures needed to make an accurate diagnosis. These may include a transvaginal ultra-sound exam, endometrial biopsy and a minor surgical procedure called dilation and curettage (D and C).

Health history

Often, the first part of an evaluation for endometrial cancer is a discussion of your health history, including any risk factors for the disease. Risk factors are discussed in Chapter 21.

You may also have other medical problems that need to be evaluated to determine their effect, if any, on your treatment. Be sure to tell your doctor about any medical problems you have, including those you've had in the past. Also tell your doctor about any medications or herbal supplements you're taking.

Physical exam

The next step is often a complete physical examination. A thorough exam allows

case of endometrial cancer. Screening by way of endometrial biopsy isn't even recommended for women taking tamoxifen — a known risk factor for endometrial cancer.

The current recommendation of the American College of Obstetricians and Gynecologists is to perform an endometrial biopsy only if a woman develops bleeding. A yearly pelvic exam can find some cancers of the female reproductive system, but it's not a very effective way of finding early endometrial cancers. A Pap test can detect some early endometrial cancers, but only a relatively small number. It's a much better tool for detecting cervical cancer.

In the absence of a routine screening test for endometrial cancer, your best defense against the disease is to be informed. Familiarize yourself with its signs and symptoms, especially if you've gone through menopause or have known risk factors for the disease. Above all, if you have any abnormal vaginal bleeding or spotting, make an appointment to see your doctor.

your doctor to feel for suspicious lymph nodes or areas within the pelvis where cancer may have spread. As part of your assessment, your doctor may order some tests. A blood test called a complete blood count (CBC) is done to make sure you can safely undergo surgery. A CBC measures red blood cells, white blood cells and blood platelets. Often, women with excessive blood loss from endometrial cancer have a low red blood cell count (anemia). Other routine blood and urine tests may be done to make sure you don't have undetected health problems.

Pelvic exam

During a pelvic exam, you lie on your back on an examining table with your knees bent. Usually, your heels rest in metal supports called stirrups (see the illustration on page 296).

Your doctor first examines your external genitals to make sure they look normal — no sores, discoloration or swelling. The internal examination is next. To see the inner walls of your vagina and your cervix, your doctor inserts an instrument called a speculum into your vagina. When the speculum is in the open position, it holds your vaginal walls apart so that your cervix can be seen. Your doctor then shines a light inside to look for lesions, inflammation, signs of abnormal discharge and anything else unusual. Looking at your cervix also helps your doctor determine whether cervical cancer might be causing your bleeding.

Your pelvic exam may or may not include a Pap test — a test in which your doctor takes a sample of cells from your cervix by gently scraping it with a small spatula, brush or cotton swab. Because endometrial cancer begins inside the body of the uterus, not the cervix, it rarely shows up in the results of a Pap test.

After removing the speculum, your doctor checks the condition of your uterus and ovaries. This is done by inserting two lubricated, gloved fingers into your vagina and pressing down on your abdomen with the other hand. Usually, this is followed by a rectovaginal exam, done with one finger in your vagina and another in your rectum. This allows your doctor to locate your uterus, ovaries and other organs, judge their size and confirm that they're in the proper position. While exploring the contours of these organs, your doctor feels for any lumps or changes in the shape of your uterus that may indicate a problem.

You may be apprehensive about having a pelvic exam. Many women are. During the exam, try to relax as much as you can by breathing slowly and deeply. If you tense up, your muscles may tighten, which can make the exam even more uncomfortable. Let your doctor know if you're experiencing a lot of discomfort. Remember, a typical pelvic exam takes only a couple of minutes.

Ultrasound

Ultrasound may be used to examine the uterus, fallopian tubes and ovaries. The procedure may be done with a device called a transducer that's placed either on your abdomen (transabdominally) or within the vagina (transvaginally). For viewing the uterine lining, transvaginal ultrasound is most often used (see the illustration on page 297).

In a transvaginal ultrasound exam, a wand-like device (transducer) is inserted into your vagina. The transducer uses sound waves to create a video image of your uterus. This test helps your doctor evaluate the size and shape of your uterus and look for abnormalities in your uterine lining. Increased thickness of the uterine lining or tissue buildup can be a predictor of endometrial cancer. In some cases, transvaginal ultrasound images can help determine if an endometrial tumor is present and if it extends into the muscular wall of the uterus (myometrium).

Sometimes, sterile saline water is inserted into your uterus by way of a thin tube during the ultrasound test. The saline water enhances the image, making any abnormalities of the uterine lining more visible on video. This procedure is called a saline infusion sonogram (sonohysterogram). With a more detailed picture of your uterine lining, your doctor is better able to determine whether your problem might be related to a noncancerous condition, such as an endometrial polyp or uterine fibroid.

Ultrasound is an important imaging tool when evaluating a woman for one of several gynecologic diseases, including endometrial cancer. Its advantages are that it's safe, relatively inexpensive and noninvasive. It can detect a suspected endometrial cancer and, sometimes, provide information about whether the cancer has spread through the muscular uterine wall or to the cervix.

But ultrasound also has limitations. Transvaginal ultrasound isn't a definitive test. It can't indicate for certain whether you have endometrial cancer. It can only highlight abnormalities in your uterine lining that look suspicious. To know for sure whether you have cancer, your doctor must obtain a sample of tissue from your endometrium, through either an endometrial biopsy or a D and C.

Biopsy

Endometrial biopsy is a procedure in which your doctor removes a small piece of tissue from your uterine lining so that it can be examined under a microscope. It's a commonly performed diagnostic test for endometrial cancer.

QUESTION & ANSWER

Q: **Is a biopsy painful?**

A: You may feel some pain during an endometrial biopsy, something similar to menstrual cramps. Some women may also have cramps and vaginal bleeding for a few days after a biopsy.

To reduce your discomfort, your doctor may recommend that you take an over-the-counter pain reliever about an hour before the biopsy. If you have pain after the procedure, your doctor may prescribe one or two doses of a pain reliever.

Biopsy procedure

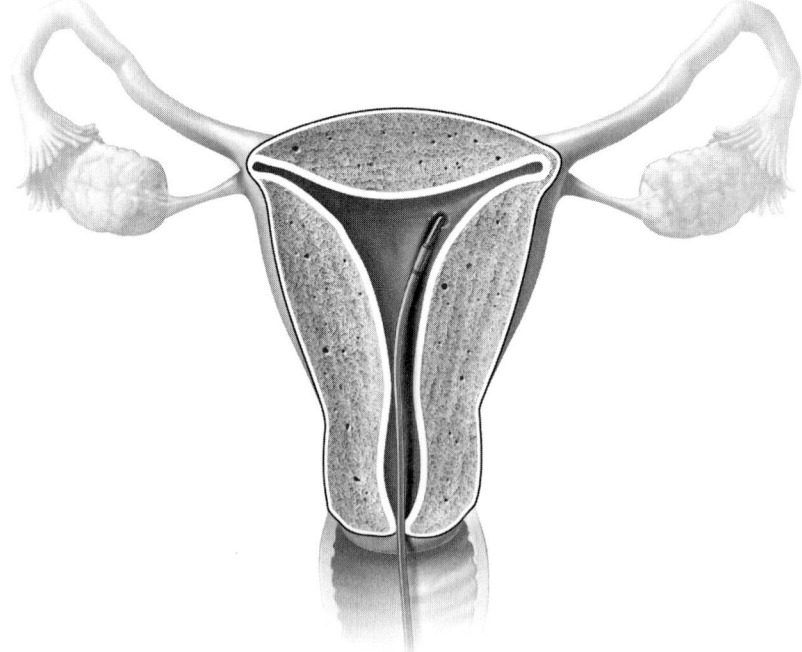

Endometrial biopsy is typically done in your doctor's office and usually doesn't require anesthesia. However, in some women who've gone through menopause, the opening into the cervical canal has closed off. The canal needs to be reopened, and therefore general anesthesia is required.

During an endometrial biopsy, your doctor uses a speculum to open your vagina and then threads the biopsy instrument — a flexible tube about the diameter of a thin straw — into your vagina, through the cervix and into the uterus. The biopsy instrument removes a small sample of your uterine lining, either through suction, scraping or both. The tissue is then sent to a laboratory, where a pathologist examines it under a micro-scope to determine whether cancer cells are present.

You may need a few minutes of rest after an endometrial biopsy, but you'll probably be able to drive yourself home and resume your normal activities right away. Before you leave your doctor's office, be sure to ask when and how you'll get the results of the biopsy.

After a biopsy, you may experience cramping, similar to menstrual cramping. And you may have some spotting for a day or two, requiring the need to wear a panty liner. If you experience heavy bleeding, call your doctor. Also call if you have any signs or symptoms that suggest infection, such as pain in your vagina or lower abdomen, foul-smelling vaginal dis-charge or fever.

D and C procedure

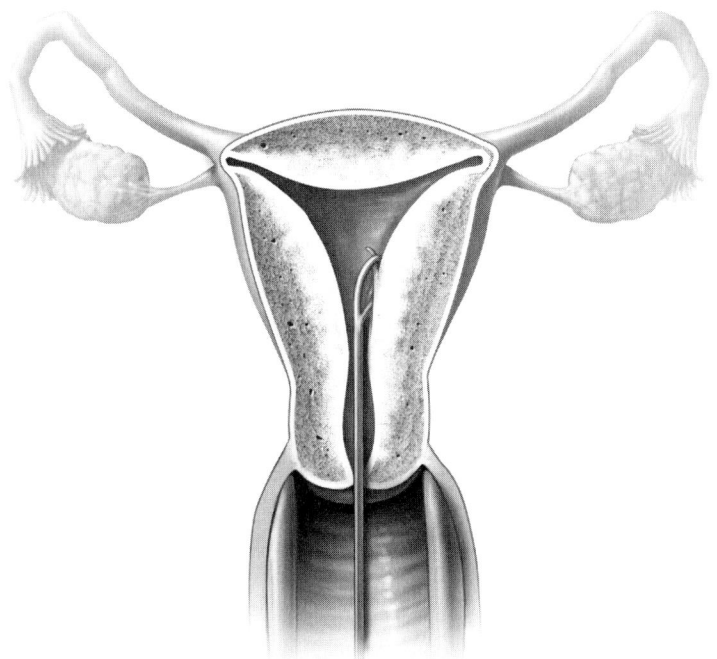

Dilation and curettage

In certain situations, a doctor wants to remove and examine the majority of cells that line the uterus. This minor surgical procedure is called dilation and curettage (D and C).

For the procedure, your doctor dilates your cervix by inserting a series of progressively enlarging rods into its opening. Once your cervix is dilated, your doctor scrapes endometrial tissue from the entire inside of your uterus using a thin, spoon-like surgical instrument called a curet, a low-pressure suction device or both. The tissue that's removed is then sent to a pathologist for analysis.

The procedure takes about an hour. You may have general anesthesia, in which

you're fully sedated, or conscious sedation, in which you're drowsy but awake.

As part of your D and C, your doctor may also insert a thin, telescope-like instrument through your vagina and cervix, directly into your uterine cavity. This procedure is called a hysteroscopy. Unlike endometrial biopsy or D and C, hysteroscopy allows your doctor to see the inside of your uterus.

Having a D and C generally doesn't require an overnight hospital stay. Most women go home the same day. You may experience some vaginal bleeding for a few days afterward, and you may have some cramps or back pain. But most women usually can resume normal activities almost immediately. However, you shouldn't have sexual intercourse or use

GYNECOLOGIC CANCERS

tampons until your cervix returns to normal and your endometrium is completely healed, which usually takes a few weeks.

Determining the Extent of the Cancer

If laboratory tests of your endometrial tissue show that you have cancer, the next step is to determine if the cancer is confined to the endometrium or if it has spread. This is known as staging. Staging typically involves imaging tests, followed by surgery. To stage your cancer, you'll likely be referred to a gynecologic oncologist — a surgeon who specializes in treating cancers of the female reproductive system.

Imaging tests

Imaging tests help provide your doctor an "inside view" of your internal organs. Imaging tests may be used to help determine if cancer has spread beyond the uterus to neighboring structures or, rarely, to the lungs or liver.

Chest X-ray

A chest X-ray is used to make an image of the lungs. It may be helpful in determining if the cancer has spread to your lungs. It can also indicate the presence of any lung or heart diseases, which could affect plans for treating your cancer.

Computerized tomography

A computerized tomography (CT) scan is a procedure that produces detailed images of your internal organs. Unlike a normal X-ray, which produces just one image of your body taken from one angle, a CT scan produces many images of your body taken at different angles. A CT scan also shows soft tissues, such as your uterus, much better than a regular X-ray does.

If pathology results from your endometrial biopsy or D and C indicate that your tumor is the least aggressive form and your uterus appears to be of normal size, your doctor may not need a CT scan before proceeding to surgical staging of your cancer. If tests show that your cancer may be a more aggressive form or your blood tests indicate abnormalities, your doctor may want you to have a CT scan or other imaging tests before surgical staging. This will help him or her determine how extensively your tumor has spread, if at all. The different types and grades of endometrial cancer are discussed later in this chapter.

During a CT scan, you lie faceup on a movable table. The table is guided into the center of the CT scanner, which looks like a giant doughnut. You lie still, holding your breath as directed, while an ultrathin X-ray beam passes through your body. Different tissues in your body absorb different amounts of the beam. An X-ray detector then measures the intensity of the beam that emerges from your body. All the measurements are processed by a computer to create a composite image.

Before your scan, you may be asked to drink a substance known as a contrast medium. It allows the radiologist to distinguish the outline of your stomach and intestines. After the first set of pictures is taken, you may receive another contrast medium — a dye that's injected into one of your veins. This injectable contrast medium can enhance the visual differences between normal tissues and abnormal cancerous areas, making small cancerous masses easier to find.

If your doctor thinks that your cancer may have spread beyond your uterus, he or she may recommend a CT-guided needle biopsy. For this procedure, you lie on a scanning table while your doctor carefully advances a biopsy needle toward any suspicious masses seen on the CT image. Once the biopsy needle is inside the mass, a small sample of tissue is removed and examined under a microscope for cancer cells.

Magnetic resonance imaging

Magnetic resonance imaging (MRI) uses magnetic fields and radio waves to create cross-sectional pictures of your body. These images display your internal organs with clarity, providing information not available with other imaging methods.

MRI is currently being investigated as a tool to determine how far an endometrial cancer has grown into the muscular wall of the uterus (myometrium). In some studies, MRI has been shown to be better than CT scanning for assessing whether cancer has spread to the cervix or the connective tissue between the uterus and pelvic side walls (parametrium).

During an MRI procedure, you're positioned on a motorized bed that's moved into the tunnel (cylinder) of the scanner. The scanner houses a powerful magnet that surrounds the cylinder. When atoms in your body are exposed to a very strong

magnetic field, they line up parallel to one another. Radio waves from a radio frequency magnet briefly knock the atoms out of their parallel alignment. As they realign, the atoms emit tiny signals, which are picked up and passed on to a computer. The computer then converts these signals into an image.

Sometimes, a contrast medium is injected into one of your veins to help improve image clarity, but this is done less often with MRIs than with CT scans.

An MRI procedure takes longer than does a CT scan — sometimes up to an hour. Some people, especially those bothered by claustrophobia, find the cylinder confining, in which case a sedating medication may be given. You may also be given headphones to wear because the MRI machine makes a thumping noise that can be disturbing.

Because of the strong magnet used, MRI may not be performed on people with certain implanted devices, such as pacemakers, inner ear (cochlear) implants and certain vascular clips. If you have an implanted device, make sure your doctor knows about it beforehand.

Surgery

The purpose of surgery in the diagnostic process is twofold. It's used to determine the extent of disease spread. Surgery is also used to treat the cancer.

Most often, a procedure called an exploratory laparotomy is done. After making an incision in the abdomen, a surgeon feels and views the pelvic and abdominal areas for signs of disease, looking especially close to see whether any

GYNECOLOGIC CANCERS

QUESTION & ANSWER

Q: **Why are all the reproductive organs removed during surgery if the cancer is just in the uterus?**

A: Endometrial cancer cells can spread to the ovaries and fallopian tubes very early in the disease. Removing the ovaries and fallopian tubes and testing them for cancer cells is the best way to tell whether this has happened.

tumors or suspicious lesions are outside the uterus. The surgeon also takes samples of fluid from the abdominal cavity (peritoneum) to test for cancer cells. This process of examining the uterus, pelvic organs and abdominal cavity for signs of cancers is referred to as surgical staging.

During the same procedure, the surgeon usually treats the cancer as well. The most common surgery is removal of the uterus, cervix, fallopian tubes and ovaries (total hysterectomy with bilateral salpingo-oophorectomy). In addition, the surgeon may remove lymph nodes from the pelvis and the area near the aorta, the large vessel supplying blood to the abdomen and pelvis. Lymph nodes are small, bean-shaped structures found throughout the body that produce and store infection-fighting cells. They're often early sites of tumor spread.

All the tissue removed during surgery is sent to a pathologist for analysis. This analysis, along with observations made during the surgery, allows your team of doctors to determine the stage of your cancer. One exception is an endometrial tumor so large that it's impossible to remove all the visible cancer. In such cases, doctors may first recommend other therapies, such as radiation therapy, with-

out removing the uterus. A hysterectomy may be performed after radiation.

As soon as the uterus is removed, the surgeon and pathologist examine it to see how far and how deep the cancer has spread. If the cancer has penetrated less than halfway through the muscular wall (myometrium), a surgeon may opt against removing any lymph nodes near the uterus or may just remove a small number of them.

In the case of a tumor that has spread more than halfway through the myometrium or if biopsy results suggest an aggressive type of endometrial cancer, a sample of lymph nodes is generally removed, even if the lymph nodes don't look suspicious. If a surgeon spots any enlarged lymph nodes, he or she will likely remove them for examination. The surgeon may also take samples of fatty tissue from the abdomen and have them sent to a pathologist for microscopic examination.

If the cancer has spread beyond the body of the uterus to the cervix, typically lymph nodes in the general area are removed so that they can be checked for cancer cells. If the cancer appears to have spread beyond the uterus, a doctor may perform a radical hysterectomy instead of a total hysterectomy. In a radical hysterectomy, the upper inch of the vagina and some surrounding tissue are removed, in addition to the uterus, cervix, fallopian tubes and ovaries.

Removal of the reproductive organs during surgery causes some women profoundly mixed feelings. Once the uterus is removed, pregnancy is no longer possible. For a woman in her childbearing years who wants to have a baby, this can be a difficult thing to accept. However, it's important to remember that surgery plays a key role in defeating endometrial cancer. In many cases, it can eliminate the cancer entirely, as well as the need for further treatment.

Pathology Report

All tissue removed during surgical staging for endometrial cancer is examined by a pathologist. He or she looks for and records a number of important factors that are essential in determining your treatment. These include the cancer's specific cell type and how aggressive it is (grade), how far it has extended into the muscular wall (myometrium) and whether it has spread to fluid in the abdominal cavity (peritoneum) or to surrounding structures or lymph nodes.

Cell type

The cells that line or cover most of your organs are called epithelial cells. Cancers that develop from these cells are called carcinomas. Therefore, the medical term for cancer that begins in the cells lining your uterus is *endometrial carcinoma.*

Within the broad category of endometrial carcinoma, different cell types have different microscopic appearances.

Endometrioid adenocarcinoma

Endometrioid adenocarcinoma is the most common type of endometrial cancer, making up 75 percent to 80 percent of all cases of the disease. Endometrioid adenocarcinoma cells resemble those that normally line the endometrium.

This cancer is typically seen in women with increased exposure to estrogen. In most cases, these cancers are diagnosed at an early stage and are less aggressive.

Papillary serous carcinoma

Papillary serous carcinoma behaves much more aggressively than does endometrioid adenocarcinoma. Fortunately, it's also less common, affecting fewer than 10 percent of women with endometrial cancer.

This cancer closely resembles the types of cells normally found in the ovary or fallopian tube. The cancer typically grows in the shape of a small mushroom.

Papillary serous carcinoma tends to occur in older and thinner women who don't have the classic estrogen-related risk factors for endometrial cancer. It tends to invade deeply into the muscular wall and spread to lymph nodes. Spread outside the uterus to the lining of the abdominal cavity (peritoneum) also is common.

Clear cell carcinoma

Clear cell carcinoma is a more rare form of endometrial cancer, affecting about 4 percent of women with the disease. However, it's another aggressive type of endometrial cancer. Under a microscope,

GYNECOLOGIC CANCERS

cells from clear cell carcinoma of the endometrium look similar to clear cell cancers that can arise in the cervix, vagina, ovaries and fallopian tubes.

Like papillary serous carcinomas, clear cell carcinomas tend to occur in older and thinner women who don't have the classic estrogen-related risk factors for endometrial cancer.

Grade

A microscopic view of the tumor cells allows a pathologist to give the cancer a grade. The grade depends on how normal or abnormal the cells appear. This determination is made in three ways:

- By looking at the growth pattern of the tumor (tumor architecture)
- By looking at the size and shape of the center portion of the cell (nucleus) that controls cellular functions
- By calculating the percentage of tumor cells that are dividing or growing

Generally, the lower the grade, the fewer the abnormalities and the better the prognosis. The higher the cancer grade, the more aggressive the cancer is and the greater the chances that it has invaded or will invade the muscular wall of your uterus and spread to lymph nodes. In fact, studies show that half of all high-grade (grade 3) endometrial cancers have spread more than halfway through the myometrium. Between 20 percent and 30 percent of these cancers spread to the pelvic and para-aortic lymph nodes.

Extent of myometrial invasion

In addition to assigning the cancer a cell type and grade, a pathologist also exam-

ines how deeply the cancer has spread into (invaded) the myometrium.

In the pathology report, the extent of myometrial invasion may be expressed as inner, middle or outer involvement. Or it may be expressed as inner half or outer half. Alternatively, the pathologist may measure the entire width of the myometrium, in millimeters, as well as the specific depth of invasion by the tumor, in millimeters. Stage I cancers can be subdivided based on how deep they penetrate the wall.

The extent of myometrial invasion is one of the most important predictors of the likelihood of a cancer recurrence. Invasion through more than half the myometrium is associated with a higher risk of spread outside the uterus, and recurrence. It's also a risk factor for spread of the cancer to the lymph nodes. Only 1 percent of women whose cancer is confined to the endometrium experience spread of the cancer to the pelvic or para-aortic lymph nodes. This number jumps to about 20 percent for women with deep myometrial invasion.

Peritoneal cytology

During surgical staging, the surgeon typically takes a sample of fluid from the abdominal (peritoneal) cavity. A pathologist tests this fluid for cancer cells.

If cancer cells are floating in your peritoneal fluid, you're said to have positive peritoneal cytology. Between 12 percent and 15 percent of women who undergo surgical staging for endometrial cancer have positive peritoneal cytology. In about 25 percent of these women, the cancer has spread to their pelvic lymph nodes, and in 19 percent the cancer has spread to lymph nodes around the aorta.

Staging

Based on the results of your surgery and laboratory tests, your doctor or team of doctors gathers all the information provided to classify the stage of your cancer.

Staging is the most important factor in selecting a treatment for endometrial cancer. The system used to stage endometrial cancer is determined by the International Federation of Gynecology and Obstetrics. It's called the FIGO system.

The FIGO system for staging endometrial cancer is based on information obtained during surgery, including the pathology. However, some women have medical problems that make them unable to undergo surgical staging. For these women, their cancer is staged based on the results of a physical exam, biopsy and imaging tests, such as a CT scan or MRI.

Similar to other staging systems, a lower number indicates that the cancer is still in its early stages, whereas a higher number indicates a more advanced, serious cancer. See page 266 for color illustrations of the endometrial cancer stages.

Stage I

Stage I cancer is limited to the main body (corpus) of the uterus. About 75 percent of endometrial cancers are diagnosed at stage I.

- In stage IA, the cancer is limited to the inner lining of the uterus (endometrium).

- In stage IB, the cancer has spread less than halfway through the muscular wall of the uterus (myometrium).
- In stage IC, the cancer has spread more than halfway through the myometrium, but not beyond the corpus.

Stage II

Stage II cancer involves both the uterine corpus and the uterine cervix. About 13 percent of endometrial cancers are diagnosed at stage II.

- In stage IIA, the cancer has spread to the glands forming the inner lining of the cervix, but not to the deeper, supporting connective tissue of the cervix.
- In stage IIB, the cancer is in the supporting connective tissue of the cervix.

Stage III

Stage III cancer has spread beyond the uterus but not beyond the pelvic area. About 9 percent of endometrial cancers are diagnosed at stage III.

- In stage IIIA, the cancer has spread to the layer of tissue on the outer surface of the uterus (serosa) or to the tissues immediately to the left and right of the uterus (ovaries, fallopian tubes, connective tissues holding the uterus in place), or to both. A stage IIIA endometrial cancer also includes cancers that have shed cells into the peritoneal fluid. The cancer hasn't spread to lymph nodes or more distant sites.
- In stage IIIB, the cancer has spread to the vagina but not to lymph nodes or more distant sites.
- In stage IIIC, the cancer has spread to pelvic or para-aortic lymph nodes but not distant sites. It can be any size.

5-year survival rates for endometrial cancer

Stage	Description	5-year survival rate
Stage I	The cancer is confined to the body of the uterus (corpus).	90%-95%
Stage II	The cancer involves both the corpus and the cervix of the uterus.	75%
Stage III	The cancer has spread beyond the uterus but not beyond the pelvic area.	60%
Stage IVA	The cancer has spread to the rectum or bladder or outside the pelvis.	Less than 26%
Stage IVB	The cancer has spread to the upper abdomen or more distant sites.	Less than 10%

Stage IV

The cancer has spread to the rectum or bladder or to sites outside the pelvis. About 3 percent of endometrial cancers are diagnosed at stage IV.

- In stage IVA, the cancer has spread to the inner lining of the rectum or bladder or both. It may have spread to lymph nodes, but not to more distant sites.
- In stage IVB, the cancer has spread outside of the pelvis, including the upper abdomen or more distant sites, such as the lungs.

Estimating Survival

In general, the chances of surviving endometrial cancer are quite good. Most women do — about 85 percent. But even this figure is a bit misleading. About three out of every four endometrial cancers are diagnosed at stage I, the earliest stage. The five-year survival rate for women who receive a diagnosis of stage I cervical cancer is even higher, over 90 percent.

Your chances of surviving endometrial cancer depend on the stage, cell type and grade of your tumor. Endometrioid adenocarcinoma, the most common form of endometrial cancer, is often diagnosed at an early stage. The more aggressive papillary serous and clear cell endometrial cancers are often at a more advanced stage when diagnosed.

Cell type also is an important factor in survival. Within a given stage and grade category, women who have the endometrioid cell type — the most common form of endometrial cancer — tend to do better. Women with the more aggressive papillary serous cell type tend to do less well.

Remember that survival statistics don't tell the whole story. They only serve to give a general picture and standard way for doctors to discuss prognosis. If you have questions about your own prognosis, discuss them with your doctor or health team members. They'll help you find out how these statistics relate, or don't relate, to you.

Treating Endometrial Cancer

How endometrial cancer is treated depends mainly on the stage of the disease and the type of cells present. Other factors, such as your age and health, also play a role in determining the best treatment plan for you.

Once your doctor has had an opportunity to review the results of your diagnostic tests, he or she will recommend one or more options for treating your cancer.

Before deciding on a course of treatment, make sure you understand the risks and side effects of the various therapies.

Surgery

Surgery is the most common treatment for endometrial cancer. If you have an unusual or aggressive form of endometrial cancer or the cancer has spread to other parts of your body, you may also need additional (adjuvant) treatments. These may include radiation or chemotherapy. The treatment you receive will depend on the type and stage of your cancer and your overall health.

Most women diagnosed with endometrial cancer have a hysterectomy. A hysterectomy is a major operation that can be performed through an incision in the abdomen (abdominal hysterectomy) or through the vagina (vaginal hysterectomy). For treatment of endometrial cancer, doctors almost always recommend an abdominal hysterectomy. An exception may be if a different approach to hysterec-

tomy is being studied in a specific clinical trial, such as minimally invasive (laparoscopic-assisted) vaginal hysterectomy.

A total abdominal hysterectomy — the removal of the uterus and cervix through an abdominal incision — allows the surgeon to closely examine the abdominal cavity for evidence that the cancer may have spread. During surgery, the surgeon will likely take fluid and tissue samples from other areas of the abdomen and have them examined to make sure the cancer hasn't spread. Because pregnancy

Treating Endometrial Hyperplasia

Most endometrial cancers evolve from a precancerous condition known as endometrial hyperplasia (see page 370). Proper evaluation and treatment of endometrial hyperplasia can prevent it from developing into cancer.

Treatment options include hormone therapy, a minor surgical procedure called dilation and curettage (D and C) and surgical removal of your uterus (hysterectomy). Treatment will depend on several factors, including your age, the type of hyperplasia you have and whether you want to preserve your ability to become pregnant.

Hormone therapy

One option for treatment of endometrial hyperplasia is progestins, which are synthetic forms of the hormone proges-

terone. Progesterone is a natural female hormone secreted by the ovaries in the second half of your monthly menstrual cycle, between ovulation and bleeding. Progestins essentially shut off increased cell growth in your endometrium. Women taking a progestin for endometrial hyperplasia typically take a pill for 10 to 14 days each month for three to four months. This treatment is then followed by an endometrial biopsy to determine whether the endometrium has returned to normal. If it has, your doctor may recommend that you stay on progestin for about a year. If endometrial hyperplasia persists, your doctor may recommend a different medication or recommend a hysterectomy.

Progestins can cause side effects, such as weight gain, headaches and irregular vaginal bleeding. However, several different forms of progestins are available. Working together, you and your doctor should be able to find a form and dosage that are right for you.

is no longer possible once the uterus has been removed, having a hysterectomy can be a difficult decision for a woman who's still in her reproductive years. However, it's important to remember that in many cases, a hysterectomy can entirely eliminate endometrial cancer — as well as the need for further treatment.

Types of hysterectomies

There are several different types of hysterectomies. The type of surgery your doctor recommends will depend mainly on the extent of your cancer. In addition to your reproductive organs, lymph nodes in the general area also may be removed so that they can be checked for cancer cells.

Total hysterectomy

During this procedure, a surgeon removes your entire uterus, including your cervix. Your other reproductive organs remain intact. This type of surgery generally isn't recommended for women with endometrial cancer, but it may be an option for

Dilation and curettage

Sometimes, a doctor will recommend a D and C to evaluate endometrial hyperplasia. In this procedure, a doctor scrapes away the overgrown cells lining the uterus (see the illustration on page 381). To perform the procedure, your doctor dilates the opening of your cervix and then uses instruments called curets to scrape the excess tissue. The tissue is sent to a pathologist for analysis. After reviewing the pathologist's report, your doctor may recommend hormone therapy or a hysterectomy.

Hysterectomy

Sometimes, a doctor will recommend a hysterectomy as treatment for endometrial hyperplasia. This is true for women whose hyperplasia doesn't respond to progesterone therapy because they're at significantly increased risk of endometrial cancer.

Hysterectomy also is often the treatment of choice for atypical hyperplasia or hyperplasia coexisting with another medical problem, such as severe uterine bleeding or an ovarian tumor. A hysterectomy not only eliminates abnormal bleeding but also protects against the chance of the condition developing into endometrial cancer.

Therapy and monitoring

Some women with persistent endometrial hyperplasia opt against having a hysterectomy, or they have severe medical problems that make them poor candidates for surgery. If you choose not to have surgery or it's not an option for you, your doctor may prescribe a regimen of hormone therapy combined with close monitoring of your condition. You will likely need to have a repeat endometrial biopsy or D and C.

GYNECOLOGIC CANCERS

Lymph Node Removal

In addition to a hysterectomy that includes removal of the fallopian tubes and ovaries, your surgeon may remove pelvic lymph nodes to check for spread of the cancer. Options include lymph node sampling or a lymphadenectomy. In lymph node sampling, the surgeon removes any nodes that feel enlarged or abnormal, along with a few normal-appearing nodes, to estimate the likelihood that cancer has spread to the lymph nodes. With a lymphadenectomy, all visible lymph nodes in the area are surgically removed.

The surgeon must also decide whether to remove the lymph nodes alongside two vessels that supply blood to the lower torso (the aorta and the vena cava). Removal of both the pelvic and para-aortic lymph nodes is typically done in women with high-grade cancers or deeply invasive cancers. There's evidence that in these women, para-aortic lymphadenectomy may be beneficial. For early-stage or lower grade tumors, pelvic lymph node sampling alone is sometimes the preferred choice. Regardless of the extent of lymph node evaluation, the goal is accurate staging of the cancer in order to have the most accurate information to guide treatment decisions after surgery.

Surgical removal of lymph nodes is not without risks, though, and the greater the extent of lymph node surgery the greater the risk. Lymph node removal requires extra time in surgery, and the longer the surgery the greater the risk of complications, including infections and blood clots. After surgery, patients sometimes have difficulty with lymph fluid collecting in pockets called lymphoceles. Many lymphoceles go away on their own or never cause problems. But some can cause pressure or pain or result in an infection, in which case drainage might be necessary. Finally, pelvic and para-aortic lymph node removal are associated with a small risk of leg swelling (lymphedema). Women who have postoperative radiation treatment in addition to lymphadenectomy are at increased risk of developing this complication.

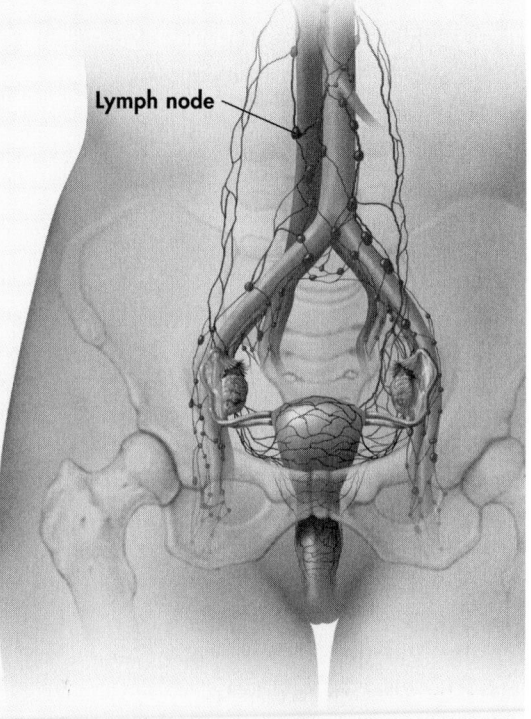

Lymph node

some women with an early-stage (stage I) endometrial cancer. If a total hysterectomy is performed in this situation, it's almost always done by way of an abdominal incision.

Total hysterectomy with bilateral salpingo-oophorectomy

This generally is the preferred surgical treatment for endometrial cancer. During this procedure, a surgeon removes the uterus, including the cervix, as well as the fallopian tubes and both ovaries (see the color illustration on page 270). If you haven't already experienced menopause, surgical removal of the ovaries initiates it.

Why remove all of your reproductive organs if the cancer is just in your uterus? Endometrial cancer cells can spread to your ovaries very early in the disease. Removing your ovaries and testing them for cancerous cells is the best way to tell whether this has happened. In addition, for younger women whose ovaries are still producing estrogen, there's concern that estrogen may stimulate the growth of any microscopic cancer cells that may remain after surgery.

Radical hysterectomy

This is the most extensive type of hysterectomy. During this procedure, a surgeon removes the uterus, including the cervix, as well as the upper inch of the vagina and some surrounding tissue. Among the tissue removed is the connective tissue between the pelvic floor and upper part of the cervix (parametrium) and the ligaments that hold the uterus in place (uterosacral ligaments). This type of surgery may be performed in situations in which the cancer has spread from the endometrium to the cervix.

What to expect

Here's a guide as to what you can expect if you need surgery:

Preparing for surgery

In the days before your surgery, you'll likely have a series of tests. These are done to make sure that you can safely undergo anesthesia and surgery, as well as to evaluate your condition and help plan the surgery.

A blood test called a complete blood count (CBC) is often done to measure the percentage of your blood composed of red blood cells, the number and kinds of white blood cells and the number of platelets. Often, women with blood loss from endometrial cancer have a low red blood cell count, indicating anemia.

Other routine blood and urine tests may be done to make sure you don't have an undetected health problem. Preparation for surgery also includes managing other medical problems you may have, such as high blood pressure or diabetes.

Before your surgery, you'll meet with the surgeon who will perform the operation. During this meeting, your surgeon will likely explain:

- Your condition and why the surgery is being done
- How the surgery will be done
- Where the incision will be
- The risks and benefits of the surgery
- The expected outcome
- What side effects you may experience
- Other options available to you

GYNECOLOGIC CANCERS

It's important that you understand all of these issues. Having a family member or friend sit in on this meeting is probably a good idea.

Before surgery, you'll be assessed by the anesthesiologist or nurse anesthetist who will provide the anesthetic during your surgery. This meeting may not take place until the day of your surgery. A hysterectomy almost always requires general anesthesia, in which you're completely unconscious. Some doctors will perform hysterectomies using regional anesthesia, in which the lower half of the body is numbed with a spinal injection. A sedative also may be given.

The night before surgery, you'll have to stop eating and drinking so that your digestive tract is empty during surgery. You may also be asked to empty your intestines by taking a laxative or having an enema.

During surgery

Just before your surgery, hospital staff will bring you to the operating room and position you comfortably on the operating table. They'll shave and disinfect the area involved in your surgery. Sometimes this is done before you're taken to the operating room.

You'll receive intravenous fluids to maintain normal levels of water in your body and to serve as an avenue for giving drugs, if necessary, during your operation. An anesthesiologist or nurse anesthetist will administer the anesthetic by having you breathe into a face mask or by injecting it into a vein in your arm. Once you're asleep, a tube is placed into your airway (trachea) through your mouth to maintain your breathing status and oxygen levels while you're unconscious.

For treatment of uterine cancer, an incision is made in the lower abdomen, vertically from the navel to the pubic hairline. The incision must be large enough to permit thorough exploration of the abdominal area, and if necessary, to remove some or all of the lymph nodes from the pelvic and para-aortic areas.

Once the surgeon cuts through to the abdominal cavity, often one of the first steps is to take fluid samples from the area for analysis to see if they contain cancer cells. Generally, the next step is a thorough examination of the abdomen and pelvis. If your surgeon spots any growths that look suspicious, tissue samples will be taken from the area and examined for cancerous cells. Your surgeon will also look closely at your uterus to determine whether the tumor has broken through to the outermost layer (serosa).

If you're having your uterus, fallopian tubes and ovaries removed — the most common surgical treatment for endometrial cancer — this process is typically done by removing the organs together, as one unit (en bloc).

Depending on your particular situation, your surgeon may also remove lymph nodes in your pelvis and lymph nodes around the aorta. Lymph nodes are small, bean-shaped structures found throughout the body. They produce and store infection-fighting cells, but they can be invaded by cancer cells, typically causing them to enlarge. After they're removed, the nodes are examined to determine whether they're cancerous.

Q: **I had my ovaries removed during surgery, and now I'm having hot flashes. Is it OK to take hormone replacement therapy to relieve them?**

A: Treatment for endometrial cancer typically involves removing both ovaries along with the uterus. With the removal of your ovaries, you stop producing female sex hormones. If you haven't already experienced menopause, removal of your ovaries initiates it immediately. This is sometimes called surgical menopause.

If your menopausal symptoms are particularly bothersome or severe, one option to treat your symptoms may be hormone replacement therapy (HRT). Whether the hormone estrogen should be prescribed to a woman who has had uterine cancer is somewhat controversial because excess estrogen is a risk factor for the disease. If dormant microscopic cancer cells remain after the sur-

gery, exposure to estrogen might stimulate them, possibly leading to recurrent disease. However, it's important to note, that there's no definite proof that taking estrogen after endometrial cancer surgery increases the risk of recurrence or reduces survival.

To address this important question, the Gynecologic Oncology Group, sponsored by the National Cancer Institute, is conducting a randomized clinical trial. Participants with early-stage endometrial cancer were randomly assigned to receive either estrogen or an inactive pill (placebo). The intent was to see if there's a difference in endometrial cancer recurrence between the two groups of women. Early follow-up results so far show no difference.

If you're concerned about taking estrogen, other types of medications are available that may effectively decrease hot flashes (see Chapter 36).

If cancer cells have reached these lymph nodes, it means the chances are higher that the disease has spread to other parts of your body. Your surgeon may also take tissue samples from the fatty tissue within your abdomen in the front of your intestines (omentum). This is another common area for endometrial cancer to spread.

Surgery for endometrial cancer generally takes one to two hours. Once your surgeon has removed all the necessary organs and tissues, the incision is closed and you're moved to a recovery room.

You'll be monitored for a couple of hours, until the anesthesia has worn off and you're breathing on your own again.

After surgery

After surgery, you may remain in the hospital for a few days to a week. During this time, you'll likely experience some pain and feel tired. You may have some difficulty emptying your bladder and having bowel movements. These bladder and bowel problems typically resolve within one to two weeks after surgery.

GYNECOLOGIC CANCERS

Your doctors will want you out of bed and walking as soon as possible. It may be hard at first, but walking helps speed your recovery. Walking after surgery also helps prevent blood clots from forming in your legs.

Once you're well enough to continue your recovery at home, you'll be discharged. Keep in mind, though, that recovery after a hysterectomy takes time. An abdominal hysterectomy usually requires six weeks for full recovery. You may need more or less time than that.

Listen to your body. If you're feeling tired, scale back your activities until you're feeling a bit stronger. Ask for help if you need it.

Side effects

Surgery can lead to some chronic problems. After surgery, you may be more prone to bowel or bladder problems, such as mild leakage of urine (urinary incontinence). If your ovaries were removed as part of your surgery, you may experience symptoms of menopause, such as vaginal dryness and hot flashes. If part of your vagina was removed, you may experience some pain during intercourse.

Talk to your doctor if you experience any of these conditions. He or she can recommend exercises or medication to help treat these problems and reduce symptoms.

Low vs. High Risk of Recurrence

After your doctor completes the staging of your cancer, your tumor may be classified into one of three groups: low risk of recurrence, intermediate risk of recurrence or high risk of recurrence.

Women considered at low risk have a high rate of cure after surgery and don't need additional (adjuvant) treatment. For endometrial cancer, additional treatment may involve radiation therapy, chemotherapy or both.

Women in the high-risk group, meanwhile, tend to have a lower rate of cure with surgery alone and generally need additional treatment to increase the chances of a cure. Women in the intermediate-risk group fall somewhere in

between. They may or may not benefit from additional therapy.

- **Low risk.** The cancer is relatively slow-growing (grade 1 or 2) and is confined to the endometrium (stage IA). There's a high rate of cure with surgery alone.
- **Intermediate risk.** The cancer is confined to the endometrium (stage IA) but is grade 3. A woman is also classified at intermediate risk if the cancer has spread to the muscular wall of the uterus (stages IB and IC) or if it has spread to the cervix (stages IIA and IIB), no matter what the grade. If cancer cells are found in a sample of peritoneal fluid, this also indicates intermediate risk. For women at intermediate risk, adjuvant therapy may be recommended.
- **High risk.** The cancer has spread through the entire uterine wall or to

Radiation Therapy

Radiation therapy is the use of high-energy radiation to destroy cancer cells. It's a local therapy, meaning that the treatment is focused on a specific area of your body, not your entire body.

If your doctor thinks that you're at high risk of a local cancer recurrence — that is, development of cancer in the pelvis or neighboring lymph nodes — he or she may suggest radiation therapy after a hysterectomy. Your doctor may recommend radiation therapy if your tumor is a fast-growing type (high-grade) or if the cancer has invaded deeply into the muscle of the uterus.

With endometrial cancer, radiation usually isn't recommended before surgery or in place of it. Your doctor might recommend radiation instead of surgery only if your health is too poor to have surgery or if the cancer has spread extensively. In some cases, radiation therapy may shrink the tumor enough to make surgery a possibility at a later date.

Two types of radiation therapy are used to treat endometrial cancer:

- **External beam.** With external beam radiation, you receive doses of radiation from a large, high-energy X-ray machine called a linear accelerator.
- **Internal radiation (brachytherapy).** With internal radiation therapy,

Risk level	Typical treatment
Low risk	• Surgery
Intermediate risk	• Surgery • Internal radiation (brachytherapy), pelvic external beam radiation or both
High risk	Surgery, plus one of the following: • Pelvic external beam radiation • Pelvic and abdominal external beam radiation, with or without internal radiation • Chemotherapy with or without radiation

the tissues immediately adjacent to the uterus (ovaries, fallopian tubes, connective tissues holding the uterus in place) or both (stage IIIA). A woman is also classified at high risk if the cancer has spread to the vagina (stage IIIB), lymph nodes (IIIC), or bladder or bowel (stage IVA). Adjuvant therapy is almost always recommended for

women classified at high risk. It's also commonly recommended if the cancer cell type is papillary serous or clear cell.

The type of treatment your doctor recommends will depend on your particular situation. The chart above reflects the treatment regimens often recommended, based on risk factors and cancer stage.

radioactive substances called radioisotopes are placed in or near the tumor or in the location from where the cancer was removed. As the radioisotopes break down, they release radiation, killing cancer cells in the area.

The type of radiation you receive depends on the extent of your cancer:

- If only the upper portion of your remaining vagina needs to be treated, your doctor may recommend internal radiation therapy only.
- For treatment of the entire pelvis, external radiation is most often used.
- For women with more advanced endometrial cancer, the entire abdominal cavity may receive radiation for the first few weeks of treatment followed by radiation to just the pelvis. Some women receive both external and internal radiation therapy.

If you have advanced-stage endometrial cancer (stage III or IVA) at the time of your diagnosis, radiation therapy may be part of your treatment. After undergoing surgery, women with advanced-stage endometrial cancer usually receive external beam radiation therapy, and some also receive internal radiation therapy to treat the upper third of the vagina.

If laboratory tests show that cancer cells are floating in your abdominal (peritoneal) fluid, the field for external beam radiation may be widened to include the entire abdomen. If the cancer has spread to the lower third of the vagina, lymph nodes in the groin area may be treated with external radiation, too. If the disease has spread to the lymph nodes near the aorta, radiation treatments to that area may be included in your treatment plan.

External beam radiation

External beam radiation therapy is much like having an X-ray taken, but the radiation emitted is higher energy. You attend radiation sessions as an outpatient in a

Getting Ready for Radiation Treatment

Before your radiation, you'll meet with a radiation oncologist who will design your radiation treatments. During this meeting, he or she will likely explain:

- Your condition and why the radiation is being done
- How the radiation will be done
- Where the radiation will be directed
- The risks and benefits of the radiation
- The expected outcome
- What side effects you may experience
- Other options available to you

It's important that you understand all these issues. Having a family member or friend sit in on this meeting is probably a good idea. If you don't understand something, ask to have it explained again.

hospital or clinic, typically five days a week for four to six weeks. The actual radiation sessions take less than a minute, but time is needed to position your body and make sure the beams are aimed correctly. During external beam radiation, different areas of your body can be treated simultaneously, such as the main tumor bed and nearby lymph nodes.

Preparing for external beam radiation

If your doctor thinks that you may benefit from external beam radiation, on the first day of treatment you'll likely undergo a process called simulation, which defines the area to be treated. This is also sometimes called a planning session.

During simulation, you lie still on a table while the radiation team uses a special diagnostic X-ray machine or a computerized tomography (CT) scanner to pinpoint the exact area of your body where the radiation will be aimed. Some people lie on their stomachs and others on their backs for their planning sessions and treatments. The area of your body to receive the radiation is called the treatment field or treatment port. Most women with endometrial cancer require more than one treatment field to minimize the amount of radiation to normal structures such as the intestines, kidneys and spinal cord.

It's important that the radiation be administered to the same place in your body during each session. To ensure accuracy, the skin covering the center of the treatment field may be marked with freckle-sized dots of semipermanent ink. More commonly, dots of injected dye, similar to a tattoo, are used. These markings are per-

manent. If they bother you, they can be removed later with a laser. Your doctor may also request that a custom-made mold be made of your pelvis and lower back or even of your upper body. This will help you lie still and ensure that you're placed in the same position during each radiation session. In addition, imaging scans of your body may be necessary.

Using information from your medical history, the simulation and other tests, your doctor — in this case, a radiation oncologist — will develop your specific radiation treatment plan. This plan will specify how much radiation will be administered, how it will be delivered and how many treatments you'll need. Your doctor will develop your plan based on your overall health, the size of your tumor, how sensitive the cancer cells are to radiation and how well normal tissues adjacent to the tumor will tolerate the radiation.

The goal of radiation therapy is to administer the strongest dose of radiation possible, while sparing as much normal tissue as possible. This will help reduce side effects. To maximize radiation to your tumor and minimize damage to normal tissues, the total radiation dose is divided into multiple smaller doses (fractions), which are usually administered once a day over several weeks.

Receiving external beam radiation

For your treatment, you'll need to remove any clothing that covers the area receiving radiation. You then lie on a treatment table positioned under the radiation machine (linear accelerator) just as you were positioned in your planning session (see the color illustration on page 271). Special shields may be placed between the machine and other parts of your body to help protect normal tissues and organs.

Once you're in the proper position, the radiation therapist goes into a nearby room to turn on the machine. During the treatment, you shouldn't see or feel anything, but you might hear the machine clicking or whirring. The machine itself won't touch you. Your therapist watches you on a TV monitor and can also hear you over an intercom system.

It's important to remain as still as possible during radiation. However, unlike during a normal X-ray, you don't have to hold your breath. If you feel ill or uncomfortable during the treatment, tell your therapist immediately. The machine can be stopped at any time.

The actual treatment takes less than a minute, but the entire session can last 15 to 30 minutes. That's because of the time it takes to set up the equipment and get you into the proper position.

Side effects

You may feel the early effects of radiation therapy a few days to a couple of weeks after starting treatment. The extent of your side effects depends on the area being treated and the type of radiation (external or internal) being delivered. Remember to ask your doctor what side effects you might expect and when.

Fatigue is a common side effect of external radiation. Talk with your doctor about strategies to minimize your fatigue.

When radiation is applied to the pelvic area, it may cause frequent and uncomfortable urination (radiation cystitis), as well as diarrhea. Diarrhea can often be controlled with medications and by avoiding spicy, fried and high-fiber foods. These side effects can occur about three to four weeks after treatment begins.

Radiation to your pelvic area can also cause tenderness and inflammation in your vagina. The lining of your vagina may become thinner, causing light bleeding after sexual intercourse. Some women develop small sores (ulcers) in the vagina. These sores may take several months to heal after external radiation therapy ends.

As your pelvic area heals, scar tissue may form in the vagina, narrowing it and interfering with its ability to stretch. This condition, called vaginal stenosis, can make sexual intercourse painful. In extreme cases, scarring after pelvic radiation shortens or narrows the vagina so much that intercourse is impossible.

To prevent scar tissue from forming in the vagina, stretch the walls of the vagina several times a week. One option is to have sexual intercourse at least three or four times a week. Another is to use a plastic or rubber tube called a vaginal dilator. Using a dilator feels a lot like putting a large tampon in the vagina for a few minutes. Besides making for more comfortable intercourse, a vagina that's normal in size makes for more comfortable pelvic exams, which are an important part of follow-up care after treatment for endometrial cancer.

To prevent infection, make sure the skin in the treatment area is kept clean and protected. Moisturizing your skin with a lotion containing aloe vera, lanolin or vitamin E may help alleviate dryness and itching.

Internal radiation

Internal radiation therapy is also known as implant radiation (brachytherapy). Other terms such as *intracavity radiation* and *interstitial radiation* refer to how and where the radioactive substances are administered.

- **Intracavity radiation.** Intracavity radiation involves the placement of an applicator, such as a tube (cylinder), into a body opening (cavity), such as the vagina. Radioactive sources are placed in the applicator and treatment begins. After completion of treatment, the applicator is removed.
- **Interstitial radiation.** Interstitial radiation involves placement of radioactive substances directly into the tissue or tumor. Temporary applicators containing radioactive material are surgically inserted into the tissue. Once the treatment is complete, the applicators are removed.

The benefit of internal radiation therapy is that you can receive a higher dose of radiation to a smaller area and in a shorter time than is possible with external beam radiation. Internal radiation may be given at either a high-dose rate (HDR) or a low-dose rate (LDR).

A common form of internal radiation therapy for endometrial cancer involves inserting tiny tubes containing radioisotopes into an applicator that's placed near the top of the vagina and left in place for a few days. This delivers radiation to the site where the cancer had been before surgery. With this form of low-dose-rate radiation, you remain in the hospital during treatment. Once the implant is removed,

you no longer have any radioactivity in your body and you can go home.

High-dose-rate internal radiation is newer and is becoming more commonly used. A sealed container of radioactive material is inserted through an applicator that's placed near the top of your vagina and left in place for an hour or two. You return weekly for three to five weeks for treatment. The treatment is done as an outpatient procedure, and most women tolerate this procedure very well.

Preparing for internal radiation
Internal radiation therapy to treat the top of the vagina (vaginal apex) typically begins four to six weeks after your hysterectomy, once you've had a chance to recover from surgery. Several treatments may be necessary.

Before beginning internal radiation, you may have some imaging tests so that your doctor has the most current information about your condition. When the time comes for your therapy to begin, you'll check into the radiation suite of your local hospital or medical center.

Receiving internal radiation
During your treatment, you may need to stay in bed and lie fairly still to keep the implant from shifting position. With a high-dose implant, you should be able to go home the same day.

In the case of a low-dose implant in which you remain hospitalized overnight, there will likely be limits on who can visit you and for how long. While the implant is in place, the radioactive substance within it may transmit rays outside your body, exposing others to radiation. For this reason, pregnant women or children under age 18 won't be allowed to visit. Adults who visit must sit at least six feet from your bed and stay no longer than 30 minutes a day. Once your treatment is complete, the implant is removed and there's no longer any radioactivity in your body.

You aren't likely to feel significant pain or become ill during implant therapy. But you may experience some discomfort. If you're in pain or having trouble relaxing, ask whether you can have medication to ease your symptoms.

Side effects

Your vagina may be sore or sensitive for some time after internal radiation therapy, but most women resume their normal activities relatively quickly. With a low-dose implant, you may be fatigued immediately after treatment. Fatigue generally isn't a problem with high-dose implants. In general, you should wait four weeks before resuming sexual intercourse.

Chemotherapy

Chemotherapy also is used to treat endometrial cancer. Chemotherapy is a systemic therapy, meaning it's delivered by the bloodstream throughout the entire body. You may receive chemotherapy medication by pill (orally) or through your veins (intravenously). The medications enter your bloodstream and travel through your body, killing cancer cells that may have spread outside your uterus.

Chemotherapy may be a part of initial treatment for endometrial cancer, or it may be used to treat recurrent disease. Treatments for recurrent endometrial cancer are discussed in the next chapter.

Types of medications

Chemotherapy medications are classified according to how they destroy cancer cells. The categories of medications commonly used to treat endometrial cancer include:

- **Alkylating agents.** These medications help prevent cancer cells from functioning by binding directly to their DNA, blocking the copying of DNA and the manufacture of ribonucleic acid (RNA). Alkylating agents used to treat endometrial cancer include cisplatin (Platinol), carboplatin (Paraplatin) and cyclophosphamide (Cytoxan, Neosar).
- **Anti-tumor antibiotics.** These drugs — different from antibiotics used to treat bacterial infections — interfere with the ability of cancer cells to copy their genetic material (DNA). Doxorubicin (Adriamycin) is a common anti-tumor antibiotic used to treat endometrial cancer.
- **Mitotic inhibitors.** These drugs can inhibit or stop cell growth and division or interfere with enzymes necessary in the cell division process. Paclitaxel (Taxol), which is derived from the Pacific yew tree, is a mitotic inhibitor used to treat endometrial cancer.

If your doctor recommends chemotherapy, you may receive a combination of drugs. Combination chemotherapy is sometimes more effective than one drug alone in treating cancer. By combining drugs that work somewhat differently, the treatment may result in the destruction of a greater number of cancer cells and might reduce your risk of the cancer's becoming resistant to one particular drug.

Examples of combination regimens include:

- Doxorubicin (Adriamycin) and cisplatin (Platinol), sometimes referred to as AP
- Cyclophosphamide (Cytoxan), doxorubicin (Adriamycin) and cisplatin (Platinol), sometimes referred to as CAP
- Paclitaxel (Taxol) and carboplatin (Paraplatin)

All these chemotherapy medications are given intravenously. Doxorubicin must be administered very carefully. If it leaks on your skin or outside the vein, it can cause a severe reaction, such as damage to and scarring of the tissue. Carboplatin is generally less toxic than cisplatin. However, it tends to inhibit bone marrow activity more than some other chemotherapy drugs do, resulting in fewer red blood cells, white blood cells and platelets. This limits its usefulness among women who previously have had pelvic radiation therapy, which also can suppress bone marrow activity.

You usually receive chemotherapy in cycles, depending on your condition and which drugs are used. A cycle refers to a treatment that's generally given once every three to four weeks, providing recovery time for your body to rest and produce new, healthy cells.

Preparing for chemotherapy

Most chemotherapy is given in an outpatient setting. Occasionally, depending on which drugs your doctor prescribes and the general state of your health, you may need to stay in the hospital during your chemotherapy session.

Receiving chemotherapy

Most women receive chemotherapy intravenously through a small catheter placed into a vein in the hand or forearm. You may be given an intravenous (IV) drip or infusion, in which a mixed drug solution flows slowly from a plastic bag into your body over a period of 30 minutes to a few hours. Some chemotherapy medications can be given rapidly over a few minutes by way of a syringe that's inserted into intravenous tubing. This method is called IV push.

Side effects

Side effects of chemotherapy depend on many factors, including the specific drugs you're taking, how much you're taking and how long you're treated. Because chemotherapy works by killing rapidly dividing cells, it can damage not only cancer cells but also normal cells that divide rapidly. Side effects you may experience include:

- Hair loss
- Nausea and vomiting
- Loss of appetite
- Diffuse aching
- Numbness and tingling in your fingers or toes or both
- Mouth sores
- Low blood counts
- Diarrhea

The blood-producing cells of your bone marrow are rapidly dividing cells, so they are innocent bystanders that can be harmed by chemotherapy. Depending on the specific agents used, white blood cells, red blood cells and blood platelets may be reduced, resulting in fatigue, increased susceptibility to infection and easy bleeding. The chemotherapy agents used to treat endometrial cancer do cause hair loss, which usually begins 10 to 14 days after the first round (cycle) of drugs. Uncommon problems include damage to your heart or kidneys or severe nerve damage.

Your doctor will prescribe medications to help prevent nausea and vomiting. In some situations, growth factors can be given to build up your blood counts. In general, most side effects of chemotherapy are temporary.

Hormone Therapy

Endometrial cells are sensitive to the female hormones estrogen and progesterone. Hormone therapy for the treatment of endometrial cancer involves administering hormonally active agents that prevent cancer cells from getting or using hormones they need to grow, ultimately slowing their growth. Hormone therapy is a systemic therapy, meaning it can attack cancer cells throughout your body.

For treatment of endometrial cancer, the hormone therapy predominantly used is one of the synthetic forms of the hormone progesterone (progestins). Some alternatives to progestins may be used as well.

Usually, hormone therapy is used to treat endometrial cancer that has

Clinical Trials

Researchers continue to look for better ways to treat endometrial cancer that cause fewer side effects. In clinical trials, possible cancer treatments are tested to see if they work as well as scientists hope they might. For more information on clinical trials, see Chapter 2.

Medications

Chemotherapy drug combinations and biologic therapies are among some of the treatments for endometrial cancer being investigated in clinical trials. Biologic therapies are treatments that:

recurred. Treatments for recurrent endometrial cancer are discussed in detail in the next chapter.

Although progestins have been used successfully in the treatment of recurrent endometrial cancer, they haven't been shown to be effective in initial treatment of the disease. Three randomized trials have addressed this issue. Women with early-stage endometrial cancer, treated with surgery alone or surgery and radiation therapy, were randomly assigned to receive a progestin or an inactive pill (placebo), which in effect means no further treatment. There was no difference in outcome between the progestin and placebo treatment groups. Much larger studies are now needed to determine with more certainty if progestins are of any benefit.

- Stimulate the immune system's ability to attack the cancer
- Block growth signals needed for the cancer to grow
- Halt new blood vessel growth in order to starve the cancer

New drugs under investigation for endometrial cancer include erlotinib (Tarceva) and trastuzumab (Herceptin). Generally speaking, these drugs interfere with growth factors that cancer cells need to grow. Studies involving these drugs are currently at an early stage in the clinical trials process. It'll likely be several years before doctors and scientists know whether they show promise as treatments.

Doctors and scientists are also comparing the effectiveness of different chemotherapy regimens, plus radiation therapy, in treating stage III and stage IV endometrial cancer. To do this, they're randomly assigning participants to receive one of the following therapies:

- Radiation therapy plus the chemotherapy drugs doxorubicin and cisplatin
- Radiation, the combination of doxorubicin (Adriamycin) and cisplatin (Platinol), plus the chemotherapy drug paclitaxel (Taxol)

This study is further along in the clinical trials process than are the Tarceva and Herceptin studies, and researchers should know relatively soon which combination chemotherapy regimen is more effective for women with advanced disease.

Surgery

Researchers are currently investigating whether hysterectomy can be performed with a less invasive surgery called laparoscopy. With laparoscopy, several small incisions are made in the abdomen instead of one large incision. A lighted tube with an attached camera (laparoscope) is inserted into one of the incisions so that the surgeon can see inside. Laparoscopy generally results in fewer side effects and a speedier recovery. The concern is whether the procedure allows an adequate view of, and access to, the abdomen to check for spread of cancer to other sites.

To evaluate the usefulness of laparoscopic hysterectomy in treating endometrial cancer, researchers are randomly assigning women with stage I or stage IIA disease — where the tumor is confined to the body of the uterus or endocervical glands — to receive either laparoscopic surgery or standard surgery. The health and quality of life of these women is evaluated six weeks after surgery, then every three months for the next two years and then every six months the following year.

Researchers are also investigating whether surgical removal of the lymph nodes (lymphadenectomy) has a role in treating early-stage endometrial cancer. It's not yet known which of the following is more effective in treating the disease at this early stage:

- Conventional surgery with or without lymphadenectomy
- Conventional surgery with radiation therapy

Radiation therapy

In Europe, researchers are addressing the question of whether radiation therapy combined with chemotherapy is more effective than radiation alone in treating high-risk endometrial cancer. For this study, factors that place a woman with endometrial cancer at high risk include a tumor that has spread through the entire uterine wall or to pelvic lymph nodes.

Surveillance and Follow-up

After treatment for endometrial cancer, your doctor will likely recommend regular follow-up examinations. Regular checkups ensure that any changes in your health, such as a recurrence of your cancer, are noticed and treated appropriately.

There's no absolute prescription for how often follow-up visits should be done. Their frequency depends to some extent on the likelihood that the disease will recur, with women at higher risk of recurrence followed more intensively.

In general, though, during the first three years after treatment, you'll probably have checkups with your doctor every three to six months. The first three years are the time when risk of recurrence is highest. Studies show that about 75 percent of endometrial cancer recurrences happen within three years after treatment. If, after three years, there's no evidence that your cancer has recurred, you may need to see your doctor less often.

What to expect

During your follow-up visits, your doctor will likely perform a pelvic exam and examine your body for any enlarged lymph nodes. A Pap test also may be done to look for cancer cells in the upper part of your vagina, near where your cervix used to be. How often this test should be done is somewhat controversial. Some research suggests that frequent Pap tests have no effect on the outcome of women whose cancer has recurred in the vagina. As a result, some doctors believe it's adequate to do Pap tests yearly rather than more frequently.

Your doctor will ask you about any signs and symptoms you're experiencing that might suggest your cancer has returned. Signs and symptoms that may be of concern include abdominal or pelvic pain, weight loss, fatigue and vaginal bleeding. Be sure to tell your doctor exactly what and how you're feeling. You'll also have a chance to discuss any lingering side effects of treatment.

More than 80 percent of endometrial cancer recurrences are detected by signs and symptoms or findings during a physical exam. If your physical exams are normal and you don't have any worrisome signs and symptoms, you probably won't need further tests or exams beyond a pelvic exam and Pap test. Studies of women with endometrial cancer have shown that imaging tests and blood tests aren't necessary among women who don't have signs or symptoms or suspicious abnormalities on their physical exams.

Endometrial Cancer Recurrence

Recurrent cancer is the term for cancer that comes back after initial treatment. A recurrence of endometrial cancer may occur in the vagina or in nearby lymph nodes, or it may occur in distant sites.

When endometrial cancer is initially diagnosed, if the cancer is still confined to the uterus, chances of successful treatment are good and recurrence is uncommon. If the cancer has already spread beyond the uterus when it's first detected, recurrence is more likely. Deep invasion of the muscular wall of the uterus (myometrium) is one possible risk factor for recurrence. Studies show that women who have tumors that have invaded more than half the thickness of the myometrium have a higher risk of cancer cells spreading outside the uterus and later recurrence. Other important risk factors for recurrence include a tumor that has spread to neighboring lymph nodes, a more aggressive type of endometrial cancer and the presence of cancer cells in your abdominal cavity fluid (peritoneal fluid).

Most recurrences of endometrial cancer occur in the first few years after diagnosis. Possible sites of recurrent disease include the vagina, lymph nodes in the pelvis and lymph nodes near the large blood vessel (aorta) that serves the lower torso. Less commonly, recurrence occurs in the lungs and liver. The probability of long-term survival (prognosis) depends on the extent of the recurrence. Studies suggest that some women who have isolated recurrences of endometrial cancer in the vagina can be cured with appropriate treatment. Otherwise, recurrent endometrial cancer typically isn't curable. However, depending on the aggressiveness of the cancer, sometimes it can be controlled for long periods, often years.

Treatment Options

Treatment options for recurrent endometrial cancer include surgery, radiation therapy, hormone therapy and chemotherapy. Depending on your situation, your doctor may recommend a combination of these approaches.

Your doctor likely will design your treatment based on the cell type of the tumor (endometrioid, serous or clear cell), where the cancer has recurred and how much time has passed from your initial diagnosis to your cancer recurrence.

Surgery

Surgery generally isn't regarded as the first line of defense against recurrent endometrial cancer. However, endometrial cancer that recurs only in the vagina can sometimes be removed through an operation called an upper vaginectomy. During this procedure, a surgeon removes the upper portion of the vagina.

Sometimes, radiation treatments are paired with surgery. This generally occurs when the cancer can be surgically removed, but the surgeon is concerned about where the tumor is located or whether he or she was able to remove all of the cancerous cells located around the tumor. External radiation may be given either before or after surgery.

Additionally, during what's known as intraoperative radiotherapy (IORT), an added dose (boost) of external radiation may be directed to a localized area during surgery. The bowel or other sensitive structures are moved out of the way while a special form of radiation known as particle radiation is delivered. Another type of IORT may be given with a special applicator containing a high-dose-rate radiation source. The applicator contains flexible tubes and is placed close to the area where the cancer has been surgically removed.

The goal of radiation in these situations is to treat the tissue adjacent to where the tumor was located.

For certain women with limited disease at the time the recurrence is diagnosed, the combination of surgery and IORT may be able to destroy the cancer. Many women receive external radiation before IORT. This combination of radiation treatments generally can be done only in specialized medical centers.

Although this approach hasn't yet been tested in large groups of women, preliminary results appear promising.

A Rare Surgery

Occasionally, endometrial cancer recurs even after a woman has been treated with both radiation therapy and traditional surgery. Some women in this situation may benefit from a relatively uncommon operation called pelvic exenteration. This is an extensive procedure, and it can involve removal of several pelvic organs, including the bladder, vagina, rectum and part of the colon.

An anterior exenteration removes the pelvic structures in the front of the body, including the bladder and vagina. A posterior exenteration removes those structures toward the back, including the rectum. During a total pelvic exenteration, all the pelvic structures are removed.

After removing these organs, the surgeon constructs new ways of storing and eliminating urine and solid waste, as well as a new vagina that can be created out of skin, intestinal tissue, or muscle and skin grafts.

Pelvic exenteration is used only for women with an isolated pelvic recurrence of endometrial cancer. For some of these women, it offers the possibility of a cure. It's also sometimes used to help control serious problems that may accompany advanced endometrial cancer, such as drainage problems, uncontrolled leakage of stool or urine, uncontrolled bleeding, or blockage of the gastrointestinal or urinary tract.

There are no large, published studies on the effectiveness of pelvic exenteration as a treatment for recurrent endometrial cancer. However, reports indicate that among women who've had the procedure, approximately 25 percent have survived for more than five years.

Radiation therapy

If endometrial cancer recurs only in your pelvic area, radiation therapy may be an option if you haven't had radiation to this area before. If the recurrence is limited to your vagina, it may still be possible to cure the disease. In very select cases, radiation can sometimes be given a second time depending on the dose you received during your initial treatment and how it was delivered.

Radiation therapy for recurrent endometrial cancer can include external beam radiation, internal radiation (brachytherapy) or a combination of these two approaches.

During external beam radiation therapy, you receive daily doses of radiation from a large X-ray machine aimed at the area of recurrence and nearby lymph nodes. During internal radiation therapy, radioactive substances called radioisotopes are placed near the tumor. As the radioisotopes break down, they release radiation, killing cancer cells in the area. See Chapter 23 for more information on internal and external radiation treatments.

The goal of radiation therapy generally is to help provide a cure. Sometimes, though, radiation is part of palliative therapy. The intent of palliative therapy isn't to cure the cancer but to relieve symptoms and improve quality of life. External beam radiation to the pelvis can reduce excessive bleeding and pain. For some women, internal radiation treatments also may relieve bleeding. If the cancer has spread to the bones, lungs, brain or lymph nodes, these areas can be treated with radiation to reduce pain and other symptoms.

Hormone therapy

The female hormones estrogen and progesterone affect the growth rate of most endometrial cancers. Hormone therapy for recurrent endometrial cancer involves administering substances that halt or help slow tumor growth. The substances work by binding to estrogen and progesterone receptors found in some endometrial cancer cells, preventing the cells from getting or using the hormones they need to grow.

Hormone therapy is a systemic therapy, meaning it affects cancer cells wherever they may be located in your body. Endometrial cancers that respond best to hormone therapy are those that are relatively slow-growing (low-grade).

Studies suggest that 50 percent to 70 percent of endometrial cancers with progesterone receptors respond to hormone therapy. Unfortunately, though, only a small number of endometrial cancers that have spread throughout the body have these receptors.

The longer the time between initial diagnosis of the cancer and its recurrence, the better your chances of responding well to hormone therapy.

For some women with recurrent endometrial cancer, hormone therapy can shrink the tumors or stop them from growing. If your disease responds favorably, treatment can continue indefinitely. In most cases of recurrent cancer, the purpose of hormone therapy is to prolong survival or improve quality of life. It doesn't provide a cure.

The duration of hormone treatment varies from woman to woman, but it typically lasts as long as the disease responds to the medication. Women with recurrent endometrial cancer who have a partial or complete response to hormone therapy — meaning that the treatment shrinks or temporarily eliminates the tumor — may have remissions lasting from six months to several years.

Drugs used in hormone therapy include progestins, tamoxifen, gonadotropin-releasing hormone (Gn-RH) analogues and aromatase inhibitors.

Progestins

For treatment of recurrent endometrial cancer, women are generally prescribed a synthetic form of the hormone progesterone, called a progestin. The medication is given in different doses for treatment of endometrial cancer from that used as part of hormone replacement therapy (HRT). There are different forms of progestins. They include megestrol (Megace) and medroxyprogesterone (Provera). The dosage varies depending on the drug.

Tamoxifen

Tamoxifen (Nolvadex), a drug often used to treat breast cancer, is sometimes used to treat recurrent endometrial cancer.

Tamoxifen is a selective estrogen receptor modulator (SERM), meaning that it can bind to an estrogen receptor and change the action of estrogen in the body.

Sometimes, tamoxifen can shrink tumors in women with recurrent endometrial cancer that hasn't responded to a progestin. It's also an alternative to progestin for women who are obese or who have diabetes or high blood pressure. Progestins stimulate the appetite and can lead to weight gain.

Scientists are investigating a newer SERM for its effectiveness against metastatic endometrial cancer. This drug, called arzoxifene, has shown promise in early clinical trials. Unlike tamoxifen — which acts as an anti-estrogen on breast cancer cells but like estrogen on uterine cells — arzoxifene appears to act as a potent anti-estrogen in both tissues.

Gonadotropin-releasing hormone analogues

Two other hormonal drugs being studied for the treatment of endometrial cancer are called leuprolide and goserelin. They're synthetic versions of a natural hormone called gonadotropin-releasing hormone (Gn-RH), which stimulates the ovaries to make estrogen and progesterone. The drugs also are known as Gn-RH analogues.

Some studies of leuprolide and goserelin have been encouraging. In one study, 25 percent of women with recurrent or metastatic endometrial cancer who were treated with Gn-RH analogues had a positive response. However, in another study of women given monthly injections of leuprolide, none of the women responded

to the therapy. More research is needed to clarify the role of these drugs in treating recurrent endometrial cancer.

Aromatase inhibitors

The female ovaries are the main source of the female hormones estrogen and progesterone, but your body can produce these hormones in other ways, even after menopause. The adrenal glands produce a variety of hormones, including androgens. Certain enzymes called aromatases, which are predominant in some body tissues, such as fat cells, convert androgens into estrogen.

Medications called aromatase inhibitors block aromatases from making estrogen. Aromatase inhibitors include the drugs anastrozole (Arimidex), letrozole (Femara) and exemestane (Aromasin). Early studies show some positive benefits among women with endometrial cancer who received the drugs over a short period, but longer-term, large-scale studies are needed to determine the medication's full effects. The drugs are effective only in women who've gone through menopause, either naturally or surgically.

Chemotherapy

Chemotherapy may be used to treat recurrent cancer, especially if the cancer is fast-growing (high-grade) and it doesn't have detectable hormone receptors. Chemotherapy may also be given as a second line of treatment when hormone therapy fails. Studies show that fast-growing tumors and tumors that are least likely to respond to hormone therapy are more likely to respond to chemotherapy.

GYNECOLOGIC CANCERS

Chemotherapy drugs used to treat recurrent endometrial cancer may include:

- Carboplatin (Paraplatin)
- Cisplatin (Platinol)
- Cyclophosphamide (Cytoxan, Neosar)
- Doxorubicin (Adriamycin)
- Paclitaxel (Taxol)

These drugs may be given alone or in combination. Combination chemotherapy is sometimes more effective in shrinking tumors. By combining drugs that work somewhat differently, the treatment may result in the destruction of a greater number of cancer cells and it might reduce your risk of the cancer becoming resistant to one particular drug.

Chemotherapy may shrink recurrent tumors and may even temporarily eliminate the cancer, but it generally doesn't provide a cure. The cancer eventually comes back or continues to grow. It's estimated that most women receiving chemotherapy for recurrent cancer live an additional seven to 10 months longer than they would have if they didn't get chemotherapy.

Clinical Trials

Women with recurrent endometrial cancer may benefit from participating in studies of experimental treatments. Several experimental treatment regimens are presently being evaluated in clinical trials:

- **Chemotherapy combinations.** Researchers are studying whether the chemotherapy drugs doxorubicin and cisplatin are more effective with or without the drug paclitaxel in treating recurrent endometrial cancer. They're also comparing the effectiveness of a chemotherapy regimen composed of doxorubicin, cisplatin, paclitaxel and filgrastim with the combination of carboplatin and paclitaxel. Filgrastim is a drug called a granulocyte colony-stimulating factor (G-CSF). It stimulates the production of white blood cells so that there's less risk of infection after chemotherapy.
- **Biologic therapies.** Biologic therapies work in unique ways. Some try to harness the body's immune system to fight the cancer. Others target specific growth factors or pathways that feed a cancer. Substances currently being studied include the drugs erlotinib and gefitinib (Iressa).
- **Hormone therapies.** One hormonal agent called fulvestrant (Faslodex) blocks estrogen activity in the body and is sometimes used to treat breast cancer. Scientists think that hormone therapy with Faslodex may be effective for recurrent endometrial cancer, blocking estrogen growth stimulation in tumor cells.
- **Hyperthermia therapy.** In this procedure, body tissues are exposed to high temperatures. High temperatures appear to damage or kill cancer cells or make them more sensitive to the effects of radiation or certain chemotherapy drugs. In one clinical trial, researchers are studying whether whole-body hyperthermia treatments combined with the chemotherapy drugs 5-fluorouracil and liposomal doxorubicin, are effective in treating women whose cancer has spread to distant sites.

Uterine Sarcomas

Endometrial cancer is the most common form of uterine cancer, but not all uterine cancers begin in the uterine lining (endometrium). Some cancers, known as sarcomas, get their start in cells that make up muscle and other supportive structures. Uterine sarcomas, which begin in uterine muscle or connective tissue, are quite rare. They're estimated to account for only 2 percent to 5 percent of all uterine cancers.

Different types of uterine sarcomas behave differently. Most are associated with vaginal bleeding. Some are slow-growing and have a good prognosis. Others are more aggressive and have a poorer prognosis.

Types of Uterine Sarcomas

Within the general category of uterine sarcomas, there are three main types, subdivided according to the tissue from which the cancer originates.

Endometrial stromal sarcomas

Endometrial stromal sarcomas develop in the supporting connective tissue (stroma) of the endometrium.

They're the least common type of uterine sarcoma, making up about 10 percent of all cases. Endometrial stromal sarcoma is a pure sarcoma, meaning that it contains only cancerous (malignant) stroma-like cells. These cancers can be either low-grade (slow-growing) or high-grade (fast-growing).

Uterine leiomyosarcomas

Uterine leiomyosarcomas develop in the muscular wall of the uterus (myometrium). They make up about 40 percent of all cases of uterine sarcomas. Uterine leiomyosarcoma also is a pure sarcoma.

Mixed sarcomas

Mixed sarcomas start in the endometrium but contain glandular cells from the endometrial lining (epithelial cells) and cells from the supporting stroma (mesodermal cells).

When the tumor contains noncancerous epithelial cells but cancerous mesodermal cells, it's called an adenosarcoma. When both epithelial and mesodermal cells are cancerous, the tumor is called a uterine carcinosarcoma, also known as malignant mixed mesodermal tumor or malignant mixed mullerian tumor (MMMT). Carcinosarcomas are the most common

Uterine Fibroids

Several types of noncancerous (benign) tumors can develop in the muscular wall of the uterus. These are often referred to as uterine fibroids, benign uterine fibroid tumors or uterine leiomyomas. Uterine fibroids can be as small as a pea or as large as a grapefruit.

Uterine fibroids are extremely common. About 20 percent of women older than age 35 have them. Most experts believe that fibroids don't become cancerous, and most women who have them have no symptoms. Sometimes, though, uterine fibroids can cause heavy or prolonged menstrual periods, which can increase the risk of iron deficiency anemia. In addition, a fibroid attached to your uterine wall can become twisted and starved for blood

and oxygen and cause pain. Bladder pressure and a feeling of heaviness in the pelvis are other common symptoms. Fibroids that cause problems are usually treated with surgery. If you have fibroids but don't have any symptoms, you may not need any treatment.

If you have symptoms and aren't planning to have children, your surgeon may recommend a hysterectomy. Or he or she might suggest removing only the fibroids, leaving the uterus intact. However, this procedure, called a myomectomy, is also a major operation and may result in complications.

Rarely, a mass first thought to be a uterine fibroid is later discovered to be cancerous, after it has been surgically removed and examined under a microscope. Between one-fifth and one-half of leiomyosarcomas are diagnosed in this way.

form of uterine sarcoma, making up half of all cases.

Others

Some uterine sarcomas don't fall into any of these categories. These cancers are described as undifferentiated or unclassified uterine sarcomas.

Risk Factors

Several risk factors are connected with uterine sarcomas.

Race
Leiomyosarcoma and carcinosarcoma tend to be more common among black women than among white women. The reason for this increased risk is unknown.

Age
Uterine sarcomas tend to occur in women who are middle-aged or older, but younger women also can develop them. The age at diagnosis tends to vary by the type of tumor. For leiomyosarcomas, the average age at diagnosis is 53. For mixed sarcomas, the usual age at diagnosis is 60 to 65. About 70 percent of low-grade (slow-growing) endometrial stromal sarcomas occur in women under age 50, but high-grade (fast-growing) stromal sarcomas tend to occur after menopause.

Prior pelvic radiation therapy
Radiation therapy to the pelvis to treat cancer can damage the DNA of normal cells. If you were previously treated with radiation for another cancer and your uterus wasn't removed, you have an increased risk of later developing uterine sarcoma. The relationship between prior pelvic radiation therapy and uterine sarcoma seems to be strongest for uterine carcinosarcomas.

Estrogen-related health history
Certain factors that increase your risk of endometrial cancer, discussed in Chapter 21, may also increase your risk of developing one type of uterine sarcoma — uterine carcinosarcoma — but not the other types.

The following risk factors reflect increased exposure to the hormone estrogen, which stimulates growth of the cells lining your uterus, increasing cancer risk. Such risk factors include the following:
• Early onset of menstruation and late menopause
• Never having been pregnant
• Infertility
• Irregular ovulation or menstruation
• Polycystic ovarian syndrome (PCOS)
• Estrogen-producing ovarian tumors
• Estrogen therapy after menopause
• Obesity
• Previous tamoxifen treatment — because tamoxifen acts like estrogen on the uterine lining
• Diabetes

Recently, use of the drug tamoxifen (Nolvadex), given for the prevention or treatment of breast cancer, has been found to cause a slightly increased risk of uterine sarcoma.

One important point to remember: Many women who have known risk factors for uterine sarcoma don't get the disease. At the same time, some who get this disease have no major risk factors for it. In most cases, doctors can't explain why one woman develops uterine sarcoma and another doesn't.

Signs and Symptoms

Signs and symptoms of uterine sarcomas tend to vary according to the type of disease. If you experience one or more of the following signs or symptoms, it doesn't necessarily mean that you have cancer, but it's important that you make an appointment to see your doctor.

Abnormal vaginal bleeding

For most women with uterine sarcoma, the first clue that something is wrong is abnormal vaginal bleeding. This occurs in up to 95 percent of women who have the disease. The bleeding can range from light spotting near menopause to heavy menstrual periods or unexplained bleeding after menopause. Abnormal bleeding is more likely to be caused by uterine carcinosarcomas or endometrial stromal sarcomas than by leiomyosarcomas.

Irregular vaginal bleeding can have a benign cause, such as a hormone imbalance or benign polyps, but it's important to have it checked as soon as possible. If you've gone through menopause, it's especially important to report to your doctor any bleeding or spotting.

Other discharge

About 10 percent of women with uterine sarcoma have a vaginal discharge that contains no visible blood. This is usually a sign of a benign condition, such as a vaginal infection, but that's not always the case.

Pelvic pain or pressure

Up to one-third of all women with uterine sarcoma experience pelvic pain or pressure, which can be fairly intense. Among women with leiomyosarcoma, up to 40 percent experience pelvic pain.

Enlarged uterus

About 20 percent to 50 percent of women with either uterine carcinosarcoma or leiomyosarcoma have an enlarged uterus or a mass that can be felt in the pelvis.

QUESTION & ANSWER

Q: **Can uterine sarcomas be detected early?**

A: If you're alert to the signs and symptoms of uterine sarcoma and see a doctor right away if they occur, it may be possible to detect the disease in an early stage.

Unfortunately, though, uterine sarcoma may reach an advanced stage before it produces signs and symptoms. Currently, there's no effective screening test or exam for detecting uterine sarcomas in women who don't have signs or symptoms. Rarely, a Pap test may pick up some early uterine sarcomas, especially carcinosarcomas and endometrial stromal sarcomas, but most uterine sarcomas aren't detected this way.

Uterine sarcoma stages

Stage	Description
Stage I	The cancer is confined to the body (corpus) of the uterus.
Stage II	The cancer involves both the corpus and the cervix of the uterus.
Stage III	The cancer has spread beyond the uterus but not beyond the pelvic area.
Stage IV	The cancer has spread beyond the pelvic area.

Diagnosing Uterine Sarcomas

If your primary care doctor suspects that you may have a uterine cancer, you'll likely be referred to a gynecologist, a doctor who specializes in conditions affecting the female reproductive system, or to a gynecologic oncologist, a surgeon who specializes in diagnosing and treating cancers of the female reproductive system.

Your doctor will want to know of any signs and symptoms you may be experiencing. A physical examination is often next. This will likely include a thorough pelvic exam, an abdominal exam and examination of the lymph nodes in your groin and above your collarbone.

To make an accurate diagnosis, additional tests will likely be needed, such as an endometrial biopsy or a dilation and curettage (D and C) procedure. For more information on these tests, see Chapter 22.

Tissue sampling procedures, such as an endometrial biopsy or D and C, detect most uterine carcinosarcomas and many endometrial stromal sarcomas. But the two procedures detect only 25 percent to 50 percent of all leiomyosarcomas. These cancers start in the muscular wall of the uterus (myometrium), and sometimes they don't spread to the lining of the uterine cavity (endometrium).

Most leiomyosarcomas are diagnosed after a hysterectomy for what were thought to be benign uterine fibroids. In examining tissue samples from the uterus after it has been removed, the pathologist detects cancerous cells.

Grading and staging

The cancer grade depends on how normal or abnormal the cells appear. Generally, the lower the grade, the fewer the abnormalities and the better the prognosis. High-grade uterine sarcomas tend to grow and spread more quickly than do low-grade ones.

The tissue samples may be tested for estrogen or progesterone receptors. Some endometrial stromal sarcomas contain estrogen and progesterone receptors and depend on these female hormones to grow. If tests indicate that you have an endometrial stromal sarcoma that contains estrogen receptors, your doctor may consider prescribing hormone therapies that prevent estrogen production or block the action of this hormone. This may help slow the growth of your cancer.

Based on the results of your surgery and laboratory tests, your doctor gathers all the information available to classify the stage of your cancer. A lower number indicates that the cancer is still in its early stages, whereas a higher number means a more advanced, serious cancer.

Treating Uterine Sarcomas

Surgery is the standard treatment for uterine sarcomas. The extent of surgery depends on the type of sarcoma present, but the procedure performed most often is removal of the uterus, including the cervix, as well as both fallopian tubes and both ovaries. The medical term for this procedure is *total abdominal hysterectomy with bilateral salpingo-oophorectomy.*

Radiation therapy or chemotherapy is sometimes recommended after surgery, depending on the stage of the disease. Because uterine sarcomas are uncommon, there isn't good data from clinical trials to guide treatment recommendations.

Surgery

For stage I, II and III uterine sarcomas, the usual surgical treatment is removal of the uterus, including the cervix, as well as both fallopian tubes and both ovaries. In a few instances with early-stage leiomyosarcoma, surgery that preserves the ovaries may be an option.

In some cases of endometrial stromal sarcoma, when disease has spread to the connective tissue between your pelvic floor and the upper part of your cervix (parametrium), a radical hysterectomy may be performed. This is the most extensive type of hysterectomy. In addition to the uterus and cervix, the upper inch of your vagina also is removed, as well as the parametrium and the ligaments that hold the uterus in place.

Sometimes, a surgeon will remove lymph nodes in the pelvis or around the main artery that travels from your heart to your lower torso (aorta) to see if the lymph nodes contain cancerous cells (see "Lymph node removal," on page 392). Lymph nodes are small, bean-shaped structures found throughout the body. They produce and store infection-fighting cells and are one of the first sites of invasion when cancer spreads.

For more detailed information on what to expect before, during and after surgery for uterine cancer, see Chapter 23.

Radiation therapy

Recurrence of uterine sarcoma in the pelvic area, even after surgery appears to have removed all the cancer, is fairly common. Many women with uterine sarcoma have microscopic spread of disease within the pelvis that, if untreated, may eventually regrow.

Two types of radiation therapy may be used to treat uterine sarcoma: external beam radiation and internal radiation (brachytherapy). The type of radiation you receive depends on the extent of your cancer. Some women with uterine sarcoma need both external and internal radiation therapies. With external beam radia-

Q: **Is hormone therapy used to treat uterine sarcomas?**

A: Some endometrial stromal sarcomas contain estrogen and progesterone receptors, and the cancers depend on these female hormones to grow. If tests show that your cancer is estrogen receptor positive and the cancer is low-grade (slow-growing), your doctor may prescribe hormone therapy to prevent estrogen production or block the action of this hormone. This may help slow the growth of your cancer. Hormone therapy is rarely used for other forms of uterine sarcomas. In general, hormone therapy is used to control more advanced (stage III or stage IV) cases of low-grade endometrial stromal sarcoma.

tion, you receive doses of radiation from a large X-ray machine aimed at the tumor area from outside the body. You attend radiation sessions as an outpatient in a hospital or clinic, typically five days a week for four to six weeks.

With internal radiation therapy, radioactive substances called radioisotopes are temporarily placed in or near the tumor or in the area where the cancer has been removed. As the radioisotopes break down, they release radiation, killing cancer cells in the area.

Radiation therapy after surgery may reduce the risk of pelvic recurrence, but unfortunately, it doesn't significantly improve a woman's chances of survival. While radiation therapy may prevent the cancer from coming back in the same location, it doesn't stop the cancer from developing in distant sites.

In some women with advanced (stage IV) disease, radiation therapy is used to reduce pain, bleeding and other symptoms caused by a particular area of disease. The purpose is not to cure the cancer but to improve quality of life.

For more information on radiation therapy, see Chapter 23.

Chemotherapy

In more than 50 percent of women diagnosed with uterine sarcoma, the cancer will recur. This is true even when the cancer is diagnosed in its earliest stage (stage I), and it's especially true for the higher grade (faster growing) uterine sarcomas. Often, the recurrence is outside the pelvic area because cancer cells can spread through the bloodstream.

To reduce the risk of recurrent uterine sarcoma, your doctor may suggest that you receive chemotherapy after surgery. With chemotherapy the medications enter your bloodstream and travel through your body, killing cancer cells that have spread outside the uterus.

Chemotherapy is generally reserved for more advanced stages of uterine sarcoma. There isn't evidence that chemotherapy is beneficial in treating early-stage disease, but this possibility is being studied in clinical trials.

5-year survival rates for uterine sarcomas

Stage	Description	5-year survival rate
Stage I	The sarcoma is confined to the body (corpus) of the uterus.	About 50 %
Stage II	The sarcoma involves both the corpus and the cervix of the uterus.	About 20 %
Stage III	The sarcoma has spread beyond the uterus but not beyond the pelvic area.	About 10 %
Stage IV	The sarcoma has spread beyond the pelvic area.	Less than 10 %

Medications used to treat uterine sarcomas may include:

- Doxorubicin (Adriamycin)
- Ifosfamide (Ifex)
- Cisplatin (Platinol)
- Paclitaxel (Taxol)
- Gemcitabine (Gemzar)

The choice of chemotherapy medications depends on the type of uterine sarcoma you have, your disease stage and your overall health.

For most women with advanced uterine sarcoma, chemotherapy can't cure the cancer. The medications may shrink the tumors for a period of time, but they aren't able to destroy the cancer.

For more information on chemotherapy as a treatment for uterine cancer, see Chapter 23.

Prognosis

One way to report cancer survival rates is to specify the percentage of patients who are still living five years after receiving their diagnoses. This doesn't mean that survivors live for only five years after being diagnosed with cancer. The five-year benchmark is simply used for consistency when talking about cancer survival.

Your likelihood of surviving uterine sarcoma depends on the stage of your cancer when it was first diagnosed, as well as the type of sarcoma (carcinosarcoma, leiomyosarcoma or endometrial stromal) and the grade of your tumor. Low-grade (slow-growing) tumors have a better prognosis than do high-grade (fast-growing) ones. Your overall health also influences your prognosis.

Keep in mind that these statistics are estimates based on prior studies of women diagnosed with uterine sarcoma. They represent the average outlook for groups of people. They can't necessarily predict the outcome in your particular case. Each woman and each case is different. If you have questions about your prognosis, discuss them with your doctor or other members of your health care team. They can help you find out how these statistics relate, or don't relate, to you.

Chapter 26: Gynecologic Cancers

Cervical Cancer Overview

Each year approximately 11,000 women in the United States learn that they have cancer of the cervix. Fortunately, this is a cancer for which there's a screening test to identify it and for which effective treatment options are available.

A simple test called the Pap test can detect cervical cancer in its early stages. Thanks in large part to this test, the death rate from cervical cancer in the United States and other developed countries has decreased dramatically over the past 50 years. Still, cervical cancer remains a leading cause of cancer deaths in women across the globe. This is likely because many women worldwide don't have access to the Pap test, or they don't have the test done.

Cervical cancer occurs in both younger and older women and is most commonly diagnosed in midlife. The main symptom is abnormal vaginal bleeding, such as bleeding after sexual intercourse or bleeding between menstrual periods. The main cause of the cancer is infection with certain strains of a common sexually transmitted virus called the human papillomavirus (HPV). Major risk factors for the disease include having intercourse at a young age and having multiple sexual partners.

If you're concerned that you may have cervical cancer or that you may be at risk of developing it, make an appointment to have a Pap test. If you've recently received a diagnosis of cervical cancer, know that it's a highly treatable — and beatable — cancer. When found and treated early, cervical cancer can usually be cured. Even when women are diagnosed at a more advanced stage, some of them can be cured.

Meanwhile, researchers continue to look for new and better ways to treat cervical cancer — and perhaps even prevent it. For example, a vaccine is being studied that may protect women from HPV infection and, as a result, from cervical cancer.

Cervical Changes

A woman's womb (uterus) is shaped like an upside-down pear. At the bottom of the uterus — behind the bladder and in front of the rectum — is the cervix, a ring-like muscular band about an inch in

The Pap Test: A Success Story

The Pap test, sometimes called a Pap smear or Pap smear test, is used to detect cervical cancer or precancerous changes of the cervix. It's named after George Papanicolaou, M.D., who in 1941 first proposed this simple test as a screening tool for cervical cancer.

The Pap test has been one of medicine's greatest success stories, ranking right up there with the development of antibiotics to treat infection and insulin to treat diabetes. Cervical cancer was once the No. 1 cancer killer of American women. But thanks to the nationwide implementation of the Pap test starting in the 1950s, the death rate from cervical cancer has dropped by more than 70 percent in the United States.

The real benefit of this test is that it can detect cellular changes that precede cervical cancer, alerting your doctor to a problem that can be treated, essentially stopping the disease before cancer actually develops. These days, many women who receive a diagnosis of cervical cancer didn't get regular Pap tests, so the test wasn't able to identify the disease in its precancerous state. In addition, the Pap test isn't perfect. It can miss precancers and even cancers. This can happen, for example, if the cancer didn't shed cells when the Pap test was done or if the Pap sample wasn't taken from the optimal location. In the United States, an estimated 4,000 women die of cervical cancer annually because the disease is caught too late.

For more information on the Pap test and screening for cervical cancer, see Chapter 27.

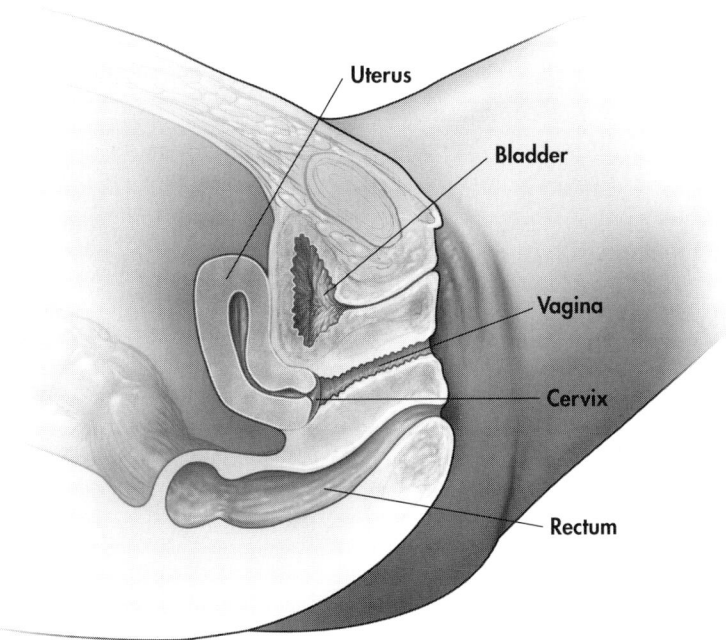

Uterus

Bladder

Vagina

Cervix

Rectum

length. *Cervix* is the Latin word for "neck." The cervix is the neck of the uterus that projects into the upper part of the vagina. A narrow canal called the cervical canal passes through the cervix. It's the cervical canal that connects a woman's uterus to her vagina.

The cervix is composed mostly of connective tissue covered by a mucous membrane layer. Most pregnant women become familiar with the anatomy of the cervix during labor and delivery. During childbirth, it's the cervix that must soften and open up (dilate) so that the baby can pass from the uterus into the birth canal (vagina).

Like other tissues in the body, the cervix is composed of several types of cells, all of which are able to divide to produce more cells when the body needs them to. If cells keep dividing when new cells aren't needed, a mass of extra cells — a growth (tumor) — forms. This mass may be noncancerous (benign) or it may be cancerous (malignant).

Cervical cancer actually begins with benign precancerous changes called cervical dysplasia, or cervical intraepithelial neoplasia (CIN). In this condition, cells begin to look abnormal in size, shape and configuration.

The three degrees of CIN are based on how abnormal the cells appear under a microscope:

- CIN 1 refers to cells that are mildly abnormal in appearance.
- CIN 2 refers to cells that are moderately abnormal in appearance.
- CIN 3 refers to cells that are severely abnormal in appearance.

CIN 3 is also known as carcinoma *in situ*. In this condition, the cells appear cancerous, but they're still limited to the surface of the cervix. They haven't invaded deeper tissues of the cervix. Precancerous changes and carcinoma *in situ* are discussed in more detail in Chapter 27.

Most of the time, mild dysplasia goes away without treatment. The body's immune system cleans up the altered cells or fights the underlying infection that's triggering the changes. In other cases, this abnormality marks the first in a series of progressive changes leading to cervical cancer, a process that likely takes years. Cervical cancer generally follows a well-known path: It starts as dysplasia, progresses to carcinoma *in situ* and finally becomes invasive cancer. Treating the disease early on can prevent cancer.

A Cervical Cancer Vaccine

Are there ways to protect yourself from human papillomavirus (HPV) infection and other sexually transmitted diseases that may put you at increased risk of cervical cancer?

You can minimize your exposure to sexually transmitted infections by practicing abstinence or, if you're sexually active, by limiting your number of sexual partners.

Birth control pills won't protect you from sexually transmitted viruses such as HPV. Even condoms can't protect you completely from HPV infection, although they can help lower your risk of contracting other sexually transmitted diseases.

What may be the best defense against HPV infection — an HPV vaccine — is the focus of current research. The vaccine under study trains a woman's immune system to recognize and eliminate one or more strains of the HPV virus. In one study, some 1,200 American women were vaccinated against HPV type 16 (HPV-16), a high-risk strain that's been implicated in roughly half of all cervical cancers in the United States. None of the vaccinated women became infected with HPV-16 over the next year and a half. In contrast, 41 young women in a similar-sized group who received inactive (placebo) injections became infected with the virus during the same period.

This particular vaccine and others like it are still being investigated in clinical trials, so none is yet available. But researchers hope that by vaccinating against HPV-16, along with other high-risk strains of HPV, they will one day further reduce rates of cervical cancer in the United States and worldwide.

In addition, researchers are studying a vaccine that helps women who are already infected with HPV mount an immune response against the infection. The goal is to stimulate the women's immune systems to destroy the virus and eliminate the infection before precancerous or cancerous cells can develop.

Types of Cervical Cancer

Two types of cells line the surface of the cervix. Cells in the middle and upper third of the cervix, which are closest to the lining of the uterus (endometrium), have a column-shaped (columnar) appearance like endometrial cells. These cells are called glandular cells. The cells lining the bottom third of the cervix are thin, flat cells, similar to those that line the vagina. These are called squamous cells.

The boundary between these two types of cells is called the transformation zone (squamocolumnar junction), and it's here that cervical dysplasia and cancer generally occur. These cells can develop into various types of cancers, including:

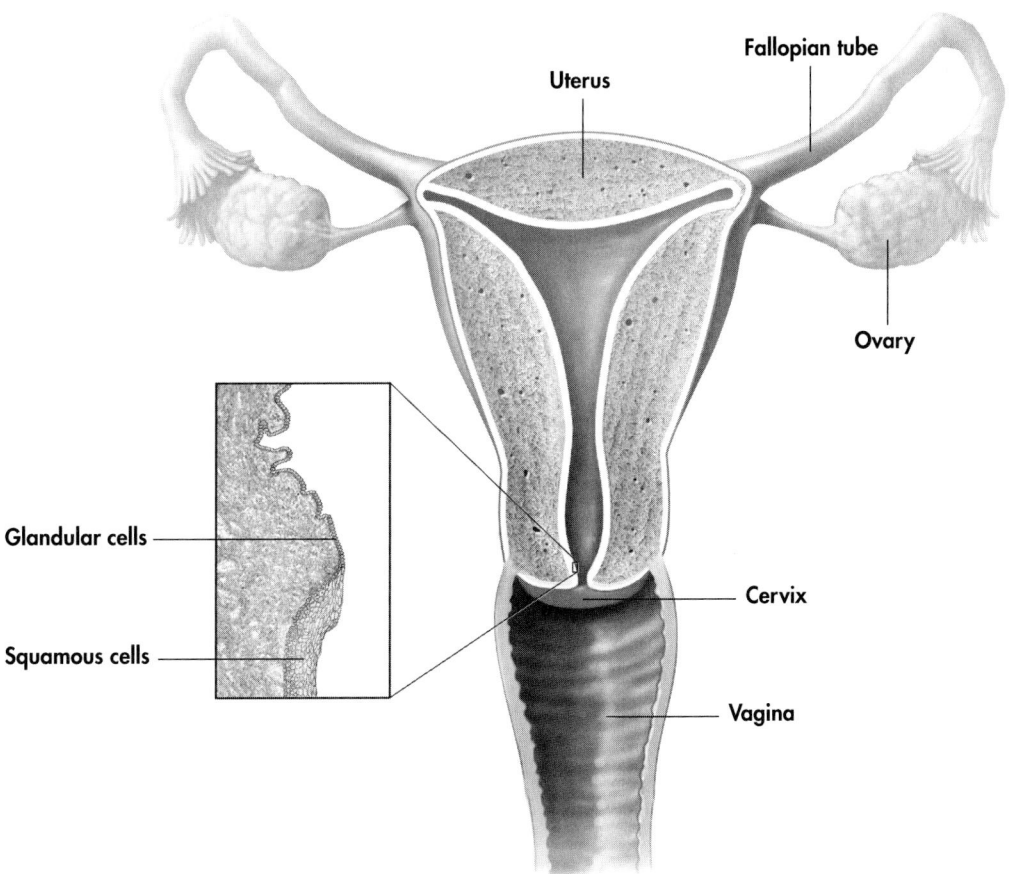

Two types of cells line the surface of the cervix. One type (glandular cells) has a column-shaped appearance. The other type (squamous cells) is thin and flat. The boundary between the two types of cells is called the transformation zone (squamocolumnar junction). It's here that precancerous changes and cancer most often occur.

- **Squamous carcinomas.** These cancers develop in squamous cells located in the lower portion of the cervix. They account for 85 percent to 90 percent of all cervical cancers.
- **Adenocarcinomas.** These cancers begin in glandular cells in the upper portion of the cervix. They account for 10 percent to 15 percent of all cervical cancers.

Rarely, the cancerous cells contain features of both squamous cell cancer and adenocarcinoma. These are called mixed cell types (adenosquamous carcinomas). Other rare cancer types that can develop in the cervix are small cell carcinoma and cervical sarcoma.

What Causes Cervical Cancer?

In recent years, scientists have made considerable progress toward understanding the possible causes of cervical cancer. Researchers believe most cervical cancers are triggered by an underlying sexually transmitted disease in the cervix. In particular, they're studying the effects of the sexually transmitted human papillomaviruses (HPVs). In almost all cervical cancers, the woman has been infected with a strain of this virus.

Human papillomaviruses

Human papillomaviruses include more than 100 types of viruses and are very common. They're called papillomaviruses because certain types cause warts (papillomas). Some types of HPV, which aren't spread through sexual contact, cause the common warts that grow on hands and feet. Other types, which are sexually transmitted, cause genital warts.

Most strains of HPV don't lead to cervical cancer. In fact, the types of HPV that cause genital warts actually carry a very low risk of cervical cancer. However, several strains of sexually transmitted HPV — so-called high-risk strains — have been linked to cervical cancer. The most common of these high-risk types — numbered 16, 18, 31, 33, 35 and 45 — account for approximately 85 percent of all HPVs found in cervical cancer samples.

Researchers have found that women who are infected with a high-risk strain of HPV or whose sexual partner is a carrier of a high-risk strain have a higher than average risk of developing cervical cancer.

HPVs may even play a role in other cancers, such as those of the anus, vulva, vagina and penis, as well some throat cancers. In addition, partners of men with penile cancer, a rare cancer, have a higher incidence of cervical cancer than do partners of men who don't have penile cancer.

Anyone who has had sexual intercourse, men as well as women, can get an HPV infection. The infection is spread by skin-to-skin contact during vaginal or anal sex. You can be infected with HPV and not know it. The infection doesn't usually produce warts or other noticeable problems, so you may be infected and pass the virus on without knowing it.

HPV infection is extremely common. In fact, studies indicate that at least half of women who've ever had sexual intercourse have been exposed to at least one strain of HPV. Among most women, though, their immune systems fight off the infection, so it doesn't persist long enough to cause problems.

Most women who are infected with HPV never develop cervical cancer. An American woman who is screened regularly for cervical cancer has a 0.8 percent lifetime risk of developing cervical cancer. In other words, fewer than one out of every 100 women in the United States develops cervical cancer. In addition, not all women who develop cervical cancer are infected with HPV.

For these reasons, scientists believe that other factors, along with HPV infection, are associated with the development of cervical cancer. Research suggests that the genital herpes virus may play a role. Evidence is also growing that the sexually transmitted disease chlamydia may increase a woman's risk of developing cervical cancer.

More research is needed to learn the exact role of sexually transmitted viruses and how they may interact with other factors in the development of cervical cancer.

Who Gets Cervical Cancer?

Lack of cancer awareness and poor access to health care each plays a significant role in the development of cervical cancer. In the United States, approximately half of all cervical cancers occur in women who don't get regular Pap tests.

Some women forgo regular Pap tests because they don't have health insurance or they don't have access to health care.

Some women may be shy about having a Pap test, or their culture may prohibit them from revealing their bodies to male doctors. Language barriers and a lack of education also keep some women from seeing a doctor for regular Pap tests. In addition, many women, especially those age 60 and older, simply don't view themselves as being at risk of developing cervical cancer, even though they may be.

Unscreened women — combined with difficulties in detecting some cancers, such as those that begin in the less accessible upper region of the cervix — account for most new cases of cervical cancer.

Geographic location

Around the world, cervical cancer is among the top three most common cancers in women, along with breast cancer and colorectal cancer. In some countries, cervical cancer is the most common female cancer. It's also one of the most deadly cancers among women living in developing countries.

The disease kills approximately 500,000 women worldwide annually. Countries with the highest number of cervical cancer cases are located in Africa, Southeast Asia and Central and South America.

Socioeconomic status

Poor, uneducated women have a higher incidence of cervical cancer than do women of higher socioeconomic status. In America, the cancer is most common in poor women living in rural areas — whites and minorities alike.

Ethnic group

In the United States, cervical cancer is more common and more likely to cause death among minorities, including Asian-Americans, Hispanics, Alaskan and Hawaiian natives, American Indians and blacks.

Age

Cervical cancer mainly affects younger women, but many older women don't realize that the risk of developing cervical cancer is still present as they get older. Research has shown that cervical cancer is diagnosed across a wide age spectrum. About 20 percent of women with cervical cancer are diagnosed when they're older than age 65.

Some data indicate that the incidence of cervical cancer peaks during two age ranges — from ages 35 to 39 and from ages 60 to 64.

Risk Factors

A risk factor is anything that increases your chances of getting a certain disease. Risk factors for any disease are based on probabilities. You may have many risk factors for cervical cancer but never develop the disease. Or a woman with no risk factors for the disease may develop it.

It's known that the most important factor contributing to cervical cancer is human papillomavirus (HPV) infection. Yet most women who are infected with the virus don't get cervical cancer. So what else may be involved?

Sexual history

Because HPV infection is spread mainly through sexual contact, a woman's sexual history plays an important role in her risk of cervical cancer.

Early sexual activity

Women who start having sexual intercourse at a young age may have a more difficult time naturally fighting off HPV infection than do women who become sexually active later on. Sexual intercourse before age 18 may also increase your risk of cervical cancer because less mature cervical cells seem to be more susceptible to the precancerous changes triggered by HPV infection.

Many sexual partners

Your chances of getting HPV increase with your number of sexual partners. The greater the number of sexual partners you've had — and the number of partners that your partners have had — the greater your chance of acquiring cancer-causing types of HPV. There also seems to be a slightly increased risk of developing cervical cancer if a male sexual partner is uncircumcised.

Other sexually transmitted diseases

If you have other sexually transmitted diseases, such as chlamydia, gonorrhea or genital herpes, you have a greater chance of having been exposed to HPV.

In addition, other sexually transmitted diseases may somehow contribute to the development of cervical cancer. Scientists don't have a clear understanding of exactly how other sexually transmitted dis-

MYTH vs. FACT

Myth: **Cancer is contagious.**

Fact: You can't catch cancer. It starts within a given person, and his or her cells can't survive in someone else. So it's OK to touch and spend time with someone who has cancer. Although cancer itself isn't contagious, sometimes infectious viruses can lead to the development of cancer. For example, human papillomavirus, a sexually transmitted disease, is associated with cervical cancer.

eases affect cervical cancer risk, but it's important they be treated promptly.

Weakened immune system

Infection with HIV, the virus that causes AIDS, is another risk factor for cervical cancer, but for a slightly different reason. Women infected with HIV have a weakened immune system. When your immune system is weakened, your body is less able to fight off HPV and other infections and, perhaps, early cancers — including cervical cancer.

In addition, and for the same reason, women who have received an organ transplant and are taking drugs to suppress their immune system may be at higher risk of cervical cancer.

Family health history

Studies suggest that if your mother or sisters had cervical cancer, you may be more likely to develop the disease. Some researchers believe that cervical cancer may run in certain families due to inherited weaknesses of the immune system that make it harder for some women to eliminate HPV infection.

Smoking

Cervical cancer is more common among women who smoke. Women who smoke are about twice as likely to develop cervical cancer as are those who don't smoke. Researchers are investigating whether smoking itself causes cervical cancer or if smoking heightens a person's vulnerability to other illnesses, such as sexually transmitted infections like HPV.

Tobacco use appears to increase a woman's risk of precancerous cervical changes, as well as cancer of the cervix. Tobacco decreases a person's ability to fight off infections, including HPV. In addition, some of the cancer-causing substances (carcinogens) in tobacco become concentrated in the cervical glands that make mucus.

Medications

Some medications have been linked to an increased risk of cervical cancer.

Exposure to DES
Women whose mothers took the drug diethylstilbestrol (DES) during pregnancy are at increased risk of a rare type of

GYNECOLOGIC CANCERS

cervical cancer called clear cell adenocarcinoma. DES was once prescribed — from about 1940 to 1970 — to prevent miscarriage, but the drug is no longer on the market. In the 1970s, it was discovered that women whose mothers took DES were at risk of this rare form of cervical cancer.

Use of birth control pills

Women who use birth control pills for five years or longer may be at slightly increased risk of cervical cancer, although it's unclear just exactly why that may be. One possibility might be that women taking birth control pills tend to be more sexually active. It's also possible that hormone medications directly affect the ability of viruses to thrive in the cervix.

Reducing Your Risk

To lower your risk of cervical cancer, undergo regular Pap testing. That's the most important step you can take. If detected and treated in its precancerous stages, cervical cancer can be prevented. Talk with your doctor about an appropriate schedule of checkups, based on your age, medical history and risk factors. If you have an abnormal Pap test result, see your doctor for follow-up care.

The second most important thing you can do to help prevent cervical cancer is to modify those risk factors for the disease that you can control, such as quitting smoking, delaying the onset of sexual activity and limiting your number of sexual partners. If you're sexually active, the use of condoms may help protect you from developing sexually transmitted diseases that could play a role in the development of cervical cancer.

Some evidence indicates that eating a healthy diet can help protect you against several cancers, possibly including cervical cancer. Some people believe that vitamin A and vitamin E, in particular, may play a role in cervical cancer prevention. But there's no strong evidence that eating foods rich in these nutrients or taking vitamins can protect you from cervical cancer.

Chapter 27: Gynecologic Cancers

Diagnosing Cervical Cancer & Precancerous Changes

In its early stages, cervical cancer generally doesn't cause signs or symptoms — you may have no warning flags that something is wrong. Signs and symptoms often don't appear until cancer cells have spread deeper into the cervix or even beyond the cervix. That's why it's so important that women — especially those with risk factors for the disease — have regular Pap tests to detect abnormal cells before they become cancerous. Cervical cancer is one of the cancers that can be prevented through screening.

The Pap test is the primary screening method used to detect cervical cancer and early changes in cells of the cervix that precede cancer development. Unfortunately, not all women have access to cervical cancer screening or make use of its availability. Women still die of cervical cancer — an oftentimes preventable disease — because it goes undiagnosed until it has advanced to an incurable stage.

Signs and Symptoms

Once the disease reaches a later stage, signs and symptoms generally appear. They may include:
- Spotting or heavy vaginal bleeding between menstrual periods
- Menstrual bleeding that's heavier and lasts longer than normal
- Vaginal bleeding after menopause
- Vaginal bleeding after sexual intercourse, douching or a pelvic exam
- Pain during sexual intercourse
- Watery or bloody vaginal discharge, which may be heavy and odorous

The longer signs and symptoms go undetected or untreated, the greater the chance of the cancer's spreading beyond the cervix, making a cure more difficult. If you have any of these signs or symptoms, see your doctor. For certain, bring to his or her attention right away any irregular vaginal bleeding. Even better, don't wait for signs and symptoms of cervical cancer to appear. Get regular Pap tests to detect precancerous changes of the cervix, which can be treated so that, in most cases, the condition won't have a chance to develop into cancer.

Screening

Regular Pap tests should be a routine part of your health care. This screening test for cervical cancer helps detect changes in cells of the cervix that precede cancer, as well as cancer cells. The development of cervical cancer is gradual and begins with abnormalities in the cells located on the surface of the cervix — a condition known as dysplasia, or cervical intraepithelial neoplasia (CIN). These changes range from mild to severe.

QUESTION & ANSWER

Q: **What does the term *dysplasia* mean?**

A: *Dysplasia* is a term used to describe abnormal cells that could become cancerous if not treated. The cells look abnormal under the microscope, but they don't invade nearby healthy tissue. The three degrees of dysplasia are mild, moderate and severe, depending on how abnormal the cells appear under the microscope. Generally, the more abnormal the cervical cells are, the more likely it is that they could become cancerous.

Doctors also refer to dysplasia as cervical intraepithelial neoplasia (CIN) or squamous intraepithelial lesion (SIL).

In addition to a Pap test, which is typically done as part of a pelvic exam, screening for cervical cancer may also include a test for human papillomaviruses (HPVs). HPVs are the most important cause of cervical cancer. These tests, which are generally done jointly, can be performed at a doctor's office, health clinic or hospital. Your primary care doctor, gynecologist or other health care professional may perform the tests.

Pelvic exam

During a pelvic examination, you lie on your back on an examining table with your knees bent. Usually, your heels rest in metal supports called stirrups.

Your doctor first examines your external genitals to make sure they look normal — no sores, discoloration, swelling or other abnormalities. To see the inner walls of your vagina and your cervix, an instrument called a speculum is inserted into the vagina. When the speculum is in the open position, it holds the vaginal walls apart so that your cervix can be seen. Your doctor shines a light inside to look for lumps, sores, inflammation, signs of abnormal discharge or anything else that's unusual. At this point, with the speculum in place, he or she will perform the Pap test.

After removing the speculum, the next step is generally to check the condition of your uterus and ovaries. This is done by inserting two lubricated, gloved fingers into your vagina and pressing down on your abdomen with the other hand. Usually, this is followed by a rectovaginal exam, which involves inserting one finger in your vagina and another in your rectum. This allows your doctor to locate your uterus, ovaries and other organs, judge their size, and confirm that they're in the proper position. He or she also feels for any lumps, changes in the shape of the uterus or other abnormalities that may indicate a problem.

Many women find a pelvic exam uncomfortable. During the exam, try to relax as much as you can. Breathe slowly and deeply. If you tense up, your abdominal and pelvic muscles may tighten, which can make the exam even more uncomfortable. Let your doctor know if you're experiencing a lot of discomfort. Remember, a typical pelvic exam takes only a couple of minutes.

Pap test

A Pap test, which takes only seconds to perform, is usually done as part of a pelvic exam. Typically, the Pap test is done in the early part of a pelvic exam, after a speculum has been placed in your vagina. After viewing the cervix with a light, your doctor inserts a small brush or spatula to collect cells from the surface of the cervix and from within the cervical canal. The cells are smeared onto a slide, preserved with a fixative and sent to a laboratory.

Cervical cell specimens can also be obtained with a liquid-based approach. The cells are gathered in the same way, but rather than smearing cells from your cervix directly onto a slide, the instrument used to collect the cells is rinsed in a vial of preservative solution. A machine is then used to filter the specimen, reducing

GYNECOLOGIC CANCERS

Pelvic exam

You lie on an examining table with your knees bent and your heels in metal supports (stirrups). After examining your external genitals, your doctor performs the following.

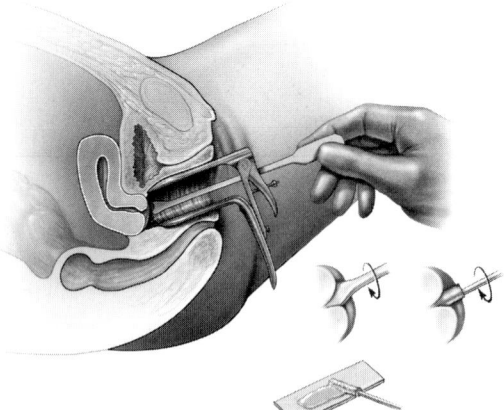

Pap test
A pelvic exam typically includes a Pap test — in which a sample of cells is taken from your cervix. For this test, a small brush or spatula is inserted to collect cells from the surface of the cervix and cervical canal.

Vaginal exam
To check the condition of your uterus and ovaries, your doctor inserts two lubricated, gloved fingers into the vagina and presses down on your abdomen with the other hand. This allows your doctor to locate your uterus, ovaries and other organs. While exploring the contours of these organs and the pelvis, your doctor feels for any lumps or changes that may signal a problem.

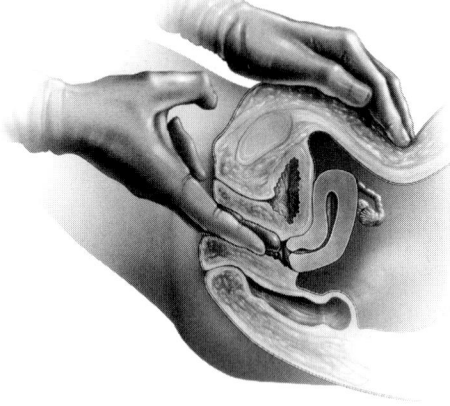

Rectovaginal exam
To feel the same organs from a different angle, your doctor will likely also perform a rectovaginal exam. For this exam, your doctor inserts one finger into your rectum while another remains in your vagina.

blood and mucus, which can obscure the cervical cells being examined. The machine applies a thin, even layer of cells to a microscope slide for examination.

With either technique, a technician called a cytotechnologist examines the slide first to make sure that an adequate sample was obtained and then looks for abnormal cells. A doctor called a pathologist further reviews the slides that contain abnormal cells before making a final diagnosis. Results of your Pap test are sent to your doctor. Your doctor's office should then provide them to you.

After you've had a Pap test, ask your doctor when you can expect the results. If you haven't heard from his or her office within a couple of weeks, contact the office for your results.

Screening Recommendations

Talk to your doctor about when and how often you should have a Pap test. The American Cancer Society's recommendations for cervical cancer screening are as follows:

- Women should have annual Pap tests beginning approximately three years after they begin to have sexual intercourse, but no later than age 21.
- Women under the age of 30 should have a Pap test every one to two years, depending on the screening method used. If a liquid-based test is used, every two years may be adequate. Otherwise, it's recommended that you have the test yearly.
- Women age 30 and older who've had three normal Pap tests in a row and have no history of cervical intraepithelial neoplasia (CIN) may extend the length of time between tests to every two to three years.
- Women who've had a hysterectomy that included removal of the cervix and who have no history of CIN or gynecologic cancers may discontinue Pap testing.

If you have a diagnosis of CIN or cervical cancer, you'll need more frequent Pap testing as part of your follow-up care.

If you have human immunodeficiency virus (HIV) infection, which weakens your immune system, frequent cancer screenings, including annual Pap tests, are important. Women of all ages who were exposed to the drug diethylstilbestrol

QUESTION & ANSWER

Q: **When I reach a certain age, can I stop having Pap tests?**

A: The American Cancer Society recommends that screening can stop at age 70, provided three or more of your recent Pap test results have been normal and you haven't had any abnormal results in the last 10 years. Keep in mind, though, that if you've had sex with a new partner, this may change your risk of the disease.

Talk with your doctor about how long you should continue to have Pap tests.

(DES) while in their mothers' wombs or who have a weakened immune system due to an organ transplant, chemotherapy or chronic steroid use should continue to have annual Pap tests for life.

Some women mistakenly believe that it's safe to discontinue cervical cancer screening after they've stopped having children. Continue having regular Pap tests even after having children, keeping to the schedule that your doctor recommends.

Women who've had a total hysterectomy — surgical removal of the uterus, including the cervix — don't need to have Pap tests, unless the surgery was done as a treatment for CIN or cancer. Women who've had a partial hysterectomy, without the removal of the cervix, should continue cervical cancer screening.

How effective is the test?

The Pap test is accurate in about 70 percent to 80 percent of cases, which means it's reliable but not foolproof. The test can produce what's known as false-positive and false-negative results. A false-positive Pap test result means that a woman is told that abnormalities were found when, in fact, the cells were normal. A false-negative Pap test result occurs when the test result is said to be normal but, in fact, the woman has cervical cancer or dysplasia.

How do inaccuracies occur? The results of a Pap test may be inaccurate if the sample cells aren't taken from the location in the cervix where precancerous changes are most likely to occur — where the glandular cells and squamous cells meet (squamocolumnar junction). This is the area of the cervix where problems typically begin. To make the test as accurate as possible, an adequate number of cells from the surface of the cervix and within the cervical canal must be collected, and the cells need to be preserved with a fixative immediately. If this doesn't happen, the sample taken may not be a satisfactory specimen.

Mistakes in Pap test results can also occur if the cytotechnologist or pathologist reviewing your slide fails to identify or correctly interpret abnormal cells. This is more often a problem when there's only a small number of abnormal cells — akin

Same Time, Next Year

To help you remember to schedule your Pap test, try making your appointment for the same time of year. Many women schedule their Pap tests near their birthdays. Or ask your doctor to send you a reminder when it's time for your next pelvic exam and Pap test.

About half the cervical cancers diagnosed in the United States occur in women who've never had a Pap test, and another 10 percent occur in women who haven't been screened within the past five years. So don't put off having the test. Like other screening tests for cancer, the small amount of time you invest can be lifesaving.

to finding a needle in a haystack. An average slide may contain more than 100,000 cells.

To ensure the accuracy of your Pap test, you can do your part by preparing for the test properly. It's recommended that you:

- Don't have sexual intercourse and don't douche for two days before the test
- Don't use spermicidal foams or jellies or vaginal creams for two days before the test, as these could wash away or hide any abnormal cells
- Try not to schedule an appointment when you're menstruating, although the test can be done during your period, if necessary

Cervical cancer takes several years to develop from its precancerous stages. If precancerous cells are missed at one Pap test, they're likely to be detected with the next test, before cancer has developed or it has spread. This is an important reason why doctors recommend regular Pap screening.

Classifying Test Results

Over the years, doctors have used a number of methods for describing Pap test results. In past decades, doctors used numbers ranging from class 1 to class 5 to describe abnormal Pap test results.

In the 1990s, a more detailed naming approach called the Bethesda system was established as the standard system. This system requires that lab technicians who read Pap test slides first report on the adequacy of each slide. Are there enough cells from the cervix on the slide to allow for an accurate reading? If not, the slide is

labeled unsatisfactory for evaluation, and your doctor should have you return for a repeat Pap test.

Under the Bethesda system, Pap tests are classified, in general terms, as:

- No abnormal cells
- Abnormal cells of undetermined significance
- Low-risk abnormal cells
- High-risk abnormal cells

Types of abnormalities

The Bethesda system further classifies abnormal Pap test results as either squamous cell abnormalities or glandular cell abnormalities.

The four categories of squamous cell abnormalities are as follows, listed in increasing order of severity:

- Atypical squamous cells of undetermined significance (ASCUS)
- Low-grade squamous intraepithelial lesion (LSIL)
- High-grade squamous intraepithelial lesion (HSIL)
- Squamous carcinoma (squamous cell cancer)

Glandular cell abnormalities are divided into two categories:

- Atypical glandular cells of undetermined significance (AGUS)
- Adenocarcinoma

Atypical squamous cells of undetermined significance

Squamous cells are flat cells that cover the surface of your cervix. *Atypical squamous cells of undetermined significance* is a catch-all term for any abnormal cells of the cervix that bear watching by your

Human Papillomavirus Testing

The human papillomavirus (HPV) has more than 100 different strains. Almost all cervical cancers are linked to infection with a sexually transmitted strain of this virus.

The types of HPVs that cause Pap test abnormalities live in cells that line the male and female genital tract and are transmitted during sexual intercourse. Some of these strains are low-risk, meaning that they aren't linked to the development of cervical cancer. Others, known as high-risk strains, are passed from one person to another during intercourse and are a major underlying cause of cervical cancer.

An HPV test is available that can check if you may be infected with a high-risk strain of the virus. This additional screening option for cervical cancer involves the same method used to collect cervical cells during a Pap test.

In fact, the test can be done at the same time as a Pap test.

If your Pap test result indicates atypical squamous cells of undetermined significance (ASCUS), ask your doctor about HPV testing. Currently, HPV testing is used by doctors mainly as a secondary test when Pap tests indicate ASCUS. However, the Food and Drug Administration recently approved use of the HPV test in conjunction with the Pap test to screen for cervical cancer in women age 30 and older.

Why the age limit? Although HPV is common in women younger than age 30, cervical cancer is rare in this age group. In most women under age 30 who have HPV, their immune systems clear the infection before it causes any serious changes to cells of the cervix. An HPV test in younger, healthy women, therefore, may not offer any additional benefits to annual Pap tests.

Although there's no known cure for HPV infection, the cervical changes that result from it can be treated.

doctor. The cells look somewhat abnormal (atypical) under the microscope, but it's not clear what the changes mean. About 5 percent of all Pap tests have cells in this category.

If your Pap test results indicate ASCUS, your doctor may advise watchful waiting and repeat Pap tests. He or she may also recommend further testing, such as a colposcopy exam, which is described later in this chapter, or a human papillomavirus (HPV) test.

Low-grade squamous intraepithelial lesion
The classification LSIL refers to the presence of abnormal cells within your cervix. This is the equivalent of mild dysplasia, which is also called cervical intraepithelial neoplasia 1 (CIN 1).

Some low-grade cervical lesions go away with time. Your body's immune system eventually destroys the abnormal cells. Other times, the cells may grow larger, or they may become more abnormal in appearance.

If your Pap test results indicate LSIL, you'll likely need additional tests.

High-grade squamous intraepithelial lesion

The classification HSIL means that you have abnormal cells in your cervix that look very different from normal, healthy cervical cells. High-grade lesions are less likely to go away without treatment than are low-grade ones, and if left untreated they're more likely to develop into cancer.

High-grade lesions typically require more evaluation, followed by removal of the irregular tissue. Doctors estimate that if these lesions are left untreated, as many as two-thirds of all cases of HSIL could progress to invasive cervical cancer.

Atypical glandular cells of undetermined significance

The glandular cells of the cervix produce mucus. The classification AGUS refers to changes in glandular cells. The cells don't appear normal, but doctors aren't sure what the cell changes mean. This type of abnormality may require more testing, including colposcopy and a biopsy, as well as a follow-up Pap test. Because it's possible that the abnormal cells may have washed down to your cervix from higher up in the uterus, your doctor may also advise an ultrasound exam or endometrial biopsy as part of your evaluation.

An AGUS result may mean nothing more than that you need a repeat Pap test. Or it may mean that the abnormal cells need to be treated to prevent cervical cancer from developing.

Cervical cancer

In addition to the precancerous changes just mentioned, a Pap test may also detect cervical cancer — squamous carcinoma or adenocarcinoma. Squamous cells lie on the surface of the cervix.

Reducing the confusion

Because doctors may use many different terms to describe an abnormal Pap test result, ask your doctor to explain the naming system used in your laboratory report. Many terms used to describe cervical abnormalities mean the same thing.

Term	Other names
Mild dysplasia	• Cervical intraepithelial neoplasia (CIN) 1 • Low-grade squamous intraepithelial lesion (LSIL)
Moderate dysplasia	• CIN 2 • High-grade squamous intraepithelial lesion (HSIL)
Severe dysplasia	• CIN 3 • HSIL • Carcinoma *in situ* • Stage 0 cervical cancer

Adenocarcinomas arise from mucus-producing glands (glandular cells) that line the cervical canal. If a Pap test indicates cervical cancer, additional tests are necessary.

This year in the United States, about 10,500 women are expected to receive a diagnosis of invasive cervical cancer. Each year approximately 300,000 women receive new diagnoses of HSILs. Another 1.25 million women are told they have a low-grade change. And each year about 2 million women are informed their Pap tests detected atypical squamous cells of undetermined significance.

Receiving an abnormal Pap test is fairly common, but it doesn't mean that you have cervical cancer.

Additional Tests

Pap tests screen women for indications of cervical cancer or precancerous changes, but they're not the final diagnostic tool. Additional tests are generally needed to clarify precancerous changes or to confirm the presence of cancer. Tests used to help diagnose cervical cancer or precancerous conditions include the following.

Colposcopy

During a colposcopy exam, your doctor is able to get a close-up view of the surface of your cervix.

At the beginning of the procedure, you lie back and place your heels in stirrups

Colposcopy exam

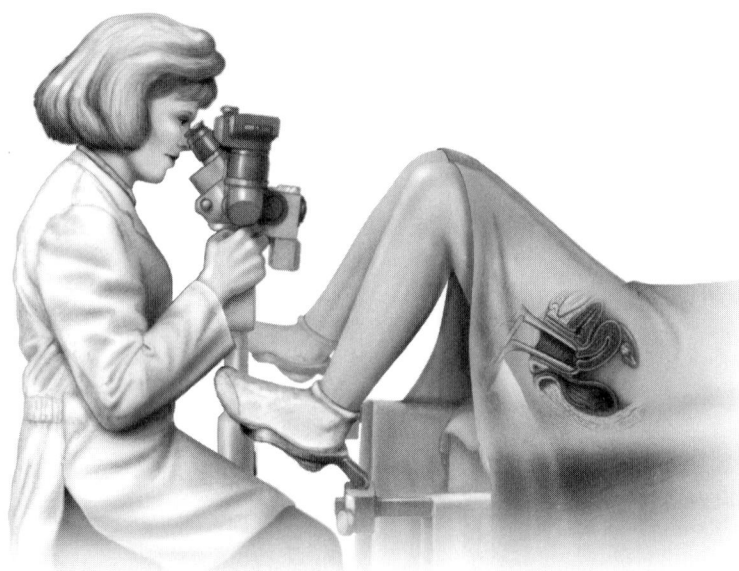

During a colposcopy examination, your doctor uses a device called a colposcope to view your cervix. The scope contains a bright light and a magnifying lens.

as you would for a Pap test. Your doctor inserts a speculum into your vagina and opens it so that he or she can see your cervix. A mild acidic solution is then applied to your cervix and vagina. This solution makes abnormal tissue on the cervix turn white so that your doctor can identify areas that need further evaluation. In addition, your doctor may coat your cervix with an iodine solution that turns healthy cells brown, a procedure called the Schiller's test. This makes abnormal areas stand out even more.

If your doctor sees areas of abnormal tissue during the colposcopy, he or she will likely also perform a biopsy procedure, removing tissue samples for examination in a laboratory.

It usually takes about 30 minutes for your doctor to complete a colposcopy with a biopsy. This procedure can be done at your doctor's office. If you have a biopsy, you may experience a little spotting for a few days afterward.

Biopsy

During a biopsy, your doctor uses a special instrument to remove small samples of abnormal tissue from your cervix. The samples are sent to a laboratory where they're examined under a microscope. A biopsy is the only way to know for certain whether you have cervical cancer.

A cervical biopsy may cause mild cramping or brief pain. Afterward, your

Cone biopsy

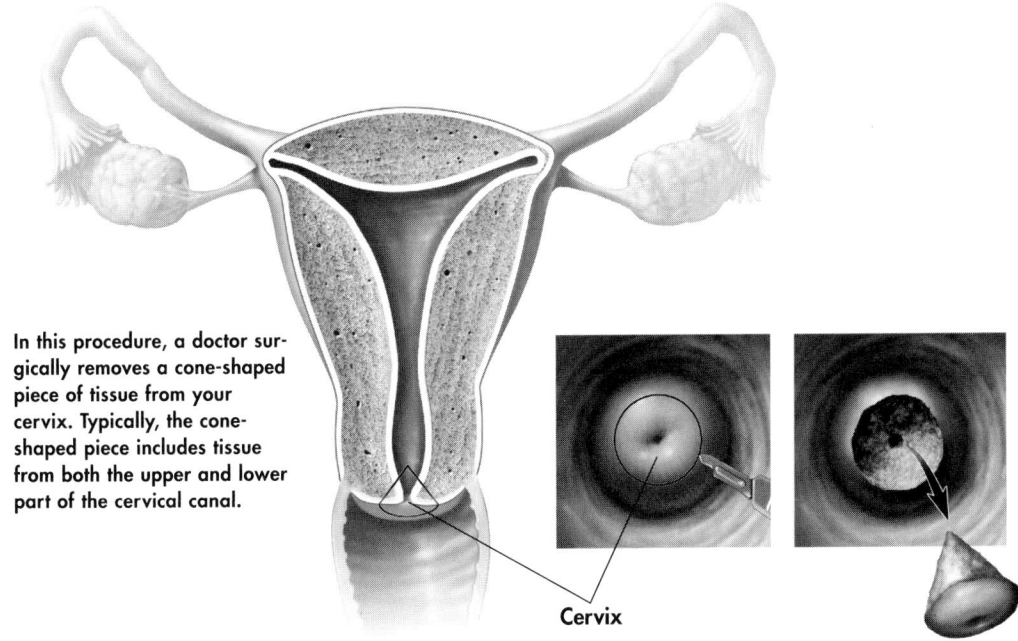

In this procedure, a doctor surgically removes a cone-shaped piece of tissue from your cervix. Typically, the cone-shaped piece includes tissue from both the upper and lower part of the cervical canal.

Cervix

doctor may place a brownish-yellow paste on the area of the cervix where the samples were taken to stop any bleeding. When this paste mixes with your blood, it can form a dark vaginal discharge. Often the discharge is accompanied by light vaginal bleeding for a few days after the biopsy.

Cone biopsy

If your colposcopy test indicates a need to look at cells that lie deep within your cervix, your doctor may perform a more extensive procedure called a cone biopsy (conization). Two methods can be used to perform a cone biopsy:

Loop electrosurgical excision procedure
This procedure, sometimes referred to as LEEP, uses an electrical current that's passed through a thin wire loop. This loop, which acts as a knife, is used to remove a piece of tissue from your cervical canal. Before this procedure, your doctor will numb your cervix using a local anesthetic. During and after the procedure, you may have some mild to moderate bleeding and cramping. LEEP is also called large loop excision of the transformation zone.

Cold conization
With this method, a doctor uses a scalpel or laser to remove a thicker piece of abnormal tissue from your cervix. You're given a general anesthetic so that you're unconscious during the procedure. LEEP can be done at your doctor's office, but cold conization, also called cold knife cone biopsy, is generally performed at a hospital. Most women are able to go home the same day. You may have some cramping and bleeding, which may last for a few weeks.

Endocervical curettage

Sometimes, a doctor wants to check for abnormal cells inside the opening of your cervix, an area that can't be seen during a colposcopy. To do this, a procedure called endocervical curettage may be used. A doctor uses a small, spoon-shaped tool (curet) or brush to scrape tissue from the cervical canal. The tissue is sent to a laboratory, where it's examined under a microscope. Endocervical curettage is usually done along with a colposcopy and biopsy. Normal results help confirm that no cancer cells have been overlooked.

You may experience menstrual-like cramping and light bleeding after the procedure. This is normal.

The Results

If your doctor recommends any of these tests, be sure to ask questions if you have some. Once you have the test results, you and your doctor can determine the next step in your care. Precancerous conditions of the cervix and cervical cancers are treated in different ways.

If, from these tests, it's clear that you have cervical cancer, it's important that you see a gynecologic oncologist, a doctor who specializes in treating cancers of a woman's reproductive system. He or she will help you determine the best course of treatment.

Precancerous Conditions & Noninvasive Cervical Cancer

If you've been told that you have a precancerous condition of the cervix — an abnormality that can precede the development of cervical cancer — you, naturally, may be worried or scared. But don't panic. Effective treatments are available to treat your condition and to prevent it from becoming cancerous.

These same treatments may also be used to treat noninvasive cervical cancer, a condition in which cancer has developed in a small area of the cervix but the cancer is still confined to the organ's surface tissues.

Your doctor will work with you to determine the best treatment plan for your particular situation.

Early Cellular Changes

Cervical cancer begins with changes in cells on the surface of your cervix that cause the cells to overgrow and take on an abnormal appearance. Regular Pap tests can detect these precancerous changes, and the abnormal tissue can be removed or destroyed to prevent cervical cancer from developing.

As discussed in earlier chapters, doctors use different medical terms to describe abnormal cells on the surface of the cervix, depending on how those cells look under a microscope. These terms include *dysplasia, squamous intraepithelial lesion (SIL)* and *cervical intraepithelial neoplasia (CIN)*. If you've had an abnormal Pap test and additional tests confirm precancerous changes, your doctor may use one or more of these terms. *Carcinoma in situ, CIN 3* and *stage 0 cervical cancer* are medical terms for noninvasive cancer. For a description of these terms, see the preceding chapter.

Treatment for precancerous changes or noninvasive cancer is usually fairly straightforward. The abnormal tissue often can be removed or destroyed without the need for major surgery.

Treatment Options

Before beginning your treatment, your doctor should discuss with you the type of abnormal cells in your cervix and the probability of these cells becoming cancerous. Abnormal cells on the surface of the cervix may be treated with one of the following procedures.

Watchful waiting

For mild conditions (CIN 1), sometimes no treatment is recommended. Your doctor may instead advise watchful waiting with repeat Pap tests and colposcopic examinations, especially if you're not at high risk of cervical cancer.

Why this approach? Over time, some abnormal cells in the cervix disappear on their own, without medical intervention. Your body's immune system cleans up the altered cells or fights off the underlying infection that's triggering the changes. Most cases of dysplasia and cervical cancer appear to be linked to infection caused by certain strains of the common human papillomavirus (HPV).

Minor surgical procedures

Many times, a precancerous condition or noninvasive cancer is treated with a minor surgical procedure. Your doctor may suggest one of the following.

Loop electrosurgical excision procedure

With the loop electrosurgical excision procedure (LEEP), a doctor uses an instrument with a thin wire loop at its tip. This wire loop is electrically charged and acts as a heated knife, allowing your doctor to remove (excise) abnormal tissue from the superficial layers of your cervix. LEEP can be used to both diagnose and to treat precancerous conditions.

Doctors also refer to LEEP as cautery or large loop excision of the transformation zone (LLETZ). The transformation zone is the area where the squamous and glandular cells of your cervix meet (see the illustration on page 425). Most cervical cancers start in this area.

Before the procedure, your doctor may apply a mild acidic or iodine solution to your cervix. This solution temporarily makes abnormal cells on the surface of your cervix more visible.

Cryotherapy

Cryotherapy, also called cryosurgery, involves destroying abnormal cells on the surface of your cervix by freezing them. Your doctor places a metal probe cooled with liquid nitrogen against areas of abnormal tissue. This freezes the outer cells of your cervix, killing them and causing them to slough off.

Laser surgery

In this procedure, a doctor uses a narrow beam of intense light to destroy abnormal cells on the surface of your cervix.

Cold conization

Cold conization involves use of a scalpel to remove a cone-shaped wedge of tissue from your cervix (see the illustration on page 441). Your doctor may also refer to this procedure as a cervical conization or cold knife cone biopsy .

Cold conization is commonly used to treat noninvasive cancer (carcinoma *in situ*). The procedure is most often used when the abnormal tissue extends into the endocervical canal, and it can't be seen completely during colposcopy.

Of the procedures described so far, cold conization is the only one that requires

general anesthesia or regional anesthesia, such as a spinal block (epidural). It's usually done in a hospital. Your doctor can also perform conization using LEEP or laser surgery.

Hysterectomy

During a hysterectomy, a woman's uterus, including her cervix, is removed. A hysterectomy may be recommended for women who aren't candidates for any of the above procedures. A hysterectomy may also be done if a woman has another condition, such as vaginal bleeding or pelvic support problems, in addition to a precancerous condition or noninvasive cervical cancer. The surgery can treat both conditions.

For more information on hysterectomy, see Chapter 29.

What to Expect

With the exception of cold knife conization and hysterectomy, each of the procedures just described can be done in a doctor's office. The goal of the treatment is to remove all abnormal cells from the surface of your cervix while leaving as much healthy tissue as possible.

Before the procedure, you'll be asked to undress from the waist down. You then will be taken to an examining table where you'll need to lie back on the table with your knees bent and your heels placed in stirrups. Your doctor gently inserts an instrument called a speculum into your vagina, to keep the vaginal walls apart and to allow access to the cervix. In addition, your doctor may use a device with a light and a magnifying lens (colposcope) to get a close-up view of your cervix and areas of abnormal tissue.

Before the procedure, you may be given a local anesthetic in the form of a shot to numb your cervix. The procedure itself generally takes less than 30 minutes to complete, and you should be able to continue with normal activities the next day.

During LEEP and laser surgery, you may feel an ache or a strong cramp. You may also see a small amount of smoke and smell a burning odor. During cryotherapy, you may hear a soft hissing sound. These are to be expected and aren't cause for alarm.

Side Effects

Side effects of these minor surgical procedures may include menstrual-like cramping, watery vaginal discharge and some vaginal bleeding for several days after the treatment. If after any of these procedures you experience unexpected pain or vaginal discharge, excessive vaginal bleeding, or a fever, contact your doctor. You may have an infection or another complication from the treatment.

Two more serious but rare complications include scarring and narrowing of your cervix (cervical stenosis), which may impair your ability to become pregnant. Some procedures just described may result in an inability of your cervix to remain closed during pregnancy (incompetent cervix). This can sometimes result in a miscarriage or premature birth. If you're pregnant or planning to become pregnant, make sure to tell your doctor about any past cervical treatments you've had. There are ways to monitor for and treat an incompetent cervix.

If you have concerns about side effects, ask your doctor about the possible risks of a treatment. Typically, these treatments, aside from a hysterectomy, shouldn't affect your fertility or your ability to carry a child to term, provided you're otherwise healthy and of childbearing age. Once your cervix has healed, you should also be able to resume sexual intercourse.

Side effects related to a hysterectomy are discussed on page 453.

Follow-up Care

If your doctor is able to treat all of the abnormal cells on the surface of your cervix, no further treatment is usually necessary. However, abnormal cells may develop again in the future, unless you had a hysterectomy. That's why regular checkups are important.

Typically, a Pap test is repeated every four to six months after treatment for precancerous conditions of the cervix or for noninvasive cancer. After the results of several tests come back normal, you and your doctor can decide how often you should have a Pap test.

If abnormal cells do reappear on your cervix, you may be re-treated with one of the minor surgical procedures just described or, possibly, with a hysterectomy. Generally, a hysterectomy isn't necessary. The goal is to prevent the abnormalities from developing into invasive cancer.

Chapter 29: Gynecologic Cancers

Treating Cervical Cancer

nvasive cervical cancer refers to the spread of cancer cells through the lining of the cervix into the structure's deeper tissues. If you've been told that you have invasive cervical cancer, you'll be relieved to hear that effective treatments are available. Today, more than ever before, for women who receive a diagnosis of invasive cervical cancer, there's hope for a cure.

Together, you and your doctor can determine the best treatment plan for your particular situation. Treatment depends on many factors, including the extent of your condition, your age and your overall health. The goal of treatment is to cure the cancer. If, however, the cancer has reached an advanced stage and a cure isn't possible, the goal then is to keep the cancer under control for as long as possible.

In this chapter, we discuss treatment options when cervical cancer is first diagnosed. In the next chapter, you'll find information on treating cancer that returns after a period of remission — a cancer recurrence.

Determining the Extent of the Cancer

Once your doctor has determined that you have cervical cancer, the next step is to learn more about the cancer to help establish a treatment plan. To gather additional information about your cancer, your doctor may use the following tests. Some of these tests may have been performed earlier, at the time of your diagnosis.

- **Physical exam.** During a physical exam, your doctor examines your reproductive organs and feels your groin and neck for swollen lymph nodes, which are indications of possible cancer spread. Lymph nodes are tiny, bean-shaped organs located throughout the body that normally help your body's immune system fight infections. Cervical cancer, like other cancers, can spread to the body's lymph nodes.
- **X-rays and other imaging tests.** Because cervical cancer may spread to your bladder, rectum, lymph nodes or lungs, your doctor may order X-rays or imaging tests to view your internal organs. A computerized tomography (CT) scan can identify the size of a cervical cancer as well as find enlarged lymph nodes in the pelvis that may contain cancer cells. X-rays may be taken of your bones and chest. Ultrasound and magnetic resonance imaging (MRI) are sometimes used to obtain detailed pictures of certain body organs or structures.
- **Cystoscopy.** In this procedure, a doctor looks inside your bladder with a thin, lighted instrument (cystoscope) for signs that the cancer may have spread to the bladder.
- **Proctosigmoidoscopy.** A lighted instrument (sigmoidoscope) is inserted into your rectum and lower large intestine (colon) to check whether the cancer may have spread to these areas.
- **Surgical examination.** This approach is described in the staging section later in this chapter. It's a surgical procedure done while you're under anesthesia, in which biopsies are taken of the tumor and surrounding tissue. Surgical examination is typically done if the cancer is going to be treated with radiation therapy. Cystoscopy and proctosigmoidoscopy may be done at the same time as the surgical examination.

Type

Cervical cancers are divided into two main types, named for the type of cell within the cervix where the cancer started. Squamous cell cancers (carcinomas) account for 85 percent to 90 percent of all cervical cancers. Squamous cells are thin, flat cells that cover the lower portion of the cervix. Adenocarcinomas account for 10 percent to 15 percent of all cervical cancers. They arise from cells that make up glands in the cervix, located in the upper portion of the cervical canal. In a small number of cases, cervical cancers have features of both squamous carcinoma and adenocarcinoma.

Generally, adenocarcinomas are more difficult to diagnose than are squamous carcinomas because they develop higher up in the cervical canal and may not be as easily detected by a Pap test.

Both types of cancers are generally treated in the same way, and survival rates for these two types of cervical cancer are fairly similar.

Grade

A microscopic view of tumor cells allows the pathologist to give it a grade. The grade depends on how normal or abnormal the cells appear under a microscope. A pathologist makes this determination by looking at the growth pattern of the tumor, by evaluating the size and shape of the center (nuclei) of cancer cells, and by calculating the percentage of cancer cells that are dividing.

Generally, the fewer the abnormalities, the lower the tumor grade and the better the prognosis. The more abnormal and aggressive the cancer cells appear, the higher the cancer grade and the greater the chances that a cancer has, or will, spread beyond the cervix to nearby organs and lymph nodes.

Stage

Staging is the system doctors use to describe how far a cancer has spread.

Cervical cancer can spread in several ways. The cancer may grow larger and invade directly into neighboring structures, such as your vagina, bladder and rectum. Or it may spread through lymphatic channels to lymph nodes in your pelvis (regional lymph nodes) or to lymph nodes along your body's major blood vessel, the aorta, as it travels down your lower back. These are known as the para-aortic lymph nodes.

The cancer can also spread through your bloodstream to distant sites, such as your lungs or bones.

Doctors first stage cervical cancer based solely on the results from a woman's clinical tests — her physical exam, cervical biopsy and imaging tests, for example. This is called clinical staging. This system often fails to identify the spread of cervical cancer to lymph nodes because clinical tests, such as imaging tests, can't detect small numbers of tumor cells in lymph nodes, but it does give doctors a basis to discuss possible treatment options.

For most women, more accurate staging is done by way of surgical examination. Surgical staging may be done at the same time as surgery to remove the cancer. Or for a woman being treated with radiation therapy, surgical staging may be performed before radiation treatment.

Doctors can use different classification systems to stage cervical cancer. The one most commonly used is the FIGO system, developed by the International Federation of Gynecology and Obstetrics. In this system, the numerals 0 to IV represent the different stages of cancer, with stage IV being the most advanced stage.

Stage 0
In stage 0, the cancer is only in the first layer of cells that cover the cervix. It hasn't invaded deeper tissues of the cervix. Doctors also refer to this stage as CIN 3, carcinoma *in situ*, or noninvasive cancer.

Stage I
In stage I cervical cancer, cancer cells have invaded into deeper tissues, but the invasion is limited to the cervix only.

Stage I is divided into two subcategories, based on the amount of cancer found.

Stage IA

The cancer cells haven't invaded any deeper than about 3 to 5 millimeters (about ¼ inch), or spread beyond an area 3 to 5 millimeters wide. Stage IA cervical cancer is also called micro-invasive cancer.

Stage IB

Abnormal cells cover an area that's deeper and wider than in stage IA, but the spread is still limited to the cervix.

Stage II

In stage II, cancer cells have spread beyond the cervix, but the cancer hasn't spread to the lower vagina or to the wall of the pelvis. Stage II is subdivided into IIA and IIB.

Stage IIA

The cancer has spread downward to the upper vagina but not to tissues around the cervix or vagina.

Stage IIB

The cancer has spread sideways to other tissues around the cervix.

Stage III

In stage III, the disease is more advanced. Cancer cells have spread to the lower vagina or to either the pelvic wall or nearby lymph nodes or both. Stage III also is divided into two subtypes.

Stage IIIA

The cancer has invaded the lower vagina.

Stage IIIB

Cancer cells have spread to the pelvic wall or to nearby lymph nodes or both. Or the tumor has become large enough to block the tubes that connect your kidneys to your bladder (ureters).

Stage IV

The cancer has spread to adjacent structures or to distant parts of the body.

Stage IVA

The cancer has spread to the bladder, rectum or both.

Stage IVB

Cancer cells have spread beyond the pelvis to other places in the body, such as the lungs or bone.

Treatment Options

As is true with other gynecologic cancers, the main methods for treating invasive cervical cancer are surgery, radiation and chemotherapy. Often, a combination of these methods is used. In addition, newer treatments may be used, including medications designed to use your body's own immune system to help fight the cancer.

Which treatment or combination of treatments you receive will depend on the stage of your cancer, your age and your overall health. Other factors that affect treatment decisions include whether you desire to have children in the future and the location of the cancer.

Most often, invasive cervical cancer is detected at an early stage, when the cancer is highly curable. Occasionally,

Treatment options by stage

You and your doctor will consider many factors when deciding upon a treatment plan for your cervical cancer, but the most important factor in this decision is the stage of your cancer.

Below are treatment options by cancer stage. Keep in mind that these are general guidelines. Every woman is different, and every cancer is different. Your doctor may recommend another treatment plan depending on your individual circumstances.

Cervical cancer stage	Treatment options
Stage IA	• Hysterectomy with removal of pelvic lymph nodes • Internal radiation with or without external radiation
Stage IB	• Radical hysterectomy and removal of lymph nodes • Radical hysterectomy and removal of lymph nodes, followed by radiation plus chemotherapy • External and internal radiation with chemotherapy • Chemotherapy followed by radical hysterectomy and removal of lymph nodes
Stage IIA	• Radical hysterectomy and removal of lymph nodes • Radical hysterectomy and removal of lymph nodes, followed by radiation plus chemotherapy • External and internal radiation with or without chemotherapy • Chemotherapy followed by radical hysterectomy and removal of lymph nodes
Stage IIB	• External and internal radiation plus chemotherapy
Stages IIIA and IIIB	• External and internal radiation plus chemotherapy
Stage IVA	• External and internal radiation plus chemotherapy
Stage IVB	• Chemotherapy • Radiation, as needed, to relieve symptoms and improve quality of life • Clinical trials of new or combination anti-cancer drugs

though, cervical cancer may reach an advanced stage before it's diagnosed. In the disease's advanced stages, treatment becomes more complicated and chances of a cure decrease. If the cancer has already spread to distant sites in the body (metastasized) before it's diagnosed, it's not considered curable.

Doctors sometimes loosely divide invasive cervical cancers into the following categories:

• Early-stage (stage IA to stage IIA tumors)
• Locally advanced (larger stage IB tumors to stage IVA tumors)
• Metastatic (stage IVB tumors)

Most early-stage cervical cancers are treated with surgery or chemoradiation. Surgery is usually used for smaller tumors, although chemoradiation is an option, too. Chemoradiation is usually used for larger tumors or for tumors that have spread beyond the cervix but remain in the pelvic area.

Chemoradiation refers to radiation therapy that's combined with lower doses of chemotherapy. The chemotherapy is used to boost the effects of the radiation. Women with locally advanced cervical cancer often are treated with chemoradiation, and women with metastatic cervical cancer are treated with chemotherapy.

Surgery

Surgery is a common treatment for invasive cervical cancer and can effectively remove small tumors. If a tumor is larger, chemoradiation, which is discussed later in this chapter, may be recommended as the primary form of treatment.

In general, surgery is used to treat cervical cancer stages IA through IIA. The goal of surgery is to remove a cancerous (malignant) tumor without leaving any cancer cells behind. Women with invasive cervical cancer may be treated with a number of surgical procedures. They include the following:

Minor surgical procedures

Minimally invasive surgical procedures such as loop electrosurgical excision procedure (LEEP) and cold conization, which are described in Chapter 28, may be used to treat some early-stage cervical cancers (stage IA cancers). These procedures are particularly useful in premenopausal women with early-stage cancer who want to retain their ability to get pregnant. They usually don't affect fertility or a woman's ability to carry a baby to term.

One drawback of the procedures is that some cancer cells could be missed, and the cancer could return. That's why follow-up care is especially important. Your doctor may recommend a Pap test every four to six months.

Total hysterectomy

Many early-stage cervical cancers are treated with a total hysterectomy. In addition to noninvasive cancer, this type of surgery is commonly used to treat stage IA cervical cancers. In a total hysterectomy, a woman's uterus, including her cervix, is removed. The procedure may be done through an abdominal incision (abdominal hysterectomy) or through the vagina (vaginal hysterectomy).

A total hysterectomy can cure early-stage cervical cancer and prevent it from coming back. The trade-off is that once your uterus has been removed, you're no longer able to bear children.

If you have a hysterectomy, tissue removed during the procedure is examined by a pathologist to determine the cell type, its grade and the extent of the cancer spread. If the cancer has spread to tissues outside your cervix, your doctor may recommend that you have a more extensive surgical procedure.

Modified radical hysterectomy or radical hysterectomy

Sometimes, more extensive types of hysterectomies are used to treat some stages

Seeing a Specialist

Women with cervical cancer should see a specialist for treatment — a gynecologic oncologist and, often, a radiation oncologist. A gynecologic oncologist specializes in the diagnosis and treatment of cancers of the female reproductive system. A radiation oncologist specializes in the treatment of cancer with radiation. Try to find a radiation oncologist with experience in treating gynecologic cancers.

Keep in mind that different doctors may recommend different treatments for your condition. That's because there may be more than one option to treat your particular stage of cervical cancer.

of cervical cancer, such as larger stage IB tumors and, occasionally, stage IIA tumors. These are called modified radical hysterectomy and radical hysterectomy.

In a modified radical hysterectomy, the surgeon removes the uterus, the cervix, some tissue surrounding the uterus (parametrium), supporting ligaments and the upper inch of the vagina, nearest the cervix. Typically, lymph nodes near the uterus also are removed.

In a radical hysterectomy, a surgeon removes a woman's uterus, including her cervix, but even more of the neighboring tissues, including the upper portion of the vagina. The surgeon typically also removes lymph nodes near the uterus to determine whether the cancer has spread to these organs.

A radical trachelectomy

A radical trachelectomy is a newer procedure that may allow some women with early-stage cervical cancers to maintain their ability to have children.

In this surgery, the cervix, the upper part of the vagina and lymph nodes in the pelvis are all removed. However,

the uterus and other reproductive structures are kept in place. The surgeon creates an artificial cervix by cinching the lower outlet of the uterus with a purse-string stitch (suture).

Radical trachelectomy may cure cervical cancers, and it doesn't affect a woman's ability to become pregnant. But the procedure is considered somewhat experimental, and pregnancies after this surgery may result in premature delivery.

Side effects of surgery

A hysterectomy of any type is major surgery. During the initial days after your operation, you may have pain in your lower abdomen, which can be treated with pain medication. Other temporary side effects may include trouble having bowel movements and difficulty emptying your bladder. For bladder problems, a narrow tube (catheter) may be inserted into your bladder to drain urine.

After surgery, you'll need to limit your activities for a while to give your body time to heal. You can usually resume your normal activities, including sexual intercourse, about six weeks after a hysterectomy or trachelectomy. Generally, the more extensive the operation, the longer the recovery time.

Radiation therapy

Radiation — usually combined with chemotherapy, called chemoradiation — also may be used to treat invasive cervical cancer.

Radiation may be used to treat all stages of cervical cancer, but in particular it's the primary treatment for larger cancers or more advanced cancers that have spread beyond the cervix to one or more of the following locations: the pelvic wall, lower vagina and urinary tract. The radiation may be accompanied by low doses of chemotherapy, which helps to boost the effects of the radiation.

Radiation may also be used to treat problems resulting from metastatic cervical cancer. In such circumstances, radiation may be used to shrink a cancerous tumor in a particular area, which can help relieve signs and symptoms of advanced cervical cancer, such as bone pain or vaginal bleeding. In this situation, the goal of radiation isn't to cure the cancer but to relieve a specific problem.

Types

Radiation therapy involves the use of X-rays to kill cancer cells. Like surgery, radiation is a local treatment, meaning it's targeted at a specific area of your body.

The two types of radiation are external radiation and internal radiation. You may receive just one form of radiation to treat your cervical cancer, or you may be given both, one type after the other.

External radiation

For treatment of cervical cancer, most women who undergo radiation receive external radiation — a procedure in which high-energy X-rays are directed at the cancer and a small margin of healthy tissue surrounding it. Specific lymph node regions also may be treated.

Before your treatments begin, you'll undergo a process called simulation. During this process, you lie very still on an examining table while a radiation specialist determines your treatment field (port), the exact location on your body where the radiation will be aimed. Simulation involves use of computerized tomography (CT) scans and other imaging scans to determine the best route to the tumor. A radiation therapist will mark the center of the treatment field on your skin with tiny dots of colored ink, which will eventually be replaced with small, permanent tattoos. It's important that the radiation be targeted at the same area each time.

Once treatment begins, a radiation therapist uses the marks on your skin to locate the treatment area and to position you correctly. You'll be in the treatment room about 15 to 30 minutes. Most of this time is spent getting you positioned. The actual treatment takes about a minute.

Right before your treatment begins, the radiation therapist will leave the treatment room. He or she will watch you on a television screen or through a window in the control room. During the treatment, the radiation machine may rotate around you, and it may give off a buzzing noise. You'll need to remain still so that the radiation reaches only the targeted area.

For treatment of cervical cancer, external radiation therapy usually is given five days a week, for five to six weeks. You're typically given the weekends off to rest and recover.

At the end of your treatment period, the site of your tumor or the tissues around it may be given an extra boost of radiation. This is to be certain that all of the cancer cells are destroyed.

For more information on simulation and external beam radiation, see page 398.

Internal radiation

With internal radiation, the source of radiation is placed inside your body. Doctors often refer to this as brachytherapy or implant therapy.

The source of the radiation is sealed within a small container called an implant. An implant can take different forms, including thin wires, plastic tubes (catheters), capsules and seeds. An implant may be placed directly into a body cavity or within a cancerous tumor itself. Sometimes, after a tumor has been surgically removed, doctors place an implant in the area where the tumor had been (tumor bed) to kill any cancerous cells that may remain.

In the case of cervical cancer, doctors usually insert an implant containing radioactive materials directly into a woman's cervix, or inside her vagina but up against her cervix. Your doctor, a radiation oncologist, will decide how long the implant is to be left in place. Internal radiation may be given at either a low-dose rate or a high-dose rate. Low-dose implants are left in place longer than are high-dose implants.

Getting Answers to Your Questions

If you're feeling overwhelmed by the information you receive from your doctors regarding treatment for cervical cancer, take the time to process what you've learned. That includes asking questions you may have about your condition.

Here are some questions that you might ask:

- What is the stage of my cancer, and what does that mean?
- Can my cancer be cured?
- What are my treatment options?
- What treatment do you recommend for me, and why?
- What are the risks and side effects of the treatment you suggest?
- How long will the treatment last?
- How often will I need to have checkups after treatment?
- How will we know whether the treatment is working?
- What are the chances of the cancer coming back again?
- Will I be able to have children after my treatment?
- Would a clinical trial be appropriate for me?

In addition to these questions, you may want to write down some of your own. For example, you may want specific information about anticipated recovery time or lingering side effects so that you can plan your schedule accordingly.

GYNECOLOGIC CANCERS

Because an implant can emit its high-energy rays outside your body, to protect others you'll be placed in a private room, and visitors may be limited. For more on internal radiation, see page 401.

Chemoradiation

Chemotherapy may be combined with radiation to enhance the effects of radiation therapy and to reduce the chance of the cancer cells surviving. This combination is known as chemoradiation.

Doctors commonly use cisplatin or cisplatin plus 5-fluorouracil, or 5-FU, along with radiation to treat invasive cervical cancer. At least five major studies have shown that when the chemotherapy drug cisplatin is administered at the same time as radiation therapy, recurrences and deaths from cervical cancer are reduced.

Combining chemoradiation with aggressive surgery increases a woman's risk of complications, including bowel toxicity, chronic diarrhea and leg edema. Therefore, in most situations, doctors will recommend either surgery or radiation as a primary form of treatment, each of which may include chemotherapy.

Side effects

To protect normal cells in your body, your doctor will carefully plan the doses of radiation that you receive. He or she will also try to shield as much healthy tissue as possible during your treatments.

Unfortunately, there's a delicate balance between attempts to cure the cancer with radiation therapy and not causing long-term damage from the therapy. Most early side effects of radiation treatment are related to the area that's being treated and will go away two to four weeks after the treatment is finished.

If you're having radiation to your pelvis to treat cervical cancer, you may experience an upset stomach, nausea or diarrhea. With both external and internal radiation treatments, you may also experience bladder irritation, which can cause discomfort or frequent urination. Drinking lots of fluids can help relieve some of this discomfort. Your doctor may also prescribe medication.

Months to years after radiation treatment to your cervix, you may experience a narrowing and tightening of your vagina, which may make intercourse difficult

---

Chemoradiation reduces cancer recurrence and death

Bulky stage IB cervical cancer	Recurrence	Deaths
Radiation alone	37%	26%
Radiation plus chemotherapy	21%	15%

One study of women with larger (bulky) stage IB cervical cancer compared the outcomes of women who received radiation alone with those of women who received radiation and the chemotherapy drug cisplatin (chemoradiation). The women who received chemoradiation had lower rates of recurrence and death.

Source: The *New England Journal of Medicine,* 340:15 (1999), pages 1154-1161

Cervical Cancer and Pregnancy

Some women discover during a pregnancy that they have cervical cancer. Treatment options in this situation depend on the severity of the disease.

If the results of a Pap test indicate abnormal cells on the surface of your cervix, or preinvasive cervical cancer, your doctor will likely recommend that treatment be delayed until after your baby is born. Most cervical cancers grow slowly, so it's generally safe to wait and treat the problem after you've delivered the baby. You may, however, have a biopsy done during the pregnancy so that you and your doctor can be certain the cancer isn't invasive.

In case of invasive cervical cancer, if the cancer has been caught at an early stage, your doctor may tell you it's safe for you to continue your pregnancy to term and that you can receive cancer treatment after you've delivered your baby. But he or she may recommend that you have a Caesarean birth, which will help reduce the risk of excessive bleeding from the cervix at delivery.

If your cancer is at a more advanced stage and immediate treatment is necessary, you and your doctor must decide whether it's safe for you to continue the pregnancy. To protect your own health and save your life, you may need to have surgery or radiation, which would mean terminating the pregnancy. If the cancer is advanced but detected in the last trimester of your pregnancy, your doctor may delay treatment until after the birth.

It's important to understand that being pregnant doesn't increase your chances of getting cervical cancer nor does it accelerate the disease if you have it. Cervical cancer itself isn't harmful to your unborn child.

or even painful. Regular sexual intercourse or devices called dilators may help keep your vagina flexible. Vaginal lubricators or moisturizers also may be used to help treat dryness. Other long-term problems that can occur from radiation therapy include diarrhea, trouble controlling your bowels, rectal bleeding, bone thinning (osteoporosis) and bone fractures.

Depending on where the radiation is directed and the dose received, premenopausal women having radiation therapy to treat cervical cancer will usually stop menstruating.

Chemotherapy

Chemotherapy refers to treatment of cancer with medications intended to kill cancer cells. Chemotherapy is a systemic therapy, meaning the medications travel through your entire body. For invasive cervical cancer, chemotherapy is used in two main ways. Low doses of chemotherapy may be combined with radiation to increase the effectiveness of the radiation. For advanced cervical cancer that may or may not be curable, chemotherapy may be given in standard doses to destroy or control the cancer and to treat its signs and symptoms.

Just one medication or a combination of chemotherapy medications may be used, depending on your situation. Examples of chemotherapy medications used to treat cervical cancer include cisplatin (Platinol), carboplatin (Paraplatin), topotecan (Hycamtin), 5-fluorouracil (Adrucil), paclitaxel (Taxol), cyclophosphamide (Cytoxan, Neosar), ifosfamide (Ifex) and hydroxyurea (Droxia, Hydrea). Chemotherapy drugs for cervical cancer are generally given through a vein (intravenously).

Depending on the regimen and situation, you may receive chemotherapy treatments daily, weekly or monthly. Chemotherapy is often given in cycles that include treatment periods alternated with rest periods. Rest periods give your body a chance to build healthy new cells and regain strength.

Side effects

Common side effects of chemotherapy — which typically last as long as you're undergoing treatment — include diarrhea and a temporary lowering of your white blood cell count, which increases your risk of infection. Whether hair loss occurs depends on the drug or drugs being used. New approaches are now being used to control many of the side effects of chemotherapy. If you're undergoing chemotherapy, ask your doctor about them.

Chemotherapy medications can affect a woman's ovaries and reduce the amount of hormones they produce. The result is that you may experience infertility and early menopause. For more information on potential side effects of chemotherapy, see pages 321 and 403.

Survival Statistics

When cervical cancer is caught early, it's highly treatable and beatable. When cervical cancer is detected at an early stage, the five-year survival rate is 80 percent to 90 percent. If you combine survival rates of women diagnosed at all stages of cervical

5-year survival rates for cervical cancer

Stage	Description	5-year survival rate
Stage I	The cancer is confined to the cervix.	About 80%-95%
Stage II	The cancer has spread beyond the cervix but is confined within the pelvis.	About 60%-80%
Stage III	The cancer has spread to your vagina, the pelvic wall or nearby lymph nodes.	About 30%-50%
Stage IVA	The cancer has spread to nearby organs.	About 15%-20%
Stage IVB	The cancer has spread to distant organs.	Less than 5%

Cervical Cancer and HIV-Positive Women

Women infected with the human immunodeficiency virus (HIV), the virus that causes AIDS, have a weakened immune system. When the immune system is weakened, the body is less able to fight off cancers, including cervical cancer.

In women with HIV, precancerous lesions in the cervix are more likely to progress to invasive cancer if left untreated than is likely in healthy women. In women with compromised immune systems, precancerous lesions

are also more likely to recur after treatment. In addition, it appears that cervical cancer tends to be more aggressive and less responsive to treatment in women with weakened immunity, often requiring more extensive treatment to eliminate the cancer.

If you're an HIV-positive woman with cervical cancer, in addition to receiving standard treatments for cervical cancer, you'll likely be treated with anti-retroviral therapy to boost your immunity. After treatment for cervical cancer, see your doctor as advised so that he or she can monitor whether the disease has persisted or returned.

cancer, the five-year survival rate — the percentage of women who live at least five years after their initial diagnosis — is about 70 percent.

In general, the farther the cancer has spread throughout the body, the more difficult it becomes to cure. But even in more advanced cases, sometimes a cure is still possible.

Follow-up Care

Once you've been treated for invasive cervical cancer, it's important that you have regular follow-up exams — including a pelvic exam, a Pap test and, perhaps, other tests. Regular follow-up exams allow your doctor to check for any sign that the cancer has returned or spread to another part of the body.

Generally, women who've been treated for cervical cancer see their doctors every three to four months during the first two to three years after treatment, and once or twice a year after that.

Follow-up care may include procedures such as X-rays, computerized tomography (CT) scans, ultrasound studies and magnetic resonance imaging (MRI). Biopsies, blood tests and other examinations also may be needed. Which tests you have and how often you have them will depend on the stage of your cancer. Report any new signs and symptoms to your doctor right away so that a cancer recurrence or delayed side effects of treatment can be treated as effectively as possible.

You can hasten your recovery and improve your quality of life by taking an active role in your care. Follow the directions of your health care team, and learn

GYNECOLOGIC CANCERS

Clinical Trials

Some women with invasive cervical cancer receive treatment as part of a clinical trial. Clinical trials help determine whether a new treatment is safe and effective. Women who take part in clinical trials for cervical cancer may be the first to receive treatments that have shown promise in laboratory research.

Today, researchers are studying new types and schedules of radiation therapy for the treatment of cervical cancer. They're also investigating new drugs, drug combinations and ways to combine various types of treatment for cervical cancer.

Immunotherapy is one newer type of treatment being studied for cervical cancer. The goal of immunotherapy is to encourage your body to use its own immune system to fight off the cancer. For example, researchers are investigating vaccines for women with advanced cervical cancer. The intent of the vaccines is to train the body's own immune system to recognize cervical cancer cells and destroy them.

Another example of an experimental treatment for cervical cancer is a class of medications called anti-angiogenics. These drugs help block the growth of a cancerous tumor by cutting off the tumor's blood supply. Tumors need a steady blood supply to grow and spread. In addition, researchers are studying how certain genes play a role in the development of cervical cancer. The hope is to devise a way to treat cervical cancer by replacing damaged genes in cancer cells with normal ones.

If you're interested in taking part in a clinical trial, talk to your doctor about trials that might be available for someone with your stage and type of disease. For more information on clinical trials, see Chapter 2.

about and watch for the side effects of treatment. If they do occur, report them to your doctor so that he or she can take steps to minimize them or shorten their duration.

After you've received a diagnosis of cervical cancer and have been treated for it, you may worry that the cancer will return. Although most women with cervical cancer recover completely and never need additional therapy, in some cases a cancer recurrence can happen months or years later. See Chapter 30 for more information on cervical cancer recurrence.

Chapter 30: Gynecologic Cancers

Cervical Cancer Recurrence

Approximately two-thirds of women diagnosed with invasive cervical cancer survive long-term without experiencing a cancer recurrence. In the remaining one-third, the cancer comes back months or years later.

If your cancer has come back, you may feel angry and wonder, "How can this be happening to me again?" You may feel that you've already been through a lot, and you worry whether treatment will work a second time. The prognosis for women with recurrent cervical cancer varies, depending on how extensive the recurrence is and how soon the disease recurred after initial therapy. In some women, recurrent cervical cancer can be cured, but in many it cannot.

Recurrent cervical cancer may be treated with surgery, radiation or chemotherapy. What treatment, or combination of treatments, is right for you depends on several factors. Your medical team will develop an individualized treatment plan that takes into account factors such as your initial treatment, the site of the recurrence and your current health.

New treatments for women with recurrent cervical cancer are continuously being developed and studied. Even if recurrent cervical cancer can't be cured, treatment can often help control the disease's symptoms.

Types of Recurrence

If cervical cancer recurs, it may be confined to the pelvis, it may appear in more distant sites, or it may recur in both of these ways.

Pelvic recurrence

Pelvic recurrence includes several possible scenarios. A woman may experience a recurrence of the cancer in one or more or the following locations:

- In the same area as the original tumor
- In neighboring structures, such as the bladder or rectum
- In the pelvic lymph nodes

Distant recurrence

In a distant recurrence, the cancer has spread (metastasized) beyond the pelvis to other locations in the body. Cervical cancer may spread to the lungs, abdominal cavity, liver, bone, brain or the lymph nodes in the neck or around the aorta. Generally, the more widespread a cancer is, the more difficult it is to treat. A distant recurrence is more common in women with cervical cancer that had already spread to the lymph nodes when the cancer was first diagnosed.

It's possible to experience more than one type of recurrence. The cancer may recur both locally and in a distant location, such as bone or the lungs.

Diagnosing Recurrent Cancer

In the initial months and years after treatment for invasive cervical cancer, see your doctor for regular follow-up exams. These exams include a pelvic exam and a Pap test to check for any sign that the cancer has returned. Cervical cancer may recur months to years after initial treatment. However, most recurrences happen within two years of receiving the initial diagnosis of the disease.

The location of the cancer recurrence generally relates to the type of treatment used to treat the cancer when it was initially diagnosed. For example, after a hysterectomy, the cancer may occur in the upper part of the vagina or the area where the cervix was located. If the cancer was initially treated with radiation therapy, the cancer is more likely to recur in the cervix, uterus, upper vagina or pelvic wall.

Recurrent cancer starts from cancer cells that weren't removed or destroyed by the original treatment. Sometimes, no matter what treatment is used, a small number of cancer cells survive. After a while, these cells divide and develop into tumors that are large enough to be detected by examination or imaging tests.

Cervical cancer that spreads to other parts of your body is still cervical cancer. For example, if you've had cervical cancer and then some time later doctors discover cervical cancer cells in your lungs, you don't have lung cancer. You have cervical cancer that has spread to the lungs.

This distinction is important because treatment for lung cancer is different from the treatment for cervical cancer that has spread to the lungs.

Signs and symptoms

Signs and symptoms of recurrent cervical cancer depend on where the cancer recurs. Cancer that recurs in the pelvis may produce:

- Abnormal vaginal bleeding
- Watery or bloody vaginal discharge
- A strange or unpleasant vaginal odor
- Pain during sexual intercourse

If cervical cancer has spread to tissues around and outside the cervix, a woman may experience:

- Painful urination, sometimes with blood in the urine
- Diarrhea
- Pain or bleeding from the rectum with bowel movements
- A dull backache or swelling in the legs
- Persistent fatigue

With distant (metastatic) cervical cancer, signs and symptoms are often related to the location where the disease has spread, such as bone, the lungs or the digestive tract. Signs and symptoms may include:

- Bone pain
- Respiratory problems
- Loss of appetite
- Weight loss

Determining the extent of the recurrence

If recurrent cancer is suspected, an accurate diagnosis is the first step in determining a treatment plan. To make an accurate diagnosis, your doctor may order many of the same tests and procedures originally used to diagnose your cancer. In addition to confirming that the cancer has returned, your doctor will also want to know the extent of the cancer spread.

Physical exam

If there's vaginal bleeding, your doctor may view the inside of your vagina for signs of cancer spread. To do this exam, called colposcopy, he or she uses a lighted instrument with a magnifying lens (colposcope).

Imaging tests

Imaging tests also can help determine if cervical cancer has recurred and where. Your doctor may recommend one or more of the following tests to look for cancerous tumors in your body: X-rays, computerized tomography (CT) scans, magnetic resonance imaging (MRI) and ultrasonography. Positron emission tomography (PET) scanning is another imaging technique under investigation for use in detecting recurrent cervical cancer.

Laboratory tests

Your doctor may request certain blood tests to help diagnose recurrent cervical cancer. Blood tests help assess the function of your liver, kidneys and bone marrow, organs that may be affected by recurrent cancer.

GYNECOLOGIC CANCERS

Biopsy

Removing suspicious tissue for examination under a microscope (biopsy) is the only way to know for certain if cancer has recurred. Your doctor may perform a biopsy during colposcopy or exploratory surgery, or by using CT scans or ultrasound tests to guide a biopsy needle.

Treatment Options

As a team, you and your doctor must weigh several factors in creating a treatment plan. The type of treatment that's right for you generally depends on the location and extent of the recurrence, the type of treatments you've received previously and your general health.

When you first received a diagnosis of cervical cancer, you were likely treated with surgery, radiation, chemotherapy or a combination of these treatments. The same types of treatment are also used to treat recurrent cervical cancer. In most instances, recurrent cervical cancer isn't considered curable. But in some circumstances, such as with an isolated pelvic recurrence, chemoradiation or aggressive surgery to remove the cancer may result in a cure.

Before you and your doctor agree on a treatment plan, make sure you understand what the likely outcome will be and why one treatment is recommended over others. Talk with your doctor about the possible benefits, risks and side effects of each treatment. By asking questions and expressing your concerns openly with your health care team, you take an active part in your overall treatment.

Surgery

In certain women, surgery may be used to treat recurrent cervical cancer or to relieve signs and symptoms of incurable cervical cancer. Whether surgery is an option in treating recurrent cervical cancer depends on where the cancer has recurred and how far it has spread.

In certain cases of pelvic recurrence, surgery may result in a cure, but this is uncommon.

Pelvic exenteration

For women whose cancer recurs in the pelvis but hasn't spread to distant sites, a procedure called pelvic exenteration may be an option. Pelvic exenteration is a very extensive operation.

During the surgery, a surgeon removes most or all of the major organs in the pelvis. This includes a woman's uterus, cervix, vagina, ovaries, fallopian tubes and pelvic lymph nodes — a more extensive excision of the same organs and structures removed in a radical hysterectomy. In addition, the surgeon may remove the bladder, the rectum and part of the large intestine if the cancer has spread to one or more of these areas.

Sometimes, surgeons are able to create a new vagina (neovagina). The new vagina is made either from muscle taken (grafted) from the inner thigh or from a skin graft taken from the back of the thigh. Vaginal reconstruction can be done at the time of a pelvic exenteration or later.

If the bladder is removed, surgeons create a new outlet for urine by using a piece of small bowel to create a sac to hold urine. The ureters are connected to the piece of bowel. Then a small opening (stoma) is created, usually on the front right side of the abdomen, for the urine to leave the body. This procedure is called a urostomy. After a urostomy, you need to wear a small, plastic bag (pouch) on the outside of your abdomen to collect the urine. Another option is to periodically drain the urine with a small tube (catheter) that's inserted into the stoma.

If your rectum needs to be removed, surgeons will create a new way for solid waste to be eliminated. To accomplish this, they may attach the remaining intestine to a stoma in your abdominal wall, usually on the lower left side of your abdomen. This procedure, called a colostomy, allows fecal matter (stool) to pass through the opening into a pouch you wear on the front of your abdomen.

Pelvic exenteration often affects how women feel sexually, and some find it challenging to resume sexual activity after a urostomy or colostomy. A member of your health care team can provide you with suggestions for garments to conceal ostomy bags and ways to resume intimate relations after recovery.

If you have a new vagina constructed, you may be given a vaginal dilator to take home with you from the hospital. The dilator, which you insert into your vagina as instructed by your doctor, helps prevent your vagina from becoming tight as it heals. Your new vagina will feel different from your original vagina.

Although pelvic exenteration is radical surgery, it offers some women with recurrent cervical cancer a chance for a cure. Of women who are found to be candidates for this procedure and who choose to

have it, approximately 30 percent are alive five years after this operation.

The prognosis is best for women who have less aggressive forms of cervical cancer and who have small tumors. Pelvic exenteration generally isn't an option for women in whom the cancer has spread to the pelvic lymph nodes, abdomen or distant places in the body. And it's not an option for women who aren't healthy enough to handle such major surgery.

Palliative care

Even if cervical cancer can't be cured, surgery may be used to control complications of the disease. For example, a large tumor in a woman's pelvis may press on part of her colon. This may lead to a blocked (obstructed) bowel, which possibly can be corrected with surgery. Or, if a vaginal recurrence is causing bleeding problems, surgery may be performed to remove the cancer in that area.

Radiation therapy

Radiation therapy may be used to treat recurrent cervical cancer as long as the same area of the body wasn't radiated during initial treatment for the cancer. Only in rare circumstances can radiation be given to the same area twice. For recurrent cervical cancer, radiation is often combined with chemotherapy.

Two types of radiation treatment may be used: external radiation and internal radiation. Your doctor may recommend one or both.

• **External radiation.** With external radiation, high-energy X-rays are directed at the cancer and a small margin of normal tissue surrounding it. In case of recurrent cervical cancer, your entire pelvic area may be treated.

- **Internal radiation.** With internal radiation (brachytherapy), the radiation source is sealed in a container and placed in the area where the tumor was removed (tumor bed). Or the radiation source may be concealed within hollow catheters and placed within the tumor itself.

For more information on external and internal radiation, including how the treatments are performed and their potential side effects, see Chapter 29.

Radiation may also be used to alleviate pain and other symptoms of metastatic cervical cancer by shrinking tumors that are pressing on nerves or growing inside bone. When radiation is used to control symptoms of cervical cancer, generally a shorter course of treatments is given, and the radiation is given alone, without chemotherapy. Chemotherapy increases the likelihood of side effects.

Chemotherapy

Chemotherapy can't cure metastatic cervical cancer, but in some women it can help to prevent or slow the progression of the disease. In addition, chemotherapy may be given to help relieve symptoms.

How well does chemotherapy work for advanced cervical cancer? A number of clinical trials have tested single-agent or combination chemotherapy regimens in women with stage IVB cervical cancer. Over the years, the single most active chemotherapy drug for cervical cancer has been cisplatin. Among women who

use cisplatin by itself, about 25 percent of them experienced significant tumor shrinkage.

A recent clinical trial compared cisplatin alone with the combination of the drug topotecan plus cisplatin in women with advanced cervical cancer. More women in the combination group responded to the treatment, and there was improvement in survival with the combination. For the women treated with cisplatin alone, the average survival was six and a half months. For women treated with both drugs, the average survival was just over nine months.

When a cancer responds to chemotherapy, it generally continues to respond for a period of months, but this can vary quite a bit from one person to another. If cancer grows again after initial chemotherapy and you're healthy enough to tolerate the side effects of additional chemotherapy, your doctor may suggest other approaches. For second-line chemotherapy, tumor shrinkage is less likely than with first-line chemotherapy.

Together with your oncologist, decide if the potential benefits may be greater than the potential side effects. Some questions you may want to ask your doctor can be found on page 455. More information on chemotherapy can be found on page 457.

Clinical Trials

Several clinical trials involving potentially new treatments for cervical cancer are currently under way.

Because of the connection between human papillomavirus (HPV) infection

---

MYTH vs. FACT

Myth: **If we can travel in outer space and put people on the moon, we should have a cure for cancer by now.**

Fact: Cancer is a large group of diseases, and each type of cancer may be associated with many different factors. Researchers are still learning about what triggers a cell to become cancerous and why some people with cancer do better than others. In addition, cancer is a moving target. Cancer cells continue to mutate and change during the course of the disease. This can cause cancer cells to no longer respond to medications or radiation treatments that initially worked well when the disease was first diagnosed.

Finding a cure for cancer is, in fact, proving to be much more complex than mastering the engineering and physics required for spaceflight.

---

and cervical cancer, one approach is to make a vaccine from HPV that, in turn, will activate the immune system to fight HPV-related substances in cervical cells. Interferon, a protein that provides the body with immunity to viral infections, is one form of immunotherapy being studied in the treatment of cervical cancer.

The intent of immunotherapy is to boost your body's own immune system to fight precancerous changes or cancer itself. Immunotherapy is being studied as a possible treatment for high-grade dysplasia, early-stage cervical cancer and recurrent disease.

Possible side effects from immunotherapy depend on the agents and approaches being used. They include fever, chills, nausea and vomiting, muscle aches and weakness. These generally subside once you complete treatment. Because flu-like side effects of immunotherapy can be severe, for some women the side effects may outweigh the possible benefits from the medication.

Other treatment approaches being studied in clinical trials include:

- High-dose implant radiation, which can be given in shorter treatment courses.
- Hyperthermia, a procedure that kills tumor cells by heating them to several degrees above body temperature. This approach is being studied in combination with chemotherapy.
- Anti-angiogenics, medications that help slow the growth and spread of cancerous tumors by cutting off the blood supply to the tumors. Most of these drugs work by blocking the action of a particular protein called vascular endothelial growth factor, which promotes the formation of new blood vessels to feed tumors. One such drug, called bevacizumab (Avastin), is now being tested in a clinical trial involving women with recurrent cervical cancer.
- Erlotinib, a medication designed to prevent cancer growth by blocking development of stimulatory pathways within cancer cells.

GYNECOLOGIC CANCERS

You can find out more about current clinical trials for treatment of cervical cancer by contacting the National Cancer Institute (see page 601). To learn more about clinical trials in general, see Chapter 2.

Chapter 31: Gynecologic Cancers

Vaginal Cancer

Cancer that begins in the vagina, known as vaginal cancer, is rare. It accounts for only 1 percent to 3 percent of all cancers of the female reproductive system. In fact, vaginal cancer is more rare than is cancer that spreads to the vagina from another location, such as endometrial cancer that spreads from the uterine lining or cervical cancer that spreads from the cervix. Researchers estimate that each year about 2,000 American women receive a diagnosis of vaginal cancer and about 800 women die of the disease.

There are different types of vaginal cancer. Prognosis depends mainly on the stage of the disease at the time it's diagnosed and the type of tumor. When caught in the earliest stages, vaginal cancer is rarely fatal. Overall five-year survival rates for the different types of vaginal cancer are around 60 percent.

Anatomy of the Vagina

The vagina is a muscular tube that connects the uterus with the outer genitals. It extends from the lower, neck-like portion of the uterus (cervix) to the folds of skin in a woman's genital area (vulva). Also known as

Layers of vaginal tissue

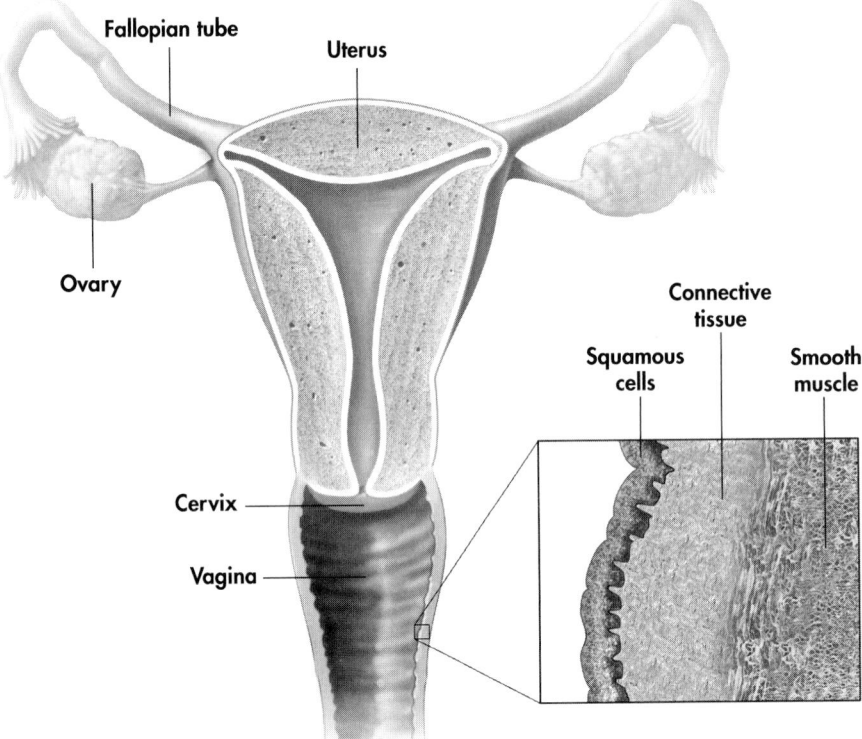

the birth canal, the vagina is important for sexual activity and reproduction. It's the passageway through which menstrual fluid leaves the body and through which a baby emerges during childbirth.

The vagina is made up of different kinds of tissue. Its walls are lined with a thin layer of cells called squamous epithelial cells. The term *epithelial* refers to cells that line most organs. Squamous cells are flat cells that cover the skin surface and the lining of many of the body's hollow organs. Beneath this layer of cells, there's some glandular tissue. The vagina's walls consist of connective tissue, smooth muscle cells, lymph vessels and nerves.

Types of Vaginal Cancer

The main type of vaginal cancer is vaginal squamous carcinoma. Other, less common forms are vaginal adenocarcinoma, malignant melanoma and vaginal sarcoma.

Vaginal squamous carcinoma

Most often — in 80 percent to 90 percent of cases — vaginal cancer begins in the cells that line the vagina. The medical name for this cancer is *squamous carcinoma* of the vagina. A rare subtype of this form of cancer is *verrucous carcinoma*. Unlike the common squamous carcinomas, which tend to occur in the upper portion of the vagina, verrucous carcinoma tends to start in the middle of the vagina. It's also less likely to invade deeply into the vaginal wall or spread to other organs, giving women who have this type of vaginal cancer a better prognosis than that of women with more common forms.

Vaginal adenocarcinoma

Vaginal adenocarcinoma begins in the glandular tissue of the vagina. A subtype of this form of cancer is clear cell adeno-carcinoma, which is more commonly diagnosed in younger women who were exposed to the drug diethylstilbestrol (DES) while they were in the womb.

Malignant melanoma

Malignant melanoma is an extremely rare and lethal form of cancer that begins in pigment-producing cells (melanocytes). It usually develops in areas of the skin that have been exposed to the sun, but it can occur in the vagina or other internal organs. Malignant melanoma can develop anywhere in the vagina, but it typically starts in the lower portion. This type accounts for about 3 percent to 5 percent of all vaginal cancers. Because of its location, malignant melanoma of the vagina is rarely detected in its early stages.

Vaginal sarcoma

Vaginal sarcoma begins deep in the walls of the vagina, in the muscle or connective tissue. The most common form of vaginal sarcoma, called leiomyosarcoma, starts in the smooth muscle cells of the vaginal wall. It typically affects women over age 50. Another type of vaginal sarcoma, called rhabdomyosarcoma, is a cancer of early childhood. Vaginal sarcomas account for 2 percent to 3 percent of all vaginal cancers.

What Causes Vaginal Cancer?

The exact cause of vaginal cancer isn't known. However, human papillomavirus (HPV), a cause of cervical cancer, appears to be involved in the development of vaginal cancer. HPVs make up a group of more than 100 viruses. Certain HPVs can infect squamous epithelial cells located in the skin of the external genitals or cells in the lining of the vagina or cervix, or both. These viruses can be passed from one person to another during sexual contact. Some types of HPV cause genital warts but nothing more serious. Other so-called high-risk types can predispose a woman to cancers of the cervix, vagina and vulva.

Studies have shown that certain high-risk HPVs produce proteins that interfere with the products of tumor suppressor genes. Tumor suppressor genes are the genes that prevent normal cells from growing too fast and becoming cancerous. For more information on tumor suppressor genes, see Chapter 2.

Because vaginal cancer is rare, relatively little research into its causes has been done. Therefore, while it's safe to say that

GYNECOLOGIC CANCERS

HPV infection seems to influence the development of some vaginal cancers, more research is needed to fully understand the cause or causes of this form of cancer.

Risk Factors

The following factors may increase your chances of developing vaginal cancer:

Human papillomavirus infection
Human papillomavirus (HPV) proteins and DNA have been found in specimens of vaginal cancers. In addition, studies have shown that women who've been exposed to the high-risk subtypes of HPV have an increased risk of vaginal cancer.

Age
Increasing age is a risk factor for the most common type of vaginal cancer, squamous carcinoma. Among women diagnosed with this cancer, about half are age 60 or older.

Exposure to diethylstilbestrol
Between 1940 and 1971, the drug diethylstilbestrol (DES) was prescribed for pregnant women to help prevent miscarriage. Women whose mothers took DES while carrying them are at increased risk of developing clear cell adenocarcinoma of the vagina, a rare form of vaginal cancer. DES is no longer used, and most DES-exposed women are now age 40 or older.

Race
Black women have three times the risk of developing vaginal cancer, compared with white women. The reasons for this are unclear.

Vaginal adenosis
Normally, the vagina is lined with flat cells called squamous cells. In some women, the vaginal lining contains one or more areas made up of gland-like cells, similar to those found in the lower uterus or uterine lining (endometrium). This condition is called vaginal adenosis, and it's a risk factor for clear cell adenocarcinoma of the vagina. Vaginal adenosis causes small bumps in the vagina that often can be seen or felt during a pelvic examination. Studies show that about one-third of the women exposed to DES in the womb develop vaginal adenosis.

Cervical cancer or precancerous cervical conditions
Cervical cancer and vaginal cancer share similar risk factors, such as HPV infection. Therefore, if you've had cervical cancer, you're also at increased risk of developing cancer of the vagina. Up to 30 percent of women with vaginal squamous carcinoma have a history of cervical cancer. Women who've had precancerous cervical conditions, such as cervical intraepithelial neoplasia or cervical dysplasia, are also at increased risk of vaginal cancer.

Chronic vaginal irritation
Some research suggests long-term irritation of the vagina, such as that caused by a pessary, may slightly increase risk of vaginal cancer. A pessary is a device used to help keep the uterus from sagging into or outside of the vagina. No studies have conclusively proved this link.

4 Ways to Help Prevent Vaginal Cancer

Vaginal cancer isn't 100 percent preventable. However, you can do some simple things to reduce your risk.

1. If you're young, put off having sexual intercourse until you're older. Sexual intercourse before age 18 is a risk factor for human papillomavirus (HPV) infection, which increases the risk of vaginal cancer.
2. Avoid having sex with multiple partners or having sex with someone who has had many partners. This, too, is a risk factor for HPV infection.
3. If you smoke, stop. If you don't smoke, don't start. Smoking increases the risk of vaginal cancer.
4. Have a yearly pelvic examination and Pap test so that precancerous conditions can be identified and treated promptly. The Pap test checks the cervix specifically, but abnormalities there can be a tip-off to problems in the vagina, too.

Smoking

Research suggests that smoking may play a role in the development of vaginal cancer, especially among younger women. Smoking probably increases risk by interfering with the body's ability to fight HPV. Other agents that suppress the immune system, such as immunosuppressant medications or the AIDS virus, also increase the risk of vaginal cancer.

Making a Diagnosis

Most vaginal cancers produce bleeding, which prompts women to seek medical attention. But some of these cancers don't bleed. The one sure way to give yourself the best chance of early detection is to have regular pelvic examinations and Pap tests. Although a Pap test is most often used to check the cervix, it's also used to check the vagina in women who've had a hysterectomy due to cervical cancer.

Signs and symptoms

Between 80 percent and 90 percent of women with vaginal cancer have one or more signs or symptoms that prompt them to seek medical care. Early medical care allows many vaginal cancers to be detected at an early stage. However, some types of vaginal cancer don't produce signs or symptoms until they've reached a more advanced stage.

Signs and symptoms of vaginal cancer may include:

- Abnormal vaginal bleeding, often after sexual intercourse
- Abnormal vaginal discharge
- A mass in the vagina
- Pain during sexual intercourse
- Painful or difficult urination
- Pelvic or vaginal pain

If you experience one or more of these signs or symptoms, it doesn't necessarily mean that you have vaginal cancer. Often such signs and symptoms stem from a

GYNECOLOGIC CANCERS

noncancerous (benign) condition, such as an infection. However, it's important to see your doctor.

Diagnostic tests

If, because of your signs and symptoms, your doctor suspects that you have vaginal cancer, he or she will likely perform a thorough pelvic exam and a Pap test. If these procedures reveal any abnormalities, more tests will likely be needed, such as a colposcopy and vaginal biopsy.

If your primary care doctor isn't a gynecologist, he or she will likely refer you to one. A gynecologist specializes in conditions of the female reproductive system. If studies confirm the presence of cancer, seek referral to a gynecologic oncologist, a surgeon who specializes in cancers of the female reproductive system.

Pelvic examination and Pap test
During a pelvic exam, you lie flat on your back on an examining table with your knees bent. Usually, your heels rest in metal supports called stirrups. Your doctor first examines your external genitals to make sure they look normal — free of sores, discoloration and swelling. An internal examination follows. To see the inner walls of the vagina and cervix, the doctor inserts into the vagina an instrument called a speculum. When in the open position, the speculum holds the vaginal walls apart so that the cervix can be seen. Your doctor then shines a light inside to look at the walls of the vagina for lesions, inflammation, signs of abnormal discharge and anything else that's unusual.

A Pap test is typically included in a pelvic exam. For this test, your doctor

VAIN: An Early Warning

Vaginal intraepithelial neoplasia (VAIN) refers to changes in the thin layer of cells that line the vaginal walls. It's the vaginal counterpart of cervical intraepithelial neoplasia, discussed in Chapter 26. VAIN is usually detected during a colposcopy exam for an abnormal Pap test.

VAIN has three categories (grades): VAIN 1, VAIN 2 and VAIN 3, with VAIN 3 being the most serious. High-grade VAIN (VAIN 3) is also classified as a stage 0 vaginal cancer, or carcinoma *in situ* of the vagina.

The goals in treating VAIN are twofold: to prevent the development of invasive cancer and to preserve vaginal function. Treatment is tailored to the severity and extent of the problem and to the woman's individual preferences.

Treatment options for VAIN include topical agents, such as a topical form of chemotherapy; laser surgery; surgical excision; and infrequently, radiation. In some cases of VAIN 3, removal of the upper portion of the vagina (upper vaginectomy) may be necessary.

Topical 5-fluorouracil cream
Applying the chemotherapy drug 5-fluorouracil, or 5-FU, directly to the

inserts a small tool — a spatula, brush or cotton swab — through the speculum (see the illustration on page 434). The tool is used to gently scrape cells from the opening of the cervix. These cells are then put onto glass slides so that they can be evaluated under a microscope. The Pap test was designed as a screening test for cervical cancer. However, in cases of suspected vaginal cancer, cells from the vagina can also be obtained for study in a laboratory.

Generally, after removing the speculum, a doctor will continue with the pelvic exam by checking the condition of the uterus and ovaries. This is done by inserting two lubricated, gloved fingers into the vagina and pressing down on your abdomen with the other hand. Usually this is followed by a rectovaginal exam, done with one finger in the vagina and another in the rectum. This allows your

doctor to locate your uterus, ovaries and other organs, judge their size and confirm that they're in the proper position. While exploring the contours of these organs, your doctor feels for any lumps or changes that may indicate a problem.

Colposcopy and biopsy

During a colposcopy test, a doctor uses an instrument with a light and special magnifying lenses (colposcope) to take a closer look at the cervix and vaginal walls (see the illustration on page 440).

A colposcopy is done much like a regular pelvic exam. You lie on your back on an examining table with your knees bent and, usually, your feet resting in metal stirrups. Your doctor inserts the speculum into the vagina and opens it slightly so that the cervix can be seen. Next your doctor applies a mild solution of acetic

vaginal lining is sometimes used to treat VAIN. The drug kills the surface layer of cells, which is then replaced with healthy cells. The drug can be applied weekly for 10 weeks or nightly for seven to 14 days. Sexual intercourse isn't recommended during therapy. This drug can cause severe irritation of the vagina or the outer skinfolds in the vaginal area (vulva).

Laser surgery

During laser surgery, a doctor uses a focused, narrow beam of high-energy light to destroy the abnormal tissue. Laser surgery is an effective treatment for VAIN, but it usually requires anesthe-

sia and outpatient surgery. More than one treatment may be needed.

Surgical excision

In some instances, a doctor may cut out the abnormal tissue from the vagina.

Radiation

Radiation is generally a last resort when all other types of localized treatment have failed and a woman doesn't want to undergo extensive surgery. Internal radiation, in which radioactive material is placed inside the vagina, is used to destroy abnormal cells. The procedure is similar to that described later in this chapter (see page 478).

acid to your cervix and vagina and views the area with the colposcope. When exposed to the solution, abnormal areas look white, making identification easier.

If abnormal areas are identified, your doctor will remove (biopsy) tissue samples from the areas and have the tissue analyzed in a laboratory to determine whether cancer or a precancerous condition is present. Before taking a biopsy sample, your doctor may numb the area with a local anesthetic. However, you may still feel some mild cramping or pinching. To reduce any discomfort, your doctor may recommend a mild pain reliever.

After a colposcopy and biopsy, you may have a dark, blood-tinged vaginal discharge for a couple of days, requiring use of a panty liner. This is normal. If you experience heavy vaginal bleeding, call your doctor. Also contact your doctor if you develop signs or symptoms that suggest infection, such as pain in your vagina or lower abdomen, fever, chills or foul-smelling vaginal discharge. Avoid using tampons and having sexual intercourse for at least a week.

Additional tests

If your biopsy results indicate you do have vaginal cancer, your doctor will likely recommend additional tests to determine the extent of the cancer. Some of the tests that may be helpful include the following:

Proctosigmoidoscopy

Proctosigmoidoscopy is a test to view the rectum and lower portion of the colon. During this test, a thin, flexible lighted tube is placed into the rectum. Any areas that look abnormal are biopsied. Doctors generally recommend proctosigmoidoscopy for women with a vaginal tumor that's large or located on the back wall of the vagina next to the colon or rectum.

Cystoscopy

Cystoscopy is a test to view the inside of the bladder. It's performed by way of a thin, flexible tube containing a lens and a fiber-optic lighting system that's inserted into the urethra and threaded up to the bladder. Your doctor may recommend cystoscopy to determine whether vaginal cancer may have spread to your bladder. If areas of concern are seen during the procedure, small samples of tissue may be removed for microscopic testing. Doctors generally recommend cystoscopy for women with a vaginal tumor that's large or located in the front wall of the vagina near the bladder.

Intravenous pyelogram

An intravenous pyelogram (IVP) is a test used to gauge kidney function and drainage of urine through the urinary tract. In some cases of vaginal cancer, the tumor spreads beyond the vagina and presses on the tubes that carry urine from your kidneys to your bladder (ureters). This can lead to kidney damage. During an IVP test, you receive an injection of a dye that passes through your bloodstream and is excreted in your urine, thus outlining your kidneys, ureters and bladder on an X-ray.

Computerized tomography scan

A computerized tomography (CT) scan of the abdomen and pelvis produces detailed images of your internal organs. Unlike a normal X-ray, which produces just one image of your body taken from one angle, a CT scan produces many images of your body taken at different levels. CT scans also show soft tissues much better than do regular X-rays.

Chest X-ray

A standard chest X-ray can help determine whether the cancer may have spread through the bloodstream to the lungs.

Staging

Staging refers to the part of the diagnostic process in which your doctors try to determine how far the cancer has spread. Cancer stages are expressed as numbers. A lower number indicates that the cancer is still in its early stages. A higher number means that the cancer is more advanced.

- **Stage 0.** The cancer is confined to the epithelial lining of the vagina. Stage 0 vaginal cancer is also called vaginal carcinoma *in situ* or grade 3 vaginal intraepithelial neoplasia (VAIN 3).
- **Stage I.** The cancer is confined to the vagina.
- **Stage II.** The cancer has grown through the vaginal wall to the connective tissues just outside the vagina, but it hasn't spread to the side wall of the pelvis or to other organs.
- **Stage III.** The cancer has spread to the pelvic side wall, to a lymph node on the same side as the tumor or both.
- **Stage IVA.** The cancer has spread to the organs next to the vagina, to lymph nodes on both sides of the pelvis or to both.

- **Stage IVB.** The cancer has spread to distant organs, such as the lungs.

Treating Vaginal Cancer

Three types of treatment may be used for vaginal cancer: radiation therapy, surgery and chemotherapy. Radiation therapy and surgery are the two main forms of treatment. Radiation therapy is the preferred treatment for most cases of vaginal cancer. Chemotherapy may be combined with external radiation (chemoradiation).

Surgical procedures are generally reserved for small, early-stage tumors or rare vaginal cancers, such as malignant melanoma and vaginal sarcoma. Surgery is also preferred for younger women who want to preserve their fertility. In addition, surgery is sometimes an option after radiation. This is uncommon and usually done only if the cancer recurs.

The type of treatment you receive is based on the type of vaginal cancer you have and how far it has spread, as well as on your age and overall health. To help you understand the pros and cons of the various treatment options, try to get the opinions of both a gynecologic oncologist and a radiation oncologist.

Radiation therapy

Radiation therapy is the use of high-energy X-rays or radioisotopes to kill cancer cells. It's a local therapy, meaning that the treatment is focused on a specific area of your body, not your entire body.

Two types of radiation therapy may be used to treat vaginal cancer: external beam radiation and internal radiation (see the color illustrations on page 271). The type of radiation you receive generally depends on the extent of your cancer. Some women with vaginal cancer — especially those with more aggressive or advanced cancers — may need both external and internal radiation therapy. Women with vaginal cancer that's still in a very early stage may be treated with internal radiation therapy alone.

In general, the goal of radiation therapy is to provide a cure. How well radiation therapy can destroy the disease depends on how advanced your cancer was at the time of your diagnosis (see the table on page 481). In some women with late-stage vaginal cancer, even when a cure isn't possible, radiation therapy may be used to help relieve pain, bleeding or other signs and symptoms.

External beam radiation

With external beam radiation, you receive doses of radiation from a high-energy X-ray machine called a linear accelerator. Treatments are generally given Monday through Friday for about five weeks. Your radiation oncologist examines you weekly to monitor the shrinkage of your tumor during treatment.

The goal of external beam radiation is to administer the strongest dose of radiation possible while sparing as much normal tissue as possible. This helps reduce side effects. Vaginal cancer often is treated with low-dose chemotherapy along with external beam radiation, to improve the response to radiation.

Side effects do occur. Common side effects of external beam radiation therapy for vaginal cancer include dry, reddened skin in the treatment area, fatigue and diarrhea. Talk with your doctor about strategies to treat or minimize these side effects.

Internal radiation therapy

With internal radiation therapy, radioactive substances called radioisotopes are placed in or near the tumor. As the radioisotopes break down, they release radiation, killing cancer cells in the area.

Internal radiation therapy is also known as brachytherapy or implant radiation. Other terms, such as *intracavitary radiation* or *interstitial radiation*, refer to how and where the radioactive substances are administered.

- **Intracavitary radiation.** Intracavitary radiation involves the placement of an applicator, such as a tube, into a body opening, such as the vagina. Radioactive sources are placed in the applicator, and treatment begins. After the treatment, the applicator is removed.

- **Interstitial radiation.** Interstitial radiation involves placement of radioactive substances directly into catheters or hollow tubes that are placed in the tissue surrounding the tumor or in the tumor itself. The catheters or hollow tubes are surgically inserted into the tissue or tumor. This is usually done in an operating room. After you recover from the anesthesia, the radioactive material is placed in the catheters or tubes. Once the treatment is complete, the applicators are removed.

A small, stage I cancer may be treated with intracavitary radiation only, but this is quite rare. If the cancer is larger but still in an early stage, external radiation therapy may be given first. If the tumor shrinks dramatically during treatment, then intracavitary treatment may be given. If the tumor doesn't shrink, interstitial radiation treatment may be used instead. Women who have more locally advanced disease may receive a combination of chemoradiation and interstitial radiation.

Internal radiation may be given at either a high-dose rate or a low-dose rate. An implant with a low-dose rate is left in place for several days. You remain in the hospital while you receive the radiation. With high-dose-rate brachytherapy, the implant is left in place a few hours to a few days, depending on whether it's an intracavitary or interstitial implant. Once the implant is removed, you can go home.

High-dose-rate brachytherapy generally involves three or four treatments. For more information on these types of implants, see Chapter 23.

Your vagina may be sore or sensitive for some time after internal radiation therapy, but most women are able to resume normal activities relatively quickly.

Surgery

Some small, early-stage — stage 0 or stage I — squamous cell cancers may be removed surgically. Surgery is also the primary treatment for more rare forms of vaginal cancer, including early-stage adenocarcinoma. These cancers can be removed with a relatively limited form of surgery, and most women do quite well.

The extent of surgery depends on the size and stage of the cancer. Several different surgical options are available.

QUESTION & ANSWER

Q: Will radiation therapy interfere with my ability to have sexual intercourse?

A: Radiation therapy for vaginal cancer can cause scar tissue to develop in your vagina, narrowing it and interfering with its ability to stretch. This condition, called vaginal stenosis, can make sexual intercourse painful. In extreme cases, scarring after radiation therapy shortens or narrows the vagina so much that intercourse is impossible.

To prevent scar tissue from forming in your vagina during radiation therapy, it's best to stretch the walls of the vagina several times a week. Talk with your doctor or a member of your health care team about how best to do this. One option is to have sexual intercourse at least three or four times a week. Another is to use a plastic or rubber cylinder called a vaginal dilator a few minutes each day. Using a dilator feels a lot like putting in a large tampon. Besides making for more comfortable intercourse later, a vagina that's normal in size makes for more comfortable pelvic exams, which are an important part of follow-up care after treatment for vaginal cancer.

Wide local excision

If you have a small stage 0 or stage I squamous cell cancer, your doctor may perform a procedure called a wide local excision. This procedure removes the cancer and some surrounding tissue, but it doesn't remove any reproductive organs.

Partial vaginectomy

Stage I squamous cell cancer may also be treated by surgically removing part of the vagina, especially if the cancer occurs in the upper portion. This procedure is called a partial (upper) vaginectomy.

Radical vaginectomy

If the cancer is in the lower portion of the vagina, the entire vagina and its adjacent tissues may be removed. This is called a radical vaginectomy. If all or most of the vagina is removed, a surgeon can reconstruct a new vagina out of skin, intestinal tissue, or muscle and skin grafts. Whether this procedure is appropriate depends on the extent of the disease.

Combination surgery

In some cases of stage I or stage II squamous cell cancer, vaginectomy may be combined with surgery to remove the uterus and its adjacent connective tissue (radical hysterectomy), as well as lymph nodes in the groin or pelvis (lymphadenectomy). This combination surgery is an option for women whose cancer has spread outside the vagina (stage II) and who have previously undergone radiation therapy, making them ineligible for additional radiation. Combination surgery is also the usual treatment for stage I adenocarcinoma of the vagina.

Pelvic exenteration

Pelvic exenteration is a relatively rare surgical procedure. It's an option for certain women with vaginal cancer who can't have radiation therapy, usually because of prior radiation for another condition. This procedure is extensive, combining removal of the uterus, ovaries, fallopian tubes and surrounding tissue with removal of the vagina, and the bladder or rectum or both (see page 464 for more information). The extent of surgery depends on the extent of the cancer. After removal of the organs, the surgeon constructs new ways of storing and eliminating urine and stool and creates a new vagina.

Chemotherapy

Little information is available on the use of chemotherapy in vaginal cancer. This is mainly because the disease is uncommon, and most women do well with radiation or surgery. However, because vaginal cancer is similar to cervical cancer in many ways, the same chemotherapy drugs used to treat cervical cancer (see page 457) are often used to treat vaginal cancer, if chemotherapy is necessary.

Surveillance and Follow-up

Treatment for vaginal cancer is generally followed by regular checkups. The checkups help ensure that any changes in your health, such as a recurrence of your cancer, are noticed early and treated appropriately.

Survival Statistics

One way to report cancer survival rates is to specify the percentage of patients who are alive five years after their diagnoses. This doesn't mean that survivors live for only five years after being diagnosed with cancer. Most cancer survivors live much longer. The five-year benchmark is simply used for consistency when talking about cancer survival.

Your likelihood of surviving vaginal cancer depends mainly on the stage of the disease at diagnosis and the type of tumor. In general, adenocarcinoma has a poorer prognosis than does squamous cell cancer, and malignant melanoma has the worst prognosis of all types.

These statistics are estimates based on studies of women with vaginal cancer. They represent the average outlook for groups of women and only serve to provide a general picture and a standard way for doctors to discuss prognoses. They don't predict the outcome in your particular case. Each woman and each case are different.

If you have questions about your own prognosis, discuss them with members of your health care team. They will help you find out how these statistics relate, or don't relate, to you.

5-year survival rates for vaginal cancer*

Stage	Description	5-year survival rate
Stage 0	The cancer is confined to the lining layer (epithelium) of the vagina.	About 95%
Stage I	The cancer has invaded through the epithelium, but it's confined to the vaginal wall.	About 75%
Stage II	The cancer has spread to the connective tissues next to the vagina, but it hasn't spread to the wall of the pelvis or to other organs.	About 60%
Stage III	The cancer has spread to the pelvic wall, to a lymph node on the same side as the tumor or both.	About 35%
Stage IVA	The cancer has spread to the organs next to the vagina, to lymph nodes on both sides of the pelvis or both.	About 10%
Stage IVB	The cancer has spread to distant organs, such as the lungs.	Less than 5%
Malignant melanoma (all stages)		About 14%

*Excluding vaginal sarcoma

Because vaginal cancer is rare, there's no standard regimen for how often follow-up visits are done. In general, during the first two to three years after treatment, you'll probably have checkups with your doctor every three to four months. This is the time when risk of recurrence is highest. Studies show that about 80 percent of vaginal cancer recurrences happen within two to three years after initial treatment. If after three years there's no evidence that your cancer has recurred, you may need to see your doctor less often, perhaps every six months.

During each follow-up visit, your doctor will ask you about any symptoms you're experiencing that might suggest your cancer has returned. Signs and symptoms that may be of concern include abdominal or pelvic pain and vaginal bleeding. Be sure to tell your doctor exactly what and how you're feeling. You'll also have a chance to discuss any lingering side effects of treatment. Your doctor will also perform a physical examination, including a pelvic exam.

If your doctor suspects that your cancer may have recurred, he or she may recommend an imaging test, such as a computerized tomography (CT) scan or magnetic resonance imaging (MRI). A biopsy is generally necessary to confirm the diagnosis.

Treating recurrent cancer

If the cancer comes back after initial treatment (recurrent vaginal cancer), how it's treated the second time depends on the site of the recurrence and how the cancer was initially treated. If the tumor recurs near the site of the original cancer and was initially treated with radiation therapy, surgery may be the best option. Depending on the extent of the recurrence, a pelvic exenteration may provide a cure. On the other hand, if the tumor recurs near the site of the original cancer and was initially treated with surgery, radiation may be the best option. Vaginal cancer that recurs outside the pelvis generally isn't considered curable.

Because recurrent vaginal cancer is so uncommon, it's difficult to conduct clinical trials needed to evaluate chemotherapy agents. It's likely that the drugs and approaches found most beneficial for the treatment of cervical cancer will continue to offer the best treatment options for women with recurrent vaginal cancer.

Chapter 32: Gynecologic Cancers

Vulvar Cancer

Vulvar cancer is a form of cancer that begins in a woman's external genitals. It's relatively uncommon, accounting for 3 percent to 5 percent of all gynecologic cancers and about 1 percent of all cancers in women. Doctors and scientists estimate that about 4,000 American women receive a diagnosis of vulvar cancer each year and that about 800 women die of the disease.

If detected early, vulvar cancer is highly curable. For women whose cancer is in an early stage, the overall five-year survival rate is more than 90 percent. Unfortunately, some women with vulvar cancer ignore, or aren't aware of, its signs and symptoms. As a result, about 40 percent of women with vulvar cancer are diagnosed when the disease is in a more advanced stage.

Anatomy of the Vulva

Several structures make up the external portion of the female reproductive system, known as the vulva. Vulvar cancer can occur in any of these structures, but it's most commonly found in the inner edges of the

Vulvar anatomy

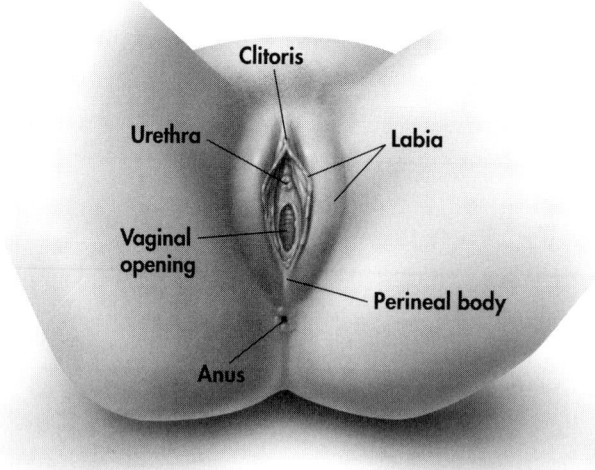

labia. Other fairly common locations for the cancer to develop are the clitoris, Bartholin's glands and perineal body.

Labia

Labia are the two sets of skinfolds that meet in the middle of the genital area, protecting the openings to the vagina and the urethra. The vagina is the muscular tube that connects the uterus with the outer genitals. The urethra is the tube that expels urine from the bladder during urination. The larger and more prominent of the folds, called the labia majora, consist of skin, connective tissue and fat. The smaller folds, called the labia minora, are located between the labia majora. They contain little or no fat.

Beneath and within the labial tissues lie small muscles that surround a vascular, spongy core. It's this core that swells to create the labial fullness associated with sexual arousal.

Clitoris

The clitoris is about three-quarters of an inch in size and is composed of highly sensitive tissue. It's this tissue that becomes swollen with blood during sexual stimulation. The clitoris is located above the vaginal and urethral openings, beneath a small overlap of skin that's called the prepuce.

Vaginal opening

The opening to the vagina, also known as the vaginal vestibule, is located in the center of the vulva. On either side of the vaginal opening are two small, mucus-secreting glands called Bartholin's glands. The ducts for these glands are located at the junction of the labia minora and vaginal opening.

Perineal body

The area between the vaginal opening and the anus is called the perineal body.

Types of Vulvar Cancer

Within the general category of vulvar cancer are several subtypes, defined according to the cell that gives rise to the cancer.

Vulvar squamous carcinoma

About 90 percent of vulvar cancers begin in the main type of skin cells known as squamous cells. The medical term for this form of cancer is *vulvar squamous carcinoma*. This form of cancer usually grows slowly over many years, often preceded by precancerous changes confined to the surface layer of the skin. These changes may persist for several years.

Vulvar adenocarcinoma

A small percentage of vulvar cancers begin in the glands of the vulva. The medical term for this form of cancer is *vulvar adenocarcinoma*. Some of these cancers develop in the Bartholin's glands, near the vaginal opening. In rare cases, these cancers may begin in the sweat glands of the vulva.

Malignant melanoma

About 4 percent of vulvar cancers begin in the pigment-producing cells of the skin (melanocytes). The medical term for this form of cancer is *malignant melanoma*. Melanoma is the most serious form of skin cancer. Malignant melanoma of the vulva typically occurs on the labia minora or clitoris.

Vulvar sarcoma

Fewer than 2 percent of vulvar cancers begin in the connective tissue beneath the vulvar skin. These cancers, called sarcomas, tend to grow rapidly.

What Causes Vulvar Cancer?

Although the exact cause of vulvar cancer isn't known, doctors and scientists are beginning to understand how certain risk factors may contribute to the disease.

Studies suggest that vulvar squamous carcinoma, the most common type of vulvar cancer, can develop in multiple ways. For up to half the women with the condition, human papillomavirus (HPV) infection appears to play a role. HPVs include a group of more than 100 viruses that can cause genital warts (papillomas) or more serious problems, such as cancer of the cervix, vagina or vulva. HPVs can infect the skin of the external genitals. These viruses can be passed from one person to another during sexual contact.

Certain high-risk HPVs produce proteins that interfere with the products of tumor suppressor genes. Tumor suppressor genes prevent normal cells from growing too fast and becoming cancerous. If these genes are inhibited, cell growth increases and damaged vulvar cells don't die on schedule as they're supposed to, leading to increased risk of vulvar cancer.

Other mechanisms possibly associated with vulvar cancer are less well understood. Some studies show that women with vulvar cancer who don't have HPV infection may have a damaged tumor suppressor gene in their vulvar skin cells. A mutation in this gene, called p53, may increase the risk of vulvar cancer.

Risk Factors

A risk factor is anything that increases your chances of getting a certain disease. Scientists determine risk factors by reviewing the medical histories and lifestyles of different groups of people. They then calculate which characteristics seem to be linked to increased incidence of a particular disease.

Some types of risk factors, such as age, race and family history, can't be changed. Others, such as smoking and sexual practices, are related to the lifestyle choices you make.

Several factors can increase your risk of developing vulvar cancer. Having one or even several of these factors doesn't necessarily mean that you'll get the disease.

VIN: An Early Warning

Vulvar intraepithelial neoplasia (VIN) is a precancerous condition of the vulva. It refers to abnormalities in the cells on the surface of the vulvar skin, called epithelial cells. VIN is most often diagnosed during a routine pelvic exam.

Doctors classify VIN depending on what proportion of epithelial cells appear to be affected. There are three categories (grades) of VIN. The lowest grade is VIN 1, and the highest grade is VIN 3. High-grade VIN (VIN 3) is also classified as carcinoma *in situ* of the vulva, or stage 0 vulvar cancer.

Treatment for VIN involves removing or destroying the abnormal area, preventing it from developing into invasive cancer. Treatment options include:

Laser surgery
During laser surgery, your doctor uses a focused, narrow beam of high-energy light to destroy abnormal tissue.

Surgical excision
During a surgical excision, your doctor removes the abnormal skin, as well as a margin of normal-appearing skin. This procedure is best suited to smaller, localized lesions and is known as vulvar local excision.

If the VIN involves a larger portion of the vulvar skin, the entire area needs to be treated. The surgical procedures used to remove larger portions of the vulvar skin are called partial skinning vulvectomy or total skinning vulvectomy, depending on the extent of tissue removed. A partial skinning vulvectomy involves removing about half of the vulvar skin. With this procedure, the wound can often be closed without the need for skin grafts. A total skinning vulvectomy, which is performed very rarely, involves removing most of the skin. Skin grafts may be used to cover the wound, thereby preserving normal vulvar folds and contour.

Two Risk Profiles

Generally, two types of women are most at risk of developing vulvar cancer. They fit what's called a risk profile for this type of disease. The more common profile is that of an older woman whose cancer may be unrelated to human papillomavirus (HPV) infection and smoking. Her main risk factor is that she's beyond the age of 50. The other profile is that of a younger woman with HPV infection who smokes. This individual has a higher likelihood of having VIN.

In fact, most women with known risk factors for vulvar cancer don't get it. At the same time, some women who get this disease have no major risk factors for it. In many cases of vulvar cancer, doctors can't point to one specific factor as the cause.

Vulvar intraepithelial neoplasia

Having a precancerous condition called vulvar intraepithelial neoplasia (VIN) increases a woman's risk of vulvar cancer. However, with treatment, most precancerous changes don't develop into cancer.

Human papillomavirus exposure or infection

Certain human papillomaviruses can infect the skin of the external genitals. These viruses are passed from one person to another during sexual contact. Risk of HPV infection is higher among women who begin sexual contact at a young age, those who've had many sexual partners and those whose partners have had many sexual partners. HPVs may be responsible for up to half the cases of vulvar cancer.

Age

Three out of four women who develop vulvar cancer are older than 50 when they receive their diagnoses. Two-thirds are older than 70. But an increasing number of women in their 30s and 40s are receiving diagnoses of VIN. It's thought that tobacco use, exposure to HPV through sexual contact and immune-suppressing diseases such as human immunodeficiency virus (HIV) infection may be contributing to the increase.

Smoking

Among women who've had HPV infection, smoking further increases the risk of vulvar cancer or a VIN recurrence.

History of genital warts

Women who've had genital warts have been exposed to HPV. The warts don't become cancerous themselves, but they indicate that HPV exposure has occurred.

HIV infection

Having an HIV infection makes you more susceptible to persistent HPV infections, increasing the risk of cancer and VIN.

Atrophic vulvar dystrophy

Atrophic vulvar dystrophy, also known as lichen sclerosus, is a condition in which the vulvar tissues become less elastic and

5 Ways to Help Prevent Vulvar Cancer

Helping to prevent vulvar cancer comes down to two things: avoiding the risk factors you can control and getting prompt treatment for precancerous conditions. To give yourself the best chance of avoiding vulvar cancer, heed these tips:

1. If you're young, put off having sexual intercourse until you're older. Sexual intercourse before age 18 is a risk factor for human papillomavirus (HPV) infection, which increases the risk of vulvar cancer.
2. Avoid having sex with multiple partners or having sex with someone who has had many partners. These, too, are risk factors for HPV infection.
3. If you smoke, stop. Ask your doctor for help. If you don't smoke, don't start. Smoking increases the risk of vulvar cancer.
4. Get to know your body. Use a mirror to look at your vulva. If you have any persistent rashes, moles, lumps or other abnormalities in your outer genitals, see your doctor. Treatment of precancerous changes can prevent many cases of vulvar cancer.
5. Have a pelvic exam and Pap test on a regular basis so that any cancerous or precancerous conditions can be identified and treated promptly. The Pap test checks the cervix specifically, but abnormalities there can be a tip-off to problems in the vulva, too.

smaller. The tissue may also feel tight and dry, and the labial inner folds may seem to shrink away. Women with this condition are at increased risk of vulvar cancer that's not associated with HPV infection.

Other genital cancers

About 15 percent of women with vulvar cancer also have another squamous cancer in the genital area, such as vaginal cancer or cervical cancer. HPV infection appears to be the underlying cause. That means that women with a confirmed case of vulvar cancer should be closely evaluated and monitored to check for a new cancer or a coexisting cancer at another site.

History of melanoma or atypical moles

Women with a family history of melanoma or atypical moles elsewhere on the body are at increased risk of malignant melanoma of the vulva.

Making a Diagnosis

Early detection of vulvar cancer increases the odds of successful treatment. Early detection is best accomplished with regular pelvic exams and being alert to signs and symptoms.

Signs and symptoms

The signs and symptoms of vulvar cancer vary according to the type of cancer. They may include:

- Persistent vulvar itching, lasting more than a month
- Areas of thicker or lighter-appearing vulvar skin

- Areas of reddish, pinkish or darker-appearing vulvar skin
- Areas of white, rough-feeling vulvar skin
- Unusual bleeding or discharge
- Areas of red, scaly vulvar skin
- In the vulvar area, red, pink or white bumps with a wart-like appearance, raw surface or both
- Cauliflower-like growths, similar to genital warts, in the vulvar area
- A vulvar sore that won't heal
- Vulvar pain, soreness or burning
- Painful urination
- Painful intercourse
- Unusual vaginal odor

More rare types of vulvar cancer may have very distinct signs and symptoms. For malignant melanoma, the most common sign is a change in the size, shape, color or texture of an existing mole in the vulvar area. The appearance of a new, darkly pigmented mole also can signal melanoma. For a cancer of the Bartholin's gland (vulvar adenocarcinoma), a new lump or mass on either side of the vaginal opening is a common sign.

If you experience one or more of these signs and symptoms, it doesn't necessarily mean that you have vulvar cancer. Many signs and symptoms associated with vulvar cancer can also be caused by noncancerous conditions, such as an infection, a cyst or another skin irritation. But that doesn't mean they should be ignored. Too often, signs and symptoms of vulvar cancer aren't taken seriously enough. A woman may spend months trying an array of over-the-counter products to relieve her discomfort. In fact, the average time between the onset of signs and

symptoms and a confirmed diagnosis of vulvar cancer is about a year.

If you have signs or symptoms of vulvar cancer, see your doctor. A biopsy is the only way to assess whether they may be the result of vulvar cancer.

Diagnostic tests

If you have signs or symptoms of vulvar cancer, it's likely your doctor will perform a thorough physical exam and pelvic exam, looking closely at your external genitals for sores or discoloration. Because women with vulvar cancer sometimes have another genital cancer, it's important to examine the vagina and cervix carefully, as well as feel the lymph nodes in your groin area to determine whether they're enlarged, signifying that the cancer may have spread to these structures.

If your primary care doctor isn't a gynecologist, he or she may refer you to one. A gynecologist specializes in conditions affecting the female reproductive system. If studies confirm the presence of cancer, seek referral to a gynecologic oncologist, a surgeon who specializes in cancers of the female reproductive system.

If your doctor detects a suspicious vulvar lesion during your pelvic exam, he or she may want you to undergo additional tests, such as colposcopy and biopsy.

Colposcopy and biopsy

During a colposcopy test, a doctor uses an instrument with a light and special magnifying lenses (colposcope) to look at the cervix, vaginal walls and vulva.

A colposcopy is done much like a regular pelvic exam. You lie on your back on an examining table with your knees bent and, usually, your feet resting in metal stirrups. Your doctor inserts a speculum into the vagina and opens it slightly so that the cervix can be seen. Next, a mild solution of acetic acid is applied to your cervix, vagina and vulva, and the area is viewed with the colposcope (see the illustration on page 440). When exposed to the solution, abnormal areas look white, allowing for ease of identification.

If abnormal areas are identified, your doctor will remove tissue samples from the areas (perform a biopsy) and have the tissue analyzed in a laboratory to determine whether cancer or a precancerous condition is present. Before taking a biopsy sample, your doctor may numb the area with a local anesthetic, but you may still feel some mild cramping or pinching. To reduce any discomfort, your doctor may recommend a mild pain reliever. If the abnormal area is very small, your doctor may cut it out entirely and stitch the wound. This is called an excisional biopsy.

After a colposcopy and biopsy, you may have a dark, blood-tinged discharge for a couple of days, requiring use of a panty liner. This is normal. If you experience heavy bleeding, call your doctor. And contact your doctor if you develop signs or symptoms that suggest infection, such as pain in your vagina or lower abdomen, fever, chills and foul-smelling vaginal discharge. Avoid using tampons and having sexual intercourse for at least a week after a colposcopy.

Additional tests

If your biopsy results show that you have vulvar cancer, your doctor may recommend additional tests to determine whether the cancer has spread to other parts of your body. This is especially true if the abnormal area is large or the results of your physical exam suggest that the cancer may have spread to other parts of the body. Additional tests may include a proctoscopy, cystoscopy, computerized tomography (CT) scan and chest X-ray.

Proctoscopy

Proctoscopy is a test to view the rectum using a lighted tube. Any areas that look abnormal are biopsied. Because some advanced vulvar cancers can spread to the rectum, doctors sometimes recommend a proctoscopic exam for women with larger vulvar tumors.

Cystoscopy

Cystoscopy is a test to view the inside of the bladder. It's done with a tiny tube with a special lens and a fiber-optic lighting system (cystoscope). By inserting it into the bladder by way of the urethra, your doctor can check the urethra and the inside of the bladder to determine whether vulvar cancer may have spread there. During the procedure, small samples of tissue may be removed for microscopic testing. Cystoscopy is usually done with a local anesthetic, but sometimes the procedure is performed using general anesthesia. Because advanced vulvar cancer can spread to the bladder, doctors sometimes recommend cystoscopy for women with larger tumors.

Computerized tomography scan

A computerized tomography (CT) scan is a procedure that produces detailed images of your internal organs and structures. Doctors use a CT scan of the abdomen and pelvis to help determine whether vulvar cancer may have spread to nearby lymph nodes or other organs.

Chest X-ray

A standard chest X-ray can help determine whether the cancer has spread through the bloodstream to the lungs.

Staging

Staging is the process of determining how far a cancer has spread. The main system used to stage vulvar cancer was developed by the International Federation of Gynecology and Obstetrics. It's called the FIGO system.

Similar to other staging systems, a lower number indicates that the cancer is still in its early stages. A higher number means the cancer is more serious and advanced. The FIGO staging system for classifying vulvar cancer is as follows:

- **Stage 0.** The cancer is confined to the surface of the vulvar skin. Stage 0 squamous cell cancer of the vulva is also known as vulvar carcinoma *in situ*, or high-grade vulvar intraepithelial neoplasia (VIN 3).
- **Stage I.** The cancer is confined to the vulva or perineum or both, and it's 2 centimeters (cm) or less in diameter. It hasn't spread to any lymph nodes.
- **Stage II.** The cancer is confined to the vulva or perineum or both, and it's larger than 2 cm in diameter. It hasn't spread to any lymph nodes.
- **Stage III.** The cancer has spread beyond the vulva or perineum to nearby tissues,

such as the urethra, vagina, anus or nearby lymph nodes on only one side of the groin.
- **Stage IVA.** The cancer has spread to the upper urethra, bladder, rectum, pubic bone or lymph nodes on both sides of the groin.
- **Stage IVB.** The cancer has spread to the pelvic lymph nodes, to distant sites or to both.

Treating Vulvar Cancer

The three treatment options for vulvar cancer are surgery, radiation therapy and chemotherapy. Traditionally, extensive (radical) surgery has been the most common treatment. More recent approaches have included less extensive surgeries combined with radiation or chemotherapy or both to preserve the function of the vulva and improve quality of life.

You may want to discuss treatment options with both a gynecologic oncologist and radiation oncologist. Your treatment options are generally based on the type of vulvar cancer you have and how far it has spread, as well as your age, overall health and personal preferences.

Surgery

For a few small, early-stage cancers, laser surgery may be used to destroy abnormal cells on the skin surface, allowing the skin to heal with minimal scarring. However, traditional surgery to remove the cancer is the preferred treatment for many stage I and stage II vulvar cancers. The amount of tissue that's removed during surgery

Vulvectomy

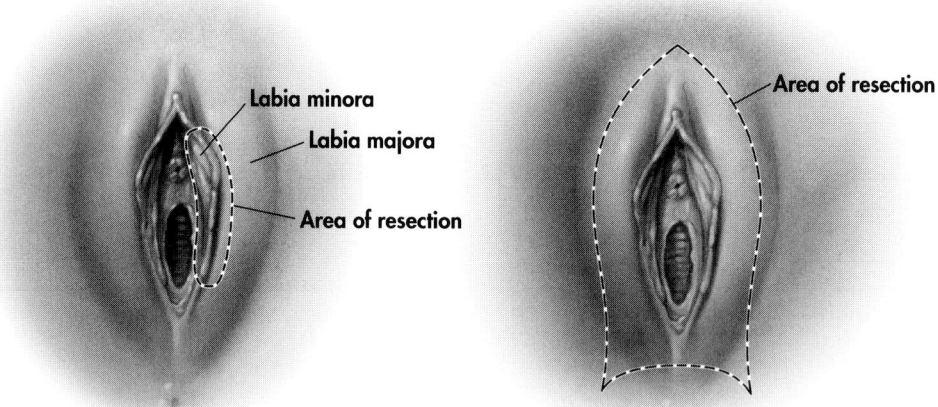

Labia minora

Labia majora

Area of resection

Area of resection

One treatment option for early-stage vulvar cancer with limited spread is partial vulvectomy (left). For more advanced early-stage cancer, radical vulvectomy (right) may be an option.

depends on the extent of the cancer and the type of surgery you receive. Researchers continue to explore whether less invasive types of surgery that help preserve more of the vulva are as effective as more extensive surgical procedures. Your doctor will try to preserve as much tissue as possible, to try to help maintain your sexual function and quality of life.

Types of surgery for vulvar cancer include the following:

Wide local excision

Wide local excision involves removal of the cancer and a margin of normal-appearing skin. This type of surgery is used for early cancers and may or may not include removal of the lymph nodes in the groin.

Partial vulvectomy

During a partial vulvectomy, a doctor removes a larger portion of the vulva and its underlying tissues. The lymph nodes in the groin are generally removed as well. Partial vulvectomy, with or without lymph node removal, is also the usual treatment for vulvar melanoma that has penetrated less than three-quarters of a millimeter into the vulva.

Radical vulvectomy

Radical vulvectomy involves removal of the entire vulva, including the clitoris, and underlying tissues. Lymph nodes in the groin area are removed as well. This surgery typically is performed only in women who have larger early-stage tumors or tumors that involve both sides of the vulva.

Another approach for larger, locally advanced cancers is a combined treatment of radiation and chemotherapy, followed by surgery.

Pelvic exenteration

Pelvic exenteration is major surgery that involves removal of the vulva and the lymph nodes of the groin and pelvic area. It may also include removal of the bladder, rectum, lower colon, vagina, cervix and uterus. This surgery is generally used only when the cancer has spread to the bladder or rectum but not distant organs. In some situations, it may be used when the cancer recurs in pelvic structures.

Surgery for vulvar cancer sometimes involves removing a large area of vulvar skin. In this case, grafts of skin taken from tissues near the vulva are used to cover the wound. A plastic (reconstructive) surgeon sometimes works with a gynecologic oncologist to provide this expertise.

With radical surgery for vulvar cancer, significant complications can occur. About 50 percent of women who have radical surgery experience some degree of difficulty with wound healing, including infection, fluid buildup under the incision or tissue death (necrosis) near the incision. Drainage tubes may need to be inserted after surgery to aid in healing.

Some women also experience groin problems, such as formation of groin cysts due to accumulation of lymphatic fluid. Some women experience swelling in the legs (lymphedema) due to an obstruction of the lymphatic drainage system that causes accumulation of fluid. Doctors are investigating steps that may be taken to help reduce the frequency and severity of groin problems and lymphedema.

In addition, with part or all of the vulvar padding gone, it can be uncomfortable to wear jeans. Your genital area may feel numb, and it may be difficult to achieve orgasm during sexual intercourse. Talk with your doctor about ways to minimize and cope with these side effects.

Radiation therapy

Radiation therapy is the use of X-rays to kill cancer. It's a local therapy, meaning that the treatment is focused on a specific area of your body, not your entire body. For vulvar cancer, radiation therapy may be used to treat advanced (stage III or stage IVA) or recurrent squamous cell cancers. It may also be used in earlier-stage vulvar cancer.

External beam radiation is the type of radiation therapy used for treatment of vulvar cancer. With external beam radiation, you receive doses of radiation from a large X-ray machine aimed at the tumor area (see the color illustration on page 271). It's much like having a diagnostic X-ray, but the radiation is higher energy and delivered over a period of a minute or two. Radiation typically is given five days a week, for about six weeks.

Your doctor may also recommend radiation therapy after surgery, to increase the chances of a cure, especially if the cancer has spread to your lymph nodes, or if cancer cells are located at or near the edge of the tissue removed during surgery (surgical margin).

Some women also benefit from radiation therapy before surgery to help shrink the tumor and lessen the amount of tissue to be removed. This includes women who have cancers in or near the clitoris, urethra or anus (midline structures) or women in whom the cancer has spread to a number of lymph nodes.

Although radiation therapy is primarily used in treating advanced disease, it can also play a role in treating certain women with earlier stage vulvar cancers.

Side effects of radiation therapy may include temporary redness in the treatment area, premature menopause (in younger women), intestinal or urinary problems, and difficulty with intercourse. If radiation is applied to the groin area, lymphedema may occur. Steps can be taken to help relieve these side effects. Sometimes, if the skin becomes very reddened, it may be necessary to take a short break from radiation treatments. Generally, though, a radiation oncologist will monitor side effects from the therapy to help make sure treatments can proceed as scheduled.

Chemotherapy

Chemotherapy is often reserved for locally advanced (stage III or stage IVA) or metastatic cancer or recurrent squamous cell cancer of the vulva. In a lower dose, chemotherapy may be paired with radiation therapy to help the radiation be more effective. Chemotherapy, with or without radiation, may also be used to shrink a large tumor before surgery. A tumor that shrinks in response to chemotherapy, radiation or both may lead to less extensive surgery, allowing the doctor to preserve more of the appearance and function of the vulva and adjacent structures. The combination of radiation therapy and chemotherapy is called chemoradiation.

The chemotherapy drugs used to treat vulvar cancer most commonly include cisplatin (Platinol), mitomycin, bleomycin and 5-fluorouracil, or 5-FU.

One clinical trial performed at multiple institutions by the Gynecologic Oncology Group studied the use of combination chemoradiation in 73 women with locally advanced cancers that couldn't be surgically removed. Treatment consisted of the chemotherapy drugs cisplatin and 5-FU combined with radiation to shrink the tumors, followed by surgical removal of the cancer and removal of lymph nodes. After chemoradiation, almost half the women had no remaining visible cancer. Most of these women went on to have surgery to remove microscopic forms of the disease, but in 70 percent of the women who had surgery, no microscopic signs of cancer were found either.

This approach of combining radiation with chemotherapy before surgery is a good alternative when women have larger, more extensive tumors that initially can't be removed with surgery. The results seen with preoperative chemoradiation also provide rationale for using a combination of chemotherapy and radiation as the primary form of treatment in some women.

Surveillance and Follow-up

After treatment for vulvar cancer, you'll see your doctor for regular follow-up examinations. Regular checkups ensure that any changes in your health, such as a recurrence of your cancer, are noticed and treated appropriately.

Because vulvar cancer is uncommon, there's no standard prescription for how often follow-up visits are done. In general, during the first two years after completion of your initial treatment, you'll prob-

Survival Statistics

One way to report cancer survival rates is to specify the percentage of patients who are alive five years after receiving their diagnoses. This doesn't mean that survivors live for only five years after being diagnosed with cancer. In fact, most cancer survivors live much longer. The five-year benchmark is simply used for consistency when talking about cancer survival.

Your likelihood of surviving vulvar cancer depends mainly on the stage of the disease at diagnosis, the type of cancer present and whether the cancer has spread to the lymph nodes in your groin. In general, spread to the lymph nodes means a poorer prognosis. Studies show that women whose cancer has spread to groin lymph nodes are about half as likely to survive vulvar cancer as are women whose cancer hasn't spread to lymph nodes in the groin.

5-year survival rates for vulvar cancer

Stage	Description	5-year survival rate
Stage 0	The cancer is confined to the surface of the vulvar skin.	Approaching 100%
Stage I	The cancer is confined to the vulva, perineum or both and measures 2 centimeters (cm) or less.	More than 90%
Stage II	The cancer is confined to the vulva, perineum or both, and it's larger than 2 cm. It hasn't spread to any lymph nodes.	75%-90%
Stage III	The cancer has spread beyond the vulva or perineum to the urethra, vagina, anus or nearby lymph nodes on one side of the groin.	50%-75%
Stage IVA	The cancer has spread to the upper urethra, bladder, rectum, pubic bone and lymph nodes on both sides of the groin.	18%-31%
Stage IVB	The cancer has spread to the pelvic lymph nodes or distant sites.	Less than 15%

ably have a checkup with your doctor every three to four months.

The first two years are the time when risk of cancer recurrence is highest. Studies show that between 20 percent and 25 percent of all women who've had surgery for vulvar cancer have a recurrence of the cancer, and that about 80 percent of these recurrences happen within two years after initial treatment. If after

Chapter 33: Living With Cancer

Feelings & Emotions

Receiving a diagnosis of cancer may be one of the most difficult challenges you'll ever face. The feelings that follow can be very powerful.

Most people know someone who has had cancer, but to have that word applied to you can be devastating. A diagnosis of cancer can dominate your thoughts and actions and produce long-lasting effects on your daily routine, your relationships with others and your view of life.

But these effects don't have to be entirely negative. Armed with the advice of health professionals and the insights of others who have dealt with cancer, you can learn to cope with cancer's impact. Life with and after cancer not only is possible but also can be fulfilling. Although cancer remains a serious illness, it's no longer the inevitable death sentence it once was. Our knowledge of cancer — its effect on the body, how to detect it as early as possible and how best to treat it — has come a long way in the past few decades.

Increasingly, cancer is becoming a tale of survivorship. According to the American Cancer Society, nearly 9 million living Americans have a history of cancer. Of the cancers that specifically affect women, most have declining death (mortality) rates. Because some forms of cancer can now be cured or controlled so well, some people have come to view cancer as more of a chronic illness, such as diabetes or heart disease.

Cancer's Emotional Toll

A cancer diagnosis often produces a roller coaster of emotions that can shake the foundations of your world. Diagnosis and treatment can cause great distress. Even follow-up care can bring feelings of anxiety or sadness, often because of the fear of a recurrence. Sometimes the feelings are overwhelming. Other times you may feel numb, even when you think you should feel something.

The important thing to remember is that there's no right way to feel if you have cancer. Feelings are simply feelings — they aren't right or wrong. Some feelings may surprise you. Others may overwhelm you at times, causing you to burst into tears or get angry about simple things. It's what you do with your feelings — recognize them and deal with them instead of bottle them up — that matters.

Certain feelings and emotions — such as disbelief, fear, anger, anxiety and depression — seem to be more common than are others in people facing cancer. You may experience all of these, just a few of them or none of them.

Disbelief

When you learn that you have cancer, shock may be one of the first feelings you experience. You can't believe this is happening to you. You may wonder if your doctor has the diagnosis right or if your test results got mixed up with someone else's. You might find yourself walking around in a dream-like state, unable to concentrate or make decisions. Or you may deny the diagnosis completely and carry on as if nothing has happened.

Fear

Next, you might experience the consuming fear that often accompanies a diagnosis of cancer. All you can think about is the cancer. You start to imagine all the terrible things cancer might do to you — some of which may be true and others not. You may be wondering if you will die from the cancer. You may be scared of the treatment procedures ahead of you and their side effects, such as nausea and pain. You may be scared for your spouse and family. You may wonder if life will ever be the same or if you'll ever be able to enjoy life again. You may even fear that you'll go crazy and that you won't be able to handle all that lies ahead of you. These fears and concerns are normal. This can be a highly stressful time, and your feelings may be new and unfamiliar.

Anger

Once the reality of your diagnosis begins to sink in, you may find yourself engulfed with anger over the unfairness of it all. You might even take out some of that anger on people who are trying to help you — your family, doctor, friends, co-workers — because they're the people most available to you. You may even be mad at yourself or at God for allowing this to happen to you. Anger can be a healthy emotion, motivating you to take action. But if it continues too long, it can become disruptive to your life.

Anxiety

The distress caused by your diagnosis or treatment or just living with cancer in general can lead to anxiety. You may be anxious or nervous about tests, treatment procedures, changes to your body, loss of control, increased dependency on others, a cancer recurrence or death. Again, these feelings are normal.

Sometimes, anxiety may be caused by medical factors such as uncontrolled pain, metabolic changes and some medications. A member of your health care team may be able to help eliminate or reduce your anxiety by addressing its cause.

Having a good relationship with your oncologist and other cancer team members can go a long way toward helping you deal with some of the fears and concerns that can fuel anxiety. Your doctor can clarify test results, explain procedures and help provide you with realistic expectations by making sure that you have accurate information. It's important that you be able to talk openly and honestly with your health care team. Let them know your fears and concerns and how they can best help you.

Family and friends also can provide support by helping to reduce the amount of stress in your life. The love and emotional support of those closest to you are invaluable. Logistically, the people around you can be of great help with tasks such as getting you to and from treatment sessions and buying groceries for the week. To effectively minimize stress and anxiety, you must be willing to accept help. Depending on others doesn't always come easily, especially if you're at the center of the family and all its activities. But sometimes you need to let others help.

Usually, feelings of anxiety tend to dissipate as you adjust to the changes you're going through. But if anxiety persists for more than a few weeks or is intense, it can affect your quality of life and interfere with your ability to function. In such a case, your anxiety may be part of a more specific disorder, such as an anxiety disorder or adjustment disorder.

You don't need to live with symptoms of persistent anxiety. Anxiety is treatable, and addressing it promptly can enhance your well-being and make your cancer treatment less worrisome. Signs and symptoms that may indicate your anxiety exceeds the "normal" threshold and for which you might benefit from specific treatment include:

- Intense fear or worry
- Restlessness or irritability
- Trouble sleeping or waking up feeling wired
- Fatigue
- Difficulty concentrating or making decisions
- A rapid pulse
- Shortness of breath
- Sweating or chills
- Trembling
- Indigestion or diarrhea
- A feeling of detachment from yourself or others

• An inability to carry on with work or social functions

Talk to your doctor if you feel that your anxiety is overwhelming. He or she can refer you to a licensed therapist, licensed counselor or other mental health specialist. Treatment for severe anxiety may include medications, receiving counseling from a licensed mental health professional or both.

Depression

Feelings of sadness, grief and loss are natural among people with cancer. A diagnosis of cancer disrupts or even shatters your life plans and may cause you to become discouraged and pessimistic about your future. Although these feelings take time to work through, they usually become more manageable over a period of weeks to months.

Among some people, though, these feelings linger and deepen. Grief and discouragement can evolve into major depression. Some studies have shown that up to 25 percent of people with cancer may be affected by major depression.

Major depression is characterized by a change in mood that lasts for more than two weeks. Signs and symptoms include:
• Persistent sadness
• Irritability or feelings of anxiety
• Loss of interest or pleasure in most activities
• Changes in appetite and sleep patterns

Adjustment Disorder

Adjustment disorder is the term used to describe a variety of emotional responses that may develop when a person encounters a major life stressor. Many people with cancer experience certain signs and symptoms of depression or anxiety. Sometimes, these signs and symptoms are considered beyond what's "normal," but they're not severe enough to be classified as an anxiety disorder or clinical depression. This in-between stage is termed an adjustment disorder.

Adjustment to cancer doesn't occur as a single event. It usually consists of multiple responses and steps throughout the course of the disease as you progress through diagnosis, treatment, follow-up, survivorship and, sometimes, recurrence.

Normal adjustment to these events involves the ability to minimize their disruption to your life, regulate emotional distress and remain actively involved in meaningful aspects of your life. In other words, even though you have fears, concerns and other difficult emotions, you remain actively engaged in coping with your cancer and still find meaning and importance in your life.

If your feelings begin to cause significant impairment to your daily functioning, whether at work, at home or in social settings, you may have an adjustment disorder. Doctors typically use these criteria in diagnosing an adjustment disorder:
• The individual's emotional or behavioral symptoms are in response to an identifiable event, such as a diagnosis

- Fatigue or loss of energy
- Mood changes
- Feelings of helplessness, hopelessness, worthlessness or guilt
- Continuous negative thinking
- Impaired concentration
- Recurrent thoughts of death or suicide

Some of these signs and symptoms, such as fatigue or a change in appetite, may be related to your cancer or treatment. But those that have to do with your thought processes and emotional responses, such as feelings of worthlessness and loss of pleasure in activities, tend to be most indicative of depression. Uncontrolled pain, metabolic abnormalities and some medications also can contribute to depression.

It's true that a diagnosis of cancer makes you lose pleasure in some activities. How do you know if what you're feeling is just a natural response to having cancer or something else, such as depression? It isn't always easy to know at first. But if the symptoms persist or are severe, discuss these concerns with your doctor. To determine whether your symptoms are within the normal range or if you're experiencing depression, your doctor may have you take one or more tests. One psychiatrist studied the usual tests given for diagnosing depression and discovered that the answer to one question in particular was highly predictive of whether a person had depression: Are you depressed most of the time? If your

of cancer or a cancer recurrence, that occurred within the last three months.
- The individual's response to the event exceeds the typical expected reaction. It's not that you cried for two hours when you were first diagnosed — it's that you keep crying for weeks.
- The individual is experiencing significant difficulty in social or work functions. You can't enjoy time with friends or accomplish tasks at work because you keep worrying about your cancer.

The person with cancer isn't the only one vulnerable to adjustment disorders. Sometimes, family members can experience an adjustment disorder.

Age can play a role in the type of adjustment disorder people experience. Adults typically become depressed or anxious. Adolescents tend to act out their

problems. This may include skipping school, vandalizing property or doing some other type of uncharacteristic behavior.

Treatment usually consists of short-term counseling or psychotherapy, which involves talking about fears and concerns, dealing with thoughts and emotions, and changing behaviors. If this doesn't work, you and your doctor may consider use of medications, such as an anti-anxiety medication or an antidepressant.

Keep in mind that an adjustment disorder is not a sign of emotional weakness. Some stressors are simply too great for many people to manage without additional professional help.

Depression and cancer myths

The topic of depression and cancer is surrounded by various myths that can stand in the way of receiving effective treatment for depression.

Myth	Fact
All people with cancer become depressed.	Only about a quarter of the people with cancer experience depression.
Depression is normal in people with cancer.	Depression is not the norm in people with cancer.
Treatment for depression isn't helpful.	Depression is among the most treatable health conditions. People with cancer who are depressed can benefit from treatment for their depression.
If you're depressed, you're weak or your faith isn't strong enough.	Any person can experience depression if faced with excessive stress.

answer to this question is yes, then you may be experiencing depression.

Similar to anxiety, depression is highly treatable. Treating depression is vital to your quality of life. If you're in the midst of active cancer treatment, eliminating depression can help you better cope with your cancer therapy and any side effects it may have. Getting help for depression is also worthwhile in terms of your relationships with your co-workers, spouse, children, other family members and friends.

Treatment for depression usually involves a combination of medication and therapy sessions with a licensed psychologist or counselor.

Dealing With Distress

Distress is an emotional, psychological or spiritual experience that can interfere with your ability to cope with a variety of things, including cancer treatment. It's different from other emotional difficulties, such as depression and anxiety disorders.

Distress evolves from mental or physical strain brought on by pain, worry or anything that presents change or a challenge. There's no question that a cancer diagnosis is one of the biggest challenges a person may face. How you handle this challenge can make a big difference in your state of mind and in your quality of life as you go through cancer treatment.

Distress may manifest itself physically, behaviorally, mentally and emotionally. Physically, you may experience headaches, digestive problems, muscle tension, shortness of breath, or other physical signs and symptoms. Behaviorally, you may bite your nails or talk faster and louder. Mentally, you may have difficulty concentrating and thinking things through. Emotionally, you may feel anxious, frustrated, sad, weepy, angry, helpless, depressed and even guilty for being sick. You may feel as if your body has betrayed you and that you have no control. In addition, surgery may alter your body image, and you may fear being unattractive and undesirable.

You may not be able to eliminate distressing or negative feelings, but you can find ways to deal with them so that they don't feel so overpowering.

Coping Skills

As you learn to cope with and adapt to the changes in your life, eventually things will become more manageable. Many people are surprised to discover reserves of strength they never thought they had. But even years later, you may have times when you struggle to conquer feelings of fear, anxiety or discouragement related to your cancer. This is normal. Everyone has distressing times. The important thing is for the balance of your emotions to lean to the positive side.

As you go through your journey with cancer — through its ups and downs and occasional plateaus — here are some strategies that may help you along the way. If these strategies aren't helpful, seek professional guidance.

Self-help strategies

Here are some suggestions for controlling or preventing distress while you come to terms with your cancer diagnosis and you go through treatment:

Educate yourself

Understanding your illness and the treatment options available to you can help you feel more in control. Decide how much information you want to know and can handle. Some people find that reading extensively about their type of cancer and the personal experiences of others helps them cope. Other people want to know only about their specific treatment. Decide which approach will work best for you.

Write down your questions and concerns and bring them with you. This can help you organize your thoughts, obtain necessary information and understand more about your cancer and treatment options. The fewer the surprises you face, the better.

But don't let your quest for knowledge become an obsession, which may cause you more stress or a need to second-guess your caregivers.

Express your feelings

Rather than holding in your feelings, find someone you can talk to, whether it's your doctor, your partner, a friend, a support group or a professional, such as a psychologist or licensed mental health counselor. Many people with a serious illness, such as cancer, find that expressing their feelings provides some relief and reduces their level of distress.

Know your fears

Either through talking, meditating or keeping a journal, try to get a grasp of what concerns you most. Are you afraid of pain? Needles? Death? The effect of your cancer on your loved ones? Recognizing what scares you is a big step in coping with your fear and reducing stress.

Learn to relax

Relaxation means eliminating tension from your body and mind. You can use numerous techniques to help you reduce and control distress. For more information on relaxation techniques, see Chapter 34.

Take good care of your body

Get enough sleep, eat a healthy diet and exercise as regularly as you're able. Exercise helps release tension in muscles and reduce stress. It's been shown to decrease depressive signs and symptoms, improve a negative mood, increase self-esteem, and have a positive effect on quality of life. Exercise also helps reduce fatigue that sometimes accompanies cancer and its treatment. See Chapter 35 for more information on exercise.

Pamper yourself

Recognize that you're going through an extremely difficult time. Nurture and pamper yourself. Listen to music you love. Light candles. It's not selfish to care for yourself — it's life-affirming. In addition, plan at least two or three enjoyable experiences a week. These might include pursuing a new hobby, playing cards with friends or going to a movie. Make it something you enjoy and look forward to.

Maintain your routine

Don't let your cancer or side effects from treatment completely control your life. Try to maintain at least some of the daily routine and lifestyle you had before learning of your cancer. Even if you're not able to resume previous work or other responsibilities, take a trip, join your children or grandchildren on an outing, or participate in social activities. It's important to have activities that give you a sense of purpose, fulfillment and meaning. If you have limitations, give yourself permission to take things easier than you did before your diagnosis.

Develop a good relationship with your health care team

One study indicated that the nature of a woman's relationship with her doctor and other members of her health care team affects how well she adjusts to being ill, how satisfied she is with her treatment, and how well she follows health care instructions.

Surround yourself with positive, supportive people

Your mind and body aren't separate. The better you feel emotionally, the better able you'll be to physically cope with your illness. Surrounding yourself with positive, caring people who want to support you will boost your spirits and give you confidence.

And don't be afraid to laugh. There may be some truth to the old saying that laughter is the best medicine. Laughing promotes the release of chemicals that help fight pain and depression. Granted, cancer is a very serious illness. Indeed, some people may feel that there can be no laughter or pleasure after a cancer diagnosis. But you may be surprised at how life goes on in spite of tears and sadness, and funny moments do take place in the midst of stress and worry. So don't be afraid to laugh — it's good for you. And if you feel free to laugh, others will take your cue and do the same.

It Helps to Laugh

You may think there's nothing funny about your situation, but humor can help you cope. In fact, some studies have shown that being able to laugh in the face of adversity may not only help you cope but also ease pain.

The first studies on the effect of humor on the body were conducted in the United States in the 1930s. But it wasn't until 1979 that humor research got a real boost. That's when *Saturday Review* editor Norman Cousins countered a diagnosis of ankylosing spondylitis, a painful and potentially crippling arthritis, with a combination of mainstream medicine and daily doses of humor.

To get his humor fix, Cousins watched Marx Brothers and Three Stooges movies and videos of *Candid Camera*. Although his doctors had given him little chance of recovery, within eight days his pain began to subside, and he returned to work.

Cousins' experience spawned a wealth of humor research. Studies have indicated that laughter relaxes the skeletal muscles of your arms and legs, exercises your heart by raising your heart rate, releases pent-up feelings like frustration and anger, lessens pain, and, for some, makes breathing more comfortable. It doesn't, however, cure disease. Laughter may help relieve your symptoms, but it won't cure your cancer.

In a small study published in 2002, women with breast cancer identified humor as an important coping skill. They said laughing helped them to relax, and it kept them from giving up and taking their situations too seriously. They reported feeling a strong need to laugh to survive low moments. The women also reported forming deeper, more-trusting relationships with health care professionals who used humor with them.

No one knows why laughter has the effects it does, but one theory is that it boosts the release of endorphins, brain chemicals that create a feeling of well-being. Whatever the reason, laughter can't hurt. So look for something to laugh about, whether it's watching comedies or finding something humorous in each day.

Look for the silver lining

Cancer doesn't have to be all negative. Good can come out of it. Confrontation with cancer may lead you to grow emotionally and spiritually, identify what really matters to you, settle long-standing disputes, and spend more time with people important to you and less time on the things that don't matter.

Maintaining a Positive Outlook

You may have heard someone who has a life-threatening illness say it's the best thing that ever happened to him or her, and you may have wondered how anyone could believe such a thing. For some people, recovering from a life-threatening illness causes them to put their lives into perspective, leads to a greater appreciation of what they have and causes them to make every moment in life count.

Maintaining a positive outlook — actively coping with your disease — may lead to greater emotional, physical and functional well-being.

A 2002 study included 98 women with endometrial, cervical or ovarian cancer that ranged from early-stage to regionally advanced disease. The study found that women who coped with their diseases by using positive thinking and acceptance had a better mood and quality of life a year after diagnosis than did women who disengaged or gave up attempts to cope.

Positive thinking means looking at a cancer diagnosis in a new way, such as using it to find new meaning in life. Acceptance means facing realities that can't be changed. The women in the study who actively attempted to cope with their diseases also tended to seek comfort and support from others. As a result, they reported better relationships with their doctors and others.

Self-help strategies

You can do things to try to make yourself feel more positive about the situation at hand and improve your ability to cope.

- **Focus on the good.** Yes, you have cancer, but that's not the entirety of your life. What's good about your life? Do you have friends and family who love and care for you? Do you have access to good medical care? What are you looking forward to? Each day, remind your-

self of the positives. This doesn't mean that you shouldn't grieve your losses. Rather, try to concentrate more on what you have than on what you've lost.
- **Don't blame yourself.** There may be things you wished you had done differently in life. But that's the past, and you can't change it. You can control only what you do from here on out. Maybe you can use your illness as a springboard to making positive life changes.
- **Pay attention to your thoughts.** You may be amazed at how many negative messages float through your head on any given day, such as "I feel awful," or "I'm tired and I can't fight this disease." Tune in to these messages. When you find yourself thinking negatively, stop the thought. Replace the negative stream with more positive thoughts, such as "Tomorrow, I'll feel better" or "I'm going to do everything I can to beat this illness."
- **Cultivate hope.** Hope keeps you going during tough times. It can motivate you to take good care of yourself and to follow the advice of your doctor. If you believe things will work out or that you can cope with whatever comes your way, you'll be more motivated to take whatever steps are needed.
- **Reward yourself.** Give yourself a pat on the back or a bubble bath or a piece of chocolate for holding on to your positive thoughts. Giving in to your fear and sadness now and then is to be expected, but try not to linger there. If you can, pull yourself away.

Maintaining a positive outlook doesn't mean that you should bottle up your emotions and pretend to be cheerful if

Myth: **A positive attitude is all you need to beat cancer.**

Fact: Although many popular books on cancer talk about fighters and optimists, there's no scientific proof that a positive attitude gives you an advantage in cancer treatment or improves your chance of being cured.

What a positive attitude can do is improve the quality of your life during cancer treatment and beyond. You may be more likely to stay active, maintain ties to family members and friends, and continue social activities. In turn, this may enhance your sense of well-being and help you find the strength to deal with your cancer. A positive attitude may also help you become a more informed and active partner with your doctor during cancer treatment.

At the same time, it's perfectly normal to feel sadness, anger or fear after a cancer diagnosis. It's a matter of degree. If you feel that negative emotions are taking up too much of your time, talk with a member of your health care team. Falsely putting on a happy face can increase your sense of isolation and hamper your ability to cope.

you're not. It does mean trying to seek out some good aspects of a difficult situation.

Communicating With Family

In some families, cancer has a way of drawing people together. Previous arguments, disagreements and pet peeves seem to fade away in the face of the illness. Family members feel united against a common enemy — the cancer — and rally around the family member who has the disease. One man felt that the years after his wife's diagnosis of cancer provided more bonding and intimacy than all the years preceding it.

Family members often learn to treasure their moments with one another. Eventually, the funny side of things starts to show up, and laughter and humor around the house sometimes increase. In essence, life becomes more real and precious than ever before. In time, the family adjusts and moves on to deal with the challenges at hand.

But illness doesn't always draw families together. In families where communication is already difficult, a crisis such as a cancer diagnosis may not improve the situation. Sometimes, it can make communication even more difficult and past conflicts even more problematic.

When cancer becomes a barrier

Even in the best of families, cancer can be a barrier to communication. Having to face this kind of illness can place tremendous stress on the family's foundations. If family relationships were strained before cancer entered the picture, they may

LIVING WITH CANCER

become even more strained. Family members may find it difficult to come to grips with the illness and may not be able to talk about important issues. A family's responses to cancer are often very similar to those of the person diagnosed. Feelings of helplessness and frustration at being powerless to solve the problem are also a common response among family members. Adjustment may be difficult for all involved.

Changing roles within the family also can exert pressure on relationships. For example, you may need to give up some of your responsibilities around the house or as an income provider in order to deal with treatment. In turn, your husband may need to pick up added responsibilities, such as making dinner, taking care of the children or working an extra job. Teenagers also may need to shoulder additional chores and duties. Young children sometimes revert to more infantile behavior in an attempt to cope with the changes.

Adjusting to everything that's going on, along with providing one another with emotional support, can be exhausting and sometimes insurmountable. Feelings of resentment and lack of appreciation can grow, and if they're not dealt with, they can harm family relationships.

Seeking help

Coping with cancer may require skills that you, your family and friends don't use on a daily basis. It's not only appropriate but often wise to seek help in the form of individual, relationship or family counseling.

A spiritual adviser or licensed mental health professional can provide you and your family an outlet for discussing fears and other feelings that may not have otherwise been expressed. He or she may also offer coping skills to help strengthen your relationships.

Many people with cancer also turn to support groups for help in coping with their disease. For more information on various types of support groups, see Chapter 36.

Individual and group counseling

Conducted by a professional, such as a psychologist, counselor or social worker, counseling provides an environment in which you can talk about what troubles you and gain support and feedback. Given the effect cancer can have on your loved ones, counseling may also include your partner and other family members. Counseling can help reduce depression and anxiety and can help you cope with your illness and learn to communicate better with loved ones and your health care providers.

Many therapeutic approaches are available, from those that focus on feelings and experiences to those that try to change behavior by addressing unhealthy — faulty or negative — thinking. To find a therapist who works with people who have cancer, talk to your doctor or other members of your health care team. Arrange to meet with the therapist to determine whether you feel comfortable with him or her and to get a sense of whether you think you'll benefit from his or her help. If you're not comfortable, find another therapist.

Communicating With Children

Parents with children still at home often find the prospect of telling them about cancer especially daunting. Besides wanting to protect them from hurt and pain, parents frequently don't know where to begin explaining the illness. It helps to come to grips with the diagnosis yourself before communicating it to your children, but at some point they must be told. Remember, too, that children, particularly younger children, may not understand cancer in the same way that adults do. The response from your children to the news may be very different from that of other family and friends. Their response will vary with their ages and their ability to grasp the concept of cancer.

In an article that appeared in the *Journal of Clinical Oncology**, a group of experts outlined a series of steps to help children cope with their parents' cancers and their fears and concerns. These suggestions may help you as you try to help your children. You know your children best. Try to recall how they may have dealt with problems in the past — they'll most likely respond in much the same way now. Respect their resilience, but remember they need you now as much as ever.

Step 1: Maximizing their support system

Allow your children to carry on as normal a schedule as possible, and assure them that it's OK to do so. Encourage your chil-

dren's relationships with other trusted adults. By letting other adults help out with events and activities, your children will see that such relationships are OK and that they're not being disloyal to you. Alert your children's teachers, counselors, coaches and spiritual teachers of what's going on.

The goal is to maintain as much stability as possible in your child's life. If you and your partner are having disagreements or difficulty communicating, it may help to rely on family members to bridge the gap for your children. Don't hesitate to seek professional help if needed.

Step 2: Talking about the illness

It's important to be open with your children and to talk with them in a way that's appropriate for their ages. Open communication with your children reassures them that they're valued members of the family, that they aren't being left out of important family matters and that the family will pull through this together. Sometimes, just spending extra time holding and talking with your children can be valuable.

Children of different ages will have different levels of understanding. Preschoolers tend to think the world revolves around them, and they may see themselves as the cause of the illness. They may exhibit their distress through anxious behavior or through angry, defiant outbursts. Find ways to reassure them that nothing they did or thought caused your cancer and that they'll continue to be

*Adapted with permission from Paula K. Rauch, Anna C. Muriel, Ned H. Cassem, "Parents with Cancer: Who's Looking After the Children?" *Journal of Clinical Oncology*, 20:21 (Nov. 1, 2002), pages 4399-4402

LIVING WITH CANCER

loved and cared for no matter what happens. Older children also may feel responsible. Try to briefly explain to them about what causes cancer so that they know it's a matter of being sick and not a result of their behavior.

Sometimes, children couch questions inside of other questions or statements, so you may need to dig a little deeper to find out what their real questions are. You may ask them, "What got you wondering about that?" or "What part did you want to know about?" You don't always need to have an immediate answer either. You may say you need to look into that question, and then get back to them when you feel you have an answer.

Children are also likely to receive misinformation from other sources. Encourage your children to share what they've heard or learned from others about cancer or having a seriously ill parent. In this way, you can help them sort out what's true and what's not, and you can reassure them that they don't have to carry these worries alone.

Step 3: Addressing common questions

It's important to be honest with your children about your diagnosis, what you're going through and what they can expect at each stage of your disease and treatment. Although you may prefer to use words like *bad cells*, *lump* or *boo-boo* instead of *cancer*, these terms are often too vague, even for children. They may begin to think that every bump or lump is serious, leading to confusion and anxiety.

Encourage your children to ask questions and express their fears. Talking about concerns allows you to dispel mis-

conceptions and ease the burden of legitimate worries. For example, some children think that cancer is contagious and that they might get it.

If you're worried about how much to share in terms of your illness, remember that overhearing information is worse than being told it directly. Inevitably, children tend to overhear the discussions of their parents. This can lead to misunderstanding and fear. If you and your husband need to talk about issues you're not ready to discuss with your children, you may wish to do it away from the home or while the children are gone. Otherwise, make sure your children are in the family loop of information.

Some kids don't want to talk about the illness. If this is the case, make yourself available for discussion, but don't force the issue. Feel free to share medical updates, but don't try to prolong the discussion if your child isn't ready to hear it.

Questions regarding death may be especially hard for both the parents and the children. Tell them that there are different types of cancer and that some people with cancer are more sick than others. Acknowledge that cancer can be life-threatening but that you and your doctors are doing your best to fight it. Or assure them that you plan on living as long as possible and that you want them to continue to be as busy and active as before. It may also be beneficial to admit that this is a time of uncertainty and that uncertainty can be hard to deal with. Ask your children if they have specific concerns about what would happen if you were to die.

You may want to avoid equating death with sleep when trying to address questions about death. Kids can become scared to go to sleep when they hear this.

Step 4: Preparing for a hospital visit

If your children want to visit you while you're in the hospital and you're in a condition to receive them, encourage them to do so. Before they come to the hospital, have your partner or another adult prepare them for the visit by describing what they'll see, such as what you may look like and items that may be attached to you — intravenous tubes, a monitor, oxygen. Let the children stay as long or as little as they want.

If one of your children doesn't want to come to the hospital, you may wish to explore why. Some fears may be alleviated, such as fear of seeing you receive an injection or fear of seeing blood. If your child still would rather not come to the hospital, don't force him or her. Other means of communication may be more appropriate, such as a card, letter or phone call. Different children, even within the same family, communicate in different ways.

Someone should follow up with the children and answer any questions or see if they wish to discuss anything that surprised them during the visit. This person might also ask them if they want to talk about what was hard or enjoyable about the visit.

Step 5: Make sure your children know they're loved

Reaffirm your love and support for each child, and help your children understand that they will always be loved no matter the outcome of your illness. If there are

things that you want your children to know and remember, tell them explicitly and repeatedly until you're sure they understand. You may wish to write each one a letter or record yourself talking to them so that they have a record of your support. Knowing you love and care for them will help them more than anything else in the times ahead.

Communicating With Friends

In some ways, friends' responses are similar to those of your family members. Some friends are quick to support you and provide any help you may need. They understand when you need to be left alone, and they're there when you need to talk. At times, the friends you least expect become the most supportive. There may also be friends who aren't able to handle the news of your illness and drift off. Other well-meaning friends — not knowing what to say or do, and not wanting to upset you — steer clear of any conversation about your health. Still others say inappropriate things or they ask more questions than you feel comfortable answering.

People with cancer usually discover soon enough the friends whose energy helps. Sometimes, you even make new friends, perhaps ones that have been through some of the same experiences you have. Learning to accept these changes and leaning on friendships that are true can help minimize some of the stress you may be feeling. Feel free to set

Telling Family, Friends and Co-workers

Telling others about your diagnosis can sometimes be difficult. Much depends on your relationships and how comfortable you feel talking about personal issues with various people.

Wait until you feel ready to communicate with family and friends. You don't have to tell everyone at once. One way to avoid repeating your story over and over is to tell a few trusted family members and friends and then have them spread the news. That way people already know about your cancer when they see you, and you may not have to face uncomfortable questions.

As far as co-workers are concerned, you need to decide whether you want them to know about your medical condition and, if so, how open you want to be. You may want your supervisor to tell your co-workers, or you may choose to do it yourself. Some people choose not to discuss their cancer with co-workers. There's no right or wrong approach. Do what's comfortable for you.

your boundaries as to how much information you want to share and how much time you're willing to spend with others or on other people's priorities. Staying connected with other people's lives is important, but you also need to learn when to say no.

Seeking Spirituality

What is spirituality, anyway? There may be as many definitions of spirituality as there are people in the world. In the past, the term *spirituality* was often used interchangeably with the word *religion*. But the two terms have different meanings. Two people can both have a heightened sense of spirituality but belong to different religions or faiths or to no religion at all.

Spirituality is the search for the sacred, and the pursuit of meaning and purpose in life. It might be described as a dynamic

process of turning inward, to reflect on our own lives, but at the same time turning outward, to seek that which is beyond our daily struggles. Spirituality is also associated with being connected — connected to yourself, to others, to a higher power, to nature, art, music or life in general. This kind of connection empowers you to be fully engaged in life's experiences from birth to death, to know life at its fullest.

Paul Rousseau, a doctor who wrote about spirituality and illness, described it even further: "Spirituality is characterized by the capacity to seek purpose and meaning, to have faith, to love and forgive, to worship, and to see beyond present circumstances, and [it] enables a person to rise above or transcend suffering."

Religion is a road map that many people use in their pursuit of meaning and purpose in life. It's usually based on a particular set of beliefs, rituals and practices and the opportunity to be part of a larger community. Religion can offer a foundation for making sense of life's mysteries and for expressing spirituality. For many, religion is a great source of comfort, particularly in times of crisis. For some people, though, a situation such as cancer can raise doubts and unanswered questions about why people suffer, even when religion has been a vital aspect of their lives in the past. For people who have had negative experiences with religion, the subject of spirituality may become even more clouded when they're confronted with a cancer diagnosis.

Spirituality and medicine

The relationship between spirituality and medicine is an important one. Once upon a time, health and spirit were inextricably linked. In many cultures, priests and shamans were the healers. As science ascended in the 19th and 20th centuries, modern medicine and spirituality became separate disciplines. Within recent years, however, there has been a renewed interest in the relationship between spirituality and medicine. The number of scientific studies regarding spirituality's effect on health has been growing since the mid-1990s. Some studies seem to suggest that spiritual well-being can help to improve physical and mental health. Spiritual well-being also appears to be closely associated with quality of life and the ability to cope with adversity and illness.

No one knows exactly how spirituality affects health. Some experts attribute the positive effect to hope, which may benefit the immune system, according to some studies. Other individuals liken spiritual activities to meditation, which can be a calming form of relaxation. In addition, spirituality often provides a form of social connectedness, which can be beneficial.

Among individuals who are seriously ill, some use their spirituality to help them cope with their illness and the distress it can cause. It's important to remember that although spirituality may be associated with healing, it isn't a cure. Spirituality may help you live life more fully despite your symptoms, but studies haven't found that it actually cures physical ailments. Medicine is targeted at healing your physical body, and spirituality aims at healing your inner self.

Author James E. Miller, who has written extensively on spirituality, illness and life changes, puts it this way in his book *When You're Ill or Incapacitated:* "This may sound contradictory, but it is true: whatever is happening or not happening to your body, you can still be healing. You can still be moving toward wholeness. In fact, you may be progressing toward the greatest sense of wholeness you have ever known."

For some people, talk of spirituality and religion isn't meaningful. If this is the case for you, think instead of what's ultimately important to you. For example, you may not believe in a higher power or life after death, but your family is important to you, as are your friends and the other people in your life. Your ultimate source of meaning, of being connected with life, may be in your relationships. Or you may find meaning in nature or in art or in your work. Sometimes, learning to live fully in spite of doubts and fears is more important than having all your questions regarding life and existence neatly answered.

Enhancing your spirituality

A person's spirituality is always evolving. It matures with life experience and is shaped by your upbringing, personality and experiences. A crisis such as cancer can affect your awareness of spiritual matters and highlight spiritual needs. In essence, spirituality is linked with self-discovery and your sense of inner worth. Thus, it's valuable to remember and share experiences that have moved you deeply or that have influenced your understanding of yourself.

Following are some questions that may help deepen your understanding of yourself and your personal experience of spirituality:

- What are your important relationships?
- Where have you found comfort in previous tough times?
- What gives your life meaning and purpose?
- What gives you hope?
- How are you connected to the religious group or to the organized faith community to which you belong?
- What are your three most memorable experiences?
- How do you get through tough times?
- How have you survived previous losses?
- What do you believe will happen to you when your physical life ends?
- Are you suffering or struggling with physical or emotional hurts? What are sources of pain for you?
- What gets you through the daily grind?

- Was there a time or instance when you felt comfortable and all was right with the world?
- Was there a time when your life was filled with a sense of meaning or when you were filled with a sense of awe?

Many people use prayer or meditation to reflect on their inner lives. Sometimes, just shutting off the television and sitting quietly can help you get in touch with your thoughts and feelings. Writing your thoughts in a journal also can help you sort things out and allow you to examine them later. Attending religious services, joining a support group and volunteering in your community are other ways to express and expand meaning in your life.

You may also wish to seek out spiritual resources in your community, such as a minister, priest, rabbi or spiritual adviser who can talk with you about the issues that concern you. Many hospitals have chaplains, counselors and volunteer cancer survivors on staff who can help you address the psychological, emotional and spiritual aspects of dealing with cancer. Even talking to a trusted friend can help.

Many people with cancer find the more in touch they feel with their spiritual being — whatever form that may take — the better able they are to cope with their cancer.

Jeanne's Story

Jeanne Greenfield has heard the popular adage many times — the one about how people fear speaking in front of a crowd more than they fear dying. She's experienced both. "Not even close!" she responds.

In 1990, Jeanne was diagnosed with advanced cervical cancer — stage IVB, about as bad as it can get. At the time of her diagnosis, she was told the survival rate for women with this type and stage of cancer was zero. Zero.

When her doctors told her she had only a short time to live, this 38-year-old single mother of three fell apart. She cried uncontrollably, beat her pillow with her fists and refused to talk with people. She was angry, she was bitter, she was scared — and she was determined. Instead of going home and getting her affairs in order, Jeanne pleaded with her doctors to try something. "I refused to believe I was going to die."

Jeanne was placed on a clinical trial of chemotherapy medications, a combination of drugs she equates to ingesting drain cleaner. The drug regimen was eventually found to have too many severe side effects. For Jeanne, though, the chemotherapy worked very well. Next came radiation. She received 30 radiation treatments.

During her treatment and the months that followed, Jeanne lived from week to week and checkup to checkup. "People would come and see me and they'd say, 'I'll see you next week,' and that gave me hope. OK. I'm going to live another week then. I would go and see my doctor for a checkup and my doctor would say, 'I'll see you in two months.' That gave me hope. I'm going to live two more months."

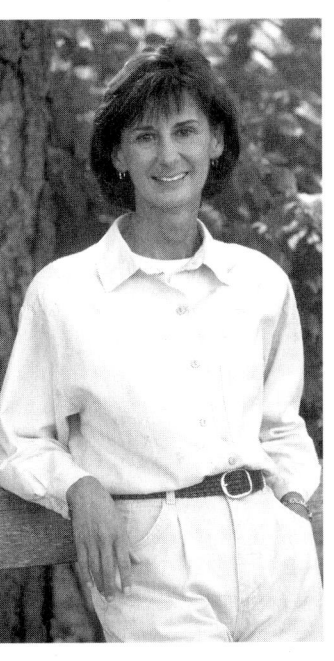

Doctors were hopeful that Jeanne's treatment would buy her some time, maybe even enough time to see her oldest son graduate from high school. But they expected the cancer to return. A few months passed, then a few more. Still, no cancer. Soon a year had gone by, which gradually turned into two and three years and kept going. The cancer never came back. Jeanne has seen all three sons graduate from high school, she has watched her oldest son get married, she has remarried, and she has celebrated the birth of two grandchildren.

So what happened? How did Jeanne survive when all odds appeared against her? The chemotherapy and long stretch of radiation treatments were undoubtedly key factors. But Jeanne, and even her doctors, feel other forces were also at play. Jeanne credits her strong faith, her unwillingness to give up and, aside from the cancer, her good physical health. Even when she was going through treatment, Jeanne would run or walk every day that she was able to. She also believes timing played a role. She began her treatment immediately upon diagnosis, at a time she believes the cancer was spreading rapidly.

Although Jeanne beat the cancer, recovery hasn't been easy. In a booklet that she wrote called *What I Learned from Having Cancer*, she writes, "The cancer did not kill me, but the cure has certainly tried to!" Jeanne has experienced shingles, blood poisoning and inflammation of the lining of her lungs. The femoral arteries in her legs closed up due to radiation damage, twice requiring bypass surgery. The same happened to the tubes leading from her kidneys to her bladder (ureters). She still experiences swelling in her lower torso, and she lives with chronic diarrhea. "Life isn't the same, but I wouldn't go back for anything. ... I've learned to appreciate life and all that I have."

Once very shy, Jeanne has become more bold and outgoing. She does mission work at her church. She acts in plays and speaks in front of groups. A speaking engagement at a cancer survivor seminar is what prompted her booklet, a lighthearted recollection of some of her experiences during treatment. Here are some excerpts:

> If you wear your best outfit and get your hair done (that is, if you have any), and polish your nails and your tennis shoes and go to the tanning booth, your doctor might still give you bad news.

> You might be in the hospital deathly ill with tubes coming out of every orifice of your body, but there's a good chance your teenager will call you up and say, "I need the car, Mom, I have a date tonight."

> My mother went with me to my local doctor each week where I was given my interim drugs. When I got there the nurse always weighed me and took my blood pressure. Each week my mother asked them to weigh her and also asked them to take her blood pressure.

> What I learned from having cancer is that if your mother volunteers to go to the doctor's office with you, it might be so that she can get a free check-up.

Today, Jeanne spends a lot of time visiting with women who have recently learned that they have cancer. She knows their fears, worries, frustrations and joys — she has experienced them all. Jeanne says it's easy to be bitter and angry, but you have to let the bitterness and anger go or they'll get the best of you. Fear, she says, is the worst pain of all. To this day, she still experiences moments of fear and anxiety, but she has learned how to deal with them and how to move on. In her booklet, Jeanne offers words of advice for women struggling to find some sort of balance during a difficult time:

> Life is simple. Don't complicate it. I think most everyone has asked themselves at one time or another," Is this all there is to life?" My answer is a resounding, "Yes, yes!" This is all there is to life. That's this life. Now the more important question: What am I going to do with that information? What am I going to do with the life that has been given me? And, in my case and maybe yours, the life that has been given back to me.

Chapter 34: Living With Cancer

Complementary & Alternative Therapies

Having cancer and undergoing treatment exacts a physical toll, but that's not all. It can also affect you emotionally and spiritually. Because cancer can turn your life upside down and leave you feeling helpless, you may look for ways to make cancer and its treatment more bearable and to restore a sense of control and emotional well-being to your life. Many people turn to complementary and alternative therapies.

There's no general agreement on what constitutes complementary and alternative medicine, but it includes a host of therapies — everything from mind-and-body interventions, such as meditation and prayer, to acupuncture, therapeutic massage, herbal preparations and dietary supplements.

The lack of an agreed-upon definition makes it difficult to determine how many people use these types of medicine, resulting in a wide variation in estimates. However, their use appears to be gradually increasing. A survey conducted in 1997 reported that

42 percent of the U.S. population —
approximately 83 million people — was
using some form of unconventional
medical treatment. The same survey
also reported that Americans spent
$32.7 billion in 1997 on complementary
and alternative therapies.

Many people experiment with alternative and complementary therapies, and
studies indicate that people with cancer
are particularly likely to try them. Anywhere from 16 percent to 72 percent of
people with cancer have tried at least
one alternative or complementary treatment. Again, the differing definitions of
complementary and alternative medicine
account, in part, for the wide variations
in estimates.

Due to the continued growth in
popularity of complementary and alternative therapies, in 1992 the National
Institutes of Health established an Office
of Alternative Medicine, now known as
the National Center for Complementary
and Alternative Medicine (NCCAM).

In 1999, NCCAM teamed up with the
National Cancer Institute to evaluate the
potential role of alternative and complementary medicine in the treatment of cancer. In addition, numerous medical
schools and universities have developed
departments, programs and courses
devoted to the study of alternative and
complementary medicine.

In this chapter, we look at some
common complementary and alternative
therapies. We discuss what the therapies
claim to do, and we cite studies that provide evidence for whether they work. In
addition, we provide some tips on how to
evaluate unconventional health practices.

Defining Complementary and Alternative Medicine

None of the many definitions of complementary and alternative medicine — also
known as integrative medicine — is uni-
formly agreed upon. The following definition came out of a 1995 conference of the
Office of Alternative Medicine: "A broad
domain of healing resources that encom-
pass all health systems, modalities and
practices, and their accompanying theories and beliefs, other than those intrinsic
to the politically dominant health system
of a particular society or culture in a given
historical period." Although comprehensive, this definition isn't practical for
determining what today's alternative and
complementary therapies are.

Another common definition classifies
treatments as either "alternative" or
"complementary." Alternative medicine
includes those therapies, such as shark
cartilage and ozone therapy, that promises
to cure disease and whose practitioners
discourage the use of conventional treatments. Complementary therapies encom-
pass treatments used in conjunction with
conventional medicine, such as meditation and music therapy. Because most
people who use complementary and
alternative medicine use it in conjunction
with conventional treatment — and only
rarely in place of it — this definition often
isn't applicable.

A more recent definition from the
National Center for Complementary and
Alternative Medicine suggests that com-

Q: **Are there any complementary or alternative treatments that cure cancer?**

A: Unfortunately, the answer is no. To date, no scientifically sound, evidence-based studies indicate that any complementary or alternative treatment has improved survival for any group of people with cancer. However, research is ongoing, with clinical trials looking at some of the more popular treatments.

Preliminary data on agents such as green tea and antioxidants suggest these products might eventually play a role in fighting cancer. Antioxidants are substances such as vitamins and minerals that remove the toxic byproducts of oxidation, a natural process that can lead to cell and tissue damage, which may contribute to some diseases, such as cancer.

plementary and alternative medicine is simply "health care practices that are not an integral part of conventional medicine." That's the definition we'll use in this chapter.

Use of Complementary and Alternative Therapies

The proliferation of complementary and alternative treatments for cancer and other diseases may seem to have been born in the United States in the past decade or two. The truth is, though, complementary and alternative therapies have their histories in Europe and Asia that go back centuries — before conventional medicine.

For hundreds of years, people have turned to alternative and complementary therapies for a host of reasons, including relieving physical distress, achieving emo-

tional well-being and controlling symptoms such as pain. Surveys of people with cancer list additional reasons why people turn to unconventional treatments:

• To boost the immune system
• To alleviate side effects of treatment, such as nausea and fatigue
• To improve quality of life
• To prevent a recurrence of cancer
• To provide a feeling of control
• To aid conventional medical treatment

If you're considering experimenting with complementary and alternative therapies, first learn all that you can about your options and the potential benefits and risks of each therapy you're considering. At the end of this chapter is a listing of sources of reliable information to help you in your quest.

Keep in mind, though, that no alternative or complementary therapy cures cancer. If a claim for a type of therapy sounds too good to be true, chances are it is. It's dangerous to pass up conventional medical treatment, such as surgery or chemotherapy, that has been shown to help treat

Talking to Your Doctor

Many people who try complementary and alternative therapies don't discuss them with their doctors. They assume their doctors will either be indifferent to or oppose their use of the therapies. Unfortunately, not cluing in your doctor to all the therapies you're using could prove dangerous. For instance, some dietary supplements and herbs can interfere with conventional medications.

When considering using a complementary or alternative therapy, talk with your doctor first. He or she may be able to provide resources to help you evaluate your options or show you studies indicating potential risks to be considered.

Whether or not your doctor agrees with your decision, it's important that he or she knows what you're doing so that you receive the best possible care.

cancer or prolong survival in favor of an unproven alternative approach.

This doesn't mean you should forgo all alternative and complementary therapies. Some therapies are known to be safe and may help improve the quality of your life by relieving symptoms or the side effects of conventional treatment.

Types of Therapies

Many different forms of complementary and alternative medicine are available, each designed to work in a different way to improve health and quality of life. In this section are some of the most commonly used therapies, beginning with those that seem to have the most support from conventional practitioners.

Mind, body and spirit interventions

For most people, having cancer and undergoing treatment causes major stress, which can have a negative effect on your

health. To make matters worse, stress affects not just you, but your loved ones as well. Fortunately, a number of safe mind, body and spiritual therapies are available that may help you relieve your stress and, in some cases, reduce some of the side effects of treatment. These include relaxation techniques, such as meditation and progressive relaxation; psychological approaches, such as counseling and support groups; and spiritual approaches, such as prayer and ritual.

Relaxation techniques

Benefits of relaxation therapy may include lower stress and anxiety, reduced depression and an improved sense of well-being. You can learn to do most of these techniques yourself. They tend to be inexpensive or free, and they're safe. Relaxation therapies include:

Meditation

Meditation techniques, which have been around for thousands of years and practiced by people of every theological bent, help you enter a deep, restful state that reduces your body's stress response.

Today, many people meditate for spiritual reasons, but meditation may have health benefits as well. Meditating regularly can help relax your breathing, slow your brain waves, and decrease muscle tension and your heart rate. Some people prefer moving meditation to sitting meditation. Walking meditation, yoga and tai chi, a Chinese martial arts form that combines gentle movement with deep breathing, are examples of moving meditation.

Progressive relaxation

This is a method by which you learn to relax your body a little bit at a time. For instance, you might start by tightening the muscles in your toes and releasing them, then working your way up your body to the top of your head, tightening and releasing muscles as you go. Progressive relaxation teaches you to identify muscle tension and release it.

Hypnosis

Hypnosis induces a state of deep relaxation while allowing your mind to remain

5 Steps to Follow

Before using a complementary or alternative therapy, do the following:

1. **Gather information.** On page 530, you'll find a list of reputable complementary and alternative health information sources and guidelines for gathering reliable information. Make sure the potential benefits of any treatment you consider outweigh the potential risks.
2. **Discuss your options.** Talk with your doctor or another member of your health care team about the therapy you're considering.
3. **Evaluate treatment providers.** If you decide on a particular treatment, find a qualified and experienced practitioner who offers it. Ask for a referral from your doctor, another trusted health care professional or someone who has undergone the treatment you're considering. Check your state

government listings for agencies that regulate and license health care providers. Contact professional organizations, such as the American Academy of Medical Acupuncture, for the names of certified practitioners in your area. Keep in mind, though, that for many complementary and alternative therapies, there are no licensure or certification standards.

4. **Consider treatment cost.** Your health insurance may not cover the complementary or alternative treatment you're considering. Check with your insurance company. If you have to pay for the treatment out of pocket, find out how much it will cost. If possible, get it in writing before you start treatment.
5. **Check your attitude.** Regard complementary and alternative medicine with an open but objective mind. Stay open to possibilities, but fully evaluate any treatment you're considering.

LIVING WITH CANCER

How to Meditate

One of the best things about meditation, other than its value as a stress reducer, is that anyone can do it. Here's how:

1. **Find a quiet place.** Experienced meditators may be able to tune out distractions, but if you're a beginner, the fewer distractions the better. So find a place where you're not likely to be disturbed. Turn off the phone; don't answer the door.

2. **Get comfortable.** Find a comfortable position, whether it's sitting on a straight-backed chair, sitting cross-legged on a cushion or kneeling on a specially designed meditation bench. Keep your back straight so that you're less likely to fall asleep, which is why lying down isn't a good idea. Close your eyes to shut out visual stimulation.

3. **Breathe.** If you're a beginner, consider starting with this technique. Simply pay attention to your breathing. Focus on how it feels when air enters or leaves your nostrils or how your chest and abdomen move in and out as you breathe. If it helps you focus your attention, count your breaths, from one to four (in, out, in, out) and then start over. Or, you might pick a word or phrase to repeat over and over with every out breath. The word can be one that has a meaning for you, or it can just be a sound you find soothing. When you become aware of your attention wandering — and it will — gently return your focus to your breathing, your counting, or your word or phrase.

narrowly focused and open to suggestion. During hypnosis, you can receive suggestions designed to decrease your perception of pain and increase your ability to cope with it. A 1995 consensus statement from the National Institutes of Health cited strong evidence that hypnosis can reduce chronic pain associated with cancer and other conditions. The success of hypnosis depends on the expertise of the practitioner and your willingness to try it. Some people eventually can be taught to hypnotize themselves. Contrary to ideas about hypnosis made popular by the film industry, while hypnotized you can't be made to do something against your will.

Biofeedback

During a biofeedback session, a trained therapist applies electrodes and sensors to various parts of your body to help you identify how your body responds to certain stimuli. Using this information, you can learn how to control certain body responses, such as decreasing muscle tension and lowering your heart rate and skin temperature, all signs of relaxation. You can receive biofeedback treatments in settings such as physical therapy clinics, medical centers and hospitals.

Guided imagery

During guided imagery, you relax by following instructions — either from a recorded voice or by someone leading you — to create a pleasant mental picture. In your mind's eye, for example, you might see yourself lying on a beach on a warm summer day listening to gentle, rhythmic waves lapping against the shore. Sometimes, guided imagery is used with progressive relaxation, to increase the relaxation effect.

Music therapy

Music has been used to supplement healing in many cultures for centuries, and it's still used today to improve quality of life for people with cancer. Listening to or playing music has many potential benefits. Music therapy may help reduce pain and, with the help of anti-nausea drugs, ease the symptoms of nausea and vomiting. More research is needed on the potential benefits of music therapy, but there's certainly no downside to its use.

More than just listening to soothing music, music therapy may involve working with a music therapist, who designs a program involving vocal or instrumental music, based on your needs.

To learn more about music therapy or to find a certified music therapist, ask a member of your health care team or check with the American Music Therapy Association (see page 599 for more information).

Dietary supplements

The type of complementary and alternative therapy perhaps used most often by people with cancer is dietary supplements, including vitamins and herbal preparations. In a 2002 survey of people with cancer, almost 65 percent said they were taking dietary supplements. Another survey found that 81 percent of respondents took vitamins and 54 percent used herbal preparations.

People tend to think of products derived from plants and herbs as "natu-ral" and, therefore, safe. Unfortunately, that's not necessarily true. Some dietary supplements may be harmful. In addition, dietary supplements aren't regulated the way medications are, and they aren't put through rigorous testing procedures. The lack of standardized manufacturing practices means that product content, purity and quality may be questionable. The relative lack of regulation of these products means you don't know what you're getting when you buy them. In addition, research hasn't established the effectiveness of most dietary supplements, or established guidelines concerning side effects or how much of a preparation is necessary for a specific claim.

Another problem with dietary supplements concerns potential interactions with medications. For example, St. John's wort, an herbal preparation used to combat mild depression, can alter the action of a number of drugs, which is a serious concern if you're receiving chemotherapy. So do your homework if you're considering taking a dietary supplement. Find out all that you can about any preparation you want to try, and discuss the information with your doctor before trying anything.

Some of the most commonly used dietary supplements among people with cancer include:

Vitamins A, E and C

These vitamins are known for their antioxidant properties and have been touted as playing a potential role in cancer prevention. But their role, if any, in altering cancer progression is unclear. The vitamins also pose risks at high doses. For example, high doses of vitamin C can

LIVING WITH CANCER

Keeping a Journal

If the thought of talking to strangers creates stress for you, consider writing your feelings in a journal. Writing gives you an outlet to express your anger, worries and fears. Writing may help you increase awareness of matters that bother you most, sort out your priorities and put things in perspective. Keeping a journal also offers a way to record your symptoms and your progress.

Perhaps the best thing about keeping a journal is that you can do it anytime you feel the need. It's as simple as taking out a piece of paper or a notebook and jotting down whatever comes to mind.

keep blood from clotting, thereby increasing the risk of bleeding.

In addition, what might be good for preventing cancer might not be good for treating it once it's established. Just because something sounds good in theory doesn't mean it'll work. For example, not too long ago, researchers hypothesized that vitamin A and beta carotene might prevent cancer, and they tried to prove it in a clinical trial. Participants were cigarette smokers at risk of lung cancer. The trial showed the opposite of what was expected. Individuals who took these substances had an increased rate of lung cancer, compared with those who received an inactive pill (placebo). Instead of preventing cancer, the substances seemed to stimulate it.

Mistletoe

In laboratory studies, extracts of mistletoe have been found to kill cancer cells and stimulate the immune system. However, almost all the studies have had weaknesses that have cast doubt on the reliability of the findings. Although mistletoe could prove to be beneficial for people with can-

cer, much more study is needed. For the time being, no one should use mistletoe extract except participants in studies.

Shark cartilage

Research indicates that protein in shark cartilage inhibits the growth of new blood vessels, preventing tumor growth. But the oral form of shark cartilage sold in stores, which has been the focus of a few studies, hasn't been shown to be effective in treating cancer. Use of shark cartilage outside of an approved research study generally isn't advised.

Manipulation and touch

From birth, the warm touch of other human beings provides comfort and pleasure. Touch and manipulation of body tissues are at the core of several complementary and alternative treatments, including massage, chiropractic treatment and osteopathy.

Massage

Benefits of massage therapy include relaxation and decreased muscle tension, so it seems reasonable to assume that massage could contribute to improved quality of life for women with cancer.

A 2002 study looked at people admitted to an oncology unit of a large, urban medical center for chemotherapy or radiation therapy. Those individuals who received therapeutic massage in addition to chemotherapy or radiation therapy had better pain control, slept better, and had less anxiety and distress. Participants in the control group, who received a nurse visit rather than massage, showed improvements only in anxiety.

Overall, few studies have looked at the effects of massage on people with cancer, and this practice does have potential risks. There's concern by some individuals that the manipulation of tissues during massage could possibly promote tumor spread (metastasis). Although there isn't any evidence to support this concern, you might want to avoid getting massaged over tumor sites. If your cancer has spread to your bones, too much pressure applied during massage could lead to fracture. Another concern is that massage may cause further harm to tissue that has already been damaged by surgery or radiation therapy.

As a result of these concerns, it's important that massage therapy be used properly. If you have a massage, make sure the massage therapist uses care in areas of your body undergoing cancer treatment or which previously received treatment. Talk with your doctor about whether massage is safe for you and what areas of your body, if any, the massage therapist should avoid. Be sure your massage therapist graduated from an accredited

program and meets state licensure requirements.

Chiropractic treatment

Many people visit a chiropractor for certain aspects of their health care. Although chiropractic treatment generally is considered safe, there's no evidence that it's beneficial for relief of cancer symptoms. For people with cancer that has spread to the bone, it can be harmful.

Osteopathic medicine

Doctors of osteopathy (D.O.s) receive training similar to that of medical doctors (M.D.s). D.O.s, like M.D.s, can perform surgery and prescribe medicine, and they specialize in all areas of medicine. But osteopathic training also involves instruction in spine and joint manipulation. In addition to providing conventional medical treatment, osteopaths may perform manipulation to release pressure in your joints, align your muscles and joints, and improve the flow of body fluids. Not all osteopaths use spinal and joint manipulation in their practices, or they may use it only in certain instances. Again, there's no evidence that manipulation is beneficial for treating cancer. For people with cancer that has spread to the bone, it could prove harmful.

Natural energy restoration

The natural energy theory centers on the belief that illness results from a blockage or disturbance of the free flow of energy through your body. According to the theory, restoring the natural energy flow restores health.

LIVING WITH CANCER

Acupuncture

One form of natural energy restoration that has been shown to have health benefits is acupuncture, although Western practitioners of acupuncture don't necessarily ascribe to the energy restoration theory.

Acupuncture is one of the most researched and accepted unconventional medical therapies. It involves inserting from one to 20 or more hair-thin needles into the skin. The needles usually are left in place 15 to 30 minutes. The practitioner may move the needles by hand or stimulate them with an electrical current.

According to a consensus statement on acupuncture by the National Institutes of Health (NIH), studies indicate that acupuncture may work, in part, because inserting needles into a person's skin releases endorphins, the body's natural painkillers, and other central nervous system chemicals. Among the potential benefits of acupuncture listed in the NIH consensus statement is relief of chronic pain associated with cancer or its treatments, as well as reduced nausea and vomiting from chemotherapy.

If you undergo acupuncture, you'll probably have several sessions. If you don't get relief after six or eight sessions, acupuncture probably isn't beneficial for you.

You should feel little or no pain from the insertion of the needles. Significant pain is a sign that the procedure isn't being performed properly. Adverse side effects are rare, but they do occur. They include transmission of hepatitis B from needles that aren't properly sterilized, possible lung puncture, tissue or nerve damage or a needle breaking off under your skin. Most adverse effects are the result of a practitioner's lack of medical knowledge or inadequate training. That's why it's important to work with an experienced practitioner.

Alternative systems

Some practices are associated with systems of health care that are very different from conventional medicine. These include practices such as homeopathy, ayurveda and naturopathy.

There's no evidence that any of these systems can cure cancer, and they may be harmful if they prevent an individual from receiving conventional treatment. However, the healthy lifestyle components of some of these practices may be beneficial if used in conjunction with conventional treatment.

Homeopathy

Homeopathy is based on two beliefs — the law of similars and the law of infinitesimals. The law of similars: A substance that causes certain symptoms in a healthy person can, when taken in tiny doses, cure someone with similar symptoms who is ill. The law of infinitesimals: The more dilute the substance, the more potent the medicine.

Substances are prepared by a series of shakings called succession. Homeopathic remedies are made from tiny amounts of plant, mineral or animal products or chemicals diluted in water or alcohol solutions. Although some of these ingredients are toxic, the amount used is typically too small to present any danger. To date, there's no scientific evidence that homeopathic remedies are effective in treating cancer.

Ayurveda

Possibly the oldest system of medicine still practiced today, ayurveda begins with the premise that people differ from one another both physically and psychologically, so treatments must take those differences into account. According to ayurveda, people are made up of three types of energy (doshas) — fire, water and air. In most people, one dosha is dominant, and different combinations cause different metabolic types. Disease is caused by energy imbalances and disharmony with nature.

The system uses a variety of therapies, including healthy eating, herbs, exercise, intestinal cleansing, meditation, massage, and breathing exercises to promote health and cure disease. Although most of the techniques promote a healthy lifestyle, some of them, such as intestinal cleansing preparations, might be harmful.

Naturopathy

Based on the healing power of nature and the body, this holistic system uses a combination of approaches, including nutrition, herbs, acupuncture and massage. Practitioners also incorporate techniques from homeopathy, ayurveda, Chinese medicine and conventional medicine. Although some of the techniques may prove harmful to someone with cancer, such as the use of certain herbal preparations and excessive dietary restrictions, most of the techniques are geared to promoting a healthy lifestyle.

Where to Get Reliable Information

Knowledge can be a powerful tool in your effort to work in partnership with your doctor and to cope with your illness. There's no shortage of books, articles and Web sites that provide health information. But when it comes to alternative and complementary medicine, hype abounds. How do you know the information you're getting is accurate? There may be no way to know for sure, but you can use certain safeguards. Here are some guidelines:

• Look for a reputable source, such as a well-known medical school or health care institution, government agency, professional medical association or familiar, disease-centered organization, such as the American Cancer Society.

• Be wary of any information that promises cures, makes claims that sound too good to be true or encourages you to give up conventional treatments.

• When using the Internet, look for a site with an editorial board or medical advisory board that reviews content.

• Check Web site dates. Outdated information can be wrong and potentially dangerous. Look for a site that reviews and updates its information regularly. Avoid sites that don't date their material.

• If you use a commercial site — which uses the ".com" suffix as opposed to an ".edu" (educational institution), ".gov" (government agency) or ".org" (organization) — look for an explanation of its policies on accepting advertising, sponsorships and commercial funding.

LIVING WITH CANCER

Where to Look

The following list offers reputable organizations that provide information about complementary and alternative therapies for cancer:

- National Center for Complementary and Alternative Medicine, *www.nccam.nih.gov* or (888) 644-6226
- American Cancer Society, *www.cancer.org*
- National Cancer Institute, *www.nci.nih.gov* or (800) 422-6237
- Mayo Clinic Health Information, *www.MayoClinic.com*
- M.D. Anderson Cancer Center's Complementary/Integrative Medicine Education Resources, *www.mdanderson.org/departments/cimer*
- Memorial Sloan-Kettering Cancer Center, About Herbs, Botanicals & Other Products, *www.mskcc.org/mskcc/html/11570.cfm*

- Look for the Health on the Net (HON) Foundation Code of Conduct symbol. Only sites that adhere to the code are allowed to display its symbol. HON sites must provide clear information from a qualified professional, unless otherwise noted, and give contact addresses. The site must spell out advertising policies.

Even if you follow these guidelines, remember that there are no guarantees. Always verify the information you get, check more than one source and talk with your doctor or other members of your health care team.

When it comes to use of complementary and alternative medicine, try to steer a middle course between uncritical acceptance and outright rejection. Learn to be open-minded and skeptical at the same time. Stay open to various treatments but evaluate them carefully. Also remember that the field is changing: What's unconventional today may well be accepted — or discredited — tomorrow.

Chapter 35: Living With Cancer

Coping With Treatment

Cancer treatment can save or extend lives. But being treated for cancer also presents a number of challenges — from changes in home or work responsibilities to side effects such as fatigue and nausea, to the ongoing stress of doing battle with a life-threatening disease.

In this chapter, we look at some of the physical and emotional challenges you may face during your treatment and discuss ways to help you cope with them. Most of the information included here applies to challenges associated with the treatment of relatively early stages of cancer. You'll find information on some of the physical and emotional challenges associated with advanced cancer in Chapter 37.

Dealing With Fatigue

When most people think of cancer treatment, often the first things that come to mind are nausea and hair loss. Fatigue, though, is probably the most common side effect of cancer treatment — not just of treatment but of cancer itself. In part, fatigue is a reaction to the physical and emotional toll that cancer takes. It can be one of the most debilitating side effects, interfering with everyday activities, including working and spending time with family and friends.

For individuals who haven't experienced cancer-related fatigue, it can be difficult to grasp what it's like. Everyone knows what it feels like to run out of steam after a hectic day, but a little rest usually helps you bounce back. Cancer-related fatigue is more pervasive, and rest may not make it better.

Among people with cancer, everyone's experience of fatigue is different. Descriptions include feeling exhausted, being worn out, running on empty, feeling weak, having heavy limbs or having absolutely no energy.

Causes of fatigue

No one knows all of the causes of cancer-related fatigue, but we do know that certain conditions can contribute to it. Cancer specialists at the National Comprehensive Cancer Network have identified the following as having a significant effect on fatigue:

- Chronic pain
- Emotional distress
- Depression or an anxiety disorder
- Reduced oxygen to the body due to a lack of hemoglobin in the blood (anemia)
- Sleep disturbances
- Low thyroid gland function (hypothyroidism)

If you're experiencing cancer-related fatigue, talk with a member of your health care team. You should be evaluated for anemia and possibly low thyroid func-

tion. If you're found to be anemic, treatments may include taking iron supplements. For severe symptoms, you may need a blood transfusion or injections of synthetic erythropoietin, a hormone normally produced by the kidneys that may help stimulate the production of red blood cells.

Low thyroid function isn't a common side effect from cancer treatment unless you received radiation therapy to your neck. However, it's a fairly common condition, caused by a number of diseases. Standard treatment for an underactive thyroid involves taking a synthetic thyroid hormone on a daily basis. This oral medication restores hormone levels to normal, easing fatigue.

Other factors that may contribute to your fatigue include medications you may be taking, such as pain relievers or antidepressants, other medical problems, poor nutrition, and inactivity. Be sure your health care team knows of any prescription or over-the-counter medications you're taking. If poor nutrition is a problem, your doctor may refer you to a registered dietitian, who can help you understand your nutritional needs. For fatigue caused by inactivity, simply getting out and walking — even for just a few minutes — can help.

Accepting your limits

Ignoring your fatigue and pushing yourself too hard may make your fatigue worse. Many people highly value their independence, and needing to ask others for help is a new and unwanted experience. But it's important to accept that you can't do it all. Call on friends and family to help with chores and errands.

In a few instances, fatigue may last for years. In fact, during the first year after cancer treatment, fatigue is one of the most common complaints.

Self-help strategies

Resting or sleeping more doesn't "cure" fatigue resulting from cancer treatment, but you can do things to help minimize it:

- Plan your activities for times when you usually have the most energy.
- Look for ways to conserve energy. For example, sit on a stool to chop vegetables or wash the dishes.
- Pace yourself. Take short naps or rest breaks when you need them.
- Work with your medical team to establish an exercise program to help lessen your fatigue. Moderate exercise after cancer treatment is strongly recommended.
- Reduce stress in your life whenever you can. Don't try to do everything. Learn to say no to some things.
- Try relaxation techniques, such as meditation or yoga.
- Ask your doctor if any of your medications could be contributing to your fatigue.
- Eat a good breakfast each morning to prepare your body for the day's demands. Then refuel every three or four hours. Limit high-fat and high-sugar foods. They tend to make you feel sluggish later.
- Make sure you're drinking enough fluids. Dehydration can contribute to fatigue.

- If fatigue remains a problem, ask your doctor about medications or other therapies that may help you.

Overcoming Nausea and Appetite Problems

Eating nutritious foods while undergoing cancer treatment can help you feel better and maintain your strength. The problem is that cancer treatment can cause nausea and vomiting, and it may affect your appetite. There are ways to avoid or reduce these problems.

Nausea medications

In just the last decade, much progress has been made in development of medications that prevent and control the nausea and vomiting that accompany cancer treatment. Anti-nausea medications (antiemetics) are routinely given before your chemotherapy treatment begins, as a preventive measure.

Chemotherapy drugs typically are rated on a scale of how likely they are to cause nausea. For drugs that tend to cause little nausea, you may not need anti-nausea medicines, or your doctor may recommend a drug such as prochlorperazine (Compazine), commonly used to treat nausea resulting from a number of causes. If your chemotherapy treatment involves medications that are more likely to cause significant nausea and vomiting, your doctor may prescribe a corticosteroid medication and one of the newer anti-nausea drugs, such as ondansetron

What to Eat

During chemotherapy treatment, it's best to avoid foods that are overly sweet, fried, spicy or fatty because they're more likely to trigger nausea. Foods that are cool or at room temperature may be more appealing because they produce less of an odor than do hot foods.

Cook and freeze meals before your treatment or have someone else prepare your food when you're not around to smell the cooking odors. Easily digested foods include crackers, dry toast, broth and broth-based soups (such as chicken noodle), hard candy, frozen fruit bars and flavored gelatin. If you tolerate those, try other mild-flavored, nonfatty foods, such as cereals, rice, plain noodles, baked potatoes, lean meats, fish, chicken, cottage cheese, fruits and vegetables.

(Zofran), granisetron (Kytril), dolasetron (Anzemet) or palonosetron (Aloxi), which may be taken with another anti-emetic called aprepitant (Emend). You take them before chemotherapy and sometimes after your treatment, as well. To boost their effectiveness, these medications may be prescribed with other anti-nausea drugs. Side effects of some anti-nausea drugs include drowsiness and constipation.

If you're taking an anti-nausea drug and still experiencing nausea, talk to your doctor. Together you can try to find a combination of medications to control your symptoms better.

Self-help strategies

In addition to medications, some self-help strategies may help:

- **Eat lightly and frequently.** Eat small amounts throughout the day rather than three large meals. A light snack a few hours before treatment may help.
- **Eat and drink slowly.** Be aware of how quickly you're eating. Pace yourself. Put your fork down between bites. During your meal, pause to visit with others at the table or to reflect.
- **Eat moderate proportions.** Stop eating when you feel comfortably satisfied. Don't overeat.
- **Eat what you like.** Avoid foods that you find displeasing because of their smell or texture. Aim for variety, but choose foods you find easiest to eat and digest. During cancer treatment, your food preferences may change. Foods you once enjoyed may no longer appeal to you. And foods you didn't care for may seem appetizing now.
- **Drink plenty of fluids.** Sip on cool beverages such as water, unsweetened fruit juice, tea and flat ginger ale. It may help to drink small amounts throughout the day rather than large amounts at one time. Limit liquids at mealtimes so that you have more room for food.
- **Make yourself comfortable after eating.** Rest after eating, but don't lie flat because doing so can hamper digestion. Wear comfortable, loosefitting

clothes and do something to help keep your mind occupied.

- **Try relaxation techniques.** Relaxation techniques such as progressive muscle relaxation, guided visualization, deep breathing and meditation may help calm your nausea. A simple form of meditation involves sitting comfortably in a straight-backed chair. You close your eyes and breathe in and out naturally. If it helps, count from one to four as you breathe. For more on relaxation techniques, see Chapter 34.

Appetite and weight changes

Cancer treatments may have two effects on your appetite and weight. They may make you lose your appetite at a time in your life when getting the proper nutrients may be more important than ever. Alternatively, chemotherapy can cause unwanted weight gain.

Weight loss

Food may not taste the way it used to before you started your cancer treatments. You may have difficulty chewing or swallowing, or your mouth may be dry. Distress, anxiety or depression also can cause you to lose your appetite.

Don't force yourself to eat, but do try to get enough nutrients. Here are some suggestions you can try to help make sure you're getting adequate nutrition:

- Think of eating a healthy diet as part of your treatment plan.
- Eat foods you like. Don't feel obligated to eat something you don't like just because someone went to the trouble of preparing it for you.

Anticipatory Nausea and Vomiting

After a few chemotherapy treatments, some people develop a reaction by which they get nauseated and vomit before chemotherapy treatment. The nausea is triggered by something connected to the treatment, such as pulling into the hospital parking lot, walking into the chemotherapy suite or smelling an alcohol swab.

This is called anticipatory nausea, and up to half of all cancer patients who undergo chemotherapy may experience this.

Chances that you'll experience anticipatory nausea are greater if:

- You had severe nausea and vomiting after your previous chemotherapy
- You have a lot of distress about your treatment
- You have a history of motion sickness
- You experienced weakness, dizziness, lightheadedness or sweating after your previous chemotherapy session

Unfortunately, standard anti-nausea drugs typically aren't very effective for anticipatory nausea and vomiting. Anti-anxiety medications, such as lorazepam (Ativan), may help a bit. Relaxation techniques and behavior modification techniques, which teach you to remain calm and relaxed when you encounter whatever triggers your nausea, also may help.

If you experience anticipatory nausea and vomiting, talk to your doctor or another member of your health care team about getting help.

- Eat when you're hungry. Don't worry about traditional mealtimes.
- Eat small meals throughout the day.

If you're having trouble chewing or swallowing, try eating soft foods, such as scrambled eggs, milkshakes, applesauce and mashed potatoes. If you're choking on your food or coughing it back up during or after your meal, tell your doctor. If your mouth is dry, sip on water, unsweetened juice and other fluids throughout the day. Try eating soups, drinking milkshakes and consuming other foods that have a high liquid content.

Maintaining your weight can be a sign that you're eating enough. If you're losing weight and need to increase the amount of calories you consume, try to take in more high-calorie foods and beverages, such as peanut butter, nuts, ice cream, malts, ice cream floats, milkshakes, nutritional drinks and eggnog. To increase protein and calories, add fortified dry milk to your beverages. Talk to your doctor if you've lost 5 or more pounds. He or she might recommend a medication to help stimulate your appetite.

Unwanted weight gain

In the 1990s, it became apparent that many women tended to gain weight following a diagnosis of breast cancer, and that weight gain was more prevalent in women who received chemotherapy. There probably are multiple causes for this weight gain:

- After diagnosis, women commonly were told that they might lose weight, so they ate more to prevent weight loss.
- Some people with nausea tend to eat more to decrease the nausea.

- Depression leads some women to overeat.
- Some women decrease their level of physical activity when receiving chemotherapy.
- Chemotherapy might affect body metabolism in a way that causes increased weight.
- Chemotherapy may induce menopause, which can result in weight gain.

What can you do if you start to gain weight? In general, two common-sense steps can lead to weight loss: First, try to reduce your daily calories either by eating less or by reducing the amount of fat in your diet. Second, increase your level of physical activity.

If you're still having trouble losing weight or maintaining your weight, talk with your doctor about making an appointment with a dietitian or enrolling in a weight-loss program.

On the upside, weight gain associated with chemotherapy is becoming less of a problem than it used to be. This is likely related to increased awareness of the potential for weight gain, better counseling of women with cancer by doctors and nurses, and shorter durations of chemotherapy.

Coping With Hair Loss

For many people, one of the more distressing side effects of cancer treatment is hair loss (alopecia). Many people find that hair loss is a very public banner that says, "I have cancer."

Most chemotherapy drugs work by destroying rapidly growing cancer cells in the body. But in addition to cancer cells, the drugs attack other rapidly growing cells, such as those that make up your hair follicles. The result is hair loss.

Hair loss from chemotherapy medications depends mostly on the drugs used and less on an individual's response to the drugs. Some women lose all of the hair on their heads in addition to their eyebrows and eyelashes. Others experience only hair thinning, and still others have no hair loss.

If you're going to lose your hair, it'll likely begin to shed 10 to 20 days after you begin chemotherapy treatment. Your hair may come out gradually or in clumps. Some women report scalp tenderness when their hair falls out. Keep in mind that your hair will grow back after treatment ends. In fact, it often grows back thicker than it was before you began chemotherapy. For some women, their hair starts to grow back before they finish treatment. It's not uncommon for the new hair to be different in color or texture.

Radiation therapy to the head also can cause hair loss. Unfortunately, if your hair loss is due to radiation, it may not grow back because the hair follicles may be permanently damaged.

Self-help strategies

Your doctor or another member of your health care team can tell you whether the chemotherapy drugs you'll be taking are likely to cause hair loss, which gives you time to make some decisions beforehand. You may opt for a wig or plan to wear

hats, turbans or scarves to cover your head. Or you may decide to leave your head bare. It's likely you'll choose different alternatives in different situations, such as when staying home or going to a social function. There's no right or wrong choice. Base your decision on what makes you feel most comfortable.

If you plan to wear a wig, consider getting it while you still have your own hair. That way, the wig maker can match it to the color and texture of your hair. Some shops specialize in creating wigs for women with cancer. To find out if such a shop is in your area, ask a member of your health care team, check the Yellow Pages or call your local American Cancer Society chapter. Many insurance companies will help pay for a wig if you have a prescription for one from your doctor.

When your hair begins to fall out, treat your remaining hair gently. Use a mild shampoo, brush it gently with a soft brush and set your blow-dryer on low heat. Don't color, perm or chemically relax your hair. Use a satin pillow case when you sleep because it won't tug on your hair the way a cotton or synthetic pillowcase might.

Some women opt to shave their heads when their hair starts falling out. If you choose to do so, have someone help you and be careful not to nick your scalp, which could lead to an infection. Be sure to apply sunscreen or wear a hat to protect your head from the sun, and cover your head when it's cold outside to protect against loss of body heat.

Talking with your health care team about your distress over losing your hair may help you manage your feelings.

LIVING WITH CANCER

Regaining Arm and Shoulder Mobility

A common concern for women who've had surgery for breast cancer is regaining arm and shoulder mobility. Depending on the type of surgery you've had, the arm and shoulder on your affected side may be stiff and sore for a time. Limited arm and shoulder mobility is most often associated with removal of lymph nodes from under the arm during surgery.

Because of the discomfort, you might be inclined to protect your arm by keeping it still and not using it. But that's not a good idea. Lack of movement can make your arm even weaker, and it can make your arm and shoulder less mobile.

Breast cancer surgery most often affects the type of arm and shoulder movement that you use when you reach upward (abduction), such as when you lift a brush to your hair. This type of movement is used in many everyday tasks, such as driving, retrieving an item from a shelf, and putting on a shirt or coat.

After breast cancer surgery, women typically are given instructions on exercises they can do at home to regain function of the affected arm and shoulder. If you haven't received instructions, ask for

Deep breathing

Shoulder rotations

Hand squeezes

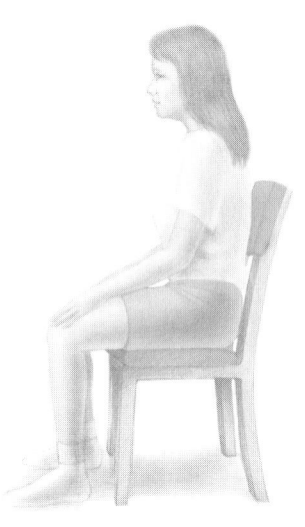

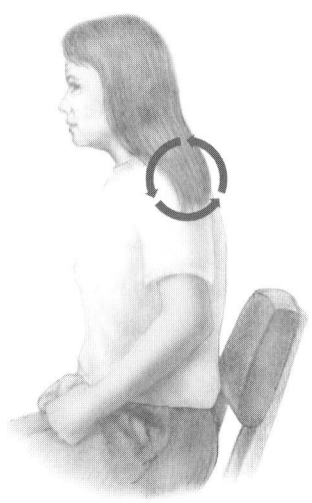

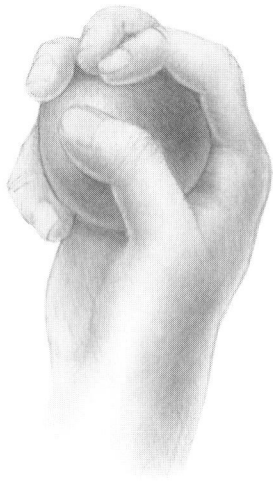

Sit in a straight-backed chair and breathe deeply in and out to expand your chest muscles.

Sit in a straight-backed chair. Gently rotate your shoulders forward, down, back and around in a smooth, circular motion to loosen your chest, shoulders and upper back muscles.

Using an object such as a rubber ball or washcloth, make a fist and squeeze tightly. Repeat several times throughout the day to strengthen your arm.

them. Exercising is generally recommended once all surgical drains are removed.

Interestingly, a study published in 2002 found that women who participated in a physical therapy program to regain arm and shoulder mobility achieved better shoulder motion than did women who were just given an instructional booklet. You might ask your health care team about enrolling in a physical therapy program and if you're able, find a physical therapist skilled at working with women recovering from breast cancer surgery.

Here are some basic exercises that you can do yourself. The most important thing is to get your arm and shoulder moving.

Recommended exercises

Inactivity following surgery can cause your arm, shoulder and upper chest muscles to become stiff and weak. When you first begin your exercises, it's important to start slowly.

Gently stretching your arm and shoulder muscles will help lessen the stiffness and the feeling of weakness. This gentle movement is the key to maintaining arm and shoulder function.

The exercises shown provide the gentle stretching necessary to keep your arm and shoulder mobile.

Arm raises

Lie on your back in bed with your arms at your sides. Slowly raise your affected arm straight above your head to stretch the muscles. Lower and repeat. If it would be helpful, fold your hands together and use your unaffected arm to help lift your affected arm.

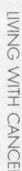

> Note: **The following exercises are a bit more strenuous. If you've had breast reconstruction, wait at least four weeks after surgery to do these.**

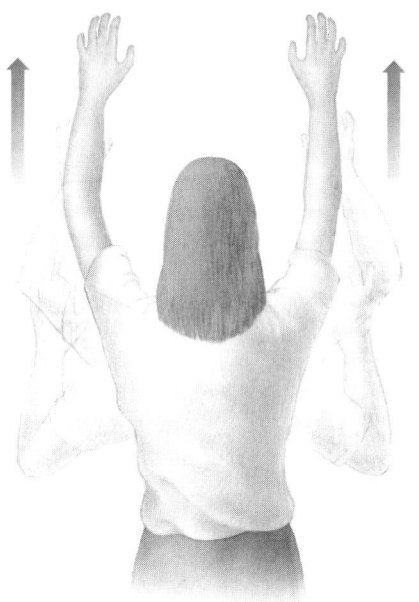

Wall climb

1. Stand facing a wall, with your toes as close to the wall as possible and your feet shoulder-width apart.

2. Bending your elbows slightly, place both your palms against the wall at shoulder level.

3. Using your fingers, work your hands up the wall — "walk up the wall" — until your arms are fully extended.

4. Work your hands back down to the starting point.

Pulley

1. Obtain a rope-and-pulley system. These are usually available at medical supply stores and hardware stores. Fasten the system to an overhead beam. Over-the-door models also are available.

2. Sit or stand with the pulley overhead but slightly behind you.

3. Grasp one end of the rope with the hand of your affected arm, or let your hand rest in a loop tied at the end of the rope. Grasp the other end of the rope with the hand of your unaffected arm.

4. With the elbow of your affected arm slightly bent, slowly raise your affected arm forward and upward by gently pulling down on the rope with your other arm.

5. Stop the motion when you feel a pinch, but before you feel any pain in your shoulder.

6. Hold for 10 seconds. Then using the pulley, slowly lower your affected arm to your side.

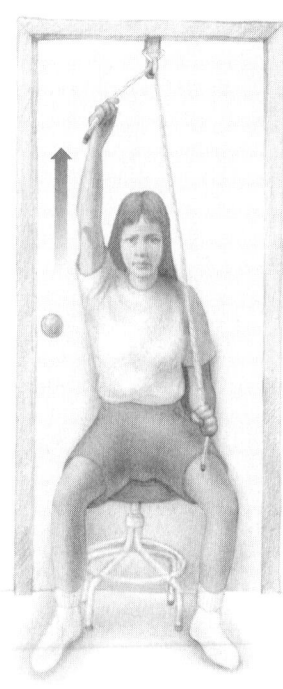

Arm swing

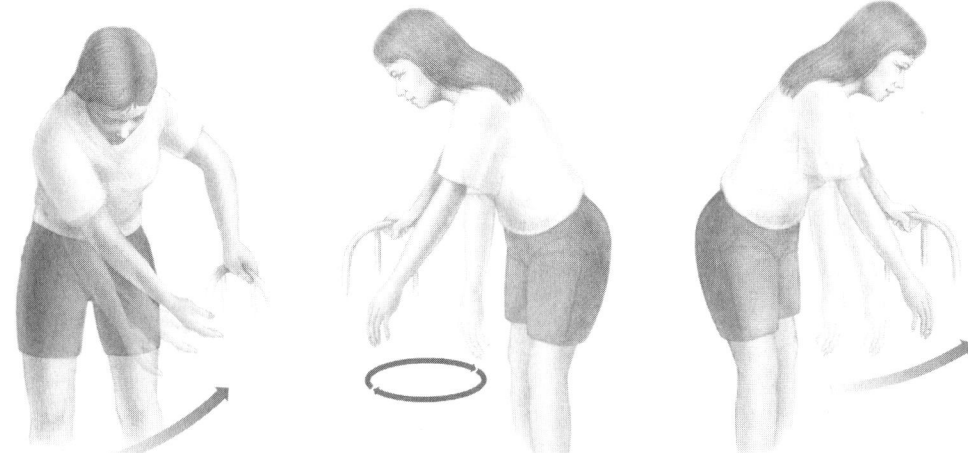

1. With your unaffected arm, hold on to the back of a sturdy chair.

2. Let your affected arm hang in a relaxed position.

3. Swing your affected arm from left to right. Be sure to move your arm from your shoulder, not your elbow.

4. Swing your affected arm in small circles, again making sure the movement comes from your shoulder. As your arm relaxes, the size of the circle will probably increase. Then circle in the opposite direction.

5. Swing your affected arm forward and backward from your shoulder, within your range of comfort.

Staying Physically and Socially Active

Having cancer and receiving treatment can alter your life significantly. One way to maintain some control and normalcy in your life is to stay active, both physically and socially. You may have to push yourself a bit, but staying active can help you cope with your disease and make a difference in how you feel about yourself.

Staying physically active

During your cancer treatment, the last thing you may feel like doing is exercis-

ing, but it's important for you to keep moving to the best of your ability. Too much rest and too little physical activity can contribute to fatigue and an inability to carry on with daily activities. Research shows that exercise can improve body image and quality of life among women with breast cancer.

Exercise has both physical and emotional benefits. Physically, it builds muscle, boosts energy, counters fatigue, strengthens the heart, improves circulation and increases the lungs' capacity to take in oxygen. If your appetite is poor, exercise may help stimulate it. It may even help cut down on nausea. Emotionally, exercise can lessen depression and anxiety, relieve stress, help you feel better about yourself and improve your quality of life.

Your ability to exercise depends on the treatment you're receiving, its side effects, the type of cancer you have, and your general health and physical condition. If you exercised regularly before your diagnosis, you may not need to be convinced of the benefits. However, you may need to exercise at a lower intensity level, especially if you've been in bed for a period of time. If you were sedentary at the time of your diagnosis, start off slowly.

If you have questions or concerns, check with your health care team before beginning any exercise program. Find out what you can and can't do. Your doctor may refer you to a physical therapist or exercise physiologist for guidance on developing an exercise program that's geared to your needs and abilities.

Types of activities

Pick an activity you enjoy so that you're more likely to stick with it. For most people, walking is the easiest type of physical activity. You can walk almost anywhere, and it requires no instruction or special equipment. All you need is a good, supportive pair of shoes. If you're limited in your ability to move, start out by exercising five minutes three times a day. Add one-minute intervals as you feel stronger, and try to work up to 20 to 30 minutes three to five times a week. Walking with someone else, such as a friend or family member, may make the activity more enjoyable.

It's important to try to include some exercises that strengthen your muscles, such as working with resistance bands,

which are large, stretchy bands that offer resistance when you pull them. Include exercises that increase your flexibility and put your joints through their full range of motion, such as yoga and tai chi. If you must stay in bed for a time, ask your doctor or physical therapist for passive or active range-of-motion exercises. Passive exercises involve having another person move your limbs for you. With active exercises, you move them yourself.

Keep in mind that anything that uses muscles and burns calories is beneficial. If you love gardening and are able to work in your garden, do so. Dance, ride a bike, rake leaves. Rest when you need to and don't push yourself too hard, but try to do a little more each time out to build your endurance.

Staying socially active

Unfortunately, some people receiving cancer treatment isolate themselves. They may feel embarrassed about their hair loss or not feel up to being with friends. But staying socially active offers many important benefits.

Staying connected to your social network of loved ones provides you with important support as you go through this difficult time. Your support network may also strengthen your ability to cope with your illness and improve your quality of life. In fact, a study of women with breast cancer concluded that the participants' social networks were critical to their physical and emotional recovery from their treatments.

Involvement with others can also help take your mind off your troubles and restore a sense of normalcy to your life. So stay connected, even if at times that means simply sending an e-mail or making a phone call. Friends are likely to ask what they can do for you. Let them help, whether that means driving you to your appointments, cooking you a meal or simply dropping by for a short visit.

If possible, keep up your involvement in volunteer, civic or religious organizations. If you can't attend meetings or do volunteer activities for a time, let the group know you want to be kept in the loop until you're able to return to more active involvement.

Continuing to Work

Many women with cancer who have jobs at the time of their diagnoses continue to work during their treatments, often with some sort of flexible arrangement they make with their employers. Working during treatment can provide a welcome distraction by focusing your attention on something other than your cancer, but it can also be exhausting if you try to do too much. Whether you can continue to work while you're going through treatment will depend largely on the type of treatment you receive, the side effects you experience, your health and the type of work you do.

Under the federal Rehabilitation Act of 1973 and the Americans With Disabilities Act of 1990, your employer is required by law to make reasonable accommodations that enable you to work while you're in treatment. However, these laws may not apply to certain organizations, such as employers with fewer than 15 employees. Under the federal Family and Medical Leave Act of 1993, which applies to employers of at least 50 people, you may be eligible for job protection and benefits for up to 12 weeks because of your illness. In addition, state and local laws and the company's own employment policies may help protect you from being discriminated against because of your illness. Learn about your company's policies regarding serious illness.

Accommodations your employer may be required to make may include:

- Flexible work hours
- The ability to work from home, if possible
- Use of earned sick and vacation leave with pay, in accordance with your company's policies
- Use of unpaid leave

Before you meet with your supervisor, make a list of what you think might be helpful to you. Do you need shorter hours or the ability to work from home? Do you need a temporary reassignment of duties or an opportunity to rest during the day? Some things you might not think about are the location of your workstation — if it's near the break room, you may need to escape the cooking smells, and you may benefit from access to a window for fresh air, assuming your office has windows that open.

If you continue working during treatment, you may want to schedule your treatments for days and times that interfere with your work as little as possible and leave you time to recuperate — either late in the day or right before the weekend.

Shirley's Story

Shirley Ruedy has stared breast cancer in the face not once, but twice. The first time she was 43. The second time — 15 years to the day after her first diagnosis — she was 58. The first time was a terrible blow. The second diagnosis "felt like a comet hitting the earth." Instead of a cancer-free anniversary celebration, Shirley sat in her doctor's office coming to grips with a nightmare of every cancer survivor — another cancer.

Unlike the first cancer, which was caught early, the second one was more advanced. It had spread to a lymph node and her chest wall. Shirley underwent a second mastectomy, followed by six rounds of chemotherapy and 35 radiation treatments. It has now been 10 years since her second breast cancer, and each day that Shirley wakes up, she knows that she's fortunate to be alive. She tries to live life to the fullest, not dwelling on the past or worrying about the future.

"I figure you do everything you absolutely can, and then you forget about it. I don't think that God has given you another chance at life to live it in misery. Worrying about it all the time is hellacious."

Shirley Ruedy knows cancer well — too well. She cared for her mother as her mother died a slow, agonizing death from colon cancer. She watched as her brother endured repeated treatments for breast cancer, until the cancer finally won. And she has stood by as good friends have received diagnoses similar to hers, and some haven't been as fortunate.

Shirley also knows cancer well because it has become her life's work. Some time after her first experience with breast cancer,

Shirley returned to her writing career, accepting a job at the local newspaper in Cedar Rapids, Iowa. She proposed a regular column on cancer, feeling readers wanted, and could benefit from, more cancer information. Twelve years later, she's still writing her award-winning "Cancer Update." The column is a platform for anything to do with cancer. Shirley shares the latest information on cancer screening and treatment. She encourages readers to be proactive — to get second opinions, to challenge doctors if they feel it's necessary and to take steps to reduce their cancer risk. She also exposes the emotional side of cancer: common fears, feelings and frustrations.

Some of Shirley's most touching and popular columns have been those in which she reflects on her own cancer battles and those of dear friends — putting into words the weighty surge of emotions in the power struggle between life and death.

Shirley Ruedy knows cancer well, but it's her sincere hope that future generations won't have to.

Here's one of Shirley's columns.

It's so good to feel good

By Shirley Ruedy
Gazette columnist

It's been a year.

A very mottled year. In a way, it seems like a lifetime since I was told, one stunning Tuesday, that the breast cancer which had beat its drum so loudly in my life 15 years ago, dying to a dim sound in the distance, now beat violently once again.

It was back, they said. A brand new one. A new one to lick, to contend with, to watch its shadow, to sleep, it seemed, with one eye open.

And in another way, it's impossible to believe that a whole year has gone by. To think how innocently I tripped into last November, thinking of the holidays, thinking of finishing the work on our newly refurbished kitchen — certainly not thinking of another cancerous visit.

So busy was I that I forgot the follow-up appointment I had made with the oncologist for that funny "blip" on my rib. After a reminder call, I went blithely off; after all, the tests had been negative so far, right?

Shirley Ruedy and her husband, George, in Washington, D.C., for a national breast cancer awareness luncheon in September 2002.

Ah, yes. So much for the "best laid plans of mice and men." Once again you are brought to your knees, made to recall that puny humankind has no firm grasp on the reins of life. What looks so leather-sturdy is as a dream, and you wake up holding only gossamer strands.

For that is, after all, all that life is: The most delicate thread (not the rope we fancy) tethering us to a final life — and we become so caught in our daily rushing about that we forget that at any given moment, the tether can reel us in to our eternal destination.

That is what I was abruptly reminded of last November. And I recalled that once there is the precedence of cancer cells in your body, in the family, one has to be forever the watchful sentinel.

REFLECTIONS: I did not have chemotherapy or radiation with my first mastectomy, as many readers know. So the "chemo" I began on Jan. 3, 1995, was a brand new world to me. My regimen, as I noted before, was not the most severe ever given, nor the lightest. I did what most of you would do: I endured, I prevailed, and I am here.

As I look back, what was most interesting, in light of the fear that so many people have worked up on the subject of chemotherapy, was simply, the chemotherapy suite.

It was, really, human nature at its best: Duty, love, compassion. The people — young, old, short, tall, fat, thin, rich, poor, men, women, white, black, brown, yellow — showed up dutifully at their appointed times. They marched like soldiers to recliner chairs or beds (their choice), sitting or lying there quietly. They thought ... or read ... or talked with companions.

The patients were on the front line, but those steadfast companions were right at their sides — husbands, wives, parents, adult children or friends, loyally accompanying their beleaguered loved ones through the weeks and months of therapy. They never asked for credit, they never sought attention, they were just there: Love aflower, love abloom, love majestic.

Mostly, it was quiet in the rooms. Whatever fears, wishes or apologies that were tucked away in the corners of souls — well, they had already been talked about before going there. Or, perhaps the thoughts would stay in their niches, never to come out. But everyone, patient and companion alike, knew why they were there. This was The Big Time. This was The Fight of Their Lives.

There was, of course, the silent drip-drip-drip of the IV — man trying anew to arrest one of the world's oldest diseases. The nurses went in and out, swiftly performing the mechanics of their trade, sometimes sensing a flagging spirit, sitting down to dispense some soft words of encouragement.

I learned that chemicals can teach you a lot about humans.

It's so good to feel good again, to see the hair on my head again. Do you want to hear something funny? It's curly! It's just a stitch! Little curls racing around my neckline. At times, I felt like the chemo was enough to curl my toes, but instead, it curled my hair.

Shirley Temple reincarnated! Wheeeee! Let a new year ring!

Reprinted with permission © 1995 *The Gazette*, Cedar Rapids, Iowa

Chapter 36: Living With Cancer

Symptoms & Conditions Following Treatment

As you complete your treatment, you're undoubtedly relieved. But the end of treatment can also mean facing some new challenges and concerns. Depending on the type of cancer and treatment you've had — and how well your body tolerated the treatment — you may continue to experience certain signs and symptoms for months or even years. Everyone is different. Some people experience few if any side effects or conditions related to cancer treatment, and others experience several.

However — as many cancer survivors will attest — you can learn to live with whatever physical changes your cancer or its treatment may have caused. This chapter covers some of the most common aftereffects of treatment for breast and gynecologic cancers, along with some tips for coping with these changes.

Lymphedema

Surgery, radiation therapy or other cancer treatment that involves removal of or damage to your lymph nodes may cause you to retain lymph fluid in the area where the lymph nodes were damaged or removed. When this happens, your arms or legs can swell, a condition called lymphedema. *Edema* is a medical term that means "swollen."

Lymph nodes are small, bean-shaped structures found throughout your body, about 350 to 500 of them in total. They produce and store infection-fighting white blood cells, called lymphocytes. Lymphocytes are distributed through your body by way of your blood vessels and also through a network of vessels called lymphatic channels. These vessels carry a clear liquid known as lymph fluid from the tissues of your body to larger lymph vessels, which eventually empty into a large vein in your upper chest, just before the vein brings blood back to your heart (see the illustration on page 260).

Surgery or radiation therapy for cancer often results in removal of or damage to lymph nodes and lymph vessels. If your remaining lymph vessels can't maintain the proper flow of lymph fluid, excess fluid can back up and accumulate in the affected limb, causing swelling.

Signs and symptoms include:
- Fullness or heaviness in an arm or leg
- Tightness of the skin
- Reduced movement or flexibility
- Difficulty fitting into your clothing, shoes or rings
- Visible pressure indentations in your affected skin, such as from wearing socks or pressing on the area with your thumb

If you were treated for breast cancer and you had radiation therapy or had your underarm lymph nodes surgically removed or both, you're at risk of lymphedema in the arm on that side. If you were treated for a gynecologic cancer, such as ovarian, endometrial or cervical cancer, and you had radiation therapy or surgery to remove lymph nodes in your pelvis or groin, you're at risk of lymphedema in one or both legs.

Sometimes, lymphedema occurs right after surgery and is mild and short-lived. At other times, it becomes a chronic problem. It might first occur months or years after treatment. The condition generally isn't painful, but it can be uncomfortable, due to the heavy feeling it causes.

Reducing your risk

There are no scientifically proven ways to prevent lymphedema, but most doctors believe you can do certain things to reduce your risk. Keep in mind, though, that the following suggestions need to be considered in the perspective of trying to live a full and active life.

Try to avoid infection
Your body responds to infection by making extra fluid to fight it. If your lymphatic system isn't operating to its full potential because of cancer treatment, this extra fluid can build up, triggering lymphedema. To avoid infection:
- Keep the skin on your arms and legs clean and moisturized with a mild lotion.

- Keep your hands and cuticles soft with moisturizer, too. Don't cut your cuticles with scissors.
- Avoid having shots or blood tests done on arms or legs that might be at risk of lymphedema because of prior surgery, radiation or both. If you need a vaccination, suggest another location, such as your hip.
- Use an electric razor for shaving your at-risk legs or the underarm area of your affected arm. This type of razor is less likely to cause cuts than is a straight razor, and it's less harsh than hair removal cream.
- Be alert to early signs of infection. These include skin redness, blotchiness or tenderness, or swelling or a feeling of warmth in an arm or leg. Fever also is a sign of infection. If you suspect that you have an infection, contact your doctor.

Try to avoid burns

Like infections, burns can lead to excess fluid in women whose lymph nodes and vessels have been damaged or removed. To avoid burns:

- When you're going to be outside in the sun, use a sunscreen labeled sun protection factor (SPF) 15 or higher. Try to avoid sun exposure during the hottest part of the day.
- Use hot tubs and saunas with caution. The excess heat they produce may cause fluid buildup.
- Use oven mitts when taking dishes out of the oven or microwave.
- Don't test the temperature of cooked food or bath water with a finger or toe of your at-risk limb.

Other tips

Suggestions include:

- Avoid wearing clothes, gloves and jewelry that are too tight. Constriction can decrease the flow of fluid, which can lead to increased swelling.
- Eat a well-balanced diet. Avoiding weight gain after cancer treatment may help prevent fluid retention.
- Use the arm or leg most affected by your cancer treatment as normally as possible, but don't overuse it.
- Avoid having your blood pressure taken in the arm at risk of lymphedema.

Treating lymphedema

Despite your best efforts, you may still develop lymphedema. If this happens, early intervention is key. It's easier to keep lymphedema from getting worse than it is to reverse the condition once it has advanced.

Treatments are available to reduce the swelling and prevent it from getting worse. Even though lymphedema has long been recognized as a chronic problem, little research demonstrates which treatment is best.

The most common way of managing this problem is to wrap the affected arm or leg with elastic bandages and, once the swelling is reduced, to wear a compression sleeve or stocking, which is a special garment made of elastic material.

There's considerable debate about the best way to get fluid out of the limb. Some doctors prescribe various compression pumps to try to help the fluid flow out of the affected arm or leg. These pumps often put pressure on the

Q: **Can lymphedema be treated with medication?**

A: In the early 1990s, researchers published a study in the *New England Journal of Medicine* reporting that a medication called coumarin (not related to Coumadin, the drug used to treat blood clots) effectively reduced lymphedema in a variety of people. Most of the participants in the study had lymphedema for reasons other than cancer treatment.

To follow up, Mayo Clinic researchers developed a clinical trial to evaluate the use of coumarin in women with lymphedema resulting from breast cancer treatment.

Unfortunately, results of this study, which included 150 women, found no benefit in taking coumarin. In fact, a few women receiving the drug developed liver toxicity, a condition that may be life-threatening.

Presently, no drug therapy is known to effectively treat lymphedema.

furthermost part of the arm or leg and try to milk the fluid up. There's some concern that this might put too much pressure on already-compromised lymphatic vessels, making the problem worse.

Some doctors suggest massage as a better means of getting the fluid out of the limb. The massage begins near the upper part of the arm or leg, working the fluid out of this area, and then proceeds down the limb, helping to get the fluid out in a stepwise fashion. Some massage therapy treatments include extensive daily therapy over two weeks. Other times, the treatments are done periodically for an indefinite period of time.

If you're seeking treatment for lymphedema, your best bet is to visit a medical facility that has staff with extensive experience in treating the condition. The doctors and therapists there can help decrease the amount of lymphedema in your limb, teach you how to keep the fluid under control, and provide appro- priately fitted elastic sleeves and stockings and ongoing therapeutic recommendations. Look for medical centers that have specialized lymphedema clinics.

Sudden Menopause

Menopause occurs naturally in women at midlife. It begins when your ovaries start making less of the hormones estrogen and progesterone, which regulate your monthly ovulation and menstruation cycles. Eventually — when hormone production ceases — your ovaries don't release any more eggs, and your menstrual periods stop.

Certain surgical or medical treatments for cancer can bring on menopause earlier than it would normally occur, which is generally about age 51.

A hysterectomy that removes your uterus but not your ovaries doesn't cause menopause. Although you no longer have periods, your ovaries still produce hormones. However, an operation that removes both your uterus and ovaries (total hysterectomy with bilateral oophorectomy) does cause menopause. This type of surgery is a common treatment for many gynecologic cancers. If you're premenopausal, your periods stop immediately and you're likely to have hot flashes and other menopausal signs and symptoms. This is known as surgical menopause.

Chemotherapy and radiation therapy to the pelvis also may induce premature menopause. In addition, many of the hormone treatments for breast cancer can cause menopausal signs and symptoms. Premenopausal women receiving chemotherapy for breast cancer may experience a relatively abrupt decline in ovarian function.

Signs and symptoms of sudden menopause are often more intense than are those of natural menopause. Unlike the more gradual hormonal changes of natural menopause, which usually occur over several years, hormone changes associated with surgical menopause are abrupt, often making the signs and symptoms much more intense. Menopause also puts you at risk of other conditions, such as the bone-thinning disease osteoporosis.

Effects of sudden menopause

Menopause can cause a number of signs and symptoms, which can range from mildly uncomfortable to severe. Some women experience several, and others experience few, if any. The most common signs and symptoms are hot flashes, sleep disturbances, night sweats, vaginal changes and emotional changes.

Hot flashes
Reduced estrogen in your bloodstream can cause abnormal regulation of your blood vessels, causing your skin temperature to rise. This can lead to a feeling of warmth that moves upward from your chest to your shoulders, neck and head. You may sweat, then feel chilled as the sweat evaporates. You may also feel slightly faint. Your face might look flushed, and red blotches may appear on your chest, neck and arms.

Sleep disturbances and night sweats
Hot flashes during the night can lead to night sweats. You may awaken from a sound sleep with your sleepwear and bed linens soaking wet, which may then cause you to feel chilled. In addition, you may have difficulty falling back to sleep, preventing you from achieving a deep, restful sleep.

Vaginal changes
Lack of estrogen can cause the tissues lining your vagina to become drier, thinner and less elastic. Decreased lubrication may cause burning or itching and may lead to increased infections of the vagina and urinary tract. These changes may make sexual intercourse uncomfortable or even painful.

Emotional changes
You may experience mood swings, be more irritable or be more prone to emotional upset. In the past, these symptoms were attributed to hormonal fluctuations.

LIVING WITH CANCER

But the stress of having cancer, menopausal sleep disturbances and other life events understandably may contribute to changes in your mood.

To relieve hot flashes

If you're bothered by hot flashes, a combination of self-help strategies and medication often can reduce their severity.

Self-help strategies
Most hot flashes last from 30 seconds to several minutes, although they can last much longer. The frequency and duration of hot flashes vary from woman to woman. You may experience them once every hour, or you may be bothered by them only occasionally.

If you're experiencing hot flashes:
- Get regular exercise. If you aren't exercising regularly, including daily aerobic exercise may reduce hot flashes.
- Dress in layers that can be easily removed and wear cotton. Cotton promotes air circulation, and it helps absorb moisture.
- Try to pinpoint what triggers your hot flashes. Common triggers are smoking, hot beverages, spicy foods, alcohol, hot weather, a warm room and a stressful event.
- Have a cold drink of water or juice and go somewhere cool when hot flashes start.

Medications
A variety of medications may reduce the effects of hot flashes. Discuss your options with your doctor, to determine what's right for you.

Hormone therapy
The most established treatment for hot flashes is the hormone estrogen, used in hormone replacement therapy (HRT). Estrogen reduces hot flashes by up to 90 percent. The hormone progesterone also can reduce hot flashes to a degree. However, because breast cancer and some gynecologic cancers are fueled by hormones, oncologists are often reluctant to prescribe HRT, and women are reluctant to take it. Many women who've had cancer don't want to take any hormone.

Clonidine
Clonidine (Catapres), a pill or patch typically used to treat high blood pressure, also may help alleviate hot flashes. Research suggests that it decreases hot flashes by about 40 percent. It does, however, have side effects, such as dry mouth, sleep disturbance, dizziness, drowsiness, lightheadedness and constipation, so doctors don't prescribe it as often as other remedies for hot flashes.

Antidepressants
Some antidepressant medications have demonstrated effectiveness in reducing hot flashes. Research indicates that a very low dose of venlafaxine (Effexor) decreases hot flashes by 40 percent. A slightly higher dose decreases hot flashes by 60 percent. Venlafaxine is well tolerated by most women, although about 5 percent to 10 percent of women taking it experience significant nausea or vomiting. For some women, the initial nausea goes away after a few days, despite continued drug use.

Venlafaxine has other side effects, such as mild dry mouth, decreased appetite

Coming to Terms With Infertility

Loss of fertility is a distinct possibility for some younger women who undergo cancer treatment. Infertility may be related to surgery, chemotherapy or radiation therapy.

If you were planning to have children, loss of fertility can be devastating. Some women experience grief and loss similar to that after the death of a loved one. When your friends and family members become pregnant, you may feel jealous and resentful — and then guilty for feeling that way.

Even women who weren't planning to have any more children may feel some grief at becoming infertile as a result of cancer. Some women feel they're less whole or less feminine. Some feel their infertility makes them less sexually appealing to their partners.

To cope with infertility caused by cancer treatment:

- **Discuss your feelings.** Talk to someone you feel close to — your doctor, a counselor, your spiritual leader, a family member or a friend. Most importantly, share your feelings with your life partner.
- **Allow yourself to feel the way you feel.** There is no right or wrong way to react.
- **Consider joining a support group.** You may find it helpful to talk with other women in the same situation. More information on support groups is available later in this chapter.

and, at higher doses than those used for hot flash treatment, constipation. If you have uncontrolled high blood pressure, your doctor may not recommend this drug because it may increase your blood pressure.

Other newer antidepressants also appear to relieve hot flashes. Paroxetine (Paxil) appears to work as well as venlafaxine. Fluoxetine (Prozac) also appears to reduce hot flashes, but not as well as the other two antidepressants mentioned. Early evidence suggests that several other newer antidepressants may also reduce hot flashes.

In addition, recent studies demonstrate that gabapentin (Neurontin), a medication typically used to treat seizures or chronic pain, can reduce hot flashes. Gabapentin appears to work about as well as venlafaxine and paroxetine. Its side effects may include lightheadedness and mild, generalized swelling.

Vitamin E

Research suggests that taking 800 international units of vitamin E a day reduces hot flashes a little bit more than does taking a placebo. What exactly does that mean? In many clinical studies, women who took a sugar pill (placebo) daily reported about a 25 percent reduction in hot flashes after four weeks. Women receiving vitamin E reported about a 40 percent reduction in hot flashes four weeks later.

LIVING WITH CANCER

Others

There's some evidence that an herbal preparation called black cohosh might help, but more study is needed. The bulk of available evidence regarding soy products, which have been studied fairly extensively, suggests that most soy products don't significantly help hot flashes.

To relieve night sweats and sleep disturbances

Night sweats are usually the nighttime equivalent of hot flashes. You may awaken from a sound sleep soaked in sweat, followed by chills. You may have difficulty falling back to sleep or achieving a deep, restful sleep. Lack of sleep may affect your mood and overall health. If you experience night sweats or have trouble sleeping, try the following strategies:

• Use cotton sheets, wear cotton clothing to bed and keep an extra set handy. Cotton allows air to flow around your skin, and it effectively absorbs moisture.
• Keep your bedroom cool.
• Avoid drinking caffeinated beverages right before bedtime. These can cause trouble sleeping.
• Avoid exercising shortly before you go to bed because it can rev up your metabolism, which can make it difficult to fall asleep.
• Try relaxation techniques, such as deep breathing, guided imagery, yoga and progressive muscle relaxation. They can help quell sleep disturbances. See Chapter 34 for more information on relaxation exercises.
• Try to follow a consistent sleep schedule, and develop a routine before you go to sleep, such as reading or writing in a journal.

To relieve vaginal dryness

As your estrogen level declines, the tissues lining your vagina and the opening to your bladder (urethra) become drier, thinner and less elastic. With decreased lubrication, you may experience burning or itching, increased risk of vaginal or urinary tract infections, and discomfort during intercourse.

For vaginal dryness:
• Use over-the-counter water-based vaginal lubricants or moisturizers. Staying sexually active also may help minimize these problems because it increases blood flow to vaginal tissues, keeping them healthier.
• Avoid use of douches. They may irritate your vagina.

If these measures don't work, you might ask your doctor about vaginal estrogen replacement therapy. Because vaginal dryness results when your ovaries no longer produce estrogen, vaginal estrogen therapy can help relieve signs and symptoms. Vaginal therapy increases the amount of estrogen in the vagina, helping to relieve vaginal dryness.

Although many doctors are concerned about giving estrogen treatment in pill form to women with breast or a gynecologic cancer, they may feel it's reasonable to use local estrogen treatment, such as a vaginal cream, for vaginal dryness.

Estrogen cream

Vaginal estrogen cream (Premarin, Estrace, others) can help relieve vaginal

Concerns About Vaginal Estrogen

Over the years, there has been much debate about the use of vaginal estrogen therapy. Most doctors and cancer survivors opt against oral estrogen therapy because of concerns about increased estrogen in the bloodstream and associated breast cancer risk. With vaginal estrogen therapy, a small amount of estrogen is absorbed and enters the bloodstream. Theoretically, this could cause some concern. However, many oncologists and gynecologists believe that breast cancer risk associated with vaginal estrogen use is likely very small, if it exists at all.

Vaginal estrogen therapy is a reasonable choice for controlling vaginal signs and symptoms associated with cancer treatment. If you're concerned about possible cancer risk from the therapy, it's OK not to use it.

dryness and itching. You insert the cream into your vagina with an applicator, daily for five to seven days. You can continue using it one to two times a week to control symptoms.

Estrogen rings

A vaginal estrogen ring (Estring) is a soft, plastic ring that you or your doctor inserts into the upper part of your vagina. The ring slowly releases estrogen over a period of 90 days.

Estrogen tablets

Another form of vaginal estrogen can be provided by a tablet (Vagifem). You use a disposable applicator to regularly place a tablet in your vagina — every day for the first two weeks and then twice a week.

All of these methods increase the amount of estrogen in your vagina and will relieve vaginal dryness for as long as you use them. Talk to your doctor about whether estrogen treatment is an option and, if so, which type might work best for you.

Sexual Changes

After treatment for cancer, your sex life may be affected in a number of ways. Studies have shown that about 25 percent to 33 percent of women diagnosed with breast cancer experience some type of sexual dysfunction. For women diagnosed with a gynecologic cancer, the numbers are about the same.

Talk with your doctor or another member of your health care team if you're experiencing sexually related problems. Many forms of sexual dysfunction can be treated.

Sexual changes that women may experience after cancer treatment include painful intercourse, difficulty reaching orgasm and decreased interest in sex.

Painful intercourse

Painful intercourse is a common sexual complaint after cancer treatment. The medical term for this problem is *dyspareunia*. It's most often caused by estrogen loss that leads to vaginal dryness, but it can also stem from other changes to the vagina, such as those that may result from pelvic radiation or gynecologic surgery. Specifically, a hysterectomy may cause some vaginal shortening, which can result in pain during intercourse. Chemotherapy and hormone therapy also can lead to sexual problems.

A more severe problem than vaginal dryness is vaginal narrowing (vaginal stenosis). Radiation treatments to the pelvis, which are sometimes used to treat gynecologic cancers, can damage the vaginal walls and the vaginal lining. Vaginal walls can scar or stick together, vaginal tissue can lose its elasticity, and the vaginal canal can narrow. Surgery to the vagina also can cause scarring and decrease the vagina's diameter or length, making intercourse painful.

Fortunately, you can do many things to help make intercourse less painful:

- Use a water-based lubricant in and around your vagina before having intercourse. Several over-the-counter creams, gels, suppositories and other lubricants are available. Experiment to find a product that you like. Avoid petroleum jelly and other oil-based lubricants.

They may make you more prone to yeast infections.

- Make sure you're fully aroused before beginning intercourse. That's when your vagina is at its longest, widest and most lubricated.
- Choose a position for intercourse that gives you control over the movement. That way, you can control the pace and depth of the thrusts.
- Tell your partner if something is causing you pain, and offer suggestions on ways to touch you that aren't painful.
- Have your partner gently stretch your vagina with a lubricated finger before intercourse. Once one finger isn't painful, have your partner add another.

If your doctor recommends a vaginal dilator to stretch your vagina, use it as directed. Vaginal dilators are latex, plastic or rubber cylinders that are made in a variety of sizes. They're lubricated and inserted into the vagina and left in place for about 10 to 15 minutes at a time, three times a week or every other day.

Difficulty reaching orgasm

Unless cancer surgery involves removal of the clitoris or the lower vagina or dam-

---

QUESTION & ANSWER

Q: **What is vaginismus?**

A: Painful intercourse, whether caused by vaginal dryness, vaginal stenosis or a shortened vagina, can sometimes trigger a condition called vaginismus. The muscles around the vaginal opening become clenched in a spasm. With vaginismus, a woman's partner can't enter the vagina with his penis. The harder he pushes, the greater her pain becomes.

Kegel Exercises

Kegel exercises can help you learn how to tense and relax your pelvic floor muscles, which may help lessen discomfort during intercourse. To do Kegel exercises, contract the muscles you use to stop urine flow, hold for a count of three, and then relax. Repeat 10 to 20 times, a couple of times a day. If you're feeling pain during intercourse, stop and take a moment to relax your pelvic floor muscles.

ages the pelvic nerves, you should still be able to achieve orgasm after cancer treatment. Almost all women who are able to reach orgasm before treatment continue to do so afterward.

However, after cancer treatment, you may find that the steps necessary for you to become sexually aroused have changed. For instance, if a part of foreplay was stroking sensitive areas that have since been affected by cancer treatment, you may need to find new areas that provoke sexual arousal when touched.

To help yourself reach orgasm:

- Communicate with your partner. Make sure your partner knows which types of touch really excite you.
- Tense and relax your vaginal muscles in rhythm with your breathing. This may help you focus on what you're feeling.
- Try a hand-held vibrator to stimulate increased blood flow to your genital area, helping to elicit arousal.
- Have a sexual fantasy during lovemaking. It may distract you from negative thoughts.

Decreased interest in sex

Just as cancer treatment causes physical changes, it often packs an emotional wal-

lop, too. You may experience several different feelings after cancer treatment or, perhaps, just a few.

A common problem following cancer treatment is loss of desire for sexual activity (libido). You may lose interest in sex for many reasons. It may be because of all the changes you're going through. You may be recovering from surgery, radiation therapy or chemotherapy, and perhaps you're tired or you don't feel well. Chemotherapy and other medications can disrupt your hormone balance, reducing your sex drive.

You may be fearful, anxious or depressed. These are common responses to a life-threatening illness. Many people find that their fears decrease with time and their libidos improve. But for some, the emotional distress becomes overwhelming and medical intervention becomes necessary. To further complicate things, some medications used to treat depression and anxiety can interfere with your sex drive.

You may also have concerns about how your body has been altered by cancer treatment and whether your partner still finds you sexually desirable.

Women who have a mastectomy for breast cancer are particularly vulnerable

LIVING WITH CANCER

QUESTION & ANSWER

Q: I've heard that testosterone may increase a woman's libido. Is this true?

A: Evidence suggests that decreased sexual desire in women may be related to lowered concentrations of the hormone testosterone. Yes, women's bodies do normally produce small concentrations of this male-associated hormone. After menopause, the levels are reduced.

The administration of testosterone has been studied as a potential treatment for decreased libido, but only to a small degree. Ongoing studies are investigating the use of testosterone in women with a history of cancer and whether its use has any potential toxicities or other unwanted side effects.

to this problem. For both women and men, the breast represents a significant aspect of sexuality. Removing an entire breast (mastectomy) or changing its look and feel (lumpectomy) can alter a woman's perception of herself as a sexual being. According to some researchers, mastectomy leads to more post-cancer sexual problems than do many other treatments.

If you have a loss of interest in sex, and if it concerns you, try these suggestions:

Talk with your partner

One of the best ways to improve sexual intimacy is to open the lines of communication. For example, your partner may think you've lost interest. You may believe your partner isn't interested in you. A conversation about the issue can clear the air and restore emotional and physical intimacy. Begin by telling your partner how you feel about your sex life and what you would like to change. Explain why you think your sex life is the way it is and how it makes you feel. Avoid blame, and try to stay positive.

Set aside time for romance

When you're ready, make a date with your partner. Create a sensual mood using lighting, music and fragrance. Go slowly at first, focusing on foreplay. Slowly reacquaint yourself with your partner. Sometimes agreeing not to include intercourse can help you relax and focus on pleasurable activities.

Focus on new ways to make yourself feel sensual and attractive. Try a new haircut or color. Buy some beautiful new pajamas or a nightgown to help you feel more desirable.

Talk with your doctor

Sexual problems may not improve on their own. If your doctor or another member of your health care team hasn't discussed sexual issues with you, take the lead. Your doctor can help determine if you need a referral to a specialist or, perhaps, suggest new ways to express sexual intimacy. If you're going to discuss your sex drive with your doctor, you might want your partner to attend the appointment, too. Having your partner with you will ensure that both of you receive the same information.

Osteoporosis

As more women survive cancer, the long-term effects of cancer treatment on bone health are becoming more apparent.

Osteoporosis is a condition in which your bones become brittle and weak, leading to an increased risk of fractures. Women who've been treated for cancer are at increased risk of osteoporosis for several reasons. Some chemotherapy drugs inhibit bone formation. And medications used to control some of the side effects of chemotherapy, such as steroids, can lead to bone loss. In some cases, the cancer itself may cause bone loss.

Cancer treatment can also have indirect effects on bone loss. Surgical removal of the ovaries — often a part of treatment for gynecologic cancers — initiates immediate menopause. Chemotherapy and radiation therapy for cancer also can cause the ovaries to stop functioning. During the first few years after this occurs, you lose calcium from your bones at a much faster rate than normal, increasing your risk of osteoporosis.

Prevention and treatment

Several options are available for preventing and treating osteoporosis.

Calcium and vitamin D
Two of the most straightforward, highly recommended strategies are to get adequate calcium and vitamin D and to take part in weight-bearing exercises. Women at risk of osteoporosis should aim for 1,500 to 2,000 milligrams a day of calcium and 400 to 800 international units of vitamin D. The calcium and vitamin D can be from food sources or from supplements.

Exercise
Weight-bearing exercise can be as simple as walking and jogging. Non-weight-bearing activities, such as swimming, are helpful for general fitness, but they're not adequate for maintaining bone strength.

Estrogen
Estrogen therapy has been shown to be useful in preventing bone loss. However, given concerns about its use in women who've survived breast cancer and some gynecologic cancers, other options are more frequently recommended for these women.

Raloxifene
Raloxifene (Evista), a medication somewhat similar to the cancer drug tamoxifen, is taken to help maintain bone strength. It may also decrease breast cancer risk. However, there's some concern about prescribing raloxifene for women who've already taken tamoxifen for five years. Therefore, raloxifene generally isn't recommended for breast cancer survivors who've had tamoxifen. Raloxifene also may cause hot flashes.

Bisphosphonates
Medications known as bisphosphonates also can help preserve bone strength. These drugs appear to be as effective as estrogen in terms of promoting bone

health. Bisphosphonates currently on the market include alendronate (Fosamax) and risedronate (Actonel). You take these medications as a pill, either once a day or once a week in a larger dose. Bisphosphonates can cause heartburn, so it's best to take them first thing in the morning, on an empty stomach. Be sure to avoid lying down for at least 30 minutes afterward to avoid acid reflux into the esophagus.

Another form of bisphosphonate, zoledronic acid (Zometa), is an intravenous medication, meaning it's administered by way of a vein. New evidence suggests that receiving intravenous doses of this drug at three-, six- or 12-month intervals may help maintain bone strength. Debate is still ongoing as to which dosing interval is the most appropriate.

Calcitonin

Calcitonin, an intranasal medication taken as an inhalant, is another option for treating osteoporosis, but it's not as effective as bisphosphonates.

Post-Chemotherapy Rheumatism

Some women who undergo chemotherapy as part of treatment for their cancers develop pain and stiffness in their muscles and joints, typically one to two months after completing treatment. This condition, which appears to be induced by chemotherapy medications, is called post-chemotherapy rheumatism.

Doctors estimate the condition may affect up to 5 percent of women who receive a combination of chemotherapy medications.

The most common complaint of post-chemotherapy rheumatism is stiffness in the morning or after periods of inactivity. The hips and knees are most often affected. In most cases, symptoms of post-chemotherapy rheumatism go away without treatment, usually within six to 12 months. Researchers theorize that the condition may be a type of withdrawal from chemotherapy. Many questions about this condition remain unanswered.

Over-the-counter pain relievers haven't been found to provide much relief for this condition. But there are some things you can do that might help. If you're experiencing musculoskeletal pain after cancer treatment:

- **Relax.** These pains don't mean that your cancer has recurred. They'll probably disappear within a matter of months.
- **Adjust your position.** Avoid long periods of sitting. If you must sit for a long time, reposition yourself often to prevent or lessen stiffness. Turn your head at different angles, shift the position of your arms, and bend and stretch your legs. These slight movements may help prevent excessive stiffness. If you're able, get up and walk from time to time.

Weight Gain

Some cancer survivors who've received chemotherapy drugs or taken certain hormone medications have problems with weight gain. Unfortunately, in many cases, the extra weight stays on even when treatment ends. If you've been treated for breast cancer with certain kinds of chemotherapy medications, you may lose muscle tissue in addition to gaining fat.

Some studies suggest that weight gain is greater among premenopausal women treated for breast cancer than among women who've already gone through menopause. This could be because chemotherapy causes premature menopause in younger women, and menopause often is accompanied by weight gain. Women who were post-menopausal when treated for cancer may have already gained the weight associated with the onset of menopause.

Reducing your risk

Most doctors point to exercise as the best way to prevent or minimize weight gain after cancer treatment. In addition to helping you lose weight, exercise helps reduce fatigue, insomnia and anxiety, all of which can be consequences of cancer diagnosis and treatment.

If you've lost muscle and gained fatty tissue in your arms and shoulders, you may find strength training exercises for your upper body to be helpful. Strength training exercises for your legs may be helpful, too.

If you've gained weight as a result of cancer treatment:

• Talk with your doctor about starting an exercise regimen that includes both aerobic exercise and strength training.

• Talk with a dietitian who can help you plan a healthy diet that won't add extra pounds.

Chronic Diarrhea

Chronic diarrhea occurs in some women who receive radiation treatments to the pelvis or abdomen. Radiation therapy can disrupt the normal lining of the bowel, causing a condition called radiation enteritis. Diarrhea associated with radiation enteritis may begin the third or fourth week after starting radiation therapy, and it typically ends two to four weeks after the last treatment. In some cases, the problem doesn't go away. It may continue for months or years after treatment ends.

Diarrhea is also sometimes a side effect of chemotherapy. The problem almost always improves once chemotherapy treatment is complete.

Treatment

Several medications are available for treating diarrhea. These include the over-the-counter medications loperamide (Imodium, Kaopectate, others) and diphenoxylate and atropine (Lofene, Lomotil, others) and prescription narcotics (opiates) such as paregoric. If necessary, these medications can be taken regularly to treat chronic diarrhea.

Anti-diarrheal medications provide relief by reducing muscle contractions in your gastrointestinal tract, slowing the transition time through your digestive system and allowing more time for absorption. For especially stubborn or severe cases of diarrhea, a prescription drug called octreotide (Sandostatin) may help. This drug must be injected under your skin, like insulin.

LIVING WITH CANCER

Avoiding some foods and focusing on others also may reduce diarrhea. Trial and error is important in determining what works for you. Some options to try:

- Limit the high-fiber foods in your diet. These include bran, whole-grain products, cooked fruits or vegetables with skins or seeds (corn, tomatoes, berries), dried fruits, dried peas and beans, raw fruits and vegetables (except bananas), nuts, popcorn, coconut, and seeds.
- Include more bland, low-fiber foods in your diet. These include white or light rye bread, refined cereals, white rice and pasta, potatoes, eggs, mild cheese, bananas, canned or cooked fruits and vegetables without skins or seeds (pears, peaches, green beans, carrots, squash), and tender meat, poultry and fish.
- Avoid greasy, fried, fatty and spicy foods.
- Avoid caffeine.
- Avoid milk products for two or three days if they seem to be contributing to your diarrhea. If you don't notice an improvement, resume using them. If milk products seem to aggravate your diarrhea, you might be lactose intolerant. Talk with your doctor. There are ways to manage this condition.
- Don't drink alcohol.

You might also try eating smaller, more frequent meals rather than two or three large ones. This puts less strain on your digestive system but still allows for adequate food intake.

Make sure that you drink plenty of fluids to replace those body fluids lost to diarrhea. Water and sports drinks are good choices.

Cognitive Changes

Some people treated for cancer report having problems with memory or concentration after chemotherapy or radiation. Studies suggest that people who've been treated with chemotherapy are at greater risk of having these problems. Higher doses of chemotherapy seem to lead to greater problems. However, even people who receive standard doses report memory or concentration difficulties. This problem has been labeled by some as "chemo brain."

It's important to note that this condition isn't prevalent. Many women who receive chemotherapy don't report cognitive changes following their treatment, and they continue to very effectively perform complex mental tasks.

The exact cause of cognitive changes and the degree to which they affect people aren't clear. Presently, most cancer experts don't consider chemo brain to be a proven side effect of chemotherapy. Researchers hope that within a few years — when results of current research become available — they'll have a better understanding of the situation.

Individuals who talk about the cognitive effects of cancer treatment tend to describe a blunting of mental sharpness, fuzziness in dealing with numbers, trouble finding the right word and short-term memory lapses. Some people report changes in memory or concentration beginning sometime during cancer treatment. Others report troubles sometime after treatment ends.

Currently, there are no proven ways to prevent or decrease cognitive changes thought to result from chemotherapy. Research is ongoing to test medications that may be useful. In the meantime, here are some things you can do to help manage the situation:

- Use a notebook or pocket calendar to help keep yourself organized. For each task, jot a quick note about what you need to do or where you need to go.
- Check your math with a calculator.
- Use a couple of reminder signs around the house to jog your memory about tasks that you tend to forget.
- Learn relaxation skills so that you can remain calm in stressful moments. Controlling stress may help improve your memory and concentration.
- If you're thinking through a problem or planning something, run your ideas by another person for feedback.
- Talk to your doctor if you suspect that your medications may be causing or contributing to your cognitive problems.

Support Groups

In the days and weeks after completing cancer treatment, you may feel as if you're suddenly all alone in the world. You may miss the emotional support you received from your health care team. Friends and family can help fill the void, but sometimes only fellow cancer survivors — people who've been there — can give you specifically what you need at this point.

Cancer support groups bring together people who've had cancer. Participants talk about their own experiences, feelings

A Tough Transition

Some people have difficulty making the transition from cancer treatment to cancer monitoring.

During your treatment, you may feel a sense of comfort in knowing that active steps are being taken to kill the cancer and that you're being checked frequently. When treatment stops, that comfort may be replaced by worry — now that "nothing is being done," will the cancer come back? This uncertainty can be difficult to accept.

In addition, during treatment, relationships with friends and family often center on your illness. Learning to refocus those relationships on the future requires a new way of thinking.

You may also find that many of the old stigmas associated with cancer still exist. You may have to remind friends and co-workers that cancer isn't contagious and that research shows cancer survivors are just as productive as other workers.

Adjusting to life after cancer treatment means moving past old fears and uncertainties. But it may also mean facing new ones. As you and others adapt to these changes, you may begin to feel completely recovered. If you feel that you need help making this transition, don't be afraid to seek help from a mental health professional, such as a psychologist or a counselor.

and concerns, they listen to the concerns of others, and they exchange practical information about how to deal with the challenges of life after cancer.

Cancer support groups can offer a variety of benefits. Simply by meeting others who've faced cancer, you may feel less isolated and gain a sense of belonging. Frank discussions can foster openness and better understanding. Shared problem-solving may help you find solutions or coping skills. And compassion and empathy can help see you through a crisis. You also may feel better about yourself by offering support and help to others.

Is a support group right for you?

It's certainly not mandatory that you join a support group. Not everyone wants or needs group support beyond family and friends. For some people, hearing other people's cancer stories makes them more anxious. But others find it helpful to turn to individuals outside their immediate circles of family and friends for help.

If you're uncertain if a support group is for you, consider these questions from the National Cancer Institute. If you answer no to most of them, a cancer support group may not be a good option for you.

- Do you enjoy being part of a group?
- Are you ready to talk about your feelings with people you don't know well?
- Do you want to hear others' stories about cancer?
- Would you like the advice of others who've gone through cancer treatment?
- Do you have helpful hints or advice to offer to other cancer survivors?

Fear of Recurrence

One of the most common fears among cancer survivors is that the cancer will come back and that the next time there may not be a cure. This fear may become more tangible at certain times, such as when a doctor's appointment is approaching, when you feel various aches or pains, on anniversary dates of your diagnosis, or when a family member or friend becomes ill.

Although it's true that cancer can recur after treatment, it's also true that many women never experience a recurrence. Thus, the challenge lies in living with uncertainty. In a world that emphasizes facts and knowledge, living with uncer-

tainty can be particularly difficult. Despite certain clues about the general outcome of a particular cancer, it's impossible to be certain of the future. Therefore, women and their doctors must learn to live with some degree of uncertainty.

Some anxiety about recurrence is healthy in the sense that it prompts you to respond to unusual signs and symptoms. As time goes on, fear of recurrence generally tends to fade, although it may never go away entirely.

Being continuously anxious about whether your cancer will come back isn't healthy. It can rob you of time that might be spent in a more worthwhile manner, such as focusing on work or family or

- Would reaching out to support other cancer survivors help you feel better?
- Can you work with people who have different approaches to cancer issues?
- Do you want to learn more about cancer and post-treatment issues?

Choosing a support group

In general, cancer support groups fall into two main categories: those led by a health professional, such as a nurse, social worker or psychologist, and those led by cancer survivors, often called peer groups or self-help groups. Some cancer support groups are for people with a specific type of cancer. Others are open to anyone who has been treated for cancer. Still others are open to cancer survivors and their family members.

Some groups are designed to be more educational and structured. They may invite a doctor to give a talk on a new cancer treatment. Others put more emphasis on emotional support and shared experience.

The key is finding a group that matches your needs and personality. You may find that you prefer a structured, moderated group that provides organized discussions and educational information. A moderator or facilitator can help ensure that all of the participants have an equal opportunity to share if they wish to and that the discussions stay on track.

Or you may prefer a group with less structure. You may feel more comfortable meeting with a small group of people at someone's home, where emotional support is the focus.

simply enjoying life. Sharing your fears and concerns with a caring family member or friend is often an effective means of dispelling these fears. Seeking the help of a licensed therapist, counselor or professional support group also can be helpful in terms of learning to control your fears and putting them in proper perspective.

One thing that many women discover as they learn to live with uncertainty is that their own feelings may be inconsistent or contradictory. For example, you may feel that you're a strong person but at the same time worry that you can't handle your cancer alone. One part of you is ready to fight, and another struggles to maintain hope.

Part of coping with uncertainty is learning to accept these paradoxes and letting go of preconceived notions of how things need to be. One study focused on 10 women who had gone through treatment for cancer. Some had had early-stage cancer, others more advanced cancer. Learning to live with uncertainty was one of the major adjustment phases the women experienced. Letting go was a big part of entering this phase. To some, letting go meant giving up control over life and death. To others, letting go of their old selves helped them adjust to their new reality. Still others used humor to let go of emotional tension, to connect with others and to put the cancer into perspective.

In addition to traditional support groups, the Internet offers online support communities. But be aware that the health information you get from online support groups may be inaccurate and even potentially harmful. Look for a group affiliated with a reputable organization or hosted by an expert.

If you decide to take part in a group, try it out. If you don't find the group useful or comfortable, you don't have to continue attending.

Making the Transition to Supportive Care

When cancer reaches an advanced stage, there comes a time when many women decide they no longer want to continue treatment to fight the cancer. Perhaps you're facing such a decision.

The decision to stop treatment aimed at killing the cancer (anti-cancer therapy) is generally considered after a woman and her doctor have discussed all remaining options, and they have determined that:

- No treatment will cure the cancer
- There's little chance any further surgery, chemotherapy or radiation therapy will change the course of the cancer
- There isn't any good evidence that continued efforts to kill the cancer will result in longer survival or better quality of life

- All evidence suggests that any positive response from continued treatment will be short-lived
- The side effects from anti-cancer treatment are significant

If this is your situation, your decision to stop cancer-killing treatments is both a logical and understandable one. The goal of treatment at this stage of your disease is to enable you to live as well as possible for as long as possible. With advanced cancer, there often comes a time when anti-cancer therapy doesn't help you achieve this goal. It's also important to remember that just because you're stopping treatment aimed at fighting the cancer doesn't mean you're ending your medical care. You'll continue to receive care from your doctor, including medications to relieve pain and other symptoms.

Accepting Your Situation

In the beginning, right after you've received a diagnosis, the emphasis of treatment typically is on curing the cancer. If the cancer isn't curable, treatments are used to slow the growth of the tumor in an attempt to allow you to live longer. When efforts to slow cancer growth are no longer effective, the emphasis shifts to alleviating discomfort and other symptoms. This is known as supportive (palliative) care. Supportive care also includes addressing any of your psychological, social, spiritual and emotional needs, as well as providing support for your family.

How do you know when the time has come to stop fighting the cancer? It's a

'How Much Time Do I Have Left?'

Many people with a terminal illness want their doctors to tell them how much time they have left. This is a hard question for doctors to answer, and many may be reluctant to respond to it directly. For one thing, they can make only an educated guess. For another, answering the question requires a difficult balance between being realistic and hoping for the best.

Because doctors can't help becoming personally connected to their patients and their patients' families, they may overestimate prognosis in order to main-

tain hope. This could mean you may not have as much time as your doctor says you do.

Independent of trying to maintain hope, a doctor may simply be wrong in his or her estimate of the manner and speed in which the cancer will progress. In one study, involving men with prostate cancer, doctors were asked to estimate survival times for the people in the study. For one of the groups, the doctors' estimated life expectancy was 13 to 18 months. In reality, the average survival was only 5.3 months. So if your doctor does give you an estimate, don't take it as gospel. Some people live longer than their doctors thought they would. Others live less time than anticipated.

difficult decision to make. It's a personal decision that only you can make with advice from your health care team, family and friends. Some women find it difficult to end treatment aimed at destroying or controlling the cancer because it feels like they're giving up. But if the cancer has become resistant to anti-cancer therapies, such treatments may do more harm than good. For many women, the quality of their lives becomes paramount because they want to enjoy the time they have left.

The time when you may fare better without anti-cancer therapy arrives when the therapy stops working and the downsides of continuing it outweigh the potential benefits. For example, for many people with cancer, there eventually comes a time when the chances that chemotherapy will make them sick — and maybe cause

potentially life-threatening side effects — may be far greater than the chances of it shrinking the cancer.

Deciding to stop treatment that's no longer helping you may be a way for you to take back control. You may feel as if your life has been out of control since you learned that you have cancer. Making the decision to stop cancer treatment and to be free of the side effects of treatment can be a powerful step in taking charge of your life.

Maintaining Hope

Even as you accept that your cancer isn't curable, you can still have hope. But hope changes as circumstances change. For example, when you first received your

---

Estimated and actual length of survival

Number of patients	Estimated length of survival, per doctor	Actual average length of survival
31	Less than 6 months	3.9 months
59	7-12 months	4.4 months
26	13-18 months	5.3 months
36	19-34 months	19.0 months

If your illness is terminal and you ask your doctor how much time you have left, keep in mind that he or she can only make an educated guess. As indicated by the estimates in this chart, doctors tend to overestimate how long individuals with advanced cancer will survive.

Source: Michael J. Fisch, et al., *Journal of Clinical Oncology*, 21:10 (2003), pages 1937-1943

Having a time frame may help you feel more in control. But no matter how much time you think, or your doctor thinks, that you have left, you have an

opportunity to make the best of that time. Try to live each day as fully as possible, doing the things you want to do.

Denying Impending Death

Some people with advanced cancer find it difficult, if not impossible, to accept that their treatments are no longer working and that their cancers are terminal. They may employ a defense mechanism known as denial.

Denial may be either harmful or beneficial. It's beneficial when it enables you to process information about your illness in your own time and in such a way that you can absorb it without being overwhelmed. But continued denial can cause you to insist on receiving anti-cancer treatments when it's clear they're no longer beneficial, and more importantly, it can keep you from getting your affairs in order, saying your goodbyes and, ultimately, dying a peaceful death. Denial can be especially problematic if your family can't accept your illness and encourages or reinforces your denial.

If you're having a difficult time accepting that your cancer is terminal, it may help you to talk with a counselor, chaplain, hospice worker or member of your health care team. An opportunity to express your fears, which can contribute to denial, may help you approach your illness more realistically so that you can make informed decisions regarding your future.

diagnosis, you may have hoped that it was a mistake. Once you accepted the diagnosis, you undoubtedly hoped to beat the cancer. When you learned the cancer wasn't curable, you may have hoped that your treatment would work well enough to extend your life for several years.

So what do you hope for now that you realize further attempts at controlling the cancer are likely to fail? That depends on your goals. This may be a time to reframe your hopes. They may include spending quality time with family, taking a trip, relieving your symptoms or living in comfort, without pain and suffering. Perhaps your hope centers on leaving a legacy for your children or grandchildren. This might involve putting your financial affairs in order, videotaping or writing family stories, or creating a document in which you write about your values, the lessons you've learned from life and your love for family and friends.

Keep in mind, though, as you set your goals, that cancer's path can be difficult to predict. The course of your cancer can change abruptly, and it may not be possible for you to meet all the goals you've set. Some people think of it this way: Hope for the best while you plan for the worst. Make time to take care of responsibilities and essentials. Sign papers you need to sign, tell friends and loved ones what you want to say to them, and write down whatever thoughts you need to express in writing.

It's fine to have some longer term projects on your list of goals, but you may also want to be sure that you have a goal for every day, such as reaching out to friends and family or writing notes to people who have touched your life.

Keep in mind that some of your loved ones will feel a strong need to express their feelings at this time, and others won't feel capable of that. This can be a beautiful time of sharing, and you are the one with the most control over this opportunity. When you're ready, you and loved ones can share many simple but important words: "I love you," "I forgive you," "I'm sorry," "Thank you" and — when the time is appropriate — "Goodbye."

When You and Your Family Disagree

Your illness affects your entire family. When you make the transition from anti-cancer treatment to supportive care, your family members may not understand. They may say that you're giving up. Maybe it's your spouse or your children or a relative who comes from out of town who hasn't been involved with your illness and treatment who wants you to "keep fighting."

Throughout your illness, you have experienced many losses. Although difficult, each loss may have caused you to establish new goals and to redefine hope. These losses, in some ways, prepare you for death. While your family members have experienced some degree of loss, too, it's different from your own. They may not be ready to let you go.

As you face the last phase of your illness, the support you receive from family and friends can influence how well you

cope. If your goals are at odds with those of family members, arrange a meeting with them and members of your health care team. Ask someone from your health care team to explain your situation so that your family understands the basis for your decision and to answer questions family members may have.

Be firm in your resolve to do what's best for you. Don't be pressured to accept treatment just to keep the peace. That may do you more harm than good. Tell your loved ones that what's most important to you now is being able to enjoy high-quality time with them.

Managing Signs and Symptoms

It's natural for people with incurable cancer to fear pain and other symptoms the disease may cause. Once you stop treatment intended to kill or slow the cancer, that doesn't mean your care will end. Your health care team will still take care of you, helping you manage your symptoms and other conditions that may arise. The goal is to help you live as comfortably as possible. Many approaches can be used to manage symptoms and conditions that may develop. Depending on your situation, your primary care doctor or oncologist may enlist the help of an individual who specializes in supportive care.

Pain

Pain can be a major factor in your ability to enjoy life, affecting your sleeping, eating and other day-to-day activities. For people with advanced cancer, pain is usually caused by the cancer spreading into organs, bone or soft tissue or by the cancer pressing on a nerve. Pain that involves an organ may be difficult to pinpoint and may be described as a dull, deep throbbing or aching or, occasionally, as sharp. Pain that involves skin, muscle or bone is usually limited to a specific area and may be described as sharp, aching, burning or throbbing. Pain that involves nerves (neuropathic pain) is often described as sharp, tingling, burning or shooting.

Pain may be severe but last a relatively short time (acute pain), or it may range from mild to severe and persist for a long time (chronic pain). Certain pain may also be associated with specific movements or activities and may be predictable (incident pain). There's also a type of pain known as breakthrough pain. It occurs when moderate to severe pain "breaks through" the medication that's controlling it. Breakthrough pain usually lasts a short time but may occur up to several times a day.

Seeing your doctor

Many medications can effectively manage pain, but your doctor needs to know the specifics of your pain to be able to treat it. To help your doctor assess your pain, provide him or her with as much information as possible, including the answers to the following questions:

- Where do you feel the pain?
- When did it start?
- What were you doing when it started?
- How does it feel — sharp, tingling, burning, aching, throbbing, shooting?

Pain scale

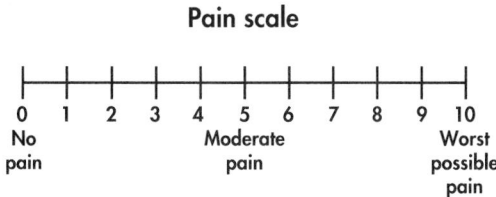

Using a pain scale can help your doctor determine how much pain you're in and measure how well your treatments are working. You rate your pain from 0 to 10. A rating of 1 to 3 generally means mild pain, while 7 or above indicates severe pain.

- Has it changed over time?
- On a scale of 0 to 10 — with 0 being no pain and 10 being worst possible pain — how bad is your pain?
- What, if anything, makes the pain better or worse?
- Have any of the medications you've taken had an effect on the pain?

It might help to keep a written record of your pain so that you can give your doctor an accurate report. Besides answering the questions above, keep track of your pain medication and the effect it has on your pain, and for how long. Let your doctor know if the medication is causing unwanted side effects, such as interfering with your activities or your ability to sleep or eat.

To assess your pain, your doctor will perform a physical examination and may request some tests, such as blood tests or X-rays, to determine the cause of the pain.

Treatment

The primary treatment for cancer pain is to treat the cause of the pain, if possible. This may include things such as radiation, surgery, chemotherapy and targeted medication. With advanced cancer, though, it's not always possible to treat the specific cause. Then treatment typically involves use of analgesic pain medications, which range from simple pain relievers to narcotics (opioids).

Simple pain relievers include acetaminophen (Tylenol, others) and nonsteroidal anti-inflammatory drugs (NSAIDs), such as aspirin and ibuprofen (Advil, Motrin,

others). Steroid medications also may be helpful in a few situations. Opioids, the strongest pain-relieving medications, include codeine, oxycodone (OxyContin, Roxicodone, others), morphine, fentanyl (Duragesic) and hydromorphone (Dilaudid), among others. For severe pain, opioids are the best medications. Sometimes, regular doses of aspirin, acetaminophen or ibuprofen may be

What About Addiction?

Studies have shown that many people with cancer are reluctant to take strong pain medications, such as narcotics (opioids), for two reasons. They're afraid of becoming addicted to the medications, and they're afraid that if they use strong medication too early in the course of their disease, it won't work for them later when their pain becomes more severe. These fears are understandable, but neither of them has a medical basis.

Addiction is a type of behavior where a person compulsively seeks drugs for the mental high they might provide. When opioid medications are used to treat cancer pain, addiction to the drugs is extremely rare.

For people who take opioids for a long time, though, it's common for them to develop tolerance to a drug. With tolerance, the effects of the drug decrease with regular use, and the person taking the drug may need higher doses to achieve the same effect. Fortunately, doses of these drugs can be increased. There's no so-called

ceiling effect. Therefore, if you become tolerant of a certain dose, your doctor can increase the dose until your pain is relieved.

In addition, your body may become used to receiving the drug at regular intervals, a condition called physical dependence. If you stop taking it abruptly, you may experience withdrawal. Withdrawal can be avoided by slowly tapering off the drug if it's no longer needed. It's important to know that tolerance and physical dependence are not the same as addiction.

Tell your doctor about any problems with pain medication you've had in the past. Follow directions for taking your medication. And let your doctor know if it isn't providing enough relief.

Pain management is vital to maintaining a good quality of life. Work with your doctor to find the medication or combination of medications that provides relief. And don't let fear of addiction keep you from taking opioids. If you aren't getting relief from your pain, ask your doctor to refer you to a pain specialist.

recommended in addition to an opioid medication to boost pain relief.

Opioids can be either long-acting or short-acting, referring to the period of time that they remain active in your system. Generally speaking, short-acting agents take effect quickly — within 30 minutes — and provide relief for two to four hours. Long-acting oral narcotics may take several hours to reach peak effectiveness, but their effects generally continue for about 12 hours.

For some people on long-acting opioids, intermittent short-acting opioids can help relieve breakthrough pain that arises between scheduled doses of the long-acting drug. If you're experiencing breakthrough pain, a rapid-onset, short-acting opioid in addition to your long-acting medication should give you relief. If you know from experience that a particular motion or activity triggers the pain, taking a short-acting opioid beforehand may block or significantly diminish the pain.

If you have continued pain, it's best to keep the pain under control by taking your pain medication at regular intervals rather than intermittently or as needed. This is especially true for the strong opioids. Steady dosing may diminish the side effects of the medication. Taking your medications on a regular schedule also provides better and more even pain control, and you actually may end up needing less medication than if you take the drugs intermittently.

Opioid medications may be given orally, by way of patches placed on the skin, by rectal suppositories or by injection.

Another method of receiving medication is by way of a pain pump. A pain pump can be implanted under the skin of your lower abdomen with a small tube placed in the spinal canal next to the spinal cord. The pump delivers a steady stream of medication to your spinal cord. Your doctor may suggest this method if you have severe pain that isn't controlled well with regular opioids or if you're experiencing excessive side effects from the medication that can't be controlled.

Opioid medications may cause side effects such as drowsiness, dizziness, nausea and confusion. Most side effects are easily managed and, with steady dosing, often diminish after a few days. One of the most common side effects is constipation. This occurs in almost all individuals who take these medications on a regular basis. Generally, only with appropriate treatment, does the condition improve. Your doctor will likely start you on a regimen of stool softeners or bowel stimulants or both, as soon as you begin taking an opioid. It's far easier to prevent constipation than to treat it.

Other medications may be useful for specific types of pain. Anti-seizure drugs or other related medications may be helpful in individuals who have nerve damage. Medications called bisphosphonates that are used to treat osteoporosis may be helpful if you're experiencing pain from bone damage. Your doctor also may suggest other means of pain control, such as nerve blocks by injections of chemicals or radiation therapy to a localized area of pain.

If you find the side effects of a drug intolerable, if your medication isn't working well enough or long enough, or if you

Controlling Pain Through Relaxation

Stress and anxiety can make your pain worse by creating tension in your body. Techniques designed to help relieve anxiety and help you relax may also help control pain. These include deep-breathing exercises, meditation, progressive relaxation and guided imagery. See Chapter 33 for more information on relaxation techniques.

In addition, try to get your mind off your pain by doing activities that you enjoy, such as listening to music or engaging in a hobby. If you're able, exercise may make you feel better and help you relax and sleep. Try to get some exercise daily, even if you only feel well enough to walk for a few minutes on the arm of a family member or friend.

have frequent breakthrough pain, you may need to try another medication or other pain control methods.

Shortness of breath

Another condition that can occur is shortness of breath (dyspnea). It has multiple causes, including cancer spreading to the lungs, heart problems, muscle weakness, anemia and generalized fatigue. Often, the underlying cause of shortness of breath is treatable. To determine the cause of this condition and how best to treat it, your doctor will likely perform a physical exam and request some tests, such as a chest X-ray, blood tests or heart tests.

If the cause can't be determined or if your doctor can't treat the underlying cause, he or she will try to relieve the discomfort of shortness of breath. Having oxygen or cool air blown across your face may be helpful. Opioid medications, such as morphine, also provide relief by blunting the sensation of being short of breath. An inhaler or nebulizer that emits medication also may provide relief.

Appetite changes and weight loss

With advanced cancer, you may find your appetite diminishing and your weight dropping. With ovarian cancer, progressive accumulation of abdominal fluid (ascites) or a bowel obstruction may interfere with your ability to eat. Your loved ones may be disturbed by your inability to eat, perhaps because of the cultural value people place on food, equating a hearty appetite with good health. There's no evidence that a person with advanced cancer will live any longer if he or she eats more. Pressuring someone to eat can cause stress and nausea, which is an unnecessary burden if he or she is already experiencing the effects of advanced cancer.

If you're bothered by your loss of appetite, try these methods to possibly stimulate appetite:

- Eat small meals more often, rather than three large meals a day.
- Eat more in the morning than in the evening, because your appetite is likely to diminish as you get tired.

LIVING WITH CANCER

- Avoid cooking smells, especially if you're nauseated.
- Try to eat foods that are cold or at room temperature because you may find them more palatable than hot foods.
- Try nutrition supplements, such as the beverages Ensure, Boost and Carnation Instant Breakfast.

In addition to trying these self-help tips, you might want to talk with your doctor about a prescription appetite stimulant. Perhaps the most widely prescribed and best studied is megestrol acetate (Megace). This drug also has an anti-nausea effect. And it's less likely to cause side effects than are corticosteroid medications, which are also used to stimulate appetite in people with advanced cancer.

Nausea and vomiting

Loss of appetite and weight may be related to nausea and vomiting. Nausea and vomiting can result from many causes, such as spread of the cancer to the liver, interference with normal digestive functioning due to cancer spread to the intestines, and use of pain medications. Eating only those foods that appeal to you and eating frequent, smaller meals instead of three large ones may help. Anti-nausea medications may help to some degree. Those commonly prescribed to stimulate appetite (megestrol acetate and corticosteroids) also may help to decrease nausea and vomiting. Some people find patches for motion sickness that contain the medication scopolamine to be helpful.

If you experienced nausea and vomiting while receiving chemotherapy, you may have gotten relief from drugs designed to treat chemotherapy-induced nausea and vomiting. But these same drugs don't appear to work as well when nausea and vomiting are caused by advanced cancer rather than chemotherapy.

Leg swelling

Swollen legs can occur in people with advanced cancer. This condition has many possible causes. Some causes, such as blood clots, may be treated, and the swelling will go down. Others, such as water retention, may be treated with prescription water pills (diuretics) to help your kidneys make more urine to get rid of some of the fluid. However, the frequent need to urinate can be bothersome. Limiting intake of salt also may help reduce the problem. Salt encourages body tissues to retain water. Keeping your legs elevated while resting — allowing gravity to help — is often the best way to decrease leg swelling. You might also want to try using compression stockings.

Hospice Care

Hospice is the term used to describe special programs in which a group of individuals — the hospice team — works together to provide optimal supportive care for terminally ill individuals and their families. The hospice team usually includes doctors, nurses, pharmacists, social workers, therapists, chaplains, volunteers and others. Hospice programs strive to enhance quality of life, while neither delaying nor hastening the dying process.

For some people, hospice care means the end of hope. Although it's true that hospice care begins only after hope of a cure is gone, the goal of hospice is to help you live well during the time you have remaining and to help you die with peace and dignity.

Hospice programs are designed to give round-the-clock support to terminally ill people and their families. The hospice team works with you and your loved ones, adjusting the services provided according to your needs and those of your family. Physical, social, spiritual and emotional needs are addressed throughout the last stages of illness and during the period of bereavement that follows a death.

Most hospice care is provided at home, but it may be provided in nursing homes and other residential settings. A few hospice programs have their own hospital or clinic facilities. In a home setting, although nurses and other members of the hospice team make visits as needed, the program is designed so that the person who's dying receives much of his or her care from loved ones, who can get advice and support from the hospice team whenever they need it.

Services offered

Hospice programs provide comprehensive services, including management of symptoms, emotional support for you and your family, and spiritual care. Emotional (psychosocial) support is intended to help you and your family members deal with issues or problems you or they may be facing, such as depression, anxiety and fear. The intent of spiritual care is to help

you maintain hope and address any questions you may have, perhaps about the meaning of your life.

Depending on the individual, hospice services may include:

- Medical services provided by your own doctor or a doctor who's affiliated with the hospice program
- Regular visits by nurses and on-call nursing support
- Chaplain services
- Counseling services
- Housekeeping and cooking services
- Medical equipment and supplies
- Medications to relieve symptoms
- Physical, speech and occupational therapy
- Relaxation therapy
- Dietary counseling
- Grief and bereavement counseling

The hospice staff generally provides bereavement services to family members for up to a year after a loved one's death.

Eligibility

You're eligible for hospice services when you stop treatment aimed at curing or controlling your cancer and your doctor indicates that — if your disease follows the expected course — you're expected to live six months or less, a criterion established by Medicare. Once enrolled in hospice, you're recertified for continuing care approximately every two months, as long as your doctor and the hospice medical director agree that your condition is appropriate for hospice services.

Although hospice care is widely acknowledged as being invaluable for people nearing the end of their lives, only

The Beginnings of Hospice

In the United States, modern-day hospice care began in Connecticut in 1974. The Connecticut Hospice in New Haven was modeled after a concept developed by Dame Cicely Saunders, a social worker who in 1967 opened the renowned St. Christopher's Hospice in Sydenham, England. Dame Cicely was so committed to providing high-quality, compassionate care for people near the end of their lives that she became a doctor to realize her goal. Her model of palliative care has since been replicated many times over in England, the United States and throughout the world.

Although hospice services initially were designed primarily for people with cancer, today they're available to people with other terminal illnesses, too.

20 percent to 50 percent of people with cancer who are eligible for hospice services receive them. For individuals who do enroll in hospice, the average time they receive hospice services is just two to three weeks, too little time for them to receive the full benefit of the range of services hospice offers. This is partly because of some people's reluctance to call hospice or because of their family member's inability to accept that they're dying. In addition, some doctors are reluctant to refer people to hospice, not because they don't see it as worthwhile but because they're hesitant to give up on treatment, or they don't want to tell individuals that they're dying.

Do-not-resuscitate status

The best time to make decisions about emergency care is before you need it. An example is when to decide on do-not-resuscitate (DNR) status. If you stop breathing or if your heart stops beating, do you want doctors to use extreme measures to try to bring you back? Extreme measures include performing cardiopulmonary resuscitation (CPR), shocking your chest to try to restart your heart or putting you on a ventilator, a machine that breathes for you.

If you decide that you don't want to be resuscitated, it's best to convey that information to your health care team as soon as you decide. Some hospice programs require that patients request DNR status to be eligible for services, in keeping with the hospice philosophy of not hastening death nor prolonging life. Requesting DNR status doesn't mean that you or your doctor will give up on your care. It simply means that you don't want extreme or heroic measures taken to extend your life, if you were to die.

Attempting resuscitation in people with advanced cancer usually is futile. It may prolong the dying process and may cause more pain and suffering. Even if a person is "successfully" resuscitated in the short term and placed on a breathing machine, he or she may not be able to breath independently again, and the family may have to decide when to stop the machine.

Doctors are mandated to discuss DNR status with all people who enter a hospital. Otherwise, the subject might not come up unless you were to initiate it. Some people hesitate to sign a DNR order because they're holding on to the hope that coming back to life will give them another chance at beating their disease. This is very unlikely for those with advanced, incurable cancer.

A Good Death

As a person faces the prospect of death, he or she is likely to experience a host of feelings, including fear, concern about those left behind and possibly anger. Some people don't understand the concept of a good death. The following true story may help.

Gayle's Story

Gayle was diagnosed with a large breast cancer that had spread beyond the breast at the time of her diagnosis. For the next two and a half years, she was treated with surgery, radiation therapy, chemotherapy and hormone therapy. At times, as part of her treatment, she needed to have catheters placed in the tubes that lead from the kidneys to the bladder (ureters).

Although the chemotherapy was hard on her, she continued to live her life, enjoying time with family and friends until her final moments. Throughout her treatment, she had open discussions with her oncologist regarding the pros and cons of various treatment approaches. She and her family were actively involved in her treatment decisions. Eventually, she reached the point where she was no longer responding to a number of anti-cancer treatments, such as hormone therapy and chemotherapy. She chose to spend her final days at home with her family, receiving hospice care.

Three weeks before her death, on the day she, her family and her doctor concluded that treatments aimed at slowing the cancer's growth were no longer working, Gayle attended a high school football game with her family. One week before her death, one of her sons and his wife invited many close friends and family members to their home for a celebration of life, to allow Gayle and her family and friends to reflect on the many good times they had shared. It was also an opportunity for words of thanks and heartfelt goodbyes.

Several days before her death, with her youngest son's encouragement, Gayle wrote to each of her three sons. Her inspiring words provide an excellent example of making sure that loved ones know what they mean to you at the end of your life. Her children, reading her words at her funeral, called it "a special gift from an incredibly special woman." This is some of what she wrote:

To Our First Born — Jeff

We've always loved you best because you were our first miracle — the fulfillment of young love, the promise of our infinity. You sustained us through the hamburger years, the first home — furnished in early poverty — the many monthly payments, trying to make ends meet.

You were new, had unused grandparents and more clothes than a Barbie doll. You were the "original model" for unsure parents trying to work the bugs out. You got the strained lamb, open pins, tiptoe treatment and three-hour naps. We have always expected a great deal from you, and you have not disappointed us. God has blessed us because you've been a fine example to your younger brothers — and we love you for it.

You were the beginning.

To Our Middle Child — Jim

We've always loved you best because you drew the dumb spot in the family, and it made you stronger. You cried less, had more patience, wore faded clothes and never did anything "first." With you, we realized you could kiss a dog or miss a nap and not get sick. You crossed the street before you went to kindergarten, and we didn't get an ulcer about your using a hammer.

You were the child of our busy, ambitious years. Without you, we never could have survived job changes and the house we couldn't afford. You've always endured the pressures of an older brother's achievements and a younger brother's gregariousness. And we've loved you for it.

You were the continuance.

To Our Baby — John

We've always loved you best because endings are generally sad, and you are such a joy. You readily accepted the milk-stained bibs and the secondhand toys, skates and bikes.

You are the one we hold on to so tightly. For, you see, you are the link with the past that gives reason to tomorrow. You quicken our steps, square our shoulders, restore our vision and give us humor that security and maturity can't give us. And we've loved you for it.

You are lucky to have two older brothers who have taught you so much and set fine examples for you. When you are older, even when your children tower over you, you will still be "the baby."

You were the culmination.

In the last week of her life, Gayle told her husband that she needed to plan her funeral. Using the excuse that he was older than she, he said they needed to plan his funeral first. So that day, they planned both of their funerals, first his, then hers.

On the day she died, she called her children and grandchildren to be with her that afternoon. They all said their goodbyes and shared some last moments with her. When her oncologist came to visit her, he found her resting comfortably, her home filled with three generations of her extended family.

Shortly after the oncologist's visit, Gayle's parish priest arrived. With Gayle's family present, the priest asked if she felt safe. He told her she was about to go to a better place and asked if she was ready to die. She replied to both questions with a smile and a nod of affirmation. She died peacefully six hours later.

Chapter 38: Living With Cancer

For Partners

Note: **This chapter is written specifically for the partners of women with breast or gynecologic cancers.**

When the woman you love learns that she has cancer, it's an intensely emotional time for both of you. It can also be a vulnerable time, bringing out both positive and negative aspects of your personality and relationship.

As the two of you come to grips with the situation and try to get your emotions in sync, your relationship will be tested. You may need to make short-term and long-term adjustments in everything from your daily routines to your sex life. There will be good days, and there will be bad days.

How you both respond to your partner's cancer diagnosis may be influenced by many factors, such as differences in temperament, family structure, communication styles and cultural expectations. Your past experiences in dealing with crises also may influence your response. You may feel additional pressure because you've been taught that you need to be strong and resilient. You may have grown up in a home where problems weren't openly discussed. You may have had relationship problems before the diagnosis.

Although each cancer situation is unique, many partners — husbands or companions of women with cancer — experience the same kinds of problems and day-to-day challenges that you may be facing. You have a special role in your partner's life during the entire process, from her cancer diagnosis to treatment to recovery. This is a time when she can benefit from your support, but at the same time you can't forget about your own needs. This chapter addresses some common concerns of partners and offers encouragement and guidance.

Dealing With Your Partner's Diagnosis

A diagnosis of cancer can be overwhelming. The first few weeks after a diagnosis often can be the most emotional and difficult time for everyone. Moods can change from moment to moment, and emotions and feelings can be intense and unpredictable as you and your partner attempt to cope with news that has changed both your lives. Usually, the intensity of emotions is temporary, and over time some of the anxiety lessens. This process varies with different individuals, and the two of you may come to terms with the diagnosis at different times.

Your emotions and feelings

It's understandable that the primary focus of everyone's attention is caring for your partner, but your feelings and emotions also are important and valid. Even though you aren't the one with cancer, you may experience feelings and emotions similar to your partner's — helplessness, anger, anxiety, fear. In addition, you may feel unappreciated if family and friends neglect to ask how you're doing.

Your role and position in your partner's life is unique because the love and level of commitment you share is different com-

pared with that of other family members or friends. You're the one who's expected to be by her side no matter what. It's normal to be unprepared for and overwhelmed by such an enormous responsibility. Don't be afraid to acknowledge your frustrations and fears so that you can find comfort, or at least learn how to persevere through this difficult time.

Common concerns

Each couple's experience is unique, but certain concerns and feelings may be universal. Three common concerns and challenges of partners of cancer patients are:
• Fearing cancer and its spread
• Knowing how to offer support
• Making adjustments to daily life

Fearing cancer and its spread
More than once, you may have found yourself asking or thinking: "Has the cancer spread?" "Will it continue to spread?" "What's the chance of it coming back?" "How many hours, months or years will she live?" Fear and worry are normal responses.

In addition to the status of the cancer, you may fear seeing your partner in pain or watching her die. You might even worry about what would happen if you became ill, especially if you feel that everyone is depending on you. You may worry about your own death and then feel guilty for thinking about yourself.

Knowing how to offer support
Many partners worry that they aren't handling the situation correctly or aren't providing enough emotional support, love

and understanding. Common questions include "How do I help?" "Am I really being helpful?" "Am I capable of being helpful and supportive?"

One of your greatest frustrations may be learning how to deal with your partner's emotions, which may be unpredictable and, at times, intense. You may feel helpless and powerless because you desperately want to fix things or at least do what you can to make your partner feel better, but you don't know how. Or perhaps you've tried to talk with your partner about her feelings and fears, but it hasn't gone well. You may question if your efforts are hurting the situation instead of helping it. This is a time to take stock of the strengths of your relationship. A diagnosis of cancer doesn't magically change a relationship. But you can build on its strengths even in difficult times.

Making adjustments to daily life

"Who's going to take care of the children?" "Who's going to cook dinner?" "What happens when my sick days and vacation days are used up?" Beyond the emotional turmoil is the day-to-day reality of living with someone who has cancer. And for some cancer patients and their families, there may be no end to the adjustments that need to be made because the situation may keep changing throughout the different stages of cancer.

Many aspects of life are affected in one way or another when a family member receives a diagnosis of cancer. You may need to take on added child-care and household responsibilities, as well as become the caregiver for your partner. For some partners, this may be especially challenging. Like many, you may not feel prepared for your new role as a caregiver. This can cause feelings of helplessness and frustration.

Perhaps you need to spend so much time at the hospital that no time is left for anything else. You might feel guilty for wanting to be free from the situation. If additional treatments are necessary, you may feel even more restricted.

What to expect from your partner

After your partner has learned that she has cancer, she may need some time before she's ready to share what she's feeling. She may distance herself from you both physically and emotionally. It's important to let her bring up the subject. If she confides in you, it's probably because she wants to share her concerns and anxieties with you. Let her know that you're available to listen to her when she's ready. There may be times when she prefers sharing her concerns with other women who've had similar experiences. This doesn't mean that your support is less important or less helpful.

Anger, fear, stress, anxiety, loneliness, depression and powerlessness are some of the emotions your partner may experience. Her feelings may be unpredictable, changing from day to day and even hour to hour. You may be on the receiving end of emotional outbursts or mood swings. Remember, even though outbursts may be directed at you, she's acting out toward the situation. These are some of the emotions you may see from your partner:

- **Anger or hostility.** Expressing anger or hostility may help your partner to reduce feelings of stress and tension. It may be your partner's way of asking, "Why me?" Unfortunately, you may have to withstand the worst of your partner's anger. Try not to take it personally.

- **Fear.** Fear is a common response to a diagnosis of cancer. Your partner may fear death, pain, an inability to work, physical changes, changes in personal relationships and uncertainty about the future. She may worry that she'll become a burden to the family.

- **Stress and anxiety.** Stress and anxiety can cause a wide range of physical symptoms, such as headaches, muscle pains and loss of appetite. Your partner may experience these.

- **Loneliness.** Many cancer patients and their loved ones may feel isolated and lonely. Friends who don't know how to deal with cancer, or simply can't deal with it, may start distancing themselves by staying away and not calling. Your partner may be surrounded by caring people but still feel that no one else can understand what she's experiencing.

- **Withdrawal.** Some people need time and space, even from those they love the most. Sometimes withdrawing is the only way to regain some control, if only temporarily. Periods of withdrawal are not uncommon. If your partner's withdrawal worries you or if your withdrawal from your partner worries her, talk about it.

- **Depression.** Your partner may be overwhelmed by feelings of deep sadness and despair. If you notice that she's experiencing a strong sense of helplessness, sadness, grief and a feeling that

life is meaningless, these could be signs of clinical depression. It's important that she share these feelings with her doctor.

- **Powerlessness.** Your partner may feel like she's losing control. She may feel a loss of independence because she has to rely on others for many of her needs. It may be difficult for her to hand over control to you or to accept help from others, especially if she's accustomed to being in charge of certain responsibilities or handling things a certain way. In addition, while your partner's body is trying to heal, it may not be functioning normally, and she may feel abandoned by her body.

How You Can Help

You're an essential part of your partner's healing. She needs your support throughout the entire process, from diagnosis to treatment to recovery. On some days, she may need emotional support or someone to talk to. On other days, she may need help with daily tasks, such as going to the grocery store or cooking dinner.

Your long-term commitment to your relationship is especially important because with some cancers, treatment can last for years. Initially, she may have strong support from family and friends, but over time these people may become less involved. Your support and encouragement may be the only constant in your partner's life.

It's important to try to focus on living as normal a life as possible. Many challenges lie ahead, and you'll probably say things or do things you regret, so patience is important. One of your ongoing challenges may be trying to balance supporting your partner while allowing her to hold on to as much independence as she can. Encourage your partner to tell you if your support is overwhelming her.

Communicating With the Team

Although doctors, nurses and other health care providers are a valuable source of information, they may assume that you understand everything they're communicating unless you ask them to explain things. Following are some ways you and your partner can establish good communication with your partner's doctor and other members of her health care team.

Keep in mind that only if your partner gives permission can her doctor or other members of her health care team talk with you or other loved ones about her condition. If she chooses not to grant this permission, you need to honor her desires, even though it may be difficult. She may have her reasons for limiting your communication with her health care team. Talk with her about such things.

Preparing questions before appointments

Ask your partner if she would like you to help write down questions to ask her doctor. If you have a long list of questions, schedule a longer appointment.

Learn as much as you can

Most people are afraid of what they don't know or understand. Knowing the facts about your partner's cancer can help both of you cope with your worries and fears.

Taking notes and asking questions during appointments

Ask your partner if she would like you to accompany her to her doctor's visits. You can help take notes and ask questions she may have forgotten to ask. This will also help you to become more knowledgeable about her situation.

It's important that both of you understand what's happening. Don't be afraid to ask the doctor to explain information you don't understand. Every question is important, and if an answer doesn't make sense to you, ask again. Make sure that you understand the available treatment options and the advantages and disadvantages of each. If your partner needs time to think about her treatment options, let her doctor know.

Supporting a second opinion

If your partner wants a second opinion, help her look for another doctor. A second opinion often confirms the options that have already been presented. However, sometimes a second opinion may bring to light a different treatment approach that your partner may want to consider. Most insurance companies cover the cost of a second opinion, but you may want to check first.

Information Gathering Checklist

Throughout the course of your partner's illness, the amount of information presented to you can be overwhelming. Keeping track of that information and learning as much as you can about the physical and emotional effects of treatment may help you support your partner.

Here's a checklist to help you gather and organize information.

Care providers
- ❑ **Primary care doctor:** _____
  Phone number: _____
- ❑ **Oncologist:** _____
  Phone number: _____
- ❑ **Surgeon:** _____
  Phone number: _____
- ❑ **Nurse:** _____
  Phone number: _____
- ❑ **Pharmacist:** _____
  Phone number: _____
- ❑ **Social worker:** _____
  Phone number: _____
- ❑ **Chaplain:** _____
  Phone number: _____
- ❑ **Other:** _____
  Phone number: _____

Testing for cancer
- ❑ Type of diagnostic procedure: _____
- ❑ Purpose of the procedure: _____
- ❑ Date test results were discussed with us: _____
- ❑ Name of the person coordinating care: _____
- ❑ Current hopes and fears: _____
  _____
- ❑ What will help us cope while we wait? _____
  _____

Surgery
- ❑ Type of surgery: _____
- ❑ Date the pathology report was discussed with us: _____

❑ Length of time in hospital: _____
❑ Home-going instructions after discharge from the hospital: _____
   _____

❑ Current hopes and fears: _____
   _____

❑ What will our family need? _____

Treatment
❑ Type of treatment: _____
❑ Number of treatments: _____
❑ Possible side effects of treatment: _____
❑ Ways to minimize side effects:_____
❑ Current hopes and fears: _____
❑ What can I do for my partner during this time? _____
❑ Support groups and other resources: _____
   _____

After treatment
❑ Next follow-up appointment: _____
❑ Current hopes and fears: _____
❑ Ways to balance the needs of my partner and family members: _____
   _____
❑ Support groups and other resources: _____

Recurrence
❑ Type of treatment: _____
❑ Number of treatments: _____
❑ Ways to minimize side effects:_____
❑ Current hopes and fears: _____
❑ What can I do for my partner during this time? _____
   _____
❑ Support groups and other resources: _____

Adapted from Laurel L. Northouse and Holly Peters-Golden, "Cancer and the Family: Strategies to Assist Spouses,"
Seminars in Oncology Nursing, 9:2 (May 1993), pages 74-82

If you know ahead of time what your partner's treatment will involve, you'll be better prepared to cope and to plan for disruptions that may occur in your daily routine.

Gathering information may be a concrete way you and your partner can regain control of the situation. It may also be an important part of the coping process as the two of you create feelings of confidence by making informed decisions together. You may gain valuable insights from each other. In addition, when visiting with your partner's health care team, the two of you may feel more confident because the information you're hearing will sound familiar to you.

Health information is available in many places, such as community, hospital and medical school libraries, and major cancer research and treatment institutions. Many organizations offer their materials online. See page 599 for a list of reliable and credible sources.

Offer to help your partner search and sort through information about her cancer. Realize that she may be overwhelmed with the amount of information you find, so let her determine when or if she's ready to read it.

But be careful not to go overboard. Some women and their partners seek out several expert opinions, try to collect all relevant materials, spend countless hours on the Internet and then try to make appropriate medical decisions themselves. This can cause considerable angst. If you find yourself in this situation, it's important to find a cancer doctor you trust and allow him or her to help you make appropriate medical decisions.

Ways to provide emotional support

You can support your partner in many ways, but what's most important is your presence. You're in a unique position to attend to her with your heart, mind and soul. Your partner needs your support to help her through a very emotional time.

- **Reaffirm your commitment.** Let her know that you intend to support her and stay by her side. She needs to know that you'll continue to love her, especially through the difficult times. It's important to remember to say, "I love you."
- **Spend quality time together.** Schedule time when the two of you can be alone without any distractions. Go on a date. If you're home, shut off the television or radio and let the answering machine answer your calls. Try to set aside at least 30 minutes every day when you and your partner can simply talk. If you find that both of you are exhausted at the end of the day, try scheduling time in the morning.
- **Listen attentively.** While your partner is sharing her frustrations and fears with you, you may not be giving her your full attention. Instead, you may be thinking about what you're going to say when it's your turn to talk. Rather than worrying about coming up with solutions or providing the right answer, give your partner your complete attention. You may not feel like you're doing much by just sitting and listening, and it may be difficult to accept what you hear, but your presence and acceptance may be exactly what your partner needs at the moment.

While being a sounding board for your partner's fears and frustrations, don't be afraid to express your own fears and frustrations — but within limits. Your partner may not be able to take on the added emotional task of comforting you.

- **Find out what her wishes are.** Ask your partner to be honest about what she wants and needs from you and others.

Ways to provide practical support

In addition to emotional support, helping out on a day-to-day basis is important. Here are some suggestions:

- **Cook dinner and clean up afterward.** If life is really hectic, now and then buy prepared foods, dine out or order food to be delivered.
- **Drive her to doctor visits.** Doctor appointments can be nerve-racking, and if she's receiving treatment, such as chemotherapy or radiation therapy, she may not feel well afterward.
- **Help keep the house in order.** If you can afford it, consider hiring a housekeeper. Or, perhaps, family members or friends can help you keep the house in order.
- **Screen telephone calls and visitors.** Family and friends may have good intentions when they call or visit, but at times your partner may not be feeling well and may not be up to seeing visitors or talking on the phone. Try to convey this to visitors in a caring way so as not to discourage them from visiting or calling in the future. You may suggest that they send a card, or you may suggest a better time to call or visit.

- **Give your partner peace and quiet.** Your partner may need some time alone to reflect, relax and emotionally recharge. Encourage your partner to do so.
- **Help out with the children.** If you previously weren't involved in packing lunches or chauffeuring the kids around, offer to help out now. It may take time for the children to adjust to relying less on mom, but it can be an opportunity for you to spend more quality time with your children. In addition, it may be time for your children to be a little more independent. Have them help with chores, too.
- **Help your partner resume her regular activities.** Don't put life on hold. Continue to enjoy spending time with friends and family and, as much as possible, doing other things you've always liked to do, such as eating out or going to the movies. Your partner may have less energy, so try to follow her cue.

Talking to Each Other

Communication is important in any relationship, but even more so during times of stress and uncertainty. Two things that can hinder communication are wrong assumptions and poor communication skills. Open and honest communication is important. In your discussions, it's OK to use the word *cancer*.

Communication barriers

A common problem among couples is making assumptions. One person simply

Don't Be Afraid to Seek Professional Help

If the cancer experience is causing problems in your relationship, it may be because you're experiencing a breakdown in communication. A trained professional may be able to help you resolve some misunderstandings and suggest ways that you can strengthen your relationship. You might consider seeking professional counseling, especially in the following circumstances:

- If you start distancing yourself from your partner because you're uncomfortable talking about cancer
- If your discussions end up as arguments
- If you and your partner are having difficulty maintaining sexual intimacy

assumes the other knows his or her needs without actually discussing the problem or situation. Because cancer is likely a new experience for both of you, be careful to not make assumptions. You won't truly know what the other needs unless you talk about it.

If your partner or you aren't the type to talk openly about difficult issues, the two of you may have trouble doing so now. A diagnosis of cancer may not instantly change the way you communicate with your partner, but it's an opportunity to make an improvement in your relationship. Just because you haven't been entirely open with each other in the past doesn't mean that you can't start now. Big changes may not occur, but small steps are possible.

Communication tips

As your partner attempts to open up to you — to share her feelings, worries, fears and hopes — keep these points in mind:

- **Respect your partner's feelings.** Your partner may want to talk about her can-

cer diagnosis one day and be silent about it the next. If she doesn't bring up the topic, you may be afraid to do so. The best thing to do is simply ask your partner if she has anything she wants to talk about, and then respect her wishes.

- **Be a good listener.** If your partner wants to talk, be attentive. Listen to what is said and how it's said. And listen without becoming defensive.
- **Be patient.** Be prepared for periods of silence and crying. Silence can be comforting because it allows your partner time to reflect. Allow your partner to cry or sigh because these behaviors help release tension and anxiety.
- **Speak from your heart.** If your partner asks you questions that you don't know how to respond to, be honest and say that you don't have an answer but that you'll try to find one. A simple touch, hug or smile is a sign of affection that shows you care.
- **Ask questions.** Your partner may want you to simply ask questions or listen. Try asking, "What are you feeling?" not just "How are you feeling?" It may be a

Keeping a Journal

Some people have difficulty expressing their feelings to others, and they tend to keep everything bottled up inside. If you happen to be such a person, you may find it therapeutic to write your thoughts in a journal.

A journal is a way to release your innermost thoughts, observations and experiences. You can be as honest as you want to be about your fears and frustrations. It's also a place where you can write about happy moments and your hopes for the future. You don't need a special notebook or to follow any special format. However, for future reference, it may be helpful to write down dates, times, your feelings at the time and other details.

You can share your writings with others if you like, but you don't have to do so. The main purpose of a journal is to release what you're feeling inside.

Throughout the cancer experience, you and your partner may find strength and comfort in your spiritual beliefs, whatever they may be. Even if your spiritual paths are different, you need to respect each other's beliefs. The strength you gain as individuals contributes to strengthening your relationship as a couple.

You may be encouraged by reading religious materials, praying or meditating. Another source of spiritual strength may be talking with spiritual advisers, who are often trained in and knowledgeable about counseling patients and families dealing with serious illness.

Dealing With Incurable Cancer

If your partner has an incurable cancer and is nearing the end of her life, you're facing many additional worries and concerns. The knowledge that death may be nearing is extremely frightening. And you may be worried about whether you can cope, whether you can make it through a long and difficult process.

It's also a profound time for your partner. She needs you close by, listening to her concerns and offering support with a smile or gentle touch. She may withdraw from life as she enters the dying process, but she still needs to know that you're present and available if she needs you.

If you don't know what to do, just simply touch her — hold her hand or rub her back — and talk. If she feels up to it, encourage your partner to talk about her life — a life review. These can be the times when marvelous stories are told. Sometimes, when adult children are present, they're amazed to find out that they've never heard these stories.

Hospice care

Don't feel guilty if you can't do it alone. No one can. This is a time when you and your partner will likely want to consider hospice care. Hospice organizations are meant to provide expert and compassionate care for people near the end of life.

Hospice care allows your partner to spend her last weeks or months in the comfortable surroundings of your home or in a homelike setting, while under the care of a team of professional and volunteer caregivers.

Oftentimes, your partner's doctor coordinates the team, and a nurse handles the details of daily care. Chaplains and social workers can offer counseling and support. Trained volunteers are available to assist with daily tasks, such as light housekeeping, cooking meals and running errands, and they can offer companionship. For more information on hospice care, see Chapter 37.

Grieving

When people are keeping a vigil for a loved one who is dying, or after a loved one has died, they often say it feels like a bad dream. You may feel the same way. Feelings of grief, loss and sadness come in waves. Emotions can be overwhelming, making even simple tasks seem difficult for a time.

This is all normal. It doesn't mean you're going to be unable to function the rest of your life. It means that right now, most of what you can do is grieve. It's all part of being human and loving. Grief is a natural response to loving and feeling loss.

If you're concerned that you have spent too much time grieving and are unable to function or if others have expressed concern about you, consider seeing a counselor. Sometimes a loss is more than a person can handle, and depression occurs.

The line between profound grief and depression is blurry. But if you're still having trouble sleeping and concentrating months after your partner's death, a visit with a counselor could help you get back on track.

When Your Loved One Is in Denial

Denial can be an important coping mechanism. Some individuals deny that they're facing death because reality is too frightening. Denial is a form of natural protection that allows a person to let reality in bit by bit. It allows a person to continue living while he or she contemplates death.

Your loved one may be in denial for a variety of reasons: She doesn't want to say goodbye. She may be afraid of the pain that might be ahead. She may be afraid of losing her bodily functions. She may be afraid of becoming a burden to others.

One of the ways you can support your partner if she's in denial is to ask her to talk about her fears. Or you might encourage your partner to visit with a member of her health care team. Sometimes, it's easier for a dying person to share what she is afraid of with someone other than a family member.

Q: **Is it wrong to tell a loved one it's OK to let go?**

A: Sometimes, it appears as though a dying person is having difficulty letting go. Perhaps the experience isn't evolving as you thought it would. Perhaps it's taking longer than you expected. People die in their own time. Whether someone really holds on until the last family member is there, for example, medical experts have no way of proving, even if it seems that way. If you think your loved one is holding on for your sake, it's OK to tell her that you'll be all right and that she can let go.

Resources

You and your partner don't have to face cancer alone. In addition to family and friends, a network of resources is available. You can begin your search by contacting organizations that offer special programs to assist cancer patients and their families or that can recommend other organizations.

Support groups

Some partners of women with cancer find support groups to be helpful. Although you may be reluctant to share your feelings with strangers, being in a support group has these advantages:
- You may find it beneficial to connect with others experiencing the same or similar cancer issues.
- You may learn something new or be encouraged by someone else's story.
- You may learn how other partners have adapted to changes and have coped.
- It may be a relief just to know that you're not alone.

As your partner may seek the camaraderie of other women with cancer, you too may find it beneficial to connect with partners in a similar situation.

You can begin your search by contacting various cancer organizations. Many types of cancer support groups exist. They're designed to meet the different needs of individuals with cancer and their loved ones. It may take you some time to find the group that meets your needs and interests.

Types
Not all support groups are the same. Following are several types of support groups for partners.

Peer support groups
Peer support groups make up the majority of support groups. Members of peer support groups help each other out by sharing similar experiences. Individuals leading the meetings may or may not have professional training.

Educational intervention groups
Educational intervention groups meet to learn about and discuss a specific topic related to cancer. The meetings often begin with a formal presentation, given

by an expert. Some women with cancer and their partners find learning more about cancer and its treatment to be an empowering experience.

Coping skill intervention groups

In this type of support group, participants learn concrete coping skills. During one class, participants might learn about relaxation techniques to help relieve stress. Another class might provide tips on mental health exercises to help keep a positive mental perspective. Coping skill intervention groups are usually led by mental health professionals with expertise leading these types of interventions.

Therapy groups

Therapy groups are led by mental health professionals trained in group therapy. These types of support groups usually focus on specific personal issues. Members are asked to share personal stories, as well as respond to others in the group. Each member is challenged to take action concerning a particular issue with which he or she needs help.

Online support groups

Online support groups allow members to communicate with others on the Internet in chat rooms and on message boards. If you participate in an online support group, be aware that chat rooms may not be reliable sources of health information.

Finding the right group

If you're searching for a support group, it may be helpful to think about what type of group would best meet your needs. Ask yourself the following questions:

Who's in the group?

Most support groups have two types of membership: open and closed. Open membership doesn't require the same level of commitment as closed membership. With open membership, you're generally not required to sign up ahead of time nor are you expected to attend all meetings. Closed membership usually requires preregistration.

Who's leading the group?

Meetings may be led by health professionals or group members, such as a partner of a person with cancer. Health professionals often are licensed and have some skill in leading groups. Although a partner may be able to empathize and share personal experiences, the discussion may not be as productive unless the facilitator has some leadership skills.

What's the format?

Some groups have a more structured program with different topics of discussion each week. Other groups have open discussions around topics members bring up.

A Time of Growth

Partners do have vital roles in the lives of women with cancer. While your experiences can be very stressful and difficult at times, they also can be rewarding. A cancer diagnosis can lead to positive growth in your relationship, as the two of you find strength in each other and as you re-explore your love for each other.

Additional Resources

This book is devoted to providing the answers you need to a wide range of health and medical questions, but no single volume can address all of the issues that may interest you and other readers. For more information about breast and gynecologic cancers and coping with cancer treatment, contact these organizations. Telephone numbers and Web addresses are subject to change.

Caregiving and Hospice

Family Caregiver Alliance
www.caregiver.org
(800) 445-8106

Hospice Web
www.hospiceweb.com

Last Acts: Campaign to Improve End-of-Life Care
www.lastacts.org

National Family Caregivers Association, Caregiving Resources
www.nfcacares.org
(800) 896-3650

Clinical Trial Information

Cancer.gov: Clinical Trials
www.cancer.gov/clinical_trials
(800) 4-CANCER, or (800) 422-6237
TTY (for hearing impaired): (800) 332-8615

Center Watch Clinical Trials Listing Service
www.centerwatch.com

Coalition of National Cancer Cooperative Groups
www.cancertrialshelp.org
(877) 520-4457

Mayo Clinic: Clinical Trials
mayoresearch.mayo.edu/mayo/research/trials/index.cfm

Complementary and Alternative Medicine

American Music Therapy Association
www.musictherpay.org

Complementary/Integrative Medicine
www.mdanderson.org
(800) 392-1611, option 3

Consumerlabs.com
www.consumerlabs.com

MedWatch
www.fda.gov/medwatch
(888) INFO-FDA (888) 463-6332

National Center for Complementary and Alternative Medicine
www.nccam.nih.gov
(888) 644-6226
TTY (for hearing impaired): (866) 464-3615

National Institutes of Health Office of Dietary Supplements
dietary-supplements.info.nih.gov

Quackwatch Home Page
www.quackwatch.org

Coping

Cancer Care
www.cancercare.org
(800) 813-HOPE, or (800) 813-4673

Cancer Hope Network
www.cancerhopenetwork.org
(877) HOPENET, or (877) 467-3638

Facing Our Risk of Cancer Empowered (FORCE)
www.facingourrisk.org

The Wellness Community
www.wellnesscolumbus.org

Español (Spanish)
Resources for Cancer Information

American Cancer Society: Informacion de referencia sobre el cancer
www.cancer.org/docroot/ESP/ESP_0.asp
(800) ACS-2345, or (800) 227-2345

Cancercare: En Espanol
www.cancercare.org/EnEspanol/EnEspanolmain.cfm
(800) 813-HOPE, or (800) 813-4673

Cancer.gov: Algunos documentos especificos estan en espanol
cancer.gov/espanol
(800) 4-CANCER, or (800) 422-6237

Espanol: Healthfinder
healthfinder.gov/espanol
(877) 696-6775

Institutos Nacionales de la Salud
salud.nih.gov

Y-Me National Breast Cancer Organization
(800) 986-9505 (Español)

Financial

Angel Flight America
www.angelflightamerica.org
(800) 446-1231

Corporate Angel Network
www.corpangelnetwork.org
(866) 328-1313

National Association of Hospital Hospitality Houses
www.nahhh.org
(800) 542-9730

Patient Advocacy Coalition
www.patientadvocacy.net

Patient Travel
www.patienttravel.org
(800) 296-1217

Pharmaceutical Research and Manufacturers of America
www.phrma.org

General Cancer Information

Association of Cancer Online Resources (ACOR)
www.acor.org

American Cancer Society
www.cancer.org
(800) ACS-2345, or (800) 227-2345

Cancer Education
www.cancereducation.com

Cancer.gov (National Cancer Institute)
cancer.gov
(800) 4-CANCER, or (800) 422-6237

Cancer Information and Cancer Resources
www.cancersource.com
(866) 234-5025

Cancer Information Service
cis.nci.nih.gov
(800) 4-CANCER, or (800) 422-6237

Centers for Disease Control and Prevention
www.cdc.gov/health/cancer.htm
(800) 311-3435

HealthWeb
healthweb.org

Mayo Clinic Cancer Center
www.mayoclinic.org/cancercenter

Mayo Clinic College of Medicine
www.mayo.edu

Mayo Clinic.com
www.MayoClinic.com

Mayo Clinic: Internet Health and Medical Resources
www.mayoclinic.org/healthinfo/resources.html

National Cancer Institute: Cancer Information Service
www.nci.nih.gov
(800) 4-CANCER, or (800) 422-6273

OncoLink
www.oncolink.com

People Living With Cancer
www.plwc.org

Research

American Institute for Cancer Research
www.aicr.org
(800) 843-8114

American Society of Clinical Oncology
www.asco.org

Cancerpage: Cancer Information and Community
www.cancerpage.com

Entrez: PubMed
www.ncbi.nlm.nih.gov/entrez/query.fcgi

MEDLINEplus
www.nlm.nih.gov/medlineplus

National Library of Medicine
www.nlm.nih.gov
(888) FIND-NLM, or (888) 346-3656

Specific Cancers

Gynecologic Cancer Foundation
www.wcn.org/gcf
(800) 444-4441

National Alliance of Breast Cancer Organizations
www.nabco.org

National Ovarian Cancer Coalition
www.ovarian.org
(888) OVARIAN, or (888) 682-7426

Susan G. Komen Breast Cancer Foundation
www.komen.org
(800) I'M-AWARE, or (800) 462-9273

Women's Cancer Network
www.wcn.org

Y-Me National Breast Cancer Organization
www.y-me.org
(800) 221-2141 (English)
(800) 986-9505 (Español)

Survivorship

Cancervive: Dedicated to the Challenge of Life After Cancer
www.cancervive.org
(800) 4-TO-CURE, or (800) 486-2873

Gilda's Club Worldwide
www.gildasclub.org
(888) GILDA-4-U, or (888) 445-3248

Living Beyond Breast Cancer
www.lbbc.org

National Coalition for Cancer Survivorship
www.canceradvocacy.org
(877) NCCS-YES, or (877) 622-7937

Treatment

American Brachytherapy Society
www.americanbrachytherapy.org

American Medical Association
www.ama-assn.org
(800) 621-8335

Center for Drug Evaluation and Research
www.fda.gov/cder
(888) INFO-FDA, or (888) 463-6332

FertileHOPE
www.fertilehope.org
(888) 994-HOPE, or (888) 994-4673

Radiofrequency Ablation
www.cc.nih.gov/drd/rfa

RadiologyInfo
www.radiologyinfo.org

Resolve: The National Infertility Association
www.resolve.org
(888) 623-0744

Glossary

A

abdominal hysterectomy. An operation to remove the uterus that's performed by way of an incision in the abdomen.

absolute risk. The actual numeric chance of developing a condition, such as cancer, during a specified time.

adenocarcinoma. Cancer that starts in glandular tissue or cancer that forms glandular-like structures.

adenosarcoma. A tumor that contains benign epithelial cells and malignant stromal cells.

adjuvant therapy. Additional treatment that's given to a person with no visible evidence of any remaining (residual) cancer after completion of the first (primary) treatment.

advanced (metastatic) cancer. Cancer that has spread to distant parts of the body, such as the bones, lungs or liver.

angiogenesis. Development of new blood vessels, allowing cells to receive nutrients.

anterior exenteration. Surgical removal of the pelvic structures in the front of the pelvis, including the bladder and vagina.

antibody. An immune system protein that binds to and eliminates a foreign substance (antigen).

anti-cancer treatment. Therapy that focuses on shrinking and killing cancer cells.

anti-emetic. A medication that prevents or lessens nausea and vomiting.

antigens. Foreign substances that elicit an immune system response.

antioxidants. Substances that protect the body's cells from the damaging effects of free radicals, highly reactive and potentially toxic oxygen molecules.

areola. The area of dark skin around a nipple.

aromatase inhibitors. Breast cancer medications that block the production of estrogen.

ascites. Accumulation of fluid in the abdomen.

axillary node dissection. Surgical removal of lymph nodes under the arm in an attempt to remove cancer cells that may have spread from a tumor in the adjacent breast.

axillary nodes. Lymph nodes located under the arm (in the axilla).

B

benign. Not cancerous.

benign tumor. A growth that doesn't invade surrounding tissue or spread to distant parts of the body.

bilateral. Affecting both sides. Bilateral breast cancer is breast cancer that occurs in both breasts. Bilateral oophorectomy is the removal of both ovaries.

biologic therapies. Nonchemotherapy approaches to treat cancer, such as immunotherapy and growth factor blockers. They target tumor cells through biologic pathways.

biopsy. Removal of a small sample of tissue for analysis in a pathology laboratory.

bone scan. A test to look for bone damage, possibly caused by spread of cancer to bone.

borderline tumor. An ovarian tumor in the epithelial cells that has some, but not all, of the features of a malignant tumor.

brachytherapy. *See* internal radiation (brachytherapy).

BRCA1 and BRCA2 genes. Genes that help govern a cell's response to DNA damage. When altered they result in a marked predisposition to breast and ovarian cancers.

breast reconstruction. A surgical procedure designed to restore a relatively natural-shaped breast mound after a mastectomy.

breast self-examination (BSE). Examination of your own breasts for lumps or changes.

C

calcifications. Calcium deposits in body tissues, including the breast. Depending on their size and clustering pattern, they may signal a benign or malignant process.

cancer. Growth of an abnormal population of cells that have acquired aggressive properties, including the ability to spread to new tissues in the body.

CA 125 blood test. A blood tumor marker test that measures the level of CA 125 in blood. CA 125 is a protein that's produced by most ovarian cancers.

carcinogen. A cancer-causing agent.

carcinoma. Cancer that originates in epithelial tissue, which covers or lines an organ or body structure.

carcinoma *in situ*. Cancer cells that are confined to the layer of cells in which they started to develop. Also known as noninvasive cancer.

cell proliferation. Cell multiplication by way of cell division.

cervix. The lower, neck-like portion of the uterus, which extends into the upper portion of the vagina.

chemoprevention. Use of medication to reduce the risk of cancer.

chemotherapy. Medications that can kill cancer cells.

choriocarcinoma. Cancer of the chorion, a layer of the placenta.

chromosome. One of 46 (23 pairs) rod-shaped structures in the nucleus of human cells that carry genetic instructions for each cell.

clinical breast examination (CBE). Examination of the breasts for lumps or changes by a health care professional.

clinical trial. A research study in humans that tests new approaches for diagnosis, treatment or prevention of a condition, or for relief of symptoms.

colposcopy. Examination of the cervix through a special magnifying telescope.

complementary and alternative therapy. Treatments used in place of or in addition to mainstream medicine.

complete blood count (CBC). A test to count levels of white and red blood cells and platelets.

complete remission. Disappearance of all evidence of cancer after treatment.

computer-aided detection (CAD). A computer technique that gives radiologists an additional tool to help them detect questionable areas on a standard mammogram.

computerized tomography (CT). An X-ray technique that produces more detailed images of the internal organs than do conventional X-ray studies.

cone biopsy. Surgical removal of a cone-shaped piece of tissue from the lower cervix.

contralateral. Referring to the opposite side of the body.

contralateral prophylactic mastectomy. A means of lowering the risk of a new breast cancer by removing the unaffected breast.

core needle biopsy. A type of biopsy in which a needle is used to withdraw a small core of tissue from a mass. A smaller needle is used for fine-needle aspiration.

corpus. The upper, larger portion of the uterus.

cryotherapy. A treatment that destroys cells by freezing them. It's often used to treat abnormal cells of the cervix. Also called cryoablation.

cyst. A fluid-filled sac that's benign.

cystadenoma. A cyst that develops on the surface of an ovary and may be filled with a watery liquid or mucous material.

cystoscopy. Examination of the inside of the bladder with a thin, lighted instrument (cystoscope).

cytokines. Immune system proteins, some of which either attack and kill cancerous cells directly or stimulate the body's immune system cells to help attack a cancer.

D

debulking (cytoreduction). Surgical removal of as much cancer as possible.

deoxyribonucleic acid (DNA). The chemical code of genes found in the nucleus of cells, which carries hereditary information.

dermoid cyst. A benign germ cell tumor that occurs as a cyst.

diagnostic mammogram. A breast X-ray used to investigate breast changes, evaluate abnormal findings on a screening mammogram or evaluate breasts with implants.

dilation and curettage (D and C). Opening (dilating) the cervix and scraping the lining of the uterus (endometrium) with an instrument called a curet.

disease-free interval. The time extending from the initial diagnosis of a cancer to the time when a recurrence becomes apparent.

distant cancer. Cancer that has spread from its original site to other parts of the body. Also called metastasis.

dosimetrist. An individual who calculates and measures radiation dosage and delivery.

doubling time. The time it takes for a tumor to become twice its size.

ductal carcinoma. Cancer that begins in the ductal cells of the breast.

ductal carcinoma *in situ* (DCIS). A noninvasive breast cancer in which the abnormal cells haven't spread through duct walls into the connective or fatty tissue of the breast.

ductal cells. Cells that line the milk ducts in the breast.

ductal lavage. Injecting saline into a breast duct through the nipple openings and then withdrawing the solution for analysis.

ductoscopy. Use of a very slender catheter with a microscopic video camera at its tip that's inserted into openings in the nipple of the breast to visualize the lining of the ducts of the breast and look for cellular changes.

ducts. Thin tubes within the breast that connect the milk-forming bulbs, lobules and lobes to the nipple.

dysplasia. A precancerous process in which normal cells begin to change in size, shape or structure.

E

endometrial hyperplasia. An increased number of cells in the lining of the uterus.

endometrioma. Endometrial tissue that attaches to the ovary and forms a cyst. It's a result of endometriosis, in which uterine lining cells grow outside the uterus.

endometrium. The thick, blood-rich inner lining of the body (corpus) of the uterus.

epithelial cells. Cells that line or cover most organs.

epithelial hyperplasia. An overgrowth of epithelial cells.

epithelial ovarian cancer. Cancer that develops in the epithelial covering of the ovary, the most common type of ovarian cancer.

epithelium. The thin layer of cells that lines the outside and inside of most organs.

estrogen. The primary female hormone. It stimulates the growth of cancer cells in hormone receptor positive tumors.

estrogen receptor. A protein found in certain cells within certain tissues, such as breast and uterine tissues, which binds to estrogen.

excisional biopsy. Surgical removal of a mass.

external beam radiation. A form of radiation therapy in which doses of radiation from a large X-ray machine located outside the body are aimed at the tumor area.

external risk factors. Outside influences on the body, including lifestyle and environmental factors. Some can contribute to cancer development.

F

fallopian tubes. The passageways for eggs to travel from the ovaries to the uterus.

fibroadenoma. A solid, benign tumor that often occurs in the breasts of women during their reproductive years.

fibrocystic breasts. The presence of benign fibrous tissue in the breasts, with or without fluid-filled sacs (cysts).

fine-needle aspiration biopsy. A type of biopsy that uses a very fine needle and syringe to collect a sample of cells from a mass.

flap surgery. Reconstructive surgery in which a section of tissue taken from one part of the body, such as the abdominal wall, is used to fashion a new breast mound.

free radicals. Highly reactive and potentially toxic oxygen molecules within cells that are created as a byproduct of normal metabolism.

frozen section. A tissue sample that's quickly frozen, sliced and analyzed under a microscope so that a surgeon can receive information on the sample within minutes.

G

Gail model. A statistical tool that allows doctors to estimate the likelihood that a woman with certain risk factors will develop invasive breast cancer in the next five years and also during her lifetime.

gene. A defined segment of DNA within a chromosome. Genes are the blueprints for how the cells of the body function.

gene therapy. The process of supplying abnormal cells with healthy copies of missing or defective genes in an effort to treat, cure or possibly prevent disease.

genetic marker. An identifiable substance associated with a normal or abnormal gene.

genetics. The study of genes and the diseases caused by gene abnormalities.

genetic testing. Testing to determine whether an individual carries a specific gene mutation that puts him or her at increased risk of a certain condition.

genomics. The study of the human genome, the complete set of approximately 40,000 genes in a human being.

germ cells. Cells in an ovary or testicle that develop into eggs and sperm, respectively.

Gn-RH analogs. Drugs resembling hormones that control production of the hormones estrogen and progesterone. Gn-RH stands for gonadotropin-releasing hormones.

grade. A measure of how much cancer cells differ from normal cells when viewed under a microscope. The grade reflects the aggressiveness of the cancer.

granulosa cell tumor. An ovarian tumor that arises from granulosa cells, which produce estrogen. This type of tumor often secretes estrogen.

H

hereditary cancer. Cancer caused by mutations in a gene, which can be passed on to a child from one or both parents.

HER-2/neu. A protein that stimulates cell growth and is overproduced in about 25 percent of breast cancers and some ovarian and endometrial cancers.

histology. The study of the microscopic appearance of tissue.

hormone receptor. A cell protein that can bind to different hormones or hormone-look-alike drugs traveling through the bloodstream.

hormone therapy. Treatment of cancer by removing, blocking or adding hormones in an attempt to inhibit cancer growth.

hospice care. A program designed to provide palliative care to people with terminal illness and supportive services to their families and significant others.

human papillomavirus (HPV). A group of viruses that may be transmitted sexually. Some have been linked to certain gynecologic cancers, particularly cervical cancer.

hyperplasia. Increased cell growth.

hyperthermia therapy. A procedure in which body tissues are exposed to high temperatures in an attempt to damage or kill cancer cells or make them more sensitive to the effects of radiation therapy or chemotherapy.

hysterectomy. Surgical removal of the uterus. *See also* radical hysterectomy.

I

immunotherapy. *See* biologic therapies.

implant, breast. A breast-shaped device placed under the skin of the chest wall and held in place by the chest muscles. It's used for cosmetic surgery or breast reconstruction.

incidence. The number of new cases of a disease within a defined time frame.

inflammatory breast cancer. Cancer that's associated with redness, warmth and swelling of the skin of the breast.

internal radiation (brachytherapy). A form of radiation therapy in which radioactive substances are placed in the tumor or near where the cancer was removed.

internal risk factors. Influences within the body that may increase the likelihood of disease, including hormonal factors, inherited genetic mutations and immune conditions.

interstitial radiation. A type of internal radiation in which radioactive material is sealed in a container and placed into or near the cancer, but not in a body cavity.

intracavitary radiation. A type of internal radiation in which the radioactive material is placed in a body cavity, such as within the uterus.

intraductal hyperplasia. A condition in which too many cells line the wall of a milk duct in the breast.

intraductal hyperplasia with atypia. A form of intraductal hyperplasia in which the cells begin to take on an abnormal appearance.

intraoperative radiation therapy (IORT). Radiation treatment during surgery in which the radiation is aimed directly toward the site intended to receive the treatment.

intraperitoneal chemotherapy. Injection of chemotherapy into the abdominal cavity.

intraperitoneal radiation. Internal radiation in which a radioactive material is delivered directly into the abdominal cavity.

invasive cancer. Cancer that has spread from its cell or cells of origin into adjacent connective tissue.

invasive mole (chorioadenoma destruens). A molar pregnancy that progresses and penetrates the muscular wall of the uterus.

ipsilateral. Referring to the same side of the body.

L

labia. Two sets of skin folds that meet in the middle of the female genital area, protecting the openings to the vagina and urethra.

laparoscopy. Use of lighted instruments and small cutting tools that are inserted through small incisions in the abdomen and pelvis to gather cell samples or perform surgery.

laparotomy. Surgery that involves opening up the abdominal cavity by way of an abdominal incision.

laser surgery. Use of a narrow beam of intense light to destroy abnormal tissue, such as precancerous cells on the surface of the cervix.

leiomyosarcoma. A type of cancer that starts in smooth muscle cells.

lifetime cancer risk. The probability that an individual will develop cancer during his or her lifetime.

lobes. Milk-forming structures within the female breast.

lobular carcinoma. Cancer that originates in the lobules of the breast.

lobular carcinoma *in situ* **(LCIS).** A condition in which lobular cells of the breast are abnormal, but the abnormal cells haven't spread beyond the breast lobules.

lobules. Glands within the lobes of the breast that can produce milk.

locally advanced breast cancer. Breast cancers with one or more of these features: larger than 5 centimeters, extensive involvement of the regional lymph nodes, or spread to breast skin or the chest wall.

local recurrence. Regrowth of cancer cells at or near the site of the original tumor.

local-regional therapy. Treatment, including surgery and radiation therapy, that's targeted directly at the tumor and nearby tissue.

loop electrosurgical excision procedure (LEEP). Use of an electrical current that's passed through a thin wire loop, which acts like a knife, to remove a piece of tissue.

lumpectomy. Removal of the portion of a breast that appears to contain cancer cells, but not the whole breast. Also known as breast-conserving surgery.

lymphadenectomy. Surgical removal of lymph nodes from a specific location.

lymphedema. Accumulation of fluid in an arm or leg from disruption of lymph vessels.

lymph node. A collection of lymphatic tissue found in many parts of the body.

lymphoma. A tumor that develops in lymphatic tissue.

lymph vessels. Vessels that carry lymph, a clear fluid that contains immune system cells and that drains waste products from tissues.

M

magnetic resonance imaging (MRI). An imaging technique that uses a magnetic field and radio waves to create a detailed, three-dimensional representation of the body.

malignant. Cancerous.

malignant tumor. Abnormal growth and multiplication of cells, causing the cells to form a mass (tumor). The cells have acquired aggressive features, including the ability to spread into other tissues. Another term for a cancer.

mammography. A procedure in which X-rays are taken of the breasts to detect any abnormalities.

margin of resection. The edge of a sample of tissue (specimen) that's removed during surgery.

mastectomy. Surgery to remove a breast. *See also* radical mastectomy.

melanoma. Cancer that typically begins in the pigment-producing cells of the body.

metaplasia. A change in tissue cells to a form that's not normal for that type of tissue, but not necessarily abnormal enough to be called cancer.

metastasis. The process by which cancer cells break away from the primary tumor and spread, usually through blood and lymph vessels, to other parts of the body.

microcalcifications. Tiny calcium deposits that can appear in the breast and often show up on a mammogram. They may suggest a benign or malignant process.

mismatch repair genes. Genes that help repair damaged DNA. When these genes are defective or damaged, mutations are more likely to accumulate.

modified radical mastectomy. Surgery that removes breast tissue, the areola and nipple, and lymph nodes under the arm near the breast.

molar pregnancy (hydatidiform mole). A condition in which an abnormal mass of cysts develops inside the uterus instead of a normal embryo.

monoclonal antibodies. One branch of the body's immune response. Monoclonal antibodies attach themselves to specific targets (antigens) in the body.

multifocal cancer. Cancer that starts within multiple areas of an organ.

mutation. An alteration in a gene.

myometrium. A layer of smooth muscle that makes up the muscular wall of the uterus.

N

negative margins. Edges (margins) of a tissue sample that are cancer-free.

neoadjuvant therapy. Chemotherapy given before surgery.

neoplasia. A new growth that may be benign or malignant.

noninvasive cancer. *See* carcinoma *in situ*.

nuclear medicine imaging. Injection of tiny amounts of radioactive tracers into the body. The tracers concentrate in given tissues and are viewed by a special camera.

O

omentum. The fatty apron in the front of the abdomen where cancer cells can collect.

oncogenes. Genes that play a role in normal cell growth and differentiation. If mutated, they can result in uncontrolled cell growth.

oncologist. A doctor trained in diagnosing and treating cancer.

oncology. The study of cancers and their treatments.

oophorectomy. Surgery to remove the ovaries.

optimal debulking. Surgery that leaves behind only minimal cancer deposits.

ovarian cysts. Benign fluid-filled pockets (sacs) within or on the surface of an ovary.

ovarian germ cell tumor. An uncommon type of ovarian cancer that originates from the egg-producing cells of the ovary.

ovarian suppression (ablation). Shut down of ovarian function by way of surgery, radiation or medication. It reduces the production of estrogen in premenopausal women.

ovary. A female reproductive organ that contains eggs and produces hormones.

P

Paget's disease of the breast. Scaling and inflammation of the nipple associated with an underlying breast cancer that may be invasive or noninvasive.

palliative care. Therapy aimed at controlling symptoms caused by a disease or treatment for a disease.

palpate. To examine a tissue or organ by feeling it.

Pap test. A screening test in which a doctor obtains a sample of cells from the cervix for examination by a pathologist.

paracentesis. A procedure by which excess fluid in the abdomen (ascites) is withdrawn with a needle.

parametrium. Part of the supporting tissue situated around the uterus.

partial remission. Reduction, but not elimination, of cancer as a result of treatment.

pathology. Study of the cause and nature of a disease, and its structural appearance.

pathology report. A detailed report that contains information about the pathologic appearance of a tissue specimen.

peau d'orange. Swollen breast skin that resembles an orange peel, caused by blocked lymph vessels in breast skin.

pedigree. A structured diagram that shows a family tree.

pelvic exam. Examination of a woman's external and internal reproductive organs.

pelvic exenteration. Removal of the bladder, vagina, rectum and part of the colon.

peritoneal implant. Tumor spread to the lining of the abdominal cavity (peritoneum).

peritoneum. The lining of the abdominal cavity.

phytoestrogens. Plant chemicals, such as those in soy, with similarities to estrogen.

placebo. A medically inactive substance that may be used as part of a clinical trial to determine if a new treatment works.

platelets. Small disc-shaped particles in the blood that aid in clotting.

pleural effusion. Accumulation of fluid within the pleural space around the lungs that may or may not be cancerous.

positive margins. Edges of a tissue sample (margins) that show signs of cancer.

positron emission tomography (PET). A nuclear medicine study in which a tracer is injected into the body and may accumulate in an area of malignant cells.

posterior exenteration. Surgery that removes the structures toward the back of the pelvis, including the rectum.

precancerous. Referring to a condition that may develop into cancer.

primary tumor. The initial site of origin of a cancer.

proctosigmoidoscopy. A procedure in which a lighted instrument (sigmoidoscope) is inserted into the rectum and lower large intestine (colon) to look for abnormalities.

progesterone. A female hormone that rises in the second half of the menstrual cycle.

progestin. A synthetic form of the hormone progesterone, used in hormone therapy.

prognosis. Prediction of the course of outcome of a disease.

prophylactic mastectomy. Surgical removal of one or both breasts in a woman at high risk of breast cancer to reduce her cancer risk.

prophylactic oophorectomy. Surgical removal of the ovaries in a woman at high risk of ovarian cancer to reduce her risk of ovarian and peritoneal cancer. In a premenopausal woman, the surgery may also reduce breast cancer risk.

prosthesis, breast. A soft device that's shaped like a breast and worn outside the body.

proteomics. The study of the body's proteins.

punch biopsy. Use of a hole-punch-type instrument to remove a sample of skin tissue.

Q

quadrantectomy. Surgical removal of the quarter of the breast that contains cancer cells. Also called partial mastectomy.

R

radiation cystitis. Bladder irritation that can develop after radiation to the pelvic region.

radiation therapy. Use of high-energy X-rays to kill cancer cells or damage them to the point where they lose their ability to grow and divide.

radical hysterectomy. Surgical removal of the uterus, including the cervix, as well as the upper inch of the vagina and some surrounding connective (supporting) tissue.

radical mastectomy. Surgical removal of the breast, chest wall muscle below the breast and all of the lymph nodes under the arm.

radical trachelectomy. Surgical removal of the cervix and upper part of the vagina.

radical vaginectomy. Surgical removal of the entire vagina and its adjacent tissues.

radical vulvectomy. Surgical removal of the entire vulva, including the clitoris, and its underlying tissues.

radioisotope. A radioactive substance.

recurrent cancer. Cancer that comes back after initial treatment.

regional recurrence. Cancer that recurs in lymph nodes or other tissues located near the original tumor.

regression. A decrease in tumor size.

relapse. Redevelopment of cancer after a cancer-free time period.

relative risk. A numeric comparison between the number of cancers or other conditions in a group of people with a particular trait and the number of cancers or other conditions in a group of people without that trait but who are otherwise similar.

remission. Disappearance of the cancer as determined by clinical evaluation, resolution of symptoms or both.

residual disease. The amount of cancer that remains after surgery.

risk factor. A factor that increases the chance of developing a condition.

S

sarcoma. A cancer that originates in connective tissue such as bone, cartilage and muscle.

screening. Being tested or observed to identify a disease or disease risk.

screening mammogram. An X-ray of the breast used to look for changes in women who have no signs or symptoms of breast cancer.

second-look laparotomy surgery. A second abdominal surgery after chemotherapy treatment for ovarian cancer to evaluate the effect of the treatment.

sentinel node biopsy. A dye or a radioactive solution is injected into the primary tumor area to determine which lymph nodes are the first to receive drainage from the cancer area (sentinel nodes). These lymph nodes are removed and examined for cancer cells.

serosa. The thin, fibrous, outermost layer of many organs.

sex cord-stromal tumor. A tumor that forms in the ovary's connective tissue cells.

simple hyperplasia. An excess of normal-appearing cells. This is the most common form of endometrial hyperplasia.

simple (total) mastectomy. Surgical removal of the breast tissue, skin, areola and nipple, but not any lymph nodes.

speculum. A device used to hold the vaginal walls apart during a pelvic exam.

squamous cells. Flat cells that cover the surface of the skin and the lining of some hollow organs of the body.

staging. Determination of the extent of the cancer or its spread. Cancer stage is based on a tumor's size and whether it has spread to lymph nodes and other areas of the body.

stroma. Connective tissue supporting the structures of an organ.

stromal sarcoma. Cancer that develops in the supporting connective tissue (stroma) of the uterus.

subcutaneous mastectomy. Removal of breast tissue, but not the nipple and areola.

supportive (palliative) care. Treatment designed to alleviate symptoms caused by cancer or anti-cancer therapy.

surgical biopsy. Surgical removal of a portion of a mass (incisional biopsy) or the whole mass (excisional biopsy) for pathologic examination.

surgical menopause. Menopause that's initiated by surgical removal of the ovaries.

systemic. Affecting the entire body.

systemic therapy. Treatment delivered to the entire body by way of the bloodstream, including chemotherapy and hormone therapy.

T

total abdominal hysterectomy. Surgical removal of the entire uterus, including the cervix, through an incision in the abdomen.

total pelvic exenteration. Pelvic surgery that removes all pelvic structures.

transvaginal ultrasound. A procedure in which a transducer is inserted into the vagina to check for suspicious masses in the pelvic region.

tubal ligation. A surgical procedure to prevent pregnancy by sealing the fallopian tubes.

tumor. An abnormal mass of tissue that results from excessive cell growth and division, which may be benign or malignant. Also called a neoplasm.

tumor marker. A substance circulating in blood that's produced by a certain tumor. The level of the tumor marker may reflect the activity or extent of the tumor.

tumor suppressor genes. Genes normally responsible for restraining cell growth.

U

ultrasound. An imaging procedure that uses high-frequency sound waves to produce images of the inside of the human body, which are displayed on a computer screen.

uterine cancer. Cancer that starts within the uterine body (corpus).

uterine carcinosarcoma. Cancer that has features of both endometrial cancer and uterine sarcoma. Also known as a malignant mixed mesodermal tumor (MMMT).

uterine fibroids. Benign tumors that develop in the muscle wall of the uterus.

uterine sarcoma. Uterine cancer that starts in muscle or connective tissues of the uterus.

uterus. A hollow organ where a baby grows and develops during pregnancy.

V

vagina. A muscular tube that connects the uterus with the outer genitals.

vaginal adenosis. Lining of the vagina that contains one or more areas made up of gland-like cells, similar to those found in the lower uterus or uterine lining.

vaginal hysterectomy. A hysterectomy that's performed through a vaginal incision.

vulva. The folds of skin in a woman's genital area.

W

wide local excision. A procedure in which a doctor removes the tumor and some surrounding tissue.

wire localization. Use of fine wires to define the area of a breast mass that can't be felt so that the mass can be removed.

Index

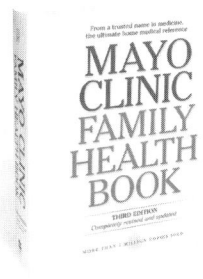

Mayo Clinic Family Health Book, Third Edition

More than 1 million copies sold!

Product # 268143 • $49.95

New! This thoroughly revised and updated edition of a classic health reference includes the latest medical information that has come to light over the past six years. Covering more than 1,000 illnesses and containing hundreds of illustrations and photos, the new edition also updates key issues in prevention, working effectively with health care professionals, the pros and cons of complementary and alternative medicine, common patient questions, end-of-life issues, and much more. It's the ultimate illustrated home medical reference!

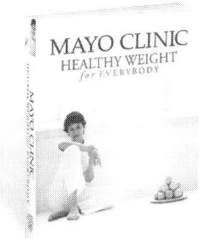

Mayo Clinic Healthy Weight for EveryBody

Maintaining a healthy weight is a vital part of staying healthy and reducing the risk of serious disease.

Product # 280400 • $22.95

Learn how to focus on the process of losing weight rather than the actual number of pounds lost by following this simple, step-by-step, 12-week program.

Other Mayo Clinic books include:	*Product #*	*Price*
• Mayo Clinic Guide to a Healthy Pregnancy	280200	$19.95
• Mayo Clinic Guide to Self-Care	270104	$21.95
• Mayo Clinic Heart Book	268150	$29.95
• Mayo Clinic on Arthritis	268502	$16.95
• Mayo Clinic on Chronic Pain	268702	$16.95
• Mayo Clinic on Depression	270500	$14.95
• Mayo Clinic on Digestive Health	268902	$16.95
• Mayo Clinic on Healthy Aging	270400	$14.95
• Mayo Clinic on Hearing	270900	$16.95
• Mayo Clinic on High Blood Pressure	268402	$16.95
• Mayo Clinic on Managing Diabetes	270300	$14.95
• Mayo Clinic on Osteoporosis	270800	$16.95
• Mayo Clinic on Prostate Health	268802	$16.95
• Mayo Clinic on Vision and Eye Health	270600	$14.95

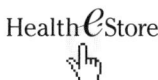

Order by calling toll-free (877) 647-6397 and mention order code 180.

Or order online at *www.Healthe-store.com.*

Price does not include shipping and handling and applicable sales tax.
All prices subject to change.

Mayo Clinic books are available at local bookstores.

When you purchase a Mayo Clinic publication, proceeds are used to further education and medical research at Mayo Clinic. You not only get answers to your questions, you become part of the solution.